Second Edition

Advanced Nutrition

Macronutrients, Micronutrients, and Metabolism

Carolyn D. Berdanier
Lynnette A. Berdanier

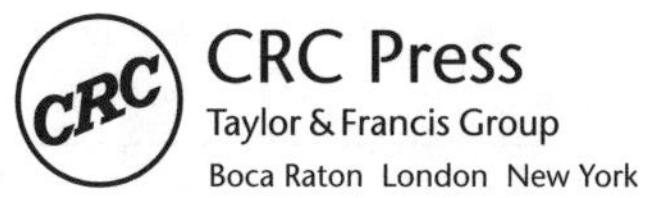

CRC Press is an imprint of the
Taylor & Francis Group, an **informa** business

CRC Press
Taylor & Francis Group
6000 Broken Sound Parkway NW, Suite 300
Boca Raton, FL 33487-2742

Printed on acid-free paper
Version Date: 20141029

International Standard Book Number-13: 978-1-4822-0517-6 (Paperback)

Library of Congress Cataloging-in-Publication Data

Berdanier, Carolyn D., author.
Advanced nutrition : macronutrients, micronutrients, and metabolism / Carolyn D. Berdanier and Lynnette A. Berdanier. -- Second edition.
p. ; cm.
Includes bibliographical references and index.
ISBN 978-1-4822-0517-6 (alk. paper)
I. Berdanier, Lynne, author. II. Title.
[DNLM: 1. Nutritional Physiological Phenomena. 2. Dietary Carbohydrates--metabolism. 3. Dietary Fats--metabolism. 4. Dietary Proteins--metabolism. 5. Micronutrients--metabolism. QU 145]

QP141
612.3--dc23 2014037992

Visit the Taylor & Francis Web site at
http://www.taylorandfrancis.com

and the CRC Press Web site at
http://www.crcpress.com

Contents

Preface

As in the first edition of this book, *Advanced Nutrition: Macronutrients, Micronutrients, and Metabolism* has been written for the advanced student who has a background in biochemistry and physiology but may or may not have a background in nutrition and dietetics. The book is divided along classical lines addressing each of the major nutrient classes. A review of nutritional biochemistry precedes the chapters on micro- and macronutrients. In addition, there are chapters on food intake, exercise, cell cycle, and nutrition and gene expression. Woven throughout the text are topics of clinical interest such as obesity, diabetes, lipemia, renal disease, hypertension, and the deficiency disorders. The second edition has been updated and revised for ease of understanding. At the end of each chapter are learning opportunities that should help the reader understand and use the information presented in the chapter. Included are problem-solving exercises, case studies, multiple-choice questions, and short-answer questions that should help the reader think about nutrition as a science that integrates knowledge gained from other disciplines.

Web addresses for food composition and Dietary Reference Intakes (DRIs) have been included so that the reader can access the most current information on these topics. The recommendations for nutrient intakes are in a state of flux. As the information base expands with respect to nutrient use and need, the DRIs are changed to reflect this newer knowledge.

It is hoped that you, the reader, will find this book an essential addition to your library.

Preface

Acknowledgments

The authors express their appreciation to all the readers of the first edition who were very kind to write to the authors with their comments. Appreciation is also extended to Reese Berdanier who put up with our many hours at the computer preparing this edition. His patience and support are much appreciated. Finally, this edition would not have been possible without the encouragement and support of Randy Brehm, our gracious editor at the Taylor & Francis Group.

Authors

Carolyn D. Berdanier, PhD, is a professor emerita of nutrition at the University of Georgia in Athens, Georgia. She earned her BS from Pennsylvania State University, University Park, Pennsylvania, and MS and PhD from Rutgers University, Piscataway, New Jersey. After a postdoctoral fellowship year with Dr. Paul Griminger at Rutgers, she served as a research nutritionist at the U.S. Department of Agriculture Human Nutrition Institute in Beltsville, Maryland. At the same time, she also served as an assistant professor of nutrition at the University of Maryland. Following these appointments, she moved to the University of Nebraska, College of Medicine, and then in 1977 moved to the University of Georgia, where she served as department head, Foods and Nutrition, for 11 years. She stepped down from this position to resume full-time research and teaching with a special interest in diabetes. Her research has been funded by a variety of funding agencies.

Dr. Berdanier has authored over 120 research articles, contributed 40 chapters in multiauthored books, prepared 45 invited reviews for scientific journals, and edited/coauthored or authored 18 books. She has served on the editorial boards of *The FASEB Journal*, *The Journal of Nutrition*, *Biochemistry Archives*, *Nutrition Research*, and the *International Journal of Diabetes Research*. She also serves as an ad hoc reviewer for articles in her specialty for a wide variety of scientific journals.

Lynnette A. Berdanier is a lecturer in the Department of Biology at the University of North Georgia, Gainesville, Georgia. She teaches biology as well as anatomy and physiology and medical microbiology. She earned her BS from the University of Nebraska, Kearney, Nebraska, and MS in physiology from the University of Georgia, Athens, Georgia. She served as a lecturer at Athens Technical College and at North Georgia College in Dahlonega prior to moving to her current position at the University of North Georgia in Gainesville, Georgia.

Abbreviations

ACAT	Acyl coenzyme A:cholesterol acyltransferase
ACE	Angiotensin-converting enzyme
ACP	Acyl carrier protein
ACTH	Adrenocorticotropic hormone
ADE	Apparent digested energy
ADH	Antidiuretic hormone, also called vasopressin
ADP	Adenosine diphosphate
AIDS	Acquired immune deficiency syndrome
AMP	Adenosine monophosphate
ANH	Atrial natruiretic hormone
ARS	Autonomously replicating sequence
ATP	Adenosine triphosphate
ATPase	A group of enzymes that catalyze the removal or addition of a single phosphate group to the high energy compound containing adenine
B cells	Lymphocytic cells produced in the bone marrow
ß cells	Cells in the islets of Langerhans in the endocrine pancreas
BAT	Brown adipose tissue
BCAA	Branched-chain amino acids
BEE	Basal energy expenditure
BMI	Body mass index = body weight (kg)/height $(cm)^2$
BMR	Basal metabolic rate
BTU	British thermal unit
cAMP (cyclic AMP)	Cyclic 3′5′ adenosine monophosphate
CCK	Cholecystokinin
CDC	Centers for Disease Control
cDNA	A single-stranded DNA molecule that is complementary to an mRNA
CDP	Cytidine diphosphate
CHO	Carbohydrate
CMP	Cytidine monophosphate
CoA	Coenzyme A
CoQ	Coenzyme Q, also called ubiquinone
COX I and COX II	Cyclooxygenase
CTP	Cytidine triphosphate
CVD	Cardiovascular disease
DE	Digestive energy
Delta (Δ)	Change; the Greek symbol is Δ
DEXA	Dual-energy x-ray absorptiometry
$\Delta G°$	Free energy that is available to do work
$\Delta G°'$	Standard free energy of biochemical reactions
DHHS	U.S. Department of Health and Human Services
DIT	Diet-induced thermogenesis
DNA	Deoxyribonucleic acid
DRI	Daily Reference Intake

ER	Endoplasmic reticulum
ESADDI	Estimated safe and adequate daily dietary intakes
FAD	Flavin adenine dinucleotide
FAO	U.S. Food and Agricultural Organization
FDA	U.S. Food and Drug Administration
FE	Fecal energy
FMN	Flavin mononucleotide
FSH	Follicle-stimulating hormone
GABA	Gamma aminobutyric acid
GDP	Guanosine diphosphate
GIP	Gastric inhibitory peptide
GMP	Guanosine monophosphate
GPE	Gaseous products of digestion
GRP	Gastrin-releasing peptide
GSH	Glutathione, reduced
GSSG	Glutathionine, oxidized
GTP	Guanosine triphosphate
$^3H^+$	Tritium (radioactive hydrogen)
HANES (NHANES I, II, III, OR HHANES)	National Health and Nutrition Examination Survey
Hb	Hemoglobin
HcE	Heat of thermal regulation
HdE	Heat of activity
HfE	Heat of fermentation; also abbreviated as GdE
HiE	Heat increment, also abbreviated HI
HLA genes	Genes that encode elements of the immune system
HMG CoA	3-Hydroxy-3-methylglutaryl coenzyme A
HNIS	Human Nutrition Information Service
HrE	Heat of product formation
HwE	Heat produced in association with the production of waste products
IBW	Ideal body weight
IE	Intake of food energy
ISF	Interstitial fluid
IU	International unit
K_m	Michaelis constant
LBM	Lean body mass
LH	Luteinizing hormone
LHA	Lateral hypothalamus
LNAA	Large neutral amino acids
M (μ)	Greek letter prefix that indicates 10^{-6} fraction of a liter
MAO	Monoamine oxidase
MCV	Mean corpuscular volume
ME	Metabolizable energy
MRI	Magnetic resonance imaging
mRNA	Messenger RNA
NAD, NADH, NADP, NADPH	Nicotine adenine dinucleotides; nicotine adenine dinucleotides, reduced; nicotine adenine diphosphate; nicotine adenine diphosphate, reduced
NCHS (U.S.)	National Center for Health Statistics
NFCS (U.S.)	Nationwide Food Consumption Survey
NIH (U.S.)	National Institutes of Health

NRC (U.S.)	National Research Council
NSF (U.S.)	National Science Foundation
ORI	Origin of replication in prokaryotes
PCR	Polymerase chain reaction
PEP	Phosphoenolpyruvic acid
PEPCK	Phosphoenolpyruvate carboxykinase
PGI, PGE	Prostaglandins in the I or E series
pH	Numerical representation of the hydrogen ion concentration in a solution
PLP	Pyridoxal phosphate
PP-Fold	Polypeptide fold hormones: polypeptide Y (PPY), pancreatic polypeptide (PP), and neuropeptide Y (NPY)
P/S ratio	Ratio of polyunsaturated fatty acids to saturated fatty acids
PTH	Parathyroid hormone
PUFA	Polyunsaturated fatty acid
PVN	Paraventricular nucleus
RBC	Red blood cell
RBP	Retinol binding protein
RDA	Recommended daily dietary allowance
RE	Recovered energy
RER	Rough endoplasmic reticulum
RIA	Radioimmunoassay
RNA	Ribonucleic acid
RQ	Respiratory quotient
SAM	S-adenosylmethionine
SDA	Specific dynamic action
SER	Smooth endoplasmic reticulum
SGOT	Serum glutamate-oxaloacetate transaminase
SGPT	Serum glutamate-pyruvate transaminase
SI units	Standard units for expressing biological values
SnRNA	Small nuclear RNA
SOD	Superoxide dismutase
T_3	Triiodothyronine
T_4	Thyroxine
T cells	Cells of the immune system that originate from the thymus gland
TCA cycle	Citric acid cycle (Krebs cycle)
TBF	Total body fat
TBG	Thyroid hormone binding globulin
TBW	Total body water
TDP, TPP	Thiamin-containing coenzyme required for decarboxylation reactions
TMP, TDP, TTP	Thymidine phosphate
TPN	Total parenteral nutrition
tRNA	Transfer ribonucleic acid
TSH	Thyroid-stimulating hormone
TXA_2	Thromboxane A2
Ubiquinone	Coenzyme Q-10
UMP, UDP, UTP	Uridine mono-, di-, or triphosphate
VIP	Vasoactive peptide
VLDL	Very low density lipoprotein

Review: Nutritional Biochemistry

The study of nutrition is an integrated one. It is based on an understanding of intermediary metabolism. In order for the body to use the nutrients in the food, it must first break the food down to usable components. Food is first digested and absorbed via a variety of mechanisms, as will be described in the chapters devoted to each nutrient. The use of food components in the macronutrient class involves both the breakdown of the macromolecules (catabolism) and the resynthesis of needed molecules (anabolism). Together, these constitute the pathways of intermediary metabolism.

Nutrient intake can affect these pathways in a variety of ways: A large intake of a given macronutrient, glucose, for example, can affect the initial reaction sequences of the glycolytic, glycogenic, and hexose monophosphate shunt pathways through substrate induction. In contrast, should the diet be deficient in glucose, the glucose synthesizing pathway, gluconeogenesis, and the glycogenolytic pathway would be stimulated. In addition to dietary effects on intermediary metabolism, there are hormonal effects that in turn can be affected by dietary status or by environmental conditions. In a number of instances, there are genetic effects on these pathways as well (see Chapter 7). Before these influences can be explained, however, the pathways themselves must be described.

GLYCOLYSIS

The glycolytic pathway for the anaerobic catabolism of glucose can be found in all cells in the body. This cytosolic pathway begins with glucose, a 6-carbon unit, and through a series of reactions produces 2 molecules of pyruvate. The pathway is shown in Figure R.1. The pathway is stimulated by insulin and is less active when glucocorticoid is present. The pathway also produces ATP by substrate phosphorylation as well as through its contribution (via the α-glycerophosphate shuttle) of reducing equivalents to the respiratory chain. Because two of the steps require ATP (the initial kinase step and the phosphofructokinase step), the net ATP production of the glycolytic sequence is 8 ATPs. The control of glycolysis is vested in several key steps. The first step is the phosphorylation of glucose through the formation of glucose-6-phosphate. In the liver and pancreatic β-cell, this step is catalyzed by the enzyme glucokinase. A molecule of ATP is used and magnesium is required. Glucose-6-phosphate is a key metabolite. It can proceed down the glycolytic pathway or move through the hexose monophosphate shunt (or shunt) or be used to make glycogen. How much glucose-6-phosphate is oxidized directly to pyruvate depends on the type of cell, the nutritional state of the animal, its genetics, and its hormonal state. Some cell types, the brain cell, for example, do not make glycogen. Some people do not have shunt activity in the red cell because the code for glucose-6-phosphate dehydrogenase has mutated to the point where the enzyme is not functional. Insulin-deficient animals likewise might have little shunt activity due to the lack of insulin's effect on the synthesis of its enzymes. All these factors determine how much glucose-6-phosphate goes in which direction.

Two enzymes are used for the activation of glucose: glucokinase and hexokinase. Both these enzymes are present in the liver. While hexokinase activity is product inhibited, that is, inhibited by glucose-6-phosphate, glucokinase is not. The hexokinase in the nonhepatic tissues must be

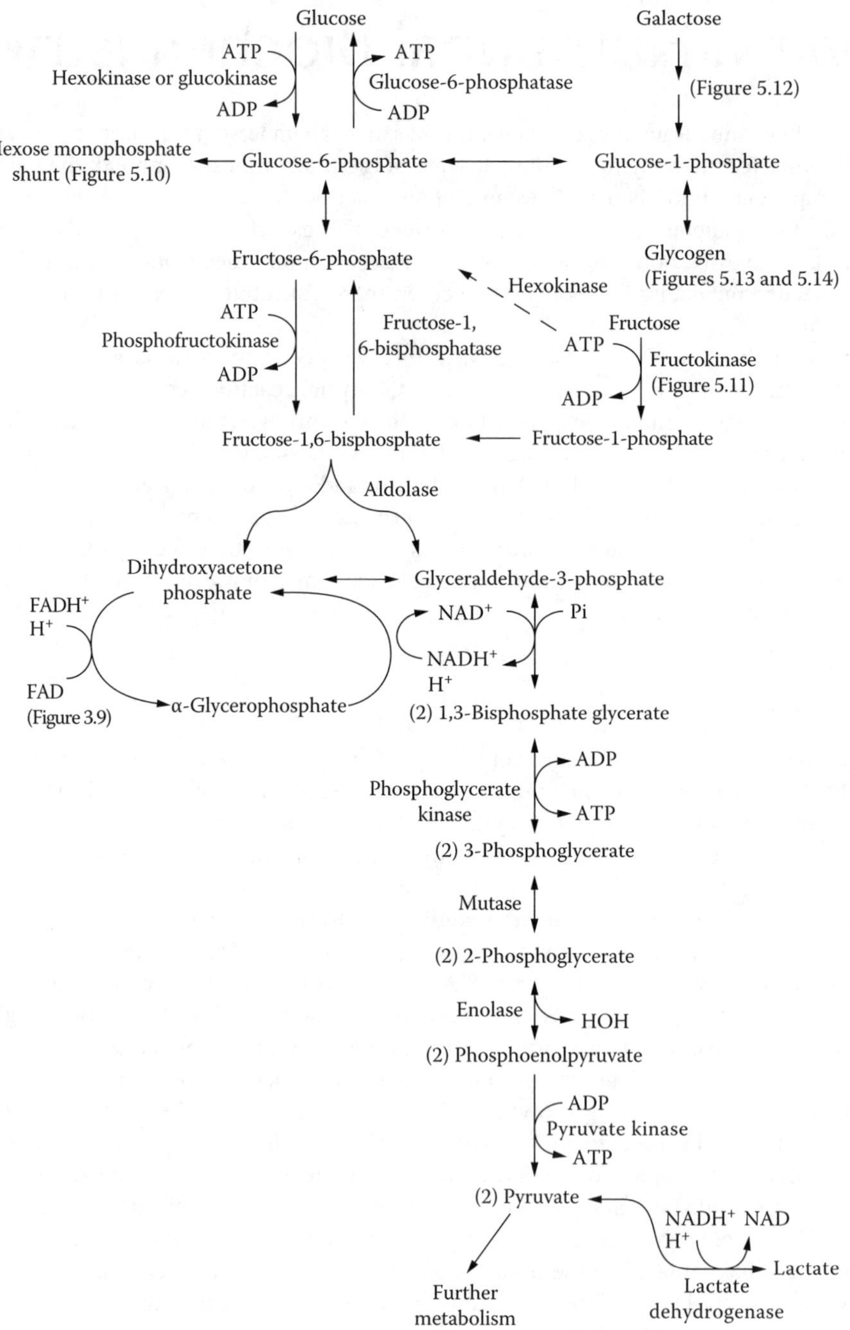

FIGURE R.1 Glycolysis.

product-inhibited to prevent the hexokinase from tying up all the inorganic phosphate in the cells as glucose-6-phosphate. The K_m for glucokinase is greater than that for hexokinase, so the former is the main enzyme for the conversion of glucose to glucose-6-phosphate in the liver. It is also the main enzyme for the phosphorylation of glucose in the pancreatic islet cells. In the islet cell, glucokinase serves as the glucose sensor that signals the need to release insulin. The other enzyme will phosphorylate not only glucose but other 6-carbon sugars as well. The amount of fructose phosphorylated by hexokinase to fructose-6-phosphate is small in comparison with the phosphorylation of fructose at the carbon 1 position catalyzed by fructokinase.

Glucose-6-phosphate is isomerized to fructose-6-phosphate and then is phosphorylated once again to form fructose-1,6-bisphosphate. Another molecule of ATP is used and again magnesium is an important cofactor. Both kinase reactions are rate-controlling reactions in that their activity determines the rate at which subsequent reactions proceed. The phosphofructokinase reaction is unique to the glycolytic sequence, while the glucokinase or hexokinase step is not. Thus, one could argue that the formation of fructose-1,6-bisphosphate is the first committed step in glycolysis. Glycolysis is inhibited when phosphofructokinase is inhibited. This occurs when levels of fatty acids in the cytosol rise, as in the instance of high rates of lipolysis and fatty acid oxidation or with the feeding of high-fat diets. Phosphofructokinase activity is increased when the fructose-6-phosphate or cAMP levels rise. Exercise stimulates the flux of fructose-6-phosphate through the phosphofructokinase reaction. Stimulation occurs also when fructose-2,6-bisphosphate levels rise. Phosphofructokinase is activated by divalent ions. In any event, glycolysis then proceeds with the splitting of fructose-1,6-bisphosphate to dihydroxyacetone phosphate (DHAP) and glyceraldehyde-3-phosphate. At this point, another rate-controlling step occurs. This step is one that shuttles reducing equivalents into the mitochondria for use by the respiratory chain. This is the α-glycerophosphate shuttle. This shuttle carries reducing equivalents from the cytosol to the mitochondria. DHAP picks up reducing equivalents when it is converted to α-glycerol phosphate. These reducing equivalents are produced when glyceraldehyde-3-phosphate is oxidized in the process of being phosphorylated to 1,3-diphosphate glyceraldehyde. The α-glycerophosphate enters the inner mitochondrial membrane, whereupon it is converted back to DHAP and releases its reducing equivalents to FAD, which in turn transfers the reducing equivalents to the mitochondrial respiratory chain. The reason that this shuttle is rate limiting is due to the need to regenerate NAD^+ in the cytosol. Without NAD^+, the glycolytic pathway ceases. NAD^+ itself cannot pass through the mitochondrial membrane, so substrate shuttles are necessary. Another means of producing NAD^+ is by converting pyruvate to lactate. This is a nonmitochondrial reaction catalyzed by lactate dehydrogenase. It occurs when an oxygen debt is developed, as happens in exercising muscle. In these muscles, oxygen consumption is more than what can be supplied. Glycolysis occurs at a rate faster than can be accommodated by the respiratory chain that joins the reducing equivalents transferred to it by the shuttles to molecular oxygen, making water. If more reducing equivalents are generated than can be used to make water, the excess is added to pyruvate to make lactate. Thus, rising lactate levels are indicative of oxygen debt.

Lactate levels are elevated in individuals with mitochondrial dysfunction due to mitochondrial DNA mutation. In this instance, the reason is due to inefficient mitochondrial oxidative phosphorylation (OXPHOS) that cannot handle all the reducing equivalents sent to it for the synthesis of water.

There are other shuttles that also serve to transfer reducing equivalents into the mitochondria. These are the malate–aspartate shuttle and the malate–citrate shuttle. Neither of these is rate-limiting with respect to glycolysis. The malate–aspartate shuttle has rate-controlling properties with respect to gluconeogenesis, while the malate–citrate shuttle is important to lipogenesis.

Once 1,3-bisphosphate glycerate is formed, it is converted to 3-phosphoglycerate with the formation of 1 ATP. The 3-phosphoglycerate then goes to 2-phosphoglycerate and then to phosphoenolpyruvate (PEP). These are all bidirectional reactions that are also used in gluconeogenesis. The PEP is dephosphorylated to pyruvate with the formation of another ATP. Because of the energy lost to ATP formation at this step, this reaction is not reversible. Gluconeogenesis uses another enzyme, phosphoenolpyruvate carboxykinase (PEPCK), to reverse this step. Glycolysis uses pyruvate kinase to catalyze the reaction. At any rate, pyruvate can now be activated to acetyl CoA, which can enter the mitochondrial citric acid cycle.

The glycolytic pathway is dependent both on ATP for the initial steps of the pathway, the formation of glucose-6-phosphate and fructose-1,6-bisphosphate, and on the ratio of ATP to ADP and inorganic phosphate, Pi. In the working muscle, the continuance of work and glycolysis depends on the cycling of the adenine nucleotides and the export of lactate. ATP must be provided at the beginning of the pathway, and ADP and Pi must be provided in the latter steps. If the tissue runs out of ATP, ADP, or Pi or accumulates lactate and H+, glycolysis will come to a halt and work cannot continue. This is what happens to the working skeletal muscle. Exhaustion sets in when the glycolytic rate is downregulated by an accumulation of lactate.

HEXOSE MONOPHOSPHATE SHUNT

The hexose monophosphate shunt (the shunt) provides an alternate pathway for the use of glucose-6-phosphate. It is an important pathway because it generates reducing equivalents carried by NADP+ and because it generates a phosphorylated ribose for use in nucleotide synthesis. It is estimated that approximately 10% of the glucose-6-phosphate generated from glucose is metabolized by the shunt.

As can be seen in Figure R.2, the shunt contains two NADP-linked dehydrogenases, glucose-6-phosphate dehydrogenase and 6-phosphogluconate dehydrogenase. The rate-limiting steps in the reaction sequence are catalyzed by these two enzymes.

In any event, as shown in Figure R.2, glucose-6-phosphate proceeds to 6-phosphoglucolactone, a very unstable metabolite, which is in turn reduced to 6-phosphogluconate. The 6-phosphogluconate is decarboxylated and dehydrogenated to form ribulose-5-phosphate with an unstable intermediate

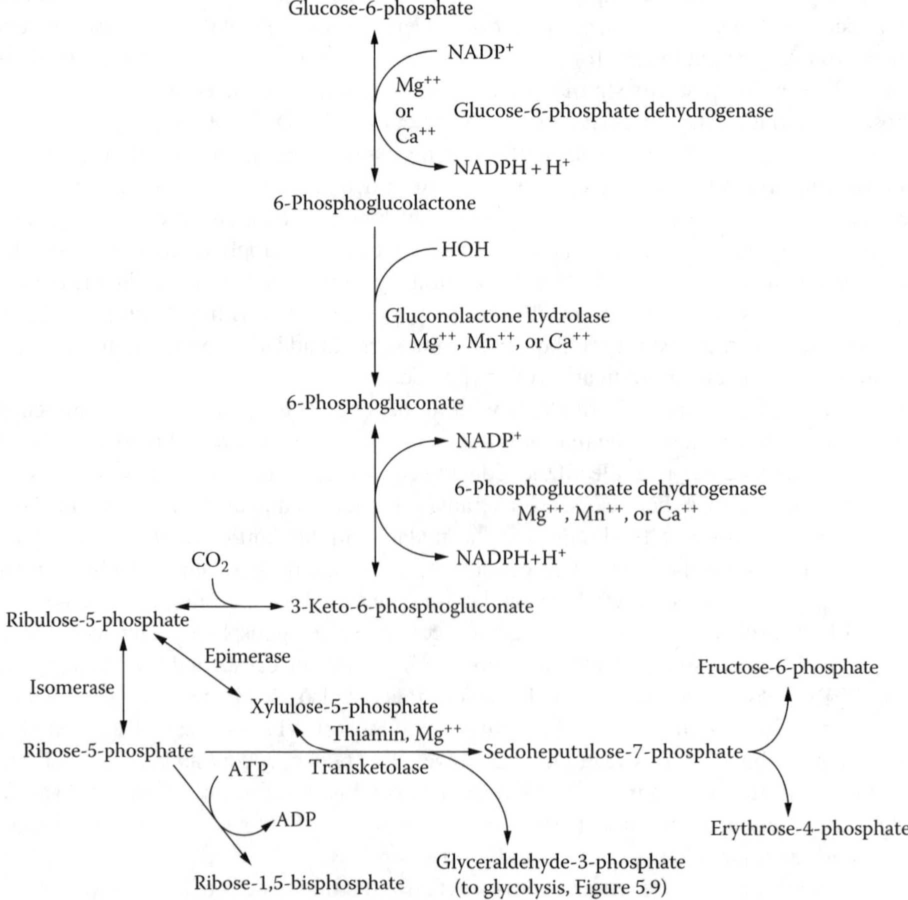

FIGURE R.2 Reaction sequence of the hexose monophosphate shunt commonly referred to as the *shunt*.

(keto-6-phosphogluconate) forming between the 6-phosphogluconate and ribulose-5-phosphate. Ribulose-5-phosphate can be isomerized to ribose-5-phosphate or epimerized to xylulose-5-phosphate. Xylulose and ribose-5-phosphate can reversibly form sedoheptulose-7-phosphate with the release of glyceraldehyde-3-phosphate. This, of course, will be recognized as a component of the glycolytic sequence.

INTERCONVERSION OF DIETARY SUGARS

Fructose

In the course of digestion, the simple sugars glucose, fructose, and galactose are released from sucrose, maltose, and lactose. The metabolism of fructose is shown in Figure R.3. Although two enzymes are available for the phosphorylation of fructose, one of these, fructokinase, is present only in the liver. Just as hexokinase has a lower K_m for glucose than glucokinase for the substrate glucose, so too does hexokinase with respect to fructose and fructokinase. The K_m for fructokinase is so high that, in fact, most of the dietary fructose that enters the portal blood is metabolized in the liver. This is in contrast to glucose, which is metabolized by all the cells in the body.

Galactose

Another monosaccharide of importance, especially to infants and children, is galactose, a component of the milk sugar lactose. In the intestine, lactose is hydrolyzed to its component monosaccharides, glucose and galactose. Galactose is converted to glucose and eventually enters the glycolytic sequence as glucose-6-phosphate. This pathway is shown in Figure R.4. Galactose is phosphorylated

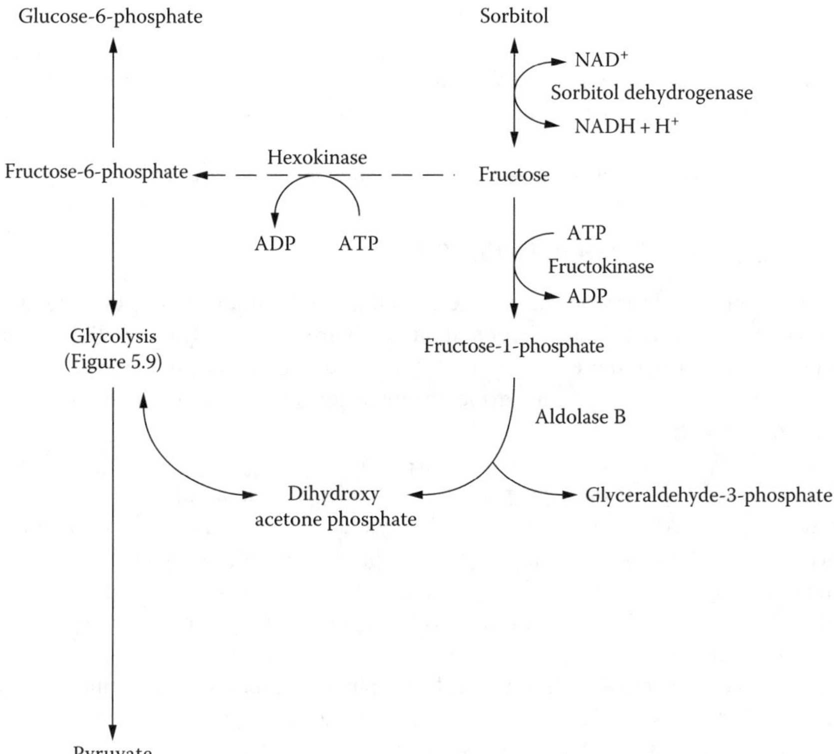

FIGURE R.3 Metabolism of fructose.

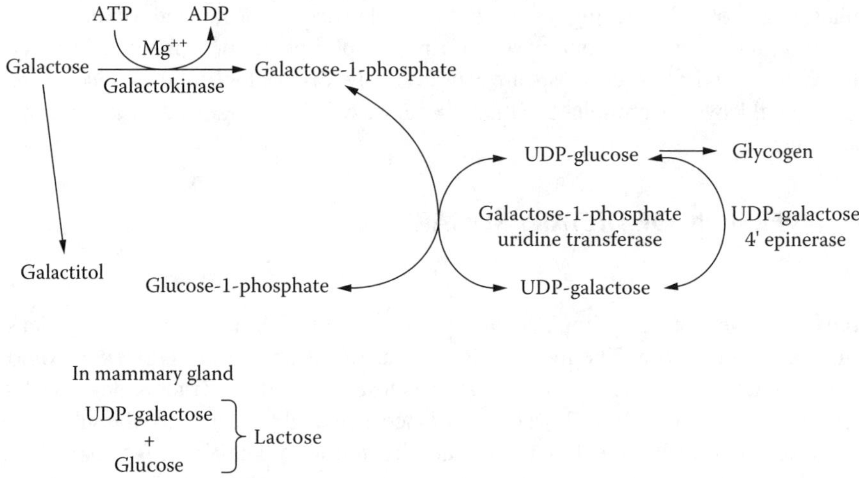

FIGURE R.4 Conversion of galactose to glucose.

at carbon 1 in the first step of its conversion to glucose. It can be isomerized to glucose-1-phosphate or converted to UDP-galactose by exchanging its phosphate group for a UDP group. This UDP-galactose can be joined with glucose to form lactose in the adult mammary tissue under the influence of the hormone prolactin. However, usually the UDP-galactose is converted to UDP-glucose and thence used to form glycogen. When glycogen is degraded, glucose-1-phosphate is released, which, in turn, is isomerized to glucose-6-phosphate and enters the glycolytic sequence.

MANNOSE

Although the main dietary monosaccharides are glucose, fructose, and galactose, mannose is also present in small amounts. Mannose found in food is converted to fructose via phosphorylation and isomerization.

Mannose → Mannose-6-phosphate → Fructose-6-phosphate → Glycolysis

GLYCOGENESIS AND GLYCOGENOLYSIS

Glucose is an essential fuel for working muscle as well as for the brain. To ensure a steady supply of this fuel, some glucose is stored in the liver and muscle in the form of glycogen. This is a ready supply of glucose accessed when these tissues are stimulated to release its glucose from its glycogen by the catabolic hormones glucagon, epinephrine, the glucocorticoids, and thyroxine or by the absence of food in the digestive tract.

An overview of glycogenesis is shown in Figure R.5.

Figure R.6 gives details of the glycogenolytic cascade. Muscle and liver glycogen stores have very different functions. Muscle glycogen is used to synthesize ATP for muscle contraction, whereas hepatic glycogen is the glucose reserve for the entire body, particularly the central nervous system. The amount of glycogen in the muscle is dependent on the physical activity of the individual. After bouts of strenuous exercise, the glycogen store will be depleted, only to be rebuilt during the resting period following exercise.

Glycogen synthesis begins with glucose-1-phosphate formation from glucose-6-phosphate through the action of phosphoglucomutase. If there are elevations in blood glucose, there will be elevations in hepatic glucose-6-phosphate and this in turn will stimulate glycogen synthesis. Thus, it could be argued that the level of glucose-6-phosphate is rate-controlling with respect to glycogenesis. Glycogen synthesis can also occur using 3-carbon precursors that traverse the gluconeogenic

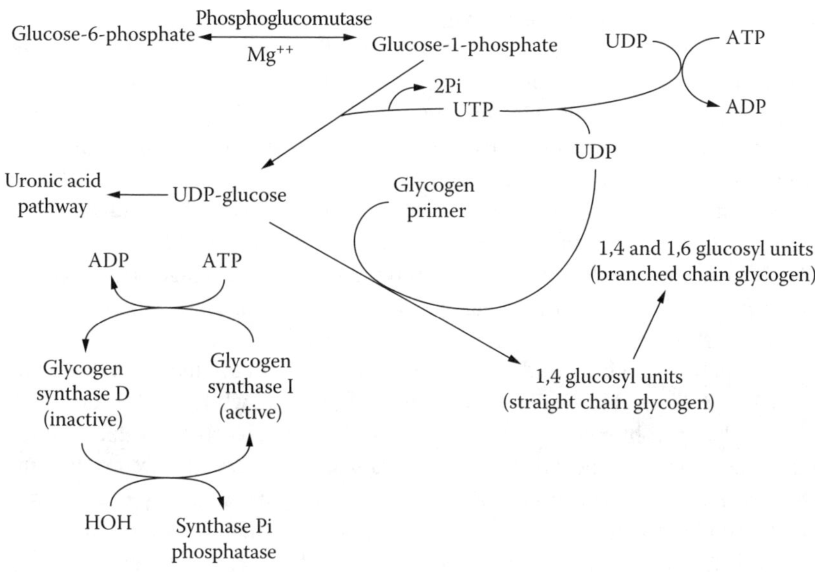

FIGURE R.5 Glycogen synthesis (glycogenesis).

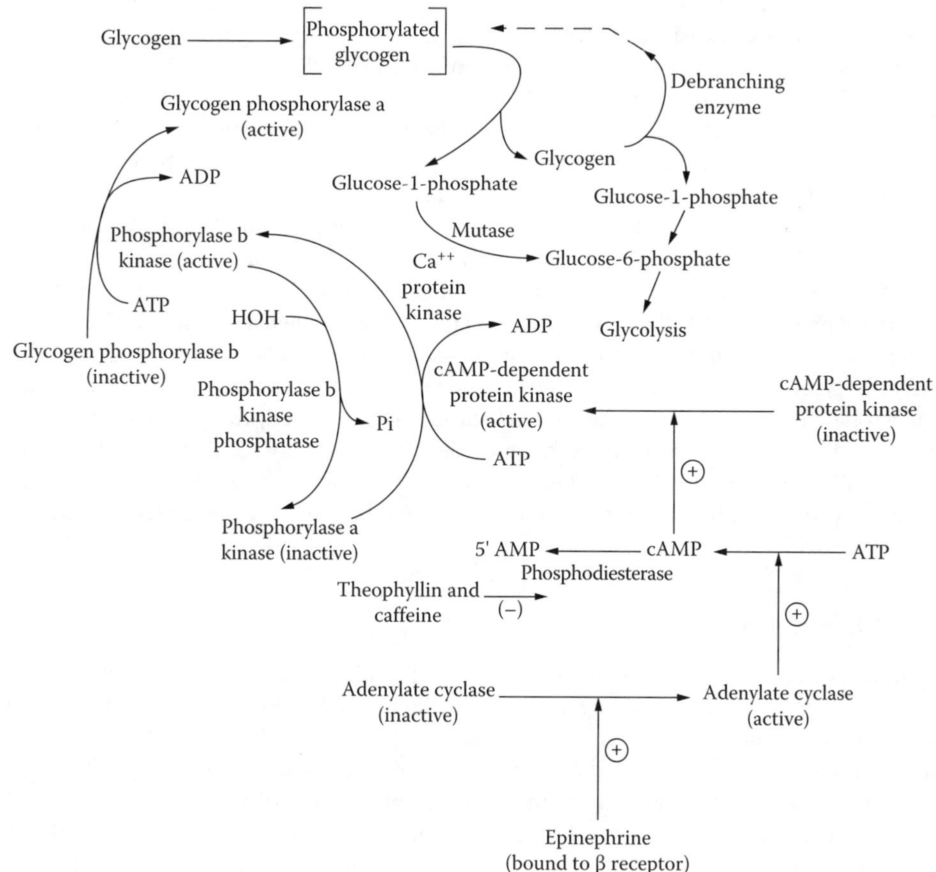

FIGURE R.6 Glycogen breakdown (glycogenolysis).

pathway before being used for glycogen synthesis. These 3-carbon intermediates are generated in the extrahepatic tissues as well as in the liver itself. The proportion of glycogen synthesis from glucose-6-phosphate compared to that from the 3-carbon intermediates depends on the amount of glucose consumed as well as the physiological state of the animal. Low-glucose diets seem to enhance the glycogen synthesis from the trios phosphates while high-glucose loads favor the direct synthesis of glycogen from glucose-6-phosphate.

In the direct path for glycogenesis, glucose-1-phosphate is converted to uridine diphosphate glucose (UDP-glucose), which can then be added to the glycogen already in storage (the glycogen primer). UDP-glucose can be added through a 1,6 linkage or a 1,4 linkage. Two high-energy bonds are used to incorporate each molecule of glucose into the glycogen. The straight chain glucose polymer is composed of glucoses joined through the 1,4 linkage and is less compact than the branched chain glycogen, which has both 1,4 and 1,6 linkages. The addition of glucose to the primer glycogen with a 1,4 linkage is catalyzed by the glycogen synthase enzyme, while the 1,6 addition is catalyzed by the so-called glycogen-branching enzyme (amylo $1 \rightarrow 4$, $1 \rightarrow 6$ transglucosidase). Once the liver and muscle cells achieve their full storage capacity, these enzymes are product-inhibited and glycogenesis is *turned off*. Glycogen synthase is inactivated by a cAMP-dependent kinase and activated by a synthase phosphatase enzyme that is stimulated by changes in the ratio of ATP to ADP. Glycogen synthesis is stimulated by the hormone insulin and suppressed by the catabolic hormones. The process does not fully cease but operates at a very low level. Glycogen does not accumulate appreciably in cells other than the liver and muscle, although all cells contain a small amount of glycogen. Note in Figure R.5 that a glycogen primer is required for glycogen synthesis to proceed. This primer is carefully guarded so that some is always available when glycogen is synthesized. This means that glycogenolysis never fully depletes the cell of its glycogen content.

Glycogenolysis is a carefully controlled series of reactions referred to as the glycogen cascade (Figure R.6). It is called a cascade because of the stepwise changes in activation states of the enzymes involved. To release glucose for oxidation by the glycogenolytic pathway, the glycogen must be phosphorylated. This is accomplished by the enzyme glycogen phosphorylase, which exists in the cell in an inactive form (glycogen phosphorylase b) and is activated to its active form (glycogen phosphorylase a) by the enzyme phosphorylase b kinase. In turn, this kinase also exists in an inactive form, which is activated by the calcium-dependent enzyme protein kinase and active cAMP-dependent protein kinase. These activations each require a molecule of ATP. Finally, the cAMP-dependent protein kinase must have cAMP for its activation. This cAMP is generated from ATP by the enzyme adenylate cyclase which, in itself, is inactive unless stimulated by a hormone such as epinephrine, thyroxine, or glucagon. As can be seen, this cascade of activation is energy dependent, with three molecules of ATP required to get the process started. Once started, the glycolytic pathway will replenish the ATP needed initially as well as provide a further supply of ATP to provide the necessary energy. As mentioned, the liver and muscle differ in the use of glycogen. This also affects how ATP is generated within the glycogen-containing cell and how much is generated by cells that do not store glycogen.

GLUCONEOGENESIS

The synthesis of glucose from nonglucose precursors is called gluconeogenesis (Figure R.7). It is a cytosolic pathway. The rate-limiting enzymes of interest are glucose-6-phosphatase, fructose-1,6-biphosphatase, and PEPCK. Pyruvate kinase and pyruvate carboxylase are also of interest because their control is a coordinated one with respect to the regulation of PEPCK. The pathway begins at the crossroads of intermediary metabolism with the use of oxaloacetate, a four-carbon skeleton. Oxaloacetate is the substrate for PEPCK, which catalyzes its conversion to PEP. This is an energy-dependent conversion that overcomes the irreversible final glycolytic reaction catalyzed by pyruvate kinase. The activity of PEPCK is closely coupled with that of pyruvate carboxylase. Whereas the pyruvate kinase reaction produces 1 ATP, the formation of PEP uses two ATPs: one

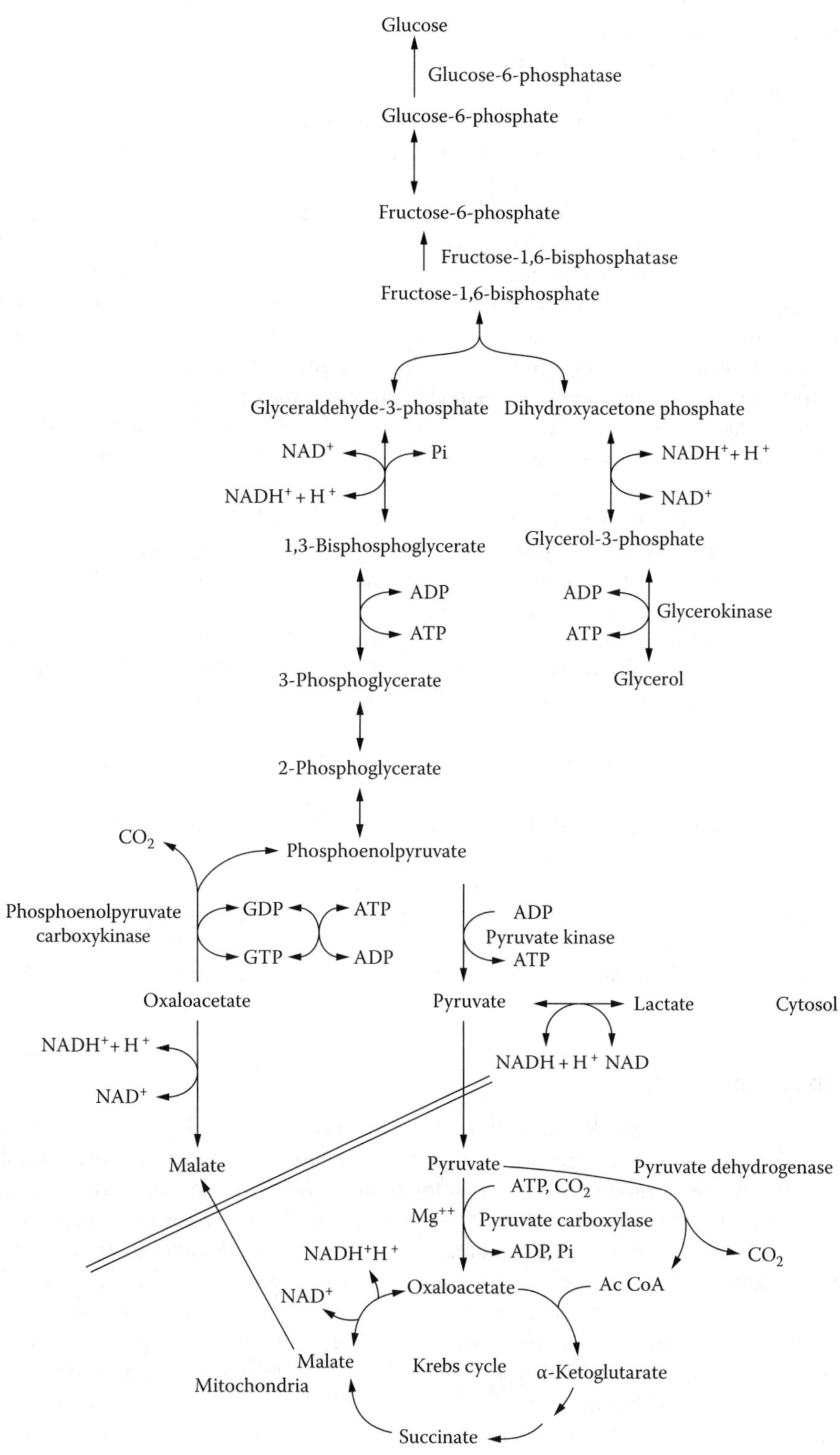

FIGURE R.7 Pathway for gluconeogenesis.

in the mitochondria for the pyruvate carboxylase reaction and one in the cytosol for the PEPCK reaction. PEPCK requires GTP provided via the nucleoside diphosphate kinase reaction, which uses ATP. ATP transfers one high-energy bond to GDP to form ADP and GTP.

The enzyme PEPCK has been studied extensively as scientists have tried to understand the gluconeogenic process. In starvation or uncontrolled diabetes, PEPCK activity is elevated, as is gluconeogenesis. Starvation elicits a number of catabolic hormones that serve to mobilize tissue energy stores as well as precursors for glucose synthesis. Uncontrolled diabetes elicits similar hormonal responses. In both instances, the synthesis of the PEPCK enzyme protein is increased. Unlike other rate-limiting enzymes, PEPCK is not regulated allosterically or by phosphorylation–dephosphorylation mechanisms. Instead, it is regulated by changes in gene transcription of its single copy gene from a single promoter site. This regulation is unique because all of the known factors (hormones, vitamins, and metabolites) act in the same place. They either turn on the synthesis of the messenger RNA for PEPCK or turn it off. What is also unique is the fact that only liver and kidney cells translate this message into active enzyme protein, which catalyzes PEP formation. Other cells and tissues have the code for PEPCK in their nuclear DNA but do not synthesize the enzyme. Instead, these cell types synthesize the enzyme that catalyzes glycerol synthesis. In effect then, only the kidney and liver have an active gluconeogenic process.

The next few steps in gluconeogenesis are identical to those of glycolysis but are in the reverse direction. When the step for the dephosphorylation of fructose-1,6-bisphosphate occurs, there is another energy barrier and instead of a bidirectional reaction catalyzed by a single enzyme, there are separate forward and reverse reactions. In the synthesis of glucose, this reaction is catalyzed by fructose-1,6-bisphosphatase and yields fructose-6-phosphate. No ATP is involved, but a molecule of water and an inorganic phosphate are produced. Rising levels of fructose-2,6-bisphosphatase allosterically inhibit gluconeogenesis while stimulating glycolysis. AMP likewise inhibits gluconeogenesis at this step.

Finally, the removal of the phosphate from glucose-6-phosphate via the enzyme complex glucose-6-phosphatase completes the pathway to yield free glucose. Again, this is an irreversible reaction that does not involve ATP. The glucose-6-phosphate moves to the endoplasmic reticulum, where the phosphatase is located.

Gluconeogenesis can use the carbon skeletons from a number of metabolites of glucose (lactate, pyruvate, and some of the triose phosphates) and also those from deaminated amino acids. Not all of the amino acids enter the gluconeogenic sequence at the same place. Some amino acids serve as substrates for glucose synthesis. Some enter as pyruvate while others enter the Krebs cycle at various points.

Cori and Alanine Cycles

The pathway shown in Figures R.8 and R.9 provides glucose to all cells in the body. Under normal dietary conditions, the glucose synthesized in the kidney is used by it as fuel to run its metabolism. Only under conditions of prolonged starvation (more than 48 h) will the kidney contribute significant amounts of glucose to the circulation. Thus, circulating glucose produced by gluconeogenesis comes from the liver. There are two important metabolite or substrate cycles that are crucial to the effective regulation of blood glucose levels. One is the Cori cycle, shown in Figure R.8, and the other is the alanine cycle, shown in Figure R.9. The Cori cycle involves the use of glucose by the red blood cell. Glucose is oxidized via glycolysis to two molecules of lactate. The lactate is delivered to the liver, which converts it back to glucose via gluconeogenesis. The red cell produces 2 ATPs through the glycolytic process while the liver uses six ATPs to resynthesize the glucose.

The alanine cycle differs from the Cori cycle in that the exchange is between muscle and the liver. Since the muscle cell has mitochondria, it can use the reducing equivalents generated by the glycolytic sequence to generate 4–6 mol of ATP. Rather than lactate, the muscle cell transaminates the surplus glycolytic product, pyruvate, to alanine and sends this alanine to the liver.

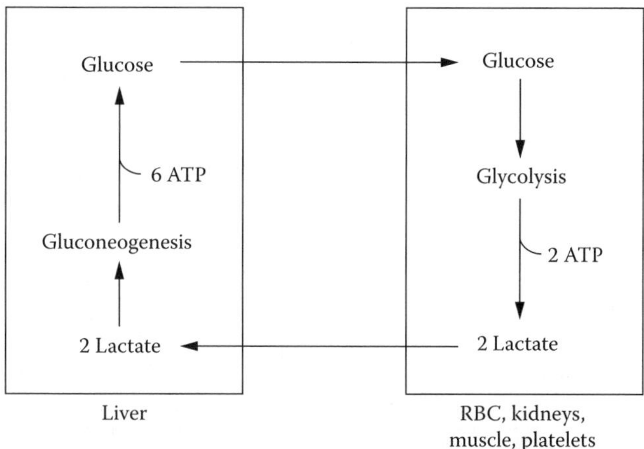

FIGURE R.8 The Cori cycle.

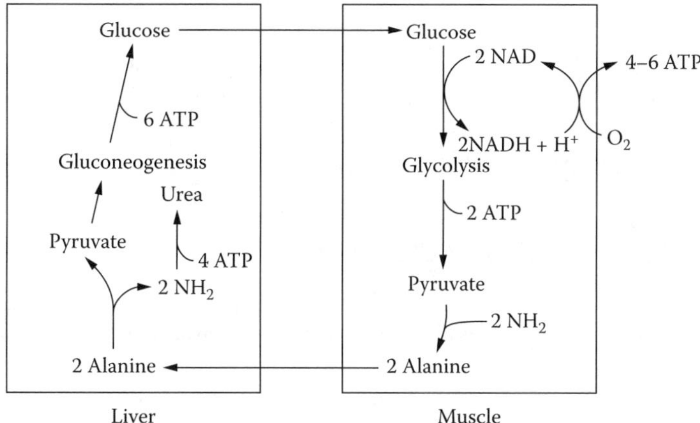

FIGURE R.9 The alanine cycle. Both the Cori cycle and the alanine cycle serve to ensure a supply of glucose to cells that require it.

Once in the hepatocyte, this alanine is deaminated (the amino group used for urea synthesis) and the resultant pyruvate used to resynthesize glucose via gluconeogenesis. These cycles are important in glucose homeostasis because they provide the means for supplying glucose to tissues that need it.

One shuttle, the malate–aspartate shuttle shown in Figure R.10, has rate-controlling properties with respect to gluconeogenesis. The malate–aspartate shuttle works to transport reducing equivalents into the mitochondria. Malate is transported into the mitochondria, whereupon it gives up two reducing equivalents and is transformed into oxaloacetate. Oxaloacetate cannot traverse the mitochondrial membrane, so it is converted to α-ketoglutarate in a coupled reaction that also converts glutamate to aspartate. Aspartate travels out of the mitochondria (along with ATP) in exchange for glutamate. Once out in the cytosol, the reactions are reversed. Aspartate is reconverted to glutamate, and α-ketoglutarate reconverted to oxaloacetate. The oxaloacetate, in turn, can be reduced to malate or decarboxylated to form PEP. Measurement of the activity of this shuttle has revealed that the more active the shuttle, the more active is gluconeogenesis. This is because the shuttle provides a steady supply of oxaloacetate via α-ketoglutarate in the cytosol. This oxaloacetate cannot get there any other way. As mentioned, it is generated by the Krebs cycle in the mitochondria but cannot leave this compartment.

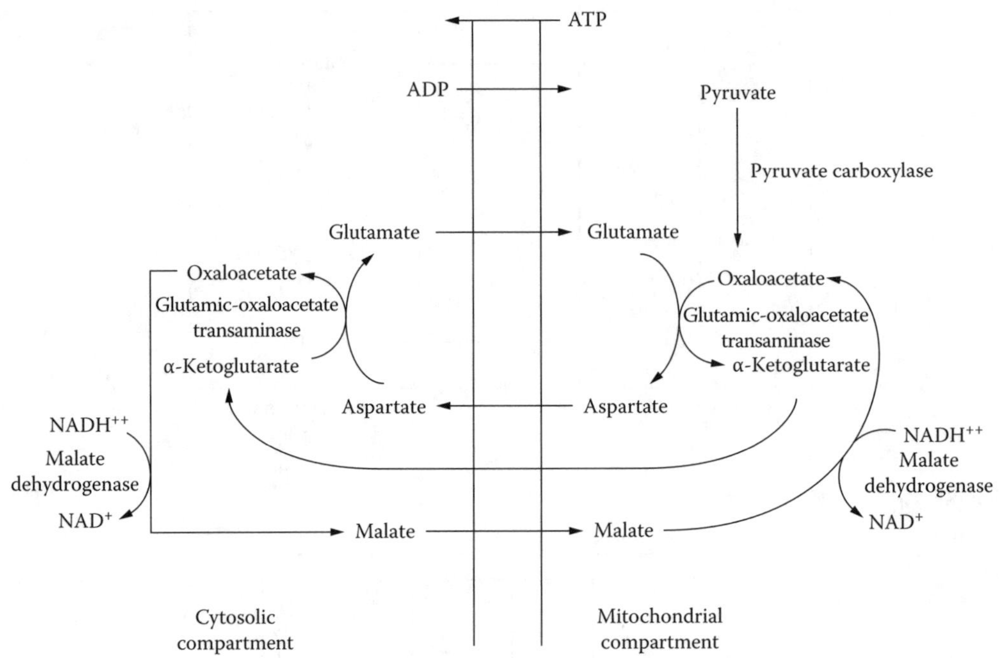

FIGURE R.10 The malate–aspartate shuttle.

RESPIRATION AND THE CITRIC ACID CYCLE

Respiration is the process by which aerobic cells obtain energy from the oxidation of fuel. When coupled with ATP synthesis, the process is called OXPHOS. Carbon dioxide, water, heat, and ATP are the products of this process.

Glycolysis, as well as fatty acid and amino acid oxidation, results in the production of an activated 2-carbon residue, acetyl CoA. This common metabolic intermediate is joined to oxaloacetate to form citrate and is then processed by the citric acid cycle. This cyclic sequence of reactions is found in every cell type that possesses mitochondria. The cycle is catalyzed by a series of enzymes and yields reducing equivalents (H^+) and carbon dioxide. It is illustrated in Figure R.11. Reducing equivalents are produced when α-ketoglutarate is produced from isocitrate, when α-ketoglutarate is decarboxylated to produce succinyl CoA, when succinate is converted to fumarate, and when malate is converted to oxaloacetate. These reducing equivalents, one pair for each step, are carried to the respiratory chain by way of either NAD or FAD. Reducing equivalents from succinate are carried by FAD to site II of the respiratory chain, while those produced by the oxidation of the other substrates are carried by NAD to site I. Once oxaloacetate is formed, it can then pick up another acetate group from acetyl CoA and begin the cycle once again by forming citrate. Thus, for every turn of the cycle, two carbon dioxide molecules and eight pairs of reducing equivalents are produced. As long as there is sufficient oxaloacetate to pick up the incoming acetate, the cycle will continue to turn and reducing equivalents will continue to be produced and these, in turn, will be joined with molecular oxygen to produce water, the end product (with carbon dioxide) of the catabolic process.

This simplistic description of the citric acid cycle implies that it is free of controls and, given adequate supplies of substrates, enzymes, and molecular oxygen, proceeds unhindered. This is not true. There are numerous controls in place that regulate the cycle. The citric acid cycle produces the reducing equivalents needed by the respiratory chain, and the respiratory chain must

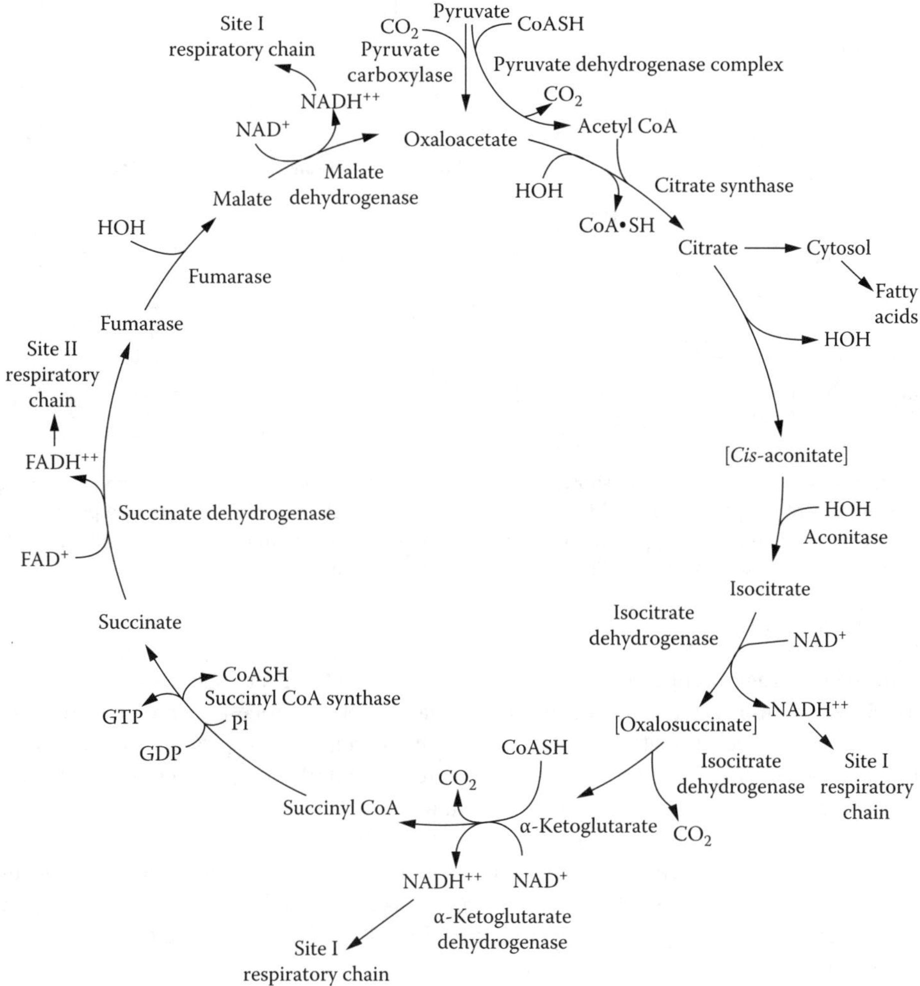

FIGURE R.11 Krebs citric acid cycle in the mitochondria. This cycle is also called the tricarboxylate cycle (TCA). Abbreviations used: HOH, water; FAD, flavin adenine nucleotide; FADH^{++}, flavin adenine nucleotide, reduced; NAD, niacin adenine dinucleotide; NADH^{++}, niacin adenine dinucleotide, reduced; GTP, guanosine triphosphate; GDP, guanosine diphosphate; CoA, coenzyme A; CO_2, carbon dioxide.

transfer these hydrogen ions and their associated electrons to the oxygen ion to produce water. In doing so, it generates the electrochemical gradient (the proton gradient) necessary for the formation of the high-energy bonds of ATP. Obviously, then, these processes, citric acid cycle, respiratory chain, and ATP synthesis, are regulated coordinately.

OXIDATIVE PHOSPHORYLATION

OXPHOS occurs in the mitochondria. Figure R.12 shows the respiratory chain and the places where energy released by the chain is trapped in the high-energy bond of ATP. OXPHOS is the coupled process used for the production of water using oxygen and the reducing equivalents released by the various metabolic steps in intermediary metabolism. Some of the energy released is trapped in the high-energy bond of ATP while the majority of this energy is released as heat.

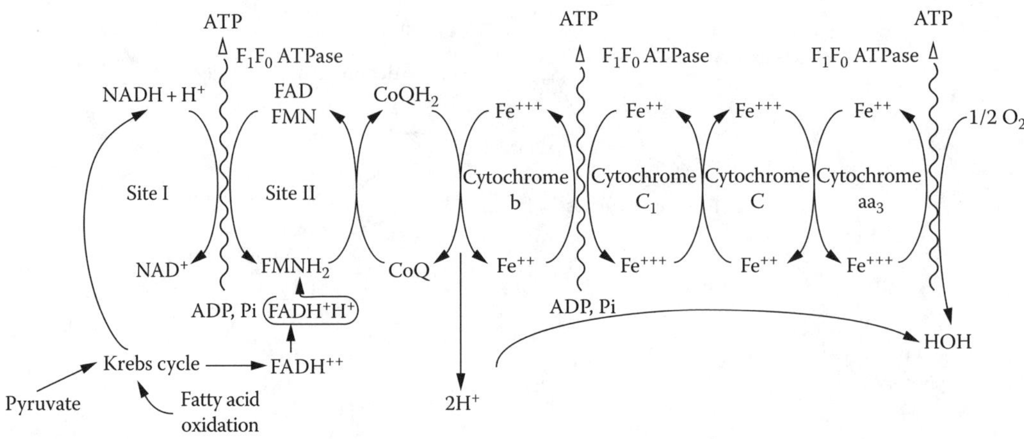

FIGURE R.12 The respiratory chain showing the points where sufficient energy has been generated to support the synthesis of 1 molecule of ATP from ADP and Pi. Each of the segments generates a proton gradient. This energy is captured by the F_0 portion of the ATPase and transmitted to the F_1 portion of the ATPase. If uncouplers are present, the proton gradient is dissipated and all of the energy is released as heat.

RESPIRATORY CHAIN

The pairs of electrons produced at the four steps described earlier in the citric acid cycle, as well as electrons transferred into the mitochondria via other processes, are passed down the respiratory chain to the ultimate acceptor, molecular oxygen. The respiratory chain is shown in Figure R.12. The enzymes of the respiratory chain are particularly complex. They are embedded in the mitochondrial inner membrane and are difficult to extract and study. They catalyze the series of oxidation–reduction reactions that together are known as the respiratory chain.

Although the respiratory chain usually proceeds in the forward direction (toward the formation of water) due to the exergonic nature of the reaction cascade, it should be realized that, except for the final reaction, all of these steps are fully reversible. In order to be reversed, sufficient energy must be provided to drive the reaction in this direction.

The overall regulation of respiration or the activity of the intact respiratory chain is vested in the availability of the phosphate acceptor, ADP. A rapid influx of ADP into the mitochondrial compartment is what is needed to ensure a rapid respiratory rate. For example, the working muscle uses the energy provided by the hydrolysis of ATP and creatine phosphate. Creatine phosphate is split to creatine and a phosphate group, and ATP is hydrolyzed to ADP and Pi. The ADP travels into the mitochondria and stimulates respiration and is used to resynthesize ATP.

ATP SYNTHESIS

As electrons pass down the respiratory chain, ATP is synthesized. The sequential reactions of the respiratory chain generate an electrochemical gradient of H^+ ions across the inner mitochondrial membrane. This gradient serves as the means for coupling the energy flow from electron transport and water formation to the formation of ATP. This involves the mitochondrial membrane. The membrane, and the enzymes and transporters that are embedded in it, couples the energy gradient of the electron flow of the respiratory chain to the synthesis of ATP. To do this, the membrane must be intact and in the form of a continuous closed vesicle. If the membrane is disrupted, coupling will not occur. Respiration may occur, but ATP synthesis will not. The enzymes of the respiratory chain are arranged so as to transport hydrogen ions from the matrix across the inner membrane so that the gradients will develop in proximity to the F_1F_0 ATPase (ATP synthase, Figure R.13) complex and provide a proton gradient sufficient to drive ATP synthesis by causing a dehydration of ADP and Pi.

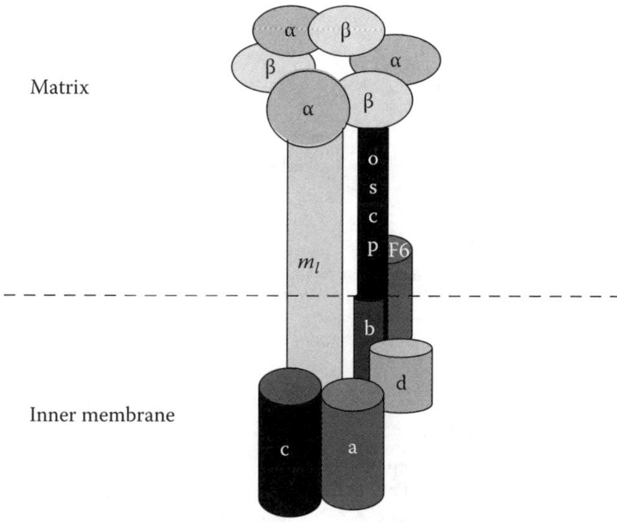

FIGURE R.13 The F_1F_0 ATPase. Note that the lower portion is embedded in the inner mitochondrial membrane while the upper part protrudes out into the matrix. The two parts can be separated. The upper part is the F_1 part.

This energy capture in the ATP molecule is only a fraction of the energy generated by the respiratory chain. The rest of the energy is released as heat.

OTHER SOURCES OF ATP

ATP can also be provided to the contracting muscle by a shuttle known as the creatine phosphate shuttle. Creatine is shuttled into the mitochondria and converted to creatine phosphate by the mitochondrial creatine kinase. The newly synthesized creatine phosphate is then shuttled back to the cytosol whereupon it is then hydrolyzed to provide energy, ATP (using cytosolic ADP) and creatine. Creatine phosphate then serves as a cytosolic source of high-energy phosphate during fast twitch muscle contraction.

FATTY ACID SYNTHESIS

Fatty acid synthesis (Figure R.14) begins with acetyl CoA, which arises from the oxidation of glucose or the carbon skeletons of deaminated amino acids. Acetyl CoA is converted to malonyl CoA with the addition of 1 carbon (from bicarbonate) in the presence of the enzyme acetyl CoA carboxylase. The reaction uses the energy from 1 molecule of ATP and biotin as a coenzyme. This reaction is the first committed step in the reaction sequence that results in the synthesis of a fatty acid. In many respects, it resembles the carboxylation of pyruvate, the first committed step in gluconeogenesis. In both reactions, activated carbon dioxide attached to the biotin–enzyme complex is transferred to the methyl end of the substrate. Although most fatty acids synthesized in mammalian cells have an even number of carbons, this first committed step yields a 3-carbon product. This results in an asymmetric molecule that becomes vulnerable to attack (addition) at the center of the molecule with the subsequent loss of the terminal carbon. The vulnerability is conferred by the fact that the carboxyl group at one end and the CoA group at the other end are both powerful attractants of electrons from the middle carbon group. This leaves the carbon in a very reactive state, and a second acetyl group carried by a carrier protein with the help of phosphopantetheine, which has a sulfur group connection, can be joined to it through the action of the enzyme malonyl transferase. Subsequently, the *extra* carbon is released via the enzyme β-ketoacyl enzyme synthase,

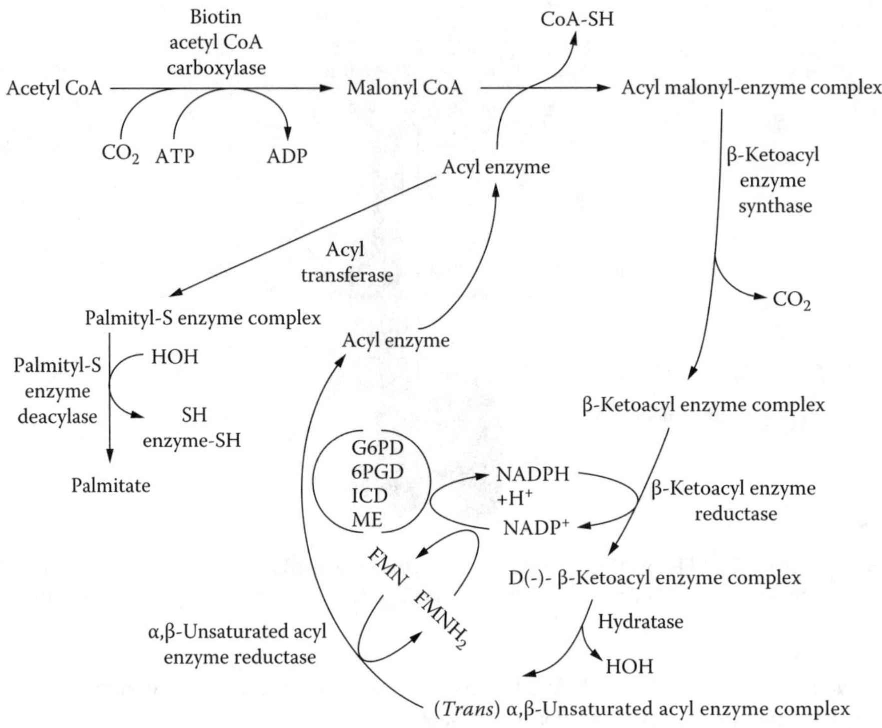

FIGURE R.14 Fatty acid synthesis from acetyl CoA.

leaving a 4-carbon chain still connected to an SH group at the carboxyl end. This SH group is the docking end for all the enzymes that the fatty acid synthase complex comprises. These enzymes catalyze the addition of two carbon acetyl groups in sequence to the methyl end of the carbon chain until the final products, palmityl CoA and then palmitic acid, are produced. Members of this fatty acid synthase complex include the aforementioned malonyl transferase and β-ketoacyl synthase, β-ketoacyl reductase, which catalyzes the addition of reducing equivalents carried by FMN, and an acyl transferase. Upon completion of these six steps, the process is repeated until the chain length is 16 carbons long. At this point, the SH-acyl carrier protein is removed through the action of the enzyme palmityl-S-enzyme deacylase, and the palmitic acid is available for esterification to glycerol to form a mono-, di-, or triacylglyceride.

Fatty acid synthesis does not occur as an uncontrolled sequence of reactions. It has a number of direct and indirect controllers. As mentioned earlier, the synthesis of malonyl CoA is the first committed step in the pathway. It is also the first rate-limiting reaction. Acetyl CoA carboxylase as a rate-limiting enzyme has been studied in detail. It is synthesized as an inactive protomer, which, when citrate levels increase, aggregates to form the active enzyme. Other tricarboxylates can stimulate aggregation but citrate is the preferred anion. Citrate, a citric acid cycle intermediate in the mitochondria, is exchanged for malate or pyruvate. The malate–citrate shuttle is very active in cells also having a very active lipogenic process. This shuttle also has rate-limiting properties. Pyruvate, from the oxidation of glucose via the glycolytic sequence, is also actively exchanged for citrate in the lipogenic cell. Citrate is cleaved through the action of the ATP-citrate lyase (citrate cleavage enzyme), producing oxaloacetate and acetyl CoA. This acetyl CoA is the beginning substrate for fatty acid synthesis. Feedback inhibition of acetyl CoA carboxylase is exerted when palmitoyl CoA accumulates.

Acetyl CoA carboxylase is sensitive to the phosphorylation state of the cytosol. High levels of ATP are needed for the carboxylation of acetyl CoA to form malonyl CoA. Thus, high phosphorylation states (high concentrations of ATP relative to ADP and inorganic phosphate) are a characteristic of high rates of lipogenesis. Acetyl CoA carboxylase is also controlled by a cAMP-mediated phosphorylation–dephosphorylation mechanism in which the phosphorylated enzyme is less active than the dephosphorylated enzyme. Insulin promotes dephosphorylation while glucagon promotes phosphorylation. Thus, when insulin levels are high, one would anticipate high rates of lipogenesis and the reverse when insulin levels are low and glucagon levels are high. One might also anticipate an increase in lipogenesis in hyperinsulinemic individuals, and, indeed, obese people as well as genetically obese experimental animals are characterized by both. As a corollary, one might also anticipate that the consumption of a high-glucose, low-fat diet that stimulates insulin release and also provides ample glucose for conversion to fatty acids would be characterized by high rates of lipogenesis, particularly in the liver. In rodents, this anticipation is justified. However, in humans, there is some discussion as to whether the human diet is sufficiently high in simple sugar and sufficiently low in fat to have the same sort of lipogenic response. Further, phosphorylated sugars have allosteric effects on this enzyme complex. An allosteric effect is one that promotes (or inhibits) the activity of an enzyme or enzyme complex by binding to a site other than the active catalytic site that promotes (or inhibits) the activity of the active catalytic site. An allosteric effector may not be involved in the reaction itself but, through its binding, causes a change in the conformation of the enzyme. In the case of inhibition, such a conformational change may *hide* the active catalytic portion of the molecule. In promotion, the reverse occurs; the *business end* of the molecule is readily accessible to substrate, cofactors, and coenzymes.

Despite the gaps in our knowledge about the details of acetyl CoA carboxylase and fatty acid synthase, the reaction sequence shown in Figure R.14 is well established, as are the effects of certain dietary ingredients and hormones on fatty acid synthesis in living creatures. We know that the fatty acid chain is continually bound to the fatty acid synthase complex and is sequentially transferred between the 4′-phosphopantetheine (pantothenic acid) group of the acyl carrier protein and the sulfhydryl group of a cysteine residue on ketoacyl-ACP synthase during the condensation step.

FATTY ACID ELONGATION

Elongation occurs in either the endoplasmic reticulum or the mitochondria. The reaction differs depending on where it occurs and in what species. Mammalian de novo fatty acid synthesis from excess dietary carbohydrate results mainly in palmitic, stearic, and oleic acid. Some longer-chain fatty acids are produced by specific tissues. Oleic acid is usually produced by the desaturation of palmitic acid, followed by elongation rather than the desaturation of stearic, although both reactions do occur. Chain elongation following desaturation of stearic acid to oleic acid will produce eicosenoic (20:1w9), erucic (22:1w9), and nervonic (24:1w9) acids. These are of the w9 series of fatty acids. Fatty acid elongation and desaturation of the w9 series in the endoplasmic reticulum essentially stops with the formation of 22:3w9. In the w7 series, elongation stops at 18:3w7. The w6 series ends with the formation of arachidonate, while the w3 series continues on up to the formation of 22:6w3. In the endoplasmic reticulum, the reaction sequence is similar to that described for the cytosolic fatty acid synthase complex. The source of the 2-carbon unit is malonyl CoA and NADPH provides the reducing power. The intermediates are CoA esters, not the acyl carrier protein 4′-phosphopantetheine. The reaction sequence in the brain can proceed to produce fatty acids containing up to 24 carbons. In the mitochondria, elongation uses acetyl CoA rather than malonyl CoA as the source of the 2-carbon unit. It uses NADH+H+ as the source of reducing equivalents and uses, as substrate, carbon chains of less than 16 carbons. Mitochondrial elongation is the reversal of fatty acid oxidation, which also occurs in this organelle.

FATTY ACID DESATURATION

Desaturation occurs in the endoplasmic reticulum and microsomes. The enzymes that catalyze this desaturation are the Δ4, Δ5, and Δ6 desaturases. Again, desaturation is species specific. Mammals, for example, lack the ability to desaturate fatty acids in the n6 or n3 position. Only plants can do this, and even among plants, there are species differences. Cold-water plants can desaturate at the n3 position while land plants of warmer regions cannot. Cold-water plants are consumed by cold-water creatures in a food chain that includes fish as well as sea mammals. These, in turn, enter the human food supply and become sources of the n3 or omega 3 fatty acids in marine oils. In animals, desaturation of de novo synthesized fatty acids usually stops with the production of a monounsaturated fatty acid with the double bond in the 9-10 position counting from the carboxyl end of the molecule. Hence, palmitic acid (16:0) becomes palmitoleic acid (16:1) and stearic acid (18:0) becomes oleic acid (18:1).

In the absence of dietary linoleic and linolenic acids, the essential fatty acids (EFAs), most mammals will desaturate eicosenoic acid to produce eicosatrienoic acid. Increases in this fatty acid with unsaturations at ω7 and ω9 positions characterize the tissue lipids of EFA-deficient animals. They are sometimes called mixed-function oxidases, because two substrates (fatty acid and NADPH) are oxidized simultaneously. These desaturases prefer substrates with a double bond in the ω6 position but will also act on ω3 fatty acid bonds and on saturated fatty acids. Desaturation of de novo synthesized stearic acid to form oleic acid results in the formation of a double bond at the ω9 position. This is the first committed step of this desaturation–elongation reaction sequence. Oleic acid can also be formed by the desaturation and elongation of palmitic acid.

Fatty acid desaturation can be followed by elongation and repeated such that a variety of mono- and polyunsaturated fatty acids can be formed. These fatty acids contribute fluidity to membranes because of their lower melting points. An increase in the activity of the desaturation pathway is a characteristic response of rats fed a diet high in saturated fatty acids. The body can convert the dietary saturated fatty acids to unsaturated fatty acids, thus maintaining an optimal P:S ratio in the tissues. Dietary fat composition can regulate desaturase activity, and this regulation correlates with the level of plasma triacylglycerides. These dietary effects are independent of weight status. That is, dietary fat effects on desaturase activity are independent of the effects of weight loss on this enzyme.

FATTY ACID ESTERIFICATION

Most fats in food, as well as those stored in the adipose tissue depots and those present in small amounts in other tissues, exist as triacylglycerides. Triacylglycerides are hydrolyzed to their component fatty acids and glycerol and reesterified at each of several points in their metabolism. The process of fat absorption by the small intestine involves hydrolysis of the dietary glycerides and reesterification prior to entry into the blood stream as either chylomicrons or VLDL. These hydrolysis and reesterification also occur when lipids arrive at the hepatocyte, the myocyte, or the adipocyte. The triacylglyceride is hydrolyzed by interstitial lipoprotein lipase, and the fatty acids are transported into the target cell and reesterified to glycerol-3-phosphate. In the fat cell, this glycerol-3-phosphate usually is a product of glycolysis rather than the glycerol liberated when the triacylglycerol is hydrolyzed. The liberated glycerol usually passes back to the liver, which has a very active glycerokinase to phosphorylate it. In the liver, the phosphorylated glycerol is either used as a substrate for glucose synthesis or recycled into hepatic phospholipids or triacylglycerides or oxidized to CO_2 and water.

The formation of triacylglycerides, regardless of the source for the glycerol-3-phosphate, follows the same pattern in all tissues. With some modification, it is the pathway used for the synthesis of phospholipids. These pathways are shown in Figure R.15.

Triacylglycerides are formed in a stepwise fashion. First, a fatty acid (usually a saturated fatty acid) is attached at carbon 1 of the glycerophosphate. The phosphate group at carbon 3 is electronegative

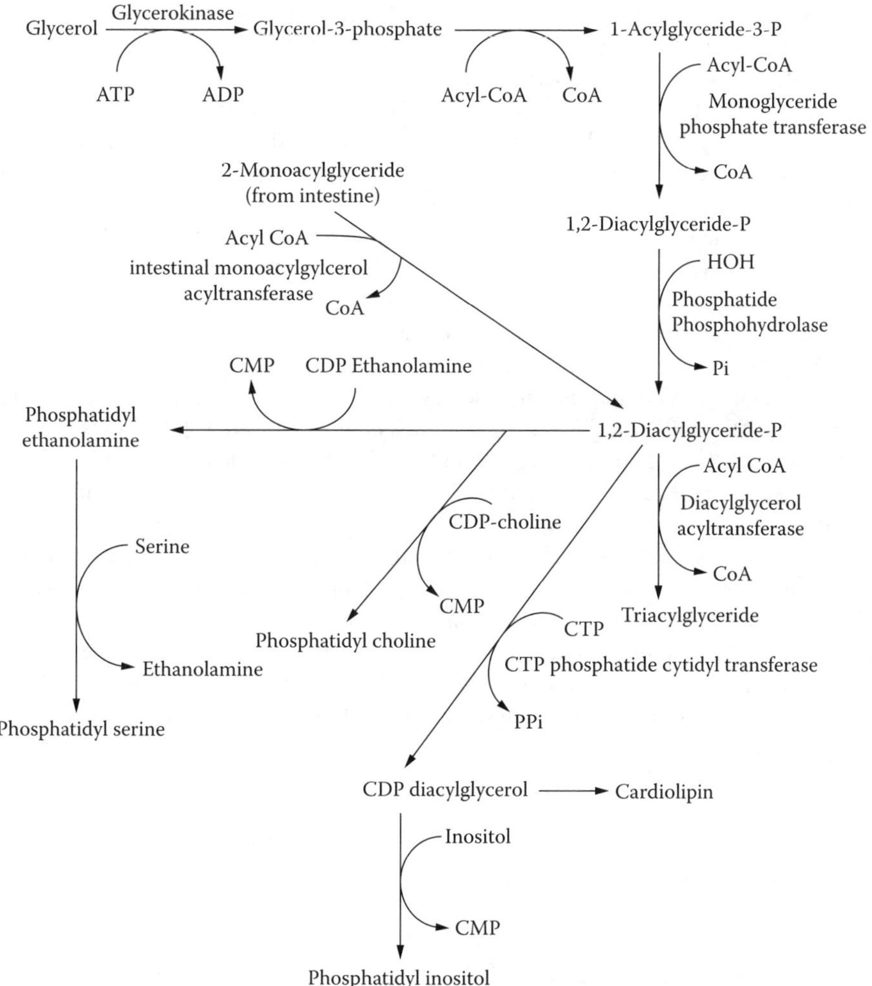

FIGURE R.15 Pathways for the synthesis of triacylglycerides and phospholipids.

and, because it pulls electrons toward it, leaves carbon 1 more reactive than carbon 2. The fatty acid (as an acyl CoA) is transferred to carbon 1 through the action of a transferase. The attachment uses the carboxy end of the fatty acid chain and makes an ester linkage releasing the CoA. Now, the molecule has electronegative forces at each end: the phosphate group on carbon 3 and the oxygen plus carbon chain at carbon 1. Now, carbon 2 is vulnerable and reactive and another carbon chain can be attached. In this instance, the fatty acid is usually an unsaturated fatty acid. At this point, the 1,2-diacylglyceride-phosphate loses its phosphate group so that carbon 3 becomes reactive. The 1,2-diacylglyceride can either be esterified with another fatty acid to make triacylglyceride or can be used to make the membrane lipids phosphatidylcholine, phosphatidylethanolamine, phosphatidylinositol, cardiolipin, and phosphatidylserine.

FATTY ACID OXIDATION

The hydrolysis of stored lipid is catalyzed in a three-step process by one of the lipases specific to mono-, di-, or triacylglycerol. Intracellular hormone-sensitive lipase hydrolyzes fatty acids one at a time from all three carbon positions of the glycerol moiety, and these fatty acids are then available for oxidation. Interstitial hormone-insensitive lipase has a similar mode of action. The lipases that act on the phospholipids to release arachidonic acid for eicosanoid synthesis or to release inositol-1,3,4-phosphate and diacylglyceride or other components of the phospholipids also provide fatty acids for oxidation—but that is not their primary role.

The lipases in the adipose tissue are the key to the regulated release of fatty acids from stored triacylglycerides. These fatty acids can be oxidized in situ by the adipocyte, but usually they are released for transport to other tissues as energy sources. The fatty acids are carried by albumin or by lipoproteins to where they are needed. At the target cell, the fatty acids are liberated from the triacylglycerides carried by the lipoproteins through the action of lipoprotein lipase or liberated from albumin by an (as-yet) undefined mechanism. The liberated fatty acids diffuse through the plasma membrane, bind to the cytosolic fatty acid–binding protein, and migrate through the cytoplasm to the outer mitochondrial membrane or to the peroxisomes, microsomes, or the endoplasmic reticulum. At each of these destinations, they are activated by conversion to their CoA thioesters. This activation requires ATP and the enzyme acyl CoA synthase or thiokinase. There are several thiokinases that differ with respect to their specificity for the different fatty acids. The activation step is dependent on the release of energy from two high-energy phosphate bonds. ATP is hydrolyzed to AMP and 2 molecules of inorganic phosphate. Figure R.16 shows the initial steps in the oxidation of fatty acids.

An important member of the system for the transfer of fatty acids into the mitochondrial or peroxisomal or endoplasmic reticulum for oxidation is the long-chain carnitine acyltransferase (Figure R.17). This is a family of enzymes that catalyze the exchange of carnitine for coenzyme A in the fatty acyl CoA. Conversion of the fatty acyl CoA to fatty acylcarnitine renders the fatty acid more permeable to the various membranes. The activity of these enzymes is regulated. Malonyl CoA inhibits their activity. However, regulation occurs at the level of mRNA transcription by a variety of transcription factors.

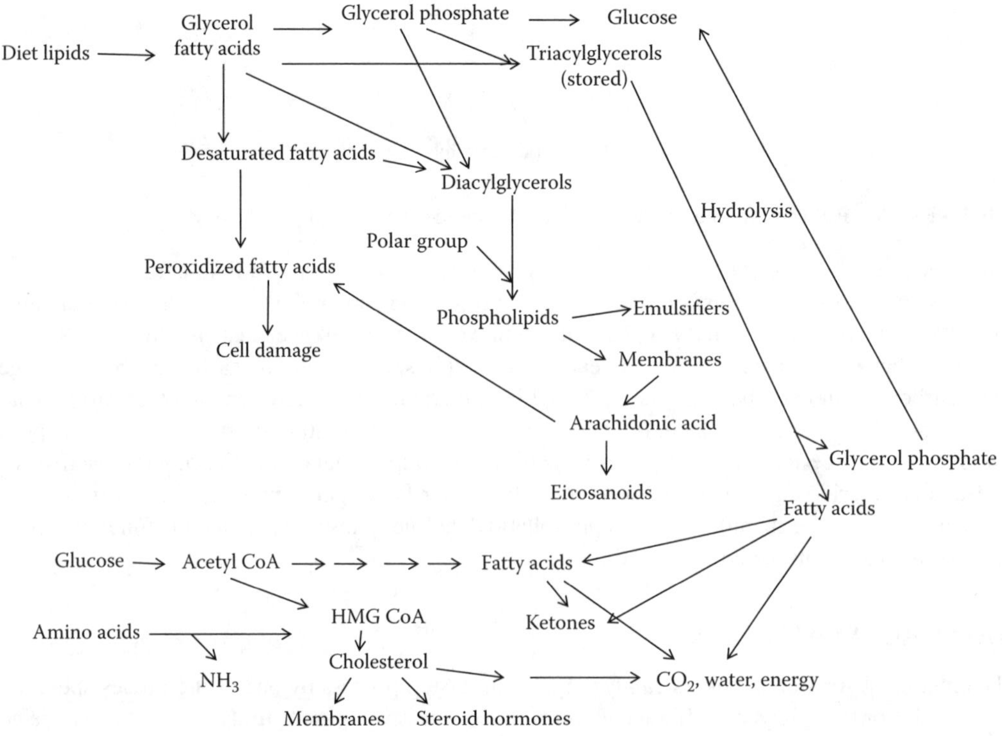

FIGURE R.16 Overview of fatty acid oxidation.

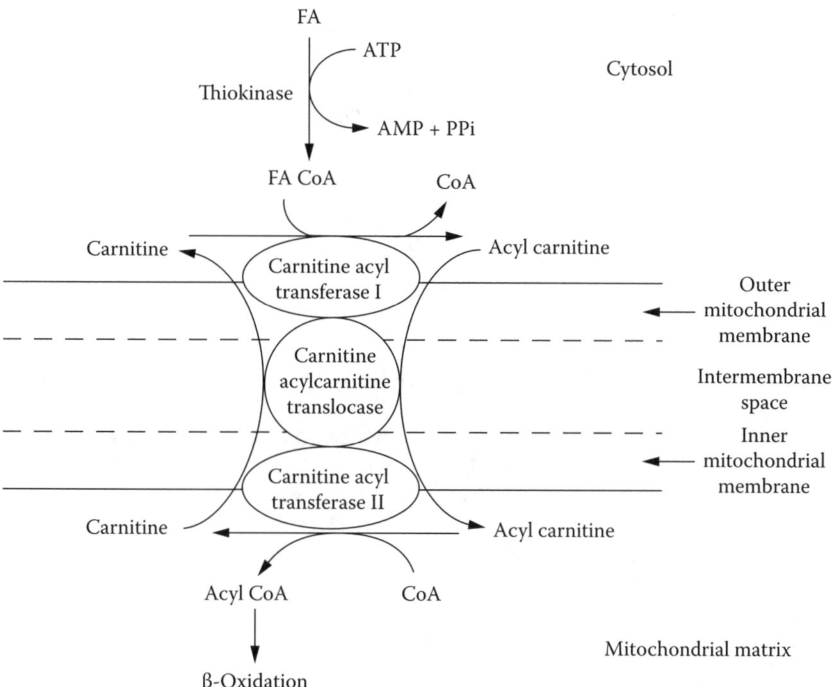

FIGURE R.17 Fatty acid oxidation—the initial steps. Mechanism for the entry of fatty acids into the mitochondrial compartment fatty acid is activated; when it is bound to carnitine with the release of CoA. The acyl carnitine is then translocated through the mitochondrial membranes into the mitochondrial matrix via the carnitine acylcarnitine translocase. As 1 molecule of acylcarnitine is passed into the matrix, 1 molecule of carnitine is translocated back to the cytosol and the acylcarnitine is converted back to acyl CoA. The acyl CoA can then enter the β oxidation pathway.

Without carnitine, the oxidation of fatty acids, especially the long-chain fatty acids, cannot proceed. Acyl CoA cannot traverse the membrane into the mitochondria and thus requires a translocase for its entry. The translocase requires carnitine. Carnitine is synthesized from methionine and lysine. While most of the fatty acids that enter the β oxidation pathway are completely oxidized via the Krebs cycle and respiratory chain to CO_2 and HOH, some of the acetyl CoA is instead converted to the ketones, acetoacetate, and β-hydroxybutyrate. The condensation of 2 molecules of acetyl CoA to acetoacetyl CoA occurs in the mitochondria via the enzyme β-ketothiolase. Acetoacetyl CoA then condenses with another acetyl CoA to form HMG CoA. At last, the HMG CoA is cleaved into acetoacetic acid and acetyl CoA. The acetoacetic acid is reduced to β-hydroxybutyrate, and this reduction is dependent on the ratio of NAD^+ to $NADH^{++}$. The enzyme for this reduction, β-hydroxybutyrate dehydrogenase, is tightly bound to the inner aspect of the mitochondrial membrane. Because of its high activity, the product (β-hydroxybutyrate) and substrate (acetoacetate) are in equilibrium. Measurements of these two compounds can thus be used to determine the redox state (ratio of oxidized to reduced NAD) of the mitochondrial compartment.

HMG CoA is also synthesized in the cytosol, however, because this compartment lacks the HMG CoA lyase; the ketones are formed only in the mitochondria. In the cytosol, HMG CoA is the beginning substrate for cholesterol synthesis. The ketones can ultimately be used as fuel but may appear in the blood, liver, and other tissues at a level of less than 0.2 mM. In starving individuals, or in people consuming a high-fat diet, blood and tissue ketone levels may rise above normal (3–5 mM). However, unless these levels greatly exceed the body's capacity to use them as fuel (as is the case in uncontrolled diabetes mellitus with levels up to 20 mM), a rise in ketone levels is not a cause for concern. Ketones are the metabolic fuels of choice for muscle and brain. Although both tissues may

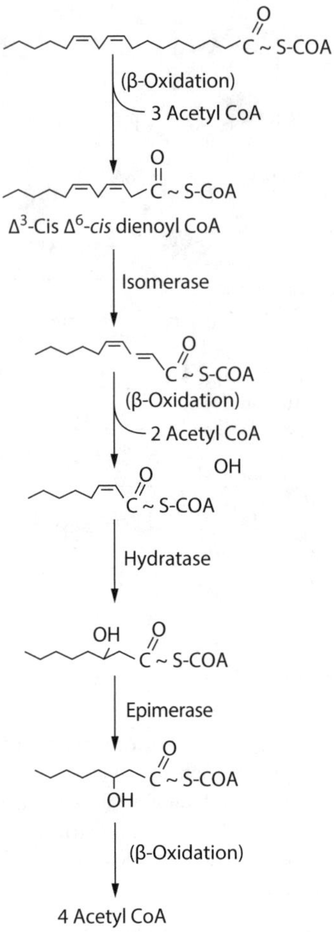

FIGURE R.18 β-Oxidation of fatty acids.

prefer to use glucose, the ketones can be used when glucose is in short supply. Ketones are used to spare glucose wherever possible under these conditions. The oxidation of unsaturated fatty acids follows the same pathway as the saturated fatty acids until the double-bonded carbons are reached. At this point, a few side steps must be taken that involve a few additional enzymes.

Linoleate has two double bonds in the *cis* configuration. β-Oxidation removes three acetyl units, leaving a CoA attached to the terminal carbon just before the first *cis* double bond (Figure R.18). At this point, an isomerase enzyme, D3 *cis* D6 *trans* enoyl CoA isomerase, acts to convert the first *cis* bond to a *trans* bond. Now, this part of the molecule can once again enter the β-oxidation sequence and two more acetyl CoA units are released. The second double bond is then opened, and a hydroxyl group is inserted. In turn, this hydroxyl group is rotated to the L position, and the remaining product can then reenter the β-oxidation pathway. Other unsaturated fatty acids can be similarly oxidized. Each time the double bond is approached, the isomerization and hydroxyl group addition takes place until all of the fatty acid is oxidized.

While β-oxidation is the main pathway for the oxidation of fatty acids, some fatty acids undergo α-oxidation so as to provide the substrates for the synthesis of sphingolipids. These reactions occur in the endoplasmic reticulum and mitochondria and involve the mixed-function oxidases because they require molecular oxygen, reduced NAD, and specific cytochromes. The fatty acid oxidation that occurs in organelles other than the mitochondria (i.e., peroxisomes) are energy-wasteful reactions because these other organelles do not have the Krebs cycle, nor do they have the respiratory chain that take the reducing equivalents released by the oxidative steps and combines them with oxygen to make water-releasing energy that is then trapped in the high-energy bonds of the ATP. Peroxisomal oxidation in the kidney and liver is an important aspect of drug metabolism. The peroxisomes are a class of subcellular organelles that are important in the protection against oxygen toxicity. They have a high level of catalase activity, which suggests their importance in the antioxidant system.

The peroxisomal fatty acid oxidation pathway differs in three important ways from the mitochondrial pathway. First, the initial dehydrogenation is accomplished by a cyanide-insensitive oxidase that produces H_2O_2. This H_2O_2 is rapidly extinguished by catalase. Second, the enzymes of the pathway prefer long-chain fatty acids and are slightly different in structure from those (with the same function) of the mitochondrial pathway. Third, β-oxidation in the peroxisomes stops at eight carbons rather than proceeding all the way to acetyl CoA. It may be that peroxisomal oxidation helps the body get rid of fatty acids that are in excess of 20 carbons in length. The peroxisomes also serve in the conversion of cholesterol to bile acids and in the formation of ether lipids (plasmalogens).

This review provides the framework for the discussion of the metabolism of the macronutrients and the micronutrients. If the reader requires further information on nutritional biochemistry, the authors suggest the following: Murray, R.K., Bender, D.A., Botham, K.M., Kennelly, P.J., Rodwell, V.W., and Weil, P.A. (2012) *Harper's Illustrated Biochemistry*, 29th edition, McGraw Hill, Lange, New York, 818 pages. Current textbooks on biochemistry and physiology will also be useful. The reader can also peruse the current literature as well as that published in the past. The literature on intermediary metabolism is immense.

1 Energy

Energy is the basis for all life. It must be provided in the food that is consumed so that all of the metabolic reactions that characterize the living creature can occur. Energy is expressed in heat units known as calories or joules. The energy that is used by living creatures or is consumed by them or is expended by them should be expressed as kjoules or kcalories; however, these units are sometimes misused.

DEFINITION

Classical nutritionists use the term Calorie or kilocalorie (kcal) to represent the amount of heat required to raise the temperature of 1 kg of water 1°C.[1] The international unit of energy is the joule. One Calorie or kcalorie is equal to 4.184 kilojoules or 4.2 kjoules (kJ). There are cogent reasons to express energy in terms of kjoules. Nutritionists have realized that the energy provided by food is used for more than heat production. It is also used for mechanical work (muscle movement) and for electrical signaling (vision; neuronal messages) and is stored as chemical energy. The joule is 107 ergs, where 1 erg is the amount of energy expended in accelerating a mass of 1 g by 1 cm/s. The international joule is defined as the energy liberated by one international ampere flowing through a resistance of one international ohm in 1 s. Even though the use of joules or kilojoules is being urged by international scientists as a means to ease the confusion in discussions about energy, students will still find the term Calorie or kcal in many texts and references. In some texts, the term calorie, spelled with a lower case *c*, is used. This heat is actually 1/1000th of the heat unit spelled with an upper case *C*. Physicists use the term calorie to represent the amount of heat required to raise the temperature of 1 g of water 1°C. Note that this definition uses 1 g, not 1 kg, as stated previously. Even though it is not correct, the term calorie is used in some nutrition literature when in fact Calorie or kcal is intended.

HOW IS ENERGY MEASURED?

The energy value of the food can be measured directly in an instrument called a bomb calorimeter (Figure 1.1). It measures the heat that is produced when a small sample (usually 1 g) of food is burned (oxidized) in the presence of oxygen. This complete oxidation represents the gross energy (GE) value of that particular food. The bomb calorimeter is a highly insulated, boxlike container. All the heat produced during the oxidation of a dried sample of food is absorbed by a weighed amount of water surrounding the combustion chamber. A thermometer registers the change in the chamber temperature. The instrument's name is derived from the design of the combustion chamber, which is, indeed, a small bomb.

Some corrections have been applied to these energy values. For example, the GE value of a protein food is higher than the actual biologic value of that food. This is because the end products of oxidation in the body must be excreted as urea, a process that costs energy. The combustion or oxidation of protein yields 5.6 Calories (23.5 kJ)/g; the energy yield from the oxidation of protein after correction for urea formation and digestive loss by the body is about 4 Calories (~16.8 kJ)/g. Corrections for digestive losses are also applied to the values obtained for the combustion of lipids and carbohydrates. The value of 4.1 Calories (17.22 kJ)/g is rounded off to 4 (16.8 kJ) for carbohydrates and the value of 9.4 (39.5 kJ) for lipids is rounded off to 9 (37.8 kJ). Listed in Table 1.1 are a few representative foods and their energy values. The energy value of a wide variety of foods can be

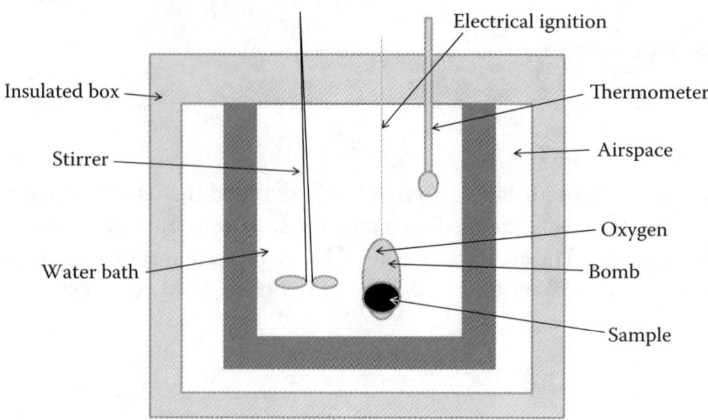

FIGURE 1.1 Cross section of a bomb calorimeter.

TABLE 1.1
Energy Content of Selected Human Foods

Item	Amount	Food Energy kcal	Food Energy kJ
Milk (3.3% fat)	8 oz	150	628
Skim milk	8 oz	85	356
Butter	1 oz	204	854
Egg	50 g	80	335
Bacon	2 slices	85	356
Hamburger, lean	3 oz	185	774
Apple	1 medium	80	335
Avocado	216 g	370	1548
Banana	119 g	100	418
Grapefruit	241 g	50	209
Orange	131 g	65	272
Bread, white	25 g (1 slice)	70	293
Brownie with nuts	20 g	95	397
Peanut butter	16 g	95	397
Green beans	1 cup, 125 g	30	126
Corn	1/2 cup, 83 g	65	272
Tomato, raw	135 g	25	105

Source: http://www.nal.usda.gov/foodcomposition
Note: 1 kcal = 4.184 kJ.

accessed using the web address http://www.nal.usda.gov/foodcomposition. The database is updated regularly. This address is for the USDA National Nutrient Database for Standard Reference, Release 25. It not only includes the energy values for a wide variety of foods but also contains the values for protein, fat, vitamins, and minerals. These data can be used to assess the nutritional adequacy of a person's food intake by comparing the nutrient content of the food eaten to the recommended daily intakes of the essential nutrients. There are a number of computer programs that are available for this assessment.[2] Some of these are listed in Table 1.2. Some of the programs provide not only nutrient analysis but also a means for calculating recipes and menu management.

TABLE 1.2
Some Software Programs for Nutrient Analysis

Name	Source	Web Address
ASA24	National Cancer Institute	www.riskfactor.cancer.gov/tools/instruments/asa24
Food Intake Analysis System	University of Texas School of Public Health	www.sph.uth.tmc.edu/research/centers/dell/fias-food-intake-and analysis-system
Food processor	SQL ESHA Research	www.esha.com
NutriGenie	NutriGenie	www.nutrigenie.biz/
NutritionistPro	Axxya Systems	www.nutritionistpro.com
Nutrition Service Suite	The CBORD Group, Inc.	http://hcl.cbord.com/products/product_193

ENERGY INTAKE

Using the values for food energy as given in the USDA Nutrient Analysis Database, one can estimate energy intake. The individual must keep a careful record of the amounts and kinds of foods and beverages consumed. The amounts can be recorded as weights or volumes and then converted to 100 g as indicated in the database. Conversions of fluid ounces or pounds or measuring amounts, that is, amounts using a measuring cup, will be needed to make best use of the database. Again, there are computer programs available to make this task easier. In order to assess food energy intake, one must make a complete and detailed record of all the foods and liquids consumed in addition to providing a description of how the food is prepared. If the chicken is fried, it will have a different energy value than chicken that is roasted or broiled. If one wishes to reduce or increase the energy intake in order to lose or gain weight, then it is important to know how much is being consumed on a regular basis. Usually, nutritionists recommend that an average of a 3-day record of intake that includes 1 weekend day can approximate the usual energy intake of an individual. If the intake is then reduced by 10% or 20% as an example, and the individual simultaneously increases his or her energy expenditure, then a net negative energy state will develop with consequent weight loss. If an increase in physical activity accompanies a decrease in energy intake, this will translate into a change in body composition (and metabolism) as weight maintained as muscle will increase the metabolic activity while energy conserved in the adipose tissue is raided and weight is lost. Similarly, if weight gain is desired, then the energy intake must be increased 10%–20% and energy expenditure decreased to have a net positive energy balance (EB). In this instance, however, it should be noted that physical activity is an important consideration because weight gained as muscle is far better than weight gained as fat. On a volume basis, muscle is more dense than adipose tissue. Weight gained as muscle will occupy less space and will be firmer than weight gained as fat. It is a delicate balance between muscle mass accretion and fat mass accretion. Chapter 3 addresses the issues of body composition in greater detail.

ENERGY NEED

The Food and Nutrition Board of the National Academy of Sciences has not made specific recommendations for the energy intakes by humans because of the variability within the human population. In contrast to the recommended intakes for the other essential nutrients, there can be no *safety factor* in the energy intake recommendation. This is because the energy need is so individualized that an intake that would result in obesity in one person might be totally inadequate for another. Instead the board has recommended a range of acceptable intakes. For children aged 1–3, a range of fat, carbohydrate, and protein intake as a percentage of the total intake of energy is 30–40, 45–65, and 5–20, respectively. For children aged 4–18, the recommendations are 25–35, 45–65, and 10–30, respectively. Lastly for adults, the ranges are 20–35, 45–65, and 10–35, respectively. Periodically, recommendations are updated by the National Research Council, Food and Nutrition Board and published by the National Academy Press (Washington, DC). For the latest information, the reader should go to the National Academy of Sciences website (www.nap.edu) or the Dietary Reference Intake (DRI) website (www.ods.od.nih.gov/Health_information/Dietary Reference Intakes). The intake recommendations are influenced by gender, age, body size, genetic background, hormonal status, and daily activity. In addition, the types of food consumed, that is, high-fiber foods or essential fatty acid–deficient foods, and prescribed medications such as corticosteroids or disease states, that is, irritable bowel syndrome, food allergies, hypertension, and diabetes (and the drugs used to control these problems), may affect energetic efficiency that in turn could influence the use of the food energy consumed. All of these factors must be considered in the development of the recommended energy intake of the individual.

ENERGY EQUATION

The objectives of digestion, absorption, and metabolism in the animal system are to convert the chemicals in foods to the chemicals in the body. The conversion of food chemicals to body chemicals is stepwise via the pathways of intermediary metabolism and not 100% efficient. Energy is lost as heat in many of the steps of this conversion. For example, energy is lost from food as it passes through the digestive system. Energy is needed to absorb the breakdown products of this digestion. Further, energy is lost as the food components are metabolized via glycolysis, the pentose phosphate shunt, glycogenolysis, glycogenesis, lipolysis, fatty acid oxidation, amino acid catabolism, and urea formation. (See the review of Nutritional Biochemistry that precedes this chapter.) The end products of these pathways include carbon fragments and reducing equivalents (H^+). The citric acid cycle takes these products and further reduces them to CO_2 and H^+. The H^+ is joined to oxygen to make water via the mitochondrial respiratory chain and the energy released by this chain is either released as heat or captured in the high-energy bond of adenosine triphosphate (ATP) via oxidative phosphorylation (OXPHOS). ATP is used in many different reactions of metabolism where it can be degraded to adenosine diphosphate (ADP) or adenosine monophosphate (AMP) or converted to some other high-energy compound such as phosphocreatine.

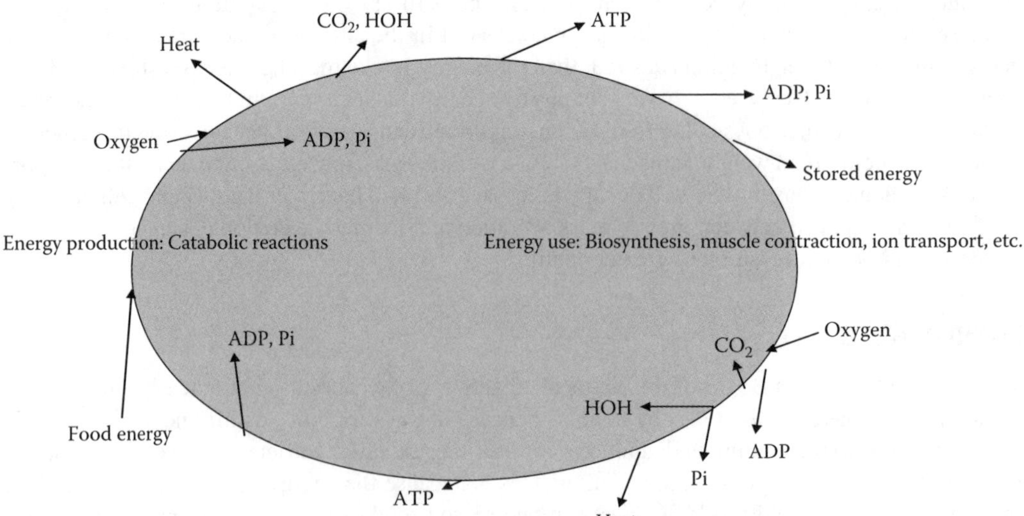

FIGURE 1.2 Overview of energy gains and losses showing the high-energy compound ATP as the medium of exchange. Other high-energy compounds, for example, GTP, UTP, and creatine phosphate, are also involved in the cycle of energy intake and expenditure.

Energy exchange and conversion are at the crossroads of the pathways that convert the food chemicals to body chemicals. As described, some of the chemical energy from food is trapped in high-energy storage compounds, but, at each step of the conversion process, much of the energy escapes as heat. This heat serves to maintain body temperature. However, because this heat is also lost from the body through radiation as well as through the various excretory processes, these losses must be replaced. Hence, the daily need for food and its associated energy content. Figure 1.2 illustrates the continuity of energy losses and gains by the living system. Energy is gained from oxidation of the fats, carbohydrates, and proteins consumed as food. This energy is transmitted via ATP (and other high-energy transfer compounds) to a variety of essential macro- and micromolecules in the body, which, in turn, are needed to sustain its optimal function. As these functions also consume and release energy, more must be provided by the diet. Over and over, this cycling occurs; this is the nature of the dynamic state of the living body. No reaction or process is ever completed and stops. The only time this happens is at death.

ENERGY TERMINOLOGY

The metabolic pathways that exist within the body have been described through the many reports of the detailed examinations of cells, tissues, and organs. However, when one is interested in the whole body, not just a particular cell, one views the energy equation in different terms that describe the losses of energy from the food as it passes from the dinner plate into the body and its metabolic end products are excreted. These terms are as follows: The energy provided by food is its GE, and it can be determined in a bomb calorimeter as already mentioned. Not all of this energy is available to the consumer. Some is lost through digestion and is assumed to appear in the feces. Corrections for this loss (GE—the energy value of the feces) are defined as the *apparent digestible energy* (abbreviated as DE). During digestion, energy is lost to the system through the breakdown of food to its appropriate absorbable components. Energy is needed for absorption (active transport) and for the excretion of metabolic end products such as urea. Together, these urinary and fecal losses amount to about 10% of the GE of the diet if that diet is a mixture of fats, proteins, and carbohydrates. Most tables giving food energy values make a correction for these losses.

Metabolizable energy (ME) consists of the energy needed to keep the body warm (the heat increment, HI) and to run the body processes.[3–10] The HI is composed of the heat released through basal work done by the body, for example, heart muscle contraction, and the heat released as food is oxidized and converted to usable body components. The latter is sometimes referred to as the specific dynamic action of food, or diet-induced *thermogenesis* (DIT). In animal nutrition, the HI is defined as the increase in heat production following the consumption of food by an animal in a thermoneutral environment. Heat production is related to the surface area of the body producing the heat and is generally expressed in terms of body size or weight to the 0.75 power ($W^{0.75}$).[3] *Utilizable energy* (UE) is that which is used for body work. *Net energy* (NE) likewise has two components: one is *basal energy* (BE) or the absolute minimum amount of energy that is needed to keep the body alive, while the other is the energy that is either available for storage or is withdrawn from storage (EB). If weight is neither gained nor lost, the body is in EB. If weight is lost, the body is in negative EB, and if weight is gained, the body is in positive EB. This concept of balance is one that is used by classical nutritionists considering a variety of essential nutrients. Methods to measure protein balance, calcium balance, and so forth have been devised. They are practical for many situations because the methodology does not usually require that the animal under study be killed.

The measurement of energy need based on energy lost as heat or on the consumption of the oxygen needed to oxidize fats, carbohydrates, and proteins to provide this energy has been well studied. The energy need is additive.[7–10] That is, energy is needed to maintain the body (BE) plus energy is needed to sustain the body's various activities, that is, voluntary movement, work, growth, reproduction, and lactation. Many methods have been developed for estimating the BE requirement. Some of these are listed in Table 1.3. The methods vary from very simplistic ones based on height

TABLE 1.3
Methods and Equations Used for Calculating BE Need

Method	Equation or Units for Expression
1. Heat production, direct calorimetry	kcal (kJ)/m^2 (surface area)
2. Oxygen consumption; indirect	O_2 cons./$W^{0.75}$
3. Heat production; indirect	Insensible water loss (IWL) = Insensible Weight loss (IW) + (CO_2 exhaled – O_2 inhaled) Heat production = IWL × 0.58 × (100/25)
4. Energy used; indirect	$\text{Basal energy} = \dfrac{\text{Creatinine } N\,(\text{mg/day})}{0.00482(W)}$
5. Estimate (energy need not be measured) (Harris–Benedict equation)[10]	BMR = 66.4730 + 13.751W + 5.0033L – 6.750A (men) BMR = 655.0955 + 9.563W + 1.8496L – 4.6756A (women)
6. Estimate (energy need not be measured)	BMR = 71.2W0.75 (men) BMR = 65.8W0.75 (women)

Notes: W, weight in kg; L, height in cm; A, age in years.

and weight to those based on actual measures of heat production, measures of oxygen consumption, or estimates of heat production based on the heat needed to evaporate water lost by the body. Each method has its advantages and disadvantages. In those methods where actual measurements are made, the BE need must be measured in the postabsorptive state and the energy needed for growth and activity added to it.[4–6,12–15] The postabsorptive state occurs after consumed food is digested and absorbed but before the state of starvation ensues. Starvation involves a series of hormonal responses that can affect the fuel used by the different tissues.

In humans, the postabsorptive state is about 12–14 h after the last meal. In the mouse, it is 10 h; rat, 17 h; guinea pig, 22 h; rabbit, 60 h; pig, 96 h; and ruminant, 5–6 days. The time needed to achieve the postabsorptive state depends on the length of the digestive tract and whether the animal is a ruminant (cow, sheep, goat) or has a sizable *fermentation vat* within the gastrointestinal tract. In some species, that is, the rat and the mouse, the cecum serves this function, while in others, that is, the horse, an enlarged intestinal tract has this function. If energy need was being assessed by measuring heat production, the postabsorptive state would be that heat released at the point (in a continuous measurement) where the slope of the line changes, as shown in Figure 1.3.

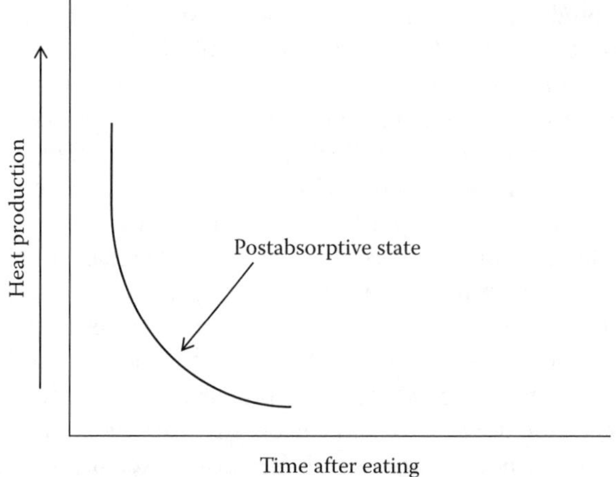

FIGURE 1.3 Changes in heat production mark the postabsorptive state.

At any rate, the postabsorptive state is characterized by a low respiratory quotient (RQ). The RQ is the ratio of CO_2 released to O_2 consumed. In the postabsorptive state, it is about 0.85, which indicates that a mixture of fat and carbohydrate is being oxidized. If only carbohydrate were being oxidized, the RQ would be 1.0 since the oxidation of glucose uses and releases equal amounts of oxygen and carbon dioxide. If only fat were being oxidized, the RQ would be about 0.7. This is because fatty acids require far more oxygen for their oxidation than they produce as carbon dioxide.

As an example, palmitic acid, $C_{16}H_{22}O_2$ when oxidized, uses 23 mol O_2. It produces 16 mol CO_2 and 16 mol water. The RQ is calculated as follows:

$$RQ = 16\ CO_2/23\ O_2 = 0.7$$

When the fatty acids are mobilized from the stored triacylglycerols and the RQ is computed on this basis, a slightly higher RQ results. For example, using a theoretical triacylglycerol consisting of two molecules of stearic acid and one of palmitic acid attached to a glycerol backbone, the equation is as follows:

$$C_{55}H_{106}O_6 + 76.5\ O_2 \rightarrow 55\ CO_2 + 53\ HOH$$

$$RQ = 55\ CO_2/76.5\ O_2 = 0.719$$

The ratio of glucose to fatty acids being oxidized will be reflected in the measured RQ. Most humans consuming a mixed diet will have an average RQ of about 0.87. It will vary throughout the typical feeding–fasting day–night cycle followed by most people who work during the day and sleep at night. Just before breakfast, the RQ will be at its lowest, while after the evening meal, it will likely be at its highest. This, of course, is dependent on the composition of the meals consumed as well as on their spacing. As mentioned in the beginning of this section, the basal heat production or oxygen consumption is usually measured in the postabsorptive state. This usually means a measurement made before breakfast, and it also usually means that the metabolic fuel mix is that of glucose (from glycogen) plus fatty acids (from the fat depots). Other species may have different patterns. For example, the rat, a nocturnal animal, will have been very active during the night and will rest during the day. The day–night cycle in RQ will therefore be reversed.

Using indirect calorimetry, the oxygen consumed and the carbon dioxide produced is measured, and it can be determined whether the subject is gaining or losing weight and whether the subject is in nitrogen balance. Nitrogen balance means that the nitrogen from the protein in the food is replacing that of the proteins being degraded in the body. (The nitrogen balance concept is discussed in greater detail in Chapter 8.) EB has a similar meaning. The energy used by the body is replaced by the energy provided by the diet. A subject in energy and nitrogen balance is neither losing nor gaining weight.

As mentioned earlier, energy released as heat can be determined directly by using a calorimeter. This instrument is similar in concept to the bomb calorimeter used to measure the GE of food. It is nothing more than a very large insulated box with sensors that can detect very small differences in temperature. It can also be designed to include measures of spontaneous activity and, in the case of small animals, can measure food and water intake. The size of the subject determines the size of the box. A small animal such as a mouse would need a very small box, while a cow or a horse would need a very large one. Using a calorimeter is extremely tedious and the instrumentation is very expensive. Much of the collected data can be computerized.[19,20]

When human heat production is assessed, the subjects live in the box for various periods of time from a few hours to several days depending on the objectives of the experiment. The heat emitted from the body is detected by sensors in the walls of the chamber and measured. There are corrections for clothing that might affect the measurement of heat released by the body. The food energy available to the subject is carefully measured before consumption, and the weight and height of the subject is known. The body weight/height measurements are used to calculate body surface area. To determine insensible body weight loss over the observation period, the subject is carefully weighed before and after the observation period. Corrections are made for food and water consumed and urine and feces excreted. In some instances, measurements of water lost through the lungs (expired air is 100% water saturated) and skin (undetected evaporative water loss) are added to the gains and losses described earlier. The weight that is lost under these conditions is considered to be the insensible weight loss. The feces and urine are collected and their energy content determined. Usually, a 24 h period of observation is used for the acquisition of basic measurements then the subject may be asked to consume different foods or different amounts of foods or engage in different activities to determine the effects these changes have on heat production. Smaller time intervals can be used to assess heat production as a result of specific treatments such as the responses to hormone treatments or specific dietary ingredients or as a result of physical activity. The BE is presumed to be that heat produced by the subject upon waking, while the heat production of a sedentary life is that measured during the interval after waking. Heat production during sleep is also measured. Usually, sleep induces a 10% decrease in heat production.

The calorimeter chamber is kept at a temperature that elicits neither sweating nor shivering. This temperature range is called the zone of thermic neutrality. Both sweating and shivering are energy-using processes. Sweating allows the individual to lose heat energy through water evaporation and loss. Shivering generates heat through surface muscle contraction and relaxation. Both processes are important to body-heat regulation at environmental temperatures above and below the zone of thermic neutrality. If one were to measure energy loss above, at, and below this zone, increased energy loss would be observed at each extreme, as shown in Figure 1.4.

The temperatures that mark the limits of the zone of thermic neutrality can vary between species as well as between individuals within a species. The zone of thermic neutrality is influenced by body covering. The winter coat of many animals is longer and thicker than the summer coat. The winter hair or fur coat traps a layer of air around the body and insulates it against the lowered environmental temperature. Humans do the same thing with their clothing choices. Heavier, more-insulating clothing is selected for winter wear keeping the human more comfortable when outside in cold weather. These strategies affect the temperature at which shivering as a heat-generating mechanism begins. In addition, many animals adopt social behaviors such as huddling that work to decrease the need to generate heat via shivering. Some animals go into hibernation (a deep long-lasting sleep) that reduces their energy need and heat output. In the summer, the reverse occurs to allow heat dissipation without the need for sweating to facilitate body-heat loss. Some species do

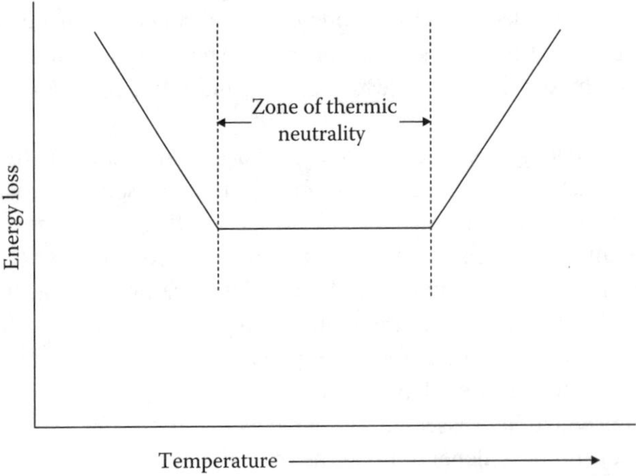

FIGURE 1.4 Zone of thermic neutrality; energy is lost when the environmental temperature is below or above this zone.

not sweat but use panting to release excess energy. With warm environmental temperatures, animals lose their heavy hair coat, while humans wear minimal clothing. Air conditioning serves to keep the environmental temperature in the thermal neutral zone. For humans, these environmental controls (heating/air conditioning) serve to decrease energy wasting and this, in turn, affects EB, adding to the amount of energy available for storage as fat and for use to maintain the body's metabolism.

Directly measuring the energy lost as heat from the body is not always convenient or possible. Few clinical settings can afford the time and expense to assess energy need in this way. There is an alternative. Because metabolic processes not only produce heat but also consume oxygen, measuring the RQ (ratio of carbon dioxide produced to oxygen consumed) provides an indirect method for determining energy need. The consumption of oxygen and the production of heat are direct correlates. The oxidation of energy-providing nutrients (fats, carbohydrates, and proteins) requires oxygen, which is used to make water and carbon dioxide. For every molecule of oxygen used to make water, there is an associated release of energy that is either trapped in the high-energy bond of ATP or released as heat.[4,5,9,11,16–20] Thus, you can measure either the heat produced or the amount of oxygen consumed and have a fairly good estimate of the energy involved. The energy need can be estimated as that needed to sustain basal metabolism (the amount of energy need to keep the body operational) plus that needed to support the body's activities. The basal oxygen consumption can be measured, as can the increase in oxygen consumption with activity.[21–23] The difference between growing and nongrowing animals can be obtained so that the energy cost of growth can be estimated.[9,16,24,25] Similarly, if a person or animal is either gaining or losing weight, the energy cost of this weight gain (or loss) can be estimated.[8,14,24,25] There are other uses for measuring oxygen consumption or respiratory rate. For example, the 24 h carbohydrate oxidation rate has been used to predict ad libitum food intake.[26]

The basal metabolic rate (BMR) is defined as the minimal amount of energy needed by the body to maintain its function. Measured as either heat production or oxygen consumption, it is the basis to which the other energy needs/uses are added. The BMR is influenced by the hormonal status of the subject. Excessive thyroid hormone production elevates the BMR and deficient thyroid production lowers it. Other hormones likewise affect the BMR. The stress hormones, epinephrine and norepinephrine, can increase oxygen consumption as can the adrenal glucocorticoids. Growth hormone, insulin, estrogen, and testosterone also influence BMR but their influence is indirect. Table 1.4 lists the effects of some of the hormones on BMR. Note that many of these hormones are those involved in the stress response. Starvation and forced food intake reduction elicits a stress response. This in turn has an effect on BMR. However, this response is short lived; as the individual adapts to starvation/food intake reduction, a variety of metabolic adjustments occur including a reduction in BE expenditure and an increase in metabolic efficiency. These adaptations or adjustments set the stage for the subsequent change in body metabolism that occurs during the recovery from such a stress. If the food restriction is released, then the body responds with an increased energetic efficiency

TABLE 1.4
Hormone Effects on BMR

Hormone	Effect
Low thyroid	Decrease
High thyroid	Increase
Epinephrine	Increase
Norepinephrine	Increase
Estrogen	Increase
Testosterone	Increase
Growth hormone	Increase
Insulin	Decrease

during the recovery period.[27] In practice, this means that if a person reduces food intake so as to lose weight, that individual might just set the stage for a weight rebound once the food restriction is lifted.

As mentioned earlier, the oxidation of metabolic fuels produces ATP, the energy coinage of the cell. ATP is a high-energy compound that serves as an intermediary in energy transfer. The major metabolic pathways are characterized by the number of ATPs used or produced.[9,16,26] Not all of the ATPs are produced by the mitochondrial OXPHOS process. Some are produced as a product of substrate oxidation. The number of ATPs used or produced by these pathways is shown in Table 1.5. This number assumes that the reducing equivalents produced enter the OXPHOS system, which produces three ATPs if site 1 is used and two ATPs if site 2 is used. Other high-energy intermediates (GTP, UTP, etc.) also play a role in the energy equation but they are not listed in this table.

Different metabolic fuels yield different amounts of ATP. For example, a molecule of glucose when oxidized to pyruvate will yield a net of six to eight molecules of ATP. Two molecules of ATP are needed to initiate the reaction sequence. The product of glycolysis is then sent to the citric acid cycle with the reducing equivalents (H^+) sent through the respiratory chain to make water and some of the energy is captured in the high-energy bond of ATP. The coupled process (respiration and ATP synthesis) is called OXPHOS. When glucose is oxidized to CO_2 and HOH under aerobic conditions, 31–33 molecules of ATP are formed. If each ATP has an energy value of 7.3 kcal (30.5 kJ)/high-energy bond, then, in theory, glucose oxidation to pyruvate should yield 7.3 kcal (30.5 kJ/mol) × 8 ATP

TABLE 1.5
ATPs Produced or Used by the Major Metabolic Pathways

Pathway	ATPs Produced or Used
Glycolysis	2 ATPs used to support hexokinase and phosphofructokinase
Glyceraldehyde-3-phosphate dehydrogenase (2 NADH)	4–6 ATPs/mol glucose[a]
Phosphoglycerate kinase	2 ATP/mol glucose
Pyruvate kinase	2 ATP/mol glucose
Total	(6–8) – 2 = 6–8 ATPs
Citric acid cycle	
Pyruvate dehydrogenase	5/mol glucose
Isocitrate dehydrogenase	5/mol glucose
α-Ketoglutarate dehydrogenase	5/mol glucose
Succinate thiokinase	2/mol glucose
Succinate dehydrogenase	3/mol glucose
Malate dehydrogenase	5/mol glucose
Total	25 ATPs
Urea synthesis	4 ATPs used for every mol of urea formed
Fatty acid synthesis	
Formation of methylmalonyl CoA	1 ATP used
Fatty acid oxidation	
Activation of fatty acid (thiokinase)	1 ATP used
Acyl CoA dehydrogenase (FADH)	2 ATPs produced/acetyl unit
β-Hydroxyacyl CoA dehydrogenase (NAD^+H^+)	3 ATPs produced
Citric acid (or TCA) cycle	24 ATPs produced/acetyl unit

[a] This number depends on whether the NADH formed during glycolysis is transported into the mitochondria via the malate–aspartate shuttle or via the α-glycerophosphate shuttle. The malate–aspartate shuttle produces 3 ATP's/NADH. If the α-glycerophosphate shuttle is used, then only 2 ATPs will be produced/NADH.

or 58.4 kcal (244.3 kJ) per molecule. Complete glucose oxidation should yield 262.8 kcal (1099.6 kJ). A fatty acid such as palmitate will yield a net of 129 molecules of ATP (2 molecules of ATP are needed for activation) and palmitate should yield 7.3 kcal × 129 ATP or 941.7 kcal (3940 kJ) trapped in the high-energy bond of ATP. However, these figures do not correct for the energy trapped in the ATP molecule through substrate phosphorylation, nor do they correct for energy lost as heat. The assumption is also made that the reducing equivalents produced by these catabolic reaction sequences will be sent to the OXPHOS system for a maximum of 3 mol ATP for every reducing equivalent. This does not always occur. When palmitate is oxidized in a bomb calorimeter, 2,609 kcal (10,958 kJ) of heat is released per molecule. Compare this to the 941.7 kcal (3940 kJ) calculated earlier for the in vivo oxidation of palmitate. Obviously, in the living system, not all of the energy of nutrient oxidation is captured in the high-energy bond of ATP, GTP, or UTP; most of it is released as heat. The difference between the in vitro and in vivo oxidation of palmitate has to do with the energetic efficiency of the living system. Some energy is lost when the carbon is joined to the oxygen to make carbon dioxide; some is lost when water is made and of course a lot is used to make the high-energy bond of ATP and its related compounds, GTP and UTP. If a ratio were to be made of the amount of energy captured in the ATP to that totally available (941.7:2609), the finding would be that about 36% of the total inherent energy of palmitate could be captured in the chemical bonds of ATP versus ~64% that is released as heat. Note that palmitate oxidation produces more than three times the amount of ATP than does glucose.

ENERGY RETAINED

After the heat production associated with exercising muscles and the inefficiency of energy capture as described earlier are accounted for, two other components must be included. These are the energy that is stored in the fat and glycogen depots and the energy needed to sustain growth or production.[28] This is quite straightforward. If weight is neither gained nor lost, then the EB is zero. If weight is gained as fat, the energy value of that fat must be accounted for. Body composition studies can provide the estimate for fat gained or lost (see Chapter 3 for details on body composition). If the fat is deposited as preformed fat, that is, the fat in the diet is hydrolyzed at the gut, transported to the depot, and re-esterified for storage, the energy cost of this storage is minimal. This is a very efficient way to accumulate body-fat stores. On the other hand, if glucose is used to make the stored triacylglycerols, the process is quite inefficient. To make 1 molecule (mol) of tripalmitin (palmitate is a 16 carbon fatty acid), 12 molecules of glucose and 45 molecules of ATP would be needed to make 3 molecules of palmitoyl CoA. Another half molecule of glucose and four ATPs would be needed to make the glycerol phosphate. Altogether, 12.5 mols of glucose plus 49 mols of ATP would be necessary to make 1 mol of tripalmitin. To generate the ATP for this synthesis, 1.3 mol glucose would have to be completely oxidized since 1 mol would give only 31–33 ATPs, and 49 are needed. Tripalmitin synthesis from glucose is energetically more expensive because only 4 of the 6 glucose carbons are used to make the 16-carbon fatty acid, palmitate. It will take 4 glucoses to make 1 palmitate and 12 glucoses to make 3 palmitates.

$$\text{12 Glucose} + \text{45 ATP} + O_2 \rightarrow \text{3 Palmityl CoA} + \text{24 } CO_2$$
$$\text{0.5 Glucose} + \text{ATP} \rightarrow \alpha \text{ glycerophosphate} + \text{ADP}$$
$$\text{3 Palmityl CoA} + \alpha \text{ glycerophosphate} \rightarrow \text{Tripalmitin}$$

1 mol glucose completely oxidized yields 36 ATP, but 49 are needed. Thus, 49/36 = 1.4 mol glucose are needed to provide the ATP or 1.4 × 294.8 = 412.72 and 12 + 0.5 + 1.4 = 13.9 mol glucose are needed to produce 1 mol tripalmitin; each glucose has a value of 294.8 kcal or 1238 kJ. Table 1.6 illustrates these calculations.

However, if this cost was computed using the energy value of tripalmitin (7,597 kcal or 31,907 kJ) corrected for the energy value of all the glucose needed to make the palmityl CoA and all the ATP used, the cost would be (7597 − 4068 − 412.72) ÷ 7597 or 41% of the total energy value of the

TABLE 1.6
Efficiency of Storing Energy from Dietary Fat versus That Using Glucose for Triglyceride Synthesis (Tripalmitin)

Cost

3 Pal + 3 ATP + 3 CoASH → 3 Pal CoA + 3 AMP (2 ATP/palmitate → pal CoA)

4 ATP + 0.5 glucose → αGP + 4 ADP

3 Pal CoA + αGP → tripalmitin

10 ATP/36 ATP per mole glucose = 0.27 mol glucose

0.5 + 0.26 = 0.76 mol glucose + 3 mol palmitate + 10 mol ATP → 1 mol tripalmitin

tripalmitin. To store preformed tripalmitin would cost 10 ATP, each with a value of 7.3 kcal or 30.5 kJ. The total cost would be 73 kcal or 305 kJ. If the total energy value of tripalmitin was 7,597 (31,907 kJ), then the efficiency of storing preformed fat would be (7,597 – 73) ÷ 7,597 or ~98%.

Using protein for energy is even more costly and less efficient because the protein that is degraded for energy must first be broken down into its constituent amino acids and these in turn must be deaminated and the amino group used to make urea. It takes five ATPs to make one molecule of urea. Approximately 20% of the GE of a typical protein is lost because of the need to synthesize urea. So, energetically, this is a very expensive process. Nonetheless, many humans overconsume food protein, and of course when this occurs, the surplus protein is degraded. The carbon skeletons of the deaminated amino acids can either be oxidized for energy or used to synthesize body fat or used to synthesize glucose (gluconeogenesis). The latter process would only use a very small number of these carbon skeletons.

Protein synthesis is likewise very expensive energetically. Each amino acid that is incorporated into a polypeptide chain requires an ATP for its activation. In a protein containing many hundred amino acids, the requirement for ATP is enormous. ATP is also required for the synthesis of the mRNA coded for the protein being synthesized. Because protein synthesis is so energy dependent, the energy requirement to support growth (protein synthesis) can be quite large.

Using dietary protein for body protein synthesis can be either very efficient or very inefficient, depending on the amino acid content of the diet and the body proteins being synthesized. This aspect of metabolism will be described in Chapter 9. However, the energetics of protein deposition using dietary protein is quite straightforward. Disregarding the energy cost of amino acid oxidation, urea formation, and the growth process, if the energetic efficiency of protein turnover is examined, an efficiency of about 82% is found. This figure is arrived at using the assumption that the dietary protein is used *completely and exclusively* to replace degraded body protein. For ease of description, let us take a hypothetical amount (100 g) of protein that is to be degraded and replaced. This 100 g would have a GE value of 570 kcal or ~2384 kJ. For every amino acid incorporated into this protein, 5 ATPs would be used plus 1.2 ATPs for rearrangements of the structure. This would mean an energy cost of about 694 kcal or ~2904 kJ. Dividing the energy value of the protein produced by the cost of its production gives an efficiency of about 82%. Practically speaking, for the average human adult in the United States, the energetic efficiency of protein turnover is of little importance. The typical U.S. diet is not limiting with respect to protein or energy.

ENERGETIC EFFICIENCY

The food that provides the energy does so by providing fuel for oxidation to provide heat, ATP, CO_2, and water. The heat produced through this oxidation is needed to keep the body warm, but it is also a measure of the energy need. That is, the heat produced (and that can be measured) is the energy that is lost from the body and must be replaced. Of the inherent energy of palmitate, 36% is trapped by the body when this fuel is used and 64% is released as heat (see previous discussion). This 40/60 (rounded figures) distribution of energy available to the body versus that released as heat is an average distribution. More or less can occur in each category. The pattern of distribution is influenced by the composition of the diet,[29–32] age or life stage,[14,15,33,34] and the genetics of the consumer.[35–42] An example of the effect of diet composition on energetic efficiency occurs when an essential fatty acid–deficient diet is fed. This deficiency state is characterized by a decrease in the efficiency of use of food for body weight gain (see Chapter 10). On the other hand, growing individuals are more efficient than nongrowing individuals. Genetically obese individuals are likely more efficient at storing fat than are genetically thin people.[35–42]

Feed efficiency is a term used to designate the efficiency with which an animal (or human) uses the food it consumes to build new tissue as it grows or rebuild body tissue that is lost through the normal conditions of life. Those animals (including humans) that can gain more body weight on less food are more efficient than those animals that require more food for the same gain. Meat-animal production research has been devoted to increasing energetic efficiency using dietary and nondietary techniques. Selective breeding, for example, of beef animals has resulted in bovines that grow rapidly and consume less food per pound of weight gained than animals used for this purpose a century ago. Whereas it used to take 3 years to produce a bovine of a size suitable for use, it now takes 2 years or less to produce a meat animal ready for market. Furthermore, the meat produced today is of higher quality in terms of tenderness, flavor, and nutrient content than that produced 100 years ago. Other meat animals (sheep, pigs, chickens, goats) likewise have been selectively bred to produce a rapidly growing, energetically efficient animal. With the growing emphasis today on the production of meat with a lower fat content, animal scientists are continuing to use genetics and dietary maneuvers to produce an animal that meets the consumers' demands.

Just as the diet and genetics of the meat animal determine its energetic efficiency, so too can these same effects be expected in humans. Genetic and dietary factors interact and, in so doing, determine the rate and extent of longitudinal growth as well as the development of muscle mass and fat mass. At present, the segregation of humans by genotype (the sequence of bases in the DNA) although possible is not practical on a population basis. However, genes that appear to be important in the development of obesity (excess fat mass) are being identified (see Chapter 5 and visit the website www.ncbi.nih.gov/OMIM). How diet, particularly the sources of energy, can affect the phenotypic expression of these obesity-related genes is being explored.

UTILIZABLE ENERGY

The energy expended to do the body's work is referred to as UE. This is the energy used by muscles as they contract in the course of voluntary activity or work. This energy is sometimes referred to as the activity increment. That is, it is the energy cost associated with body movement, which is added to the BE need when the energy requirement is estimated.[22,23] For sedentary persons, only a small increment is needed, but for very active persons, a large increment will be needed to sustain activity. As much as a 200% increment above BE need may be required to sustain a high level of activity and maintain body weight. Shown in Table 1.7 are some representative activities and their associated energy cost given as heat units per kilogram body weight per hour. These data were acquired decades ago using a mobile respirometer.[22] The researchers actually followed the subjects around holding (in some cases) the respirometer so that the subject could perform the stated tasks. Some of the activities listed may seem out of date. For example, the activity of dishwashing means washing dishes in the sink by hand in sudsy water followed by rinsing and then stacking the dishes in a drainboard. It was not the task of rinsing the dishes prior to loading them into a dishwashing machine.

The various activities used different muscles and body parts and elicited different respirometer values that in turn were translated into the energy cost of that activity. Note that this cost is in addition to that of the BE need. The energy cost is the result of the activities of the whole body, but in practical terms, it reflects the activity of the musculoskeletal system. In the course of muscle contraction, oxygen is used for the oxidation of metabolic fuels by the

TABLE 1.7
Energy Cost of Activities Exclusive of Basal Metabolism and the Influence of Food

Activity	kcal/kg/h	kJ	Activity	kcal/kg/h	kJ
Bed making	3.0	12.6	Paring potatoes	0.6	2.5
Bicycling (century run)	7.6	31.9	Playing cards	0.5	2.1
Bicycling (moderate speed)	2.5	10.5	Playing ping-pong	4.4	18.4
Boxing	11.4	47.9	Piano playing (Mendelssohn's *Song*	0.8	3.3
Carpentry (heavy)	2.3	9.7	*Without Words*)	1.4	5.9
Cello playing	1.3	5.5	Piano playing (Beethoven's *Appassionata*)	2.0	8.4
Cleaning windows	2.6	10.9	Piano playing (Liszt's *Tarantella*)	0.4	1.7
Crocheting	0.4	1.7	Reading aloud	9.8	41.0
Dancing, moderately active	3.8	16	Rowing	16.0	66.9
Dancing, rhumba	5.0	21	Rowing in race	7.0	29.3
Dancing, waltz	3.0	12.6	Running	5.7	23.8
Dishwashing	1.0	4.2	Sawing wood	0.4	1.7
Dressing and undressing	0.7	2.9	Sewing, hand	0.6	2.5
Driving car	0.9	3.8	Sewing, foot-driven machine	0.4	1.7
Eating	0.4	1.7	Sewing, electric machine	0.8	3.3
Exercise			Singing in loud voice	0.4	1.7
Very light	0.9	3.8	Sitting quietly	3.5	14.6
Light	1.4	5.6	Skating	10.3	43.1
Moderate	3.1	13	Skiing (moderate speed)	0.6	2.5
Severe	5.4	22.7	Standing at attention	0.5	2.1
Very severe	7.6	31.9	Standing relaxed	1.4	5.9
Fencing	7.3	30.7	Sweeping with broom, bare floor	1.6	6.7
Football	6.8	28.6	Sweeping with carpet sweeper	2.7	11.3
Gardening, weeding	3.9	16.4	Sweeping with vacuum sweeper	7.9	33.1
Golf	1.5	6.3	Swimming (2 miles/h)	0.9	3.8
Horseback riding, walk	1.4	5.9	Tailoring	5.0	20.9
Horseback riding, trot	4.3	18.0	Tennis	1.0	4.2
Horseback riding, gallop	6.7	28.0	Typing, rapidly	0.5	2.1
Ironing (5 lb iron)	1.0	4.2	Typing, electric typewriter	0.6	2.5
Knitting sweater	0.7	2.9	Violin playing	2.0	8.4
Laboratory work	2.1	8.8	Walking (3 miles/h)	3.4	14.2
Laundry, light	1.3	5.4	Walking rapidly (4 miles/h)	8.3	34.7
Lying still, awake	0.1	0.4	Walking at high speed (5.3 miles/h)	1.2	5.0
Office work, standing	0.6	2.5	Washing floors	0.4	1.7
Organ playing (1/3 handwork)	1.5	6.3	Writing		
Painting furniture	1.5	6.3			

working muscle. Heat is released and water and carbon dioxide are produced. The more active a person is, the more oxygen is needed for the oxidation of metabolic fuel by the muscle. It is the measurement of the oxygen consumed and carbon dioxide released that allows for the calculation of the energy cost of the activity. In some instances, the energy cost is reduced because the individual has undergone extensive training in that activity. Trained athletes are more efficient in their use of metabolic fuels than are nontrained, sedentary individuals. Training involves an increase in use of specific muscle groups as well as an increase in lung and heart action. With training, the muscles can use fatty acids as metabolic fuels in addition to the glucose

TABLE 1.8
Summary of the Effects of Training on Metabolism and Body Composition

Decreased RQ during exercise
Decreased fat mass
Increased muscle mass[a]
Increased fatty acid mobilization during exercise
Increased glucose synthesis by the liver
Increased aerobic capacity of muscle
Improved glucose tolerance
Decreased need for insulin to facilitate glucose use
Decreased heat production via activation of UCPs in muscle[a]

[a] May be localized; depends on the types of muscles used for the activity.

from glycogen and of course circulating blood glucose. During exercise, the RQ in the trained individual decreases. This indicates fatty acids are being metabolized. Fatty acid oxidation by working muscle will spare glucose and will decrease the rate of lactate production. The muscle does not store large amounts of lipid for use during work, but it can use fatty acids liberated from fat depots through the action of the catabolic hormones. Part of the training is to increase muscle fatty acid oxidation while also increasing the glycogen–glucose reserve in the muscle. The so-called glycogen-loading technique used in training endurance athletes dictates the exhaustion of the muscle glycogen store followed by rest and glycogen repletion just prior to the competitive event. During the rest/repletion period, a high-carbohydrate diet is consumed. This exhaustion/repletion routine results in an increased supply of glucose from glycogen within the muscle. Since the first phase of glycolysis is anaerobic, an enlarged supply of glucose from glycogen can be oxidized in the absence of oxygen, and thus exhaustion, which is characterized by an oxygen debt, is delayed. Training or adaptation to exercise or work is thus characterized by decrease in RQ due to both an increase in the oxidation of fatty acids and an increase in the anaerobic use of glucose from glycogen. Table 1.8 summarizes the effects of exercise on metabolism, while Table 1.9 gives some typical results of a comparison of trained and untrained subjects with respect to their oxygen and glucose use during a bout of exercise. Note that the untrained and trained subjects consumed the same amount of oxygen, but the trained subjects had a lower RQ. This means that the trained subjects were oxidizing some fatty acids. That fatty acids were used is seen in the last column, showing that the trained subjects consumed less glucose per minute than did the untrained subjects. Exercise is further discussed from the clinical perspective in Chapter 5.

Training also has effects on a number of hormones. One study by Jurimae et al.[43] reported that plasma ghrelin levels were significantly increased following exercise by trained male athletes. Ghrelin is a small peptide involved in growth hormone secretion and in energy homeostasis. It is a gut hormone produced by the stomach and signals satiety information to the hypothalamus and also

TABLE 1.9
Effect of Training on Oxygen Uptake and Fuel Use

Subject	O_2 (L)	RQ (CO_2/O_2)	Glucose (mmol/min)
Trained	3.0	0.90	10.6
Untrained	3.0	0.95	13.3

signals the release of growth hormone. Growth hormone stimulates protein synthesis and lipolysis. Plasma ghrelin levels are often reduced in obese individuals and substantially elevated in starving or malnourished people. It is likely that the increased muscle mass of the trained athlete can be explained in part by the exercise effect on not only ghrelin but also on the increased release of leptin, growth hormone, testosterone, and insulin-like growth factor (IGF-1). All of these hormones play a role in energy homeostasis as well as on the partitioning of energy and nutrients toward body protein and fat.

THERMOGENESIS

Another way energy is lost from the body as heat is the heat lost as one or more of the uncoupling proteins (UCPs) are activated. In early years, it was thought that this heat was associated with the degradation of the food components in preparation for its use by the body for its maintenance. Hence, it was called DIT. Now, however, there seems to be another explanation having to do with the production and release of proteins called UCPs.[44–54]

Uncoupling Proteins

UCPs are inner mitochondrial membrane transporters that dissipate the proton gradient, thus releasing heat.[45] The UCPs are similar in size and homologous in both amino acid sequence and gene sequence for the majority of their structures. Three distinct UCPs have been identified so far: UCP_1, UCP_2, and UCP_3. Each of these is found in different cell types. UCP_1 is uniquely expressed in brown adipose tissue. It uncouples OXPHOS in this tissue, and this action can be stimulated by norepinephrine.[44–46] Cold exposure and starvation, two events characterized by an initial rise then fall in norepinephrine, stimulate UCP_1 release and heat production by the brown fat.[51,52]

The brown fat depots are located at the base of the neck, along the backbone and, in males, across the shoulders. The brown fat cell differs from the white fat cell in that it contains many more mitochondria in the cytosol than does the white cell.[45,51] Both cell types have stored lipid droplets that, if sufficiently large, can push all of the other organelles off to the side of the cell. In contrast to the white cell depots, the brown fat depots are highly innervated and vascularized. This increase in vascularization gives the depot its brownish color and name, brown fat.

As described earlier, much of the structure of the white cell is similar to that of the brown fat cell.[48,49,51] Whereas white depots are distributed throughout the body, brown depots are found in just a few locations. Brown fat cells, if allowed to accumulate lipid, may change in appearance and look like white fat cells. Histochemical studies have failed to reveal any qualitative differences between the fat depots of the two cell types. More brown fat can be observed in newborns than in adults, and it is thought that thermoregulation in the immature animal is dependent on the activity of the brown fat depot with respect to its ability to generate heat. Both cell types can store lipid and this lipid can be readily mobilized. However, when it mobilizes its stored lipid, the brown fat oxidizes its lipid in situ rather than releasing it for utilization by other tissues. When stimulated, the brown fat can produce more heat during metabolism than can the white fat cell. The heat produced through the action of the UCPs is especially important to newborns because they lack the insulation provided by the subcutaneous fat store. This fat layer helps conserve body heat. Additional heat production is provided by the newborn's metabolic processes, which are relatively immature with respect to energy conservation. Heat loss from these processes can be quite large. As the newborn matures biochemically as well as physiologically, the importance of these UCPs in EB subsides. The baby begins to accumulate a subcutaneous fat layer that insulates it from heat loss. Glycogen accumulation and utilization patterns mature as well, so that the infant and young child can be fed less frequently.

The brown fat depot is not the only tissue that contributes to thermoregulation.[47,48,50] Heat production due to the UCPs also occurs in muscle and white adipose tissue. UCPs 2 and 3 (UCP_2 and UCP_3) have been identified. UCP_3 is found in skeletal muscle, while UCP_2 is found both in brown fat pads and white fat pads as well as muscle.[44,46–49] The expression of these UCPs is downregulated by fasting and endurance exercise training.[50–54] UCP_2 not only has a role in thermogenesis but also, in an inverse relationship, regulates hydrogen peroxide generation, mitochondrial reactive species, and therefore the redox state and oxidative state of the cell.[49] As UCP_2 rises, peroxide levels fall. If muscle UCP_2 rises in skeletal muscle, utilization of lipid by that muscle falls.[45] Dietary fat type can affect brown fat thermogenesis.[54] Diets rich in polyunsaturated fats are less thermogenic than diets rich in saturated fats.

UCP_2 is subject to dietary manipulation and, as well, probably functions in body weight regulation. UCP_3 is found in skeletal muscle and is downregulated during energy restriction or starvation. Actually, this downregulation probably explains the increased metabolic efficiency that occurs in the food-restricted individual. Following refeeding, some of this increased efficiency is lost. During the starvation period, the mRNAs for these UCPs are upregulated, but the message is not translated.[48,52–54] Translation does not occur immediately when food is restored but takes up to 10 days to appear, thus allowing for maximum food efficiency during the immediate recovery period. This upregulation of the UCP mRNA may also play a role in the rapid weight regain following food restriction.

Long-chain free fatty acids can act as partial uncoupling agents.[54] A large influx of fatty acids increases the volume of the mitochondrion and this in turn serves to spatially separate the respiratory chain and the ATPase. Other naturally occurring compounds can also reduce coupling efficiency. These agents increase body-heat production. This is an important defense reaction against invading pathogens. Increased body heat (fever) serves to reduce the viability of these pathogens. Some of these compounds are catabolic hormones and their effect on coupling is dose dependent. These include the thyroid hormones, glucocorticoids, sex hormones, catecholamines, insulin, glucagon, parathyroid hormone, and growth hormone. Some of these hormones have direct effects on mitochondrial respiration and coupling through affecting the synthesis and activation of the various protein constituents of the five complexes. Other hormones have their effects on the exchange of divalent ions, notably calcium, and/or on the phospholipid fatty acid composition of the inner mitochondrial membrane. Some hormones, thyroid hormones, for example, influence enzyme synthesis/activation, calcium flux, *and* membrane lipid composition. Clearly, this is a very carefully regulated system with checks and balances to ensure the continuity of life. Without this careful control, survival during times of energy stress could not be assured.

SUMMARY

1. Energy is expressed in kcalories or kjoules. It can be measured directly using a calorimeter or indirectly through measuring oxygen consumption.
2. EB refers to the amount of energy expended versus that consumed. Negative EB means that more energy is expended than is consumed; positive energy means that more energy is consumed than is expended.
3. The RQ is an indication of the fuels being oxidized. It is the ratio of CO_2 produced to O_2 consumed.
4. The BMR is defined as the minimal amount of energy needed to sustain life. It can be affected by gender, age, and hormonal status.
5. Energetic efficiency, thermogenesis (heat production), UE, and energy retention are terms used to describe the energetics of life.
6. Brown fat thermogenesis (BAT) contributes to the expenditure of energy after consuming food. Thermogenesis is related to the production and release of the UCPs.

LEARNING OPPORTUNITIES

1. Using the Harris–Benedict equation, calculate your BMR.
2. Keep a 3-day record of your food intake. Calculate your energy intake.
   Keeping a food diary
   The simplest way is to keep a food diary for 3 days. Write down everything you eat and drink. Record the quantities of these foods. Start with breakfast and include all meals plus snacks and beverages. At first, you will have to use a measuring cup and maybe a food scale. A food scale can be purchased very cheaply at a drug store or grocery store pharmacy. They usually cost \$3–\$4. After a while, your eye will be trained and you will be able to very closely estimate the quantity of what you are eating. After you have made a 3-day record, write down all the energy values of these foods. You can use the web to acquire this information from tables of food composition. There are also computer programs available, and if your college has these, use them. You should then add up all the energy values of the foods you have consumed over the 3-day period and divide by three. That will give you a pretty good estimate of what you usually consume. Do not forget to include a weekend day in your 3-day record. Sometimes weekends differ. Perhaps you like to sleep late and go to brunch around 11 am. This might mean you skip both breakfast and lunch then go out with friends for supper. This would be different from your Monday through Friday routine. After you have done this, you will see how much you are eating, and if you are gaining or losing weight, you might want to adjust your food intake accordingly.

Record	Meal	Food Item	Quantity	Energy Content (kcal)
Day 1	Breakfast			
	Lunch			
	Dinner			
	Snacks			
Day 2	Breakfast			
	Lunch			
	Dinner			
	Snacks			
Day 3	Breakfast			
	Lunch			
	Dinner			
	Snacks			

3. Calculate your energy output: Keep a 3-day record of all your activities including time spent sleeping. Again include 1 weekend day in your 3-day record. Average these figures to obtain a daily value for each. Add the energy attributable to activity to that for your estimated BMR. Are you in EB? Why/why not?

MULTIPLE-CHOICE QUESTIONS

1. Energy is expressed as
   a. kcal
   b. kJ
   c. Both
   d. Neither

2. A bomb calorimeter measures
   a. Food energy
   b. Excreta energy
   c. Oxygen consumption
   d. None of the above
3. RQ is an estimate of
   a. Oxygen consumption
   b. Carbon dioxide use
   c. Ratio of carbon dioxide production and oxygen consumption
   d. Energy need
4. UCP is
   a. Undetermined energy use
   b. UCP
   c. A metabolic inhibitor
   d. An additive to BMR
5. The genetic background of an individual can determine
   a. Energy need
   b. Energy expenditure
   c. Energetic efficiency
   d. All of the above

REFERENCES

1. Hargrove, J.L. (2006) History of the calorie in nutrition. *J. Nutr.* 136: 2957–2961.
2. Ashley, J., Kulick, D. (2013) Computerized nutrient analysis systems. In: *Handbook of Nutrition and Food* (C. Berdanier, J. Dwyer, D. Heber, eds.), 3rd edn. Taylor & Francis, Boca Raton, FL, pp. 115–124.
3. Heusner, A.A. (1982) Energy metabolism and body size. 1. Is the 0.75 mass exponent of Kleibers equation a statistical artifact? *Respir. Physiol.* 48: 1–12.
4. Webb, P. (1991) The measurement of energy expenditure. *J. Nutr.* 121: 1897–1901.
5. Webb, P., Annis, J.F., Troutman, S.J. (1980) Energy balance in man measured by direct and indirect calorimetry. *Am. J. Clin. Nutr.* 33: 1287–1298.
6. Westerterp, K.R. (1993) Food quotient, respiratory quotient and energy balance. *Am. J. Clin. Nutr.* 57: 759S–765S.
7. Ravussin, E., Harper, I.T., Rising, R., Bogardus, C. (1991) Energy expenditure by doubly labeled water: Validation in lean and obese subjects. *Am. J. Physiol.* 261: E402–E409.
8. Hegsted, D.M. (1974) Energy needs and energy utilization. *Nutr. Rev.* 32: 3338.
9. Welch, G.R. (1991) Thermodynamics and living systems: Problems and paradigms. *J. Nutr.* 121: 1902–1906.
10. Harris, J.A., Benedict, F.G. (1918) A biometric study of human basal metabolism. *Proc. Natl. Acad. Sci. USA* 4: 370.
11. Webb, P. (1981) Energy expenditure and fat-free mass in men and women. *Am. J. Clin. Nutr.* 34: 1816–1826.
12. Schoeller, D.A., Ravussin, E., Schutz, Y., Acheson, K.J., Baertschi, P., Jequier, E. (1986) Energy expenditure by doubly labeled water: Validation in humans and proposed calculations. *Am. J. Physiol.* 250: R823–R830.
13. Bitz, C., Toubro, S., Larsen, T.M., Harder, H., Rennie, K.L., Jebb, S.A., Astrup, A. (2004) Increased 24 h energy expenditure in type 2 diabetes. *Diabetes Care* 27: 2416–2421.
14. Donato, K.A. (1987) Efficiency and utilization of various energy sources for growth. *Am. J. Clin. Nutr.* 45: 164–167.
15. Poehlman, E.T. (1992) Energy expenditure and requirements in aging humans. *J. Nutr.* 122: 2057–2065.
16. Aw, T.Y., Jones, D.P. (1989) Nutrient supply and mitochondrial function. *Annu. Rev. Nutr.* 9: 229–251.
17. Rumpler, W.Y., Seale, J.L., Conway, J.M., Moe, P.W. (1967) Repeatability of 24-hour energy expenditure measurements in humans by indirect calorimetry. *Am. J. Clin. Nutr.* 51: 147–152.

18. Weyer, C., Snitker, S., Rising, R., Bogardus, C., Ravussin, E. (1999) Determinants of energy expenditure and fuel utilization in man: Effects of body composition, age, sex, ethnicity, and glucose tolerance in 916 subjects. *Int. J. Obes. Relat. Metab. Disord.* 23: 715–722.
19. Schadewaldt, P., Nowotny, B., Strabburger, K., Kotzka, J., Roden, M. (2013) Indirect calorimetry in humans: A postcalorimetric evaluation procedure for correction of metabolic monitor variability. *Am. J. Clin. Nutr.* 97: 763–773.
20. Gullickson, P.S., Flatt, W.P., Dean, R.G., Hartzell, D.L., Baile, C.A. (2002) Energy metabolism and expression of UCP1, 2, and 3 after 21 days of recovery from intracerebroventricular mouse leptin in rats. *Physiol. Behav.* 75: 473–482.
21. Papakonstantinow, E., Flatt, W.P., Huth, P.J., Harris, R.B. (2003) High dietary calcium reduces body fat content, digestibility of fat and serum vitamin D in rats. *Obes. Res.* 11: 387–394.
22. Sherman, H. (1952) *Chemistry of Food and Nutrition*, 8th edn. Macmillan Co., New York, pp. 179–187.
23. Hervey, G.R., Tobin, G. (1982) The part played by variation of energy expenditure in the regulation of energy balance. *Proc. Nutr. Soc.* 41: 137–153.
24. Alpert, S. (1990) Growth, thermogenesis and hyperphagia. *Am. J. Clin. Nutr.* 52: 782–792.
25. Jakobsen, K., Thorbek, G. (1993) The respiratory quotient in relation to fat deposition in fattening-growing pigs. *Brit. J. Nutr.* 69: 333–343.
26. Pannacciulli, N., Salbe, A.D., Ortega, E., Venti, C.A., Bogardus, C., Krakoff, J. (2007) The 24-h carbohydrate oxidation rate predicts ad libitum food intake. *Am. J. Clin. Nutr.* 86: 625–632.
27. Stice, E., Durant, S., Burger, K.S., Schoeller, D.A. (2011) Weight suppression and risk of future increases in body mass: Effects of suppressed resting metabolic rate and energy expenditure. *Am. J. Clin. Nutr.* 94: 7–11.
28. Baldwin, R.L. (1978) Metabolic functions affecting the contribution of adipose tissue to total energy expenditure. *Fed. Proc.* 29: 1277–1283.
29. McCargar, L.J., Baracos, V.E., Clandinin, M.T. (1989) Influence of dietary carbohydrate to fat ratio on whole body nitrogen retention and body composition in adult rats. *J. Nutr.* 119: 1240–1245.
30. Kreitzman, S.N. (1992) Factors influencing body composition during very low calorie diets. *Am. J. Clin. Nutr.* 56: 2175–2235.
31. Jones, P.J.H., Schoeller, D.A. (1988) Polyunsaturated: Saturated ratio of diet fat influences energy substrate utilization in the human. *Metabolism* 37: 145–151.
32. Livesey, G. (1991) Modifying energy density in human diets. *Proc. Nutr. Soc.* 50: 371–382.
33. Dulloo, A.G., Girardier, L. (1993) Adaptive role of energy expenditure in modulating body fat and protein deposition during catch-up growth after early undernutrition. *Am. J. Clin. Nutr.* 58: 614–621.
34. Roberts, S.B., Fuss, P., Evans, W.J., Heyman, M.B., Young, V.R. (1993) Energy expenditure, aging and body composition. *J. Nutr.* 123: 474–482.
35. Allison, D.B., Kaprio, J., Korkeila, M., Koskenvuo, M., Neale, M.C., Hayakawa, K. (1996) The heritability of body mass index among an international sample of monozygotic twins reared apart. *Int. J. Obes.* 20: 501–506.
36. Bouchard, C. (1989) Genetic factors in obesity. *Med. Clin. North Am.* 73: 67–81.
37. Wang, C., Baumgartner, R.N., Allison, D.B. (2007) Genetics of human obesity. In: *Handbook of Nutrition and Food* (C.D. Berdanier, E. Feldman, J. Dwyer, eds.). CRC Press, Boca Raton, FL, pp. 833–846.
38. Gibney, E.R., Murgatroyd, P., Wright, A., Jebb, S., Elia, M. (2003) Measurement of total energy expenditure in grossly obese women: Comparison of the bicarbonate-urea method with whole body calorimetry and free living doubly labeled water. *Int. J. Obes. Relat. Metab. Disord.* 27: 641–647.
39. Prentice, A.M., Black, A.E., Coward, W.A., Davies, H.L., Goldberg, G.R., Murgatroyd, P.R., Ashford, J., Sawyer, M., Whitehead, R.G. (1986) High levels of energy expenditure in obese women. *Br. J. Nutr.* 292: 983–987.
40. Chong, P.K., Jung, R.T., Rennie, M.J., Scrimgeour, C.M. (1993) Energy expenditure in lean and obese diabetic patients using doubly labeled water method. *Diab. Med.* 10: 729–735.
41. Ravussin, E., Burnand, B., Schutz, Y., Jequier, E. (1985) Energy expenditure before and during energy restriction in obese patients. *Am. J. Clin. Nutr.* 41: 753–759.
42. de Boer, J.O., van Es, A.J.H., Roovers, L., van Raaij, J.M.A., Hautvast, J.G.A.J. (1986) Adaptation of energy metabolism of overweight women to low-energy intake, studied with whole-body calorimeters. *Am. J. Clin. Nutr.* 44: 585–595.
43. Jurimae, J., Jurimae, T., Purge, P. (2007) Plasma ghrelin is altered after maximal exercise in elite male exercise. *Exp. Biol. Med.* 232: 904–909.
44. Geloen, A., Trayhurn, P. (1990) Regulation of the level of uncoupling protein in brown adipose tissue by insulin requires mediation of the sympathetic nervous system. *FEBS* 267: 265–267.

45. Recquier, D., Casteilla, L., Bouillaud, F. (1991) Molecular studies of the uncoupling protein. *FASEB J.* 5: 2237–2242.
46. Himms-Hagen, J. (1995) Brown adipose tissue thermogenesis in the control of thermoregulatory feeding in rats: A new hypothesis that links thermostatic and glucostatic hypothesis for control of food intake. *Proc. Soc. Exp. Biol. Med.* 208: 159–169.
47. Samec, S., Seydoux, J., Dulloo, A.G. (1998) Role of UCP homologues in skeletal muscles and brown adipose tissue: Mediations of thermogenesis or regulators of lipids as fuel substrate? *FASEB J.* 12: 715–724.
48. Simoneau, J.-A., Kelly, D.E., Neverova, M., Warden, C.H. (1998) Overexpression of muscle uncoupling protein 2 content in human obesity associates with reduced skeletal muscle lipid utilization. *FASEB J.* 12: 1739–1745.
49. Negre-Salvayre, A., Hirtz, C., Cabbera, G., Cazenave, R., Troly, M., Salvayre, R., Penicaud, L., Casteilla, L. (1997) A role for uncoupling protein-2 as a regulator of mitochondrial hydrogen peroxide generation. *FASEB J.* 11: 809–815.
50. Boss, O., Samec, S., Desplanches, D., Mayet, M.-H., Seydoux, J., Muzzin, P., Giacobino, J.-P. (1998) Effect of endurance training on mRNA expression of uncoupling proteins 1, 2 and 3 in the rat. *FASEB J.* 12: 335–339.
51. Geloen, A., Collet, A.J., Guay, G., Bukowiecki, L.J. (1990) In vivo differentiation of brown adipocytes in adult mice: An electron microscopic study. *Am. J. Anat.* 188: 366–372.
52. Trayhurn, P., Jennings, G. (1986) Evidence that fasting can induce a selective loss of uncoupling protein from brown adipose tissue mitochondria of mice. *Biosci. Rep.* 6: 805–810.
53. Champigny, O., Recquier, D. (1990) Effects of fasting and refeeding on the level of uncoupling protein mRNA in brown adipose tissue: Evidence for diet induced and cold induced responses. *J. Nutr.* 120: 1730–1736.
54. Ide, T., Sugano, M. (1988) Effects of dietary fat types on the thermogenesis of brown adipocytes isolated from rat. *Agric. Biol. Chem.* 52: 511–518.

2 Negative Energy Balance

In the previous chapter, the basic concepts of energy were discussed. In this chapter, energy balance and abnormal energy states will be described. These include inadequate energy intake, starvation, the effects of trauma on energy balance, anorexia nervosa, bulimia, and pica. Obesity will be discussed in Chapter 3.

The concept of energy balance is a simple one. An adult animal in energy balance is neither losing nor gaining weight. The concept does not apply to immature, growing animals nor does it apply to pregnant or lactating females. By definition, an animal (including humans) in energy balance is consuming enough energy to offset that which is expended. Mathematically, it is expressed as follows:

$$\Sigma \text{ kcals consumed} = \Sigma \text{ kcals expended}$$

Within the framework of energy balance, there are day-to-day variations in both intake and expenditure, but these are of little importance when the long-term energetic efficiency of the individual is maintained. Should long-term perturbations occur on either side of the equation, then energy balance will shift such that weight is either gained or lost and a new balance is established. If weight is lost, the individual is in negative energy balance, while if weight is gained, the individual is in positive energy balance. If weight is lost or gained with no change in energy expenditure, the weight loss or gain will affect the adipose tissue fat store. If expenditure is also changed (adding or reducing physical activity), then the body composition will change as well. Increased physical activity will stimulate muscle development, while a reduction in activity will result in reduced muscle mass. Body composition change affects the energy balance because muscle and adipose tissue consume fuel sources differently.

In the United States, there has been a trend toward increasing the consumption of energy-rich foods that correspond to the trend toward increasing body weight.[1,2] Comparing the 1971 National Health and Nutrition Examination Survey (NHANES) data on food consumption to those from the 2006 survey showed an increase in total energy intake with the carbohydrate kcalories contributing more to this increase than fat or protein kcalories. That segment of the population, ages 20–39, that included exercise as part of their lifestyle did not increase their energy intake as did their sedentary cohorts. Indeed, this group had a small decrease in their energy intake. The relationship of food intake (energy intake) to body weight has been well studied, yet there are aspects of this relationship that has eluded scientists for generations. One theory that describes this relationship is called the set-point theory.

SET-POINT THEORY IN BODY WEIGHT REGULATION

The idea that each body has its own unique size and weight has been discussed, denied, and supported by a wide variety of researchers. The hypothesis that adult body weight is closely regulated at its own unique level was developed from observations of both humans and animals.[3–7] The mechanism(s) that serve to regulate this steady-state body weight are not fully known. Some of this effect is related to the internal controls of food intake while some is attributed to increases in physical activity, and some is related to the unique energy-wasting capacity of the brown adipose tissue (brown fat thermogenesis).

Healthy adult humans do not vary very much in their body weight. They may be underweight, normal weight, overweight, and/or overfat but, for most humans, that weight is maintained for years until some event occurs that results in a body weight change. In women, pregnancy or menopause, two normal physiological events, may perturb the system sufficiently to establish a new steady-state body weight (or new set point), which, again, will be defended tenaciously. A change in the endocrine system, an insult to the body, and a conscious decision to eat more (or less) over a prolonged period (months to years) are other examples of events that might perturb the system sufficiently to result in a new set point—a new body weight that is maintained from that time on.

Similarly, animals appear to regulate their body weight within fairly tight limits. Much of the research on the set-point hypothesis has used rats and mice. Studies using rats that were either over- or underfed revealed that they had a body weight that was related to their food intake. That is, if they were forced to consume more energy than they would voluntarily consume, they would become overfat. If they were underfed, they would be leaner than normal. After these feeding treatments were discontinued, the rats that were overfed significantly reduced their food intake and used their fat stores to provide their energy needs, while those rats that were underfed dramatically increased their voluntary food intake until they gained the weight they would have gained had they not been food restricted. When both these groups of rats attained the weight of their untreated controls, they resumed normal feeding behavior.

Although the body weight returned to normal in these over- or underfed rats after the treatment was terminated, the composition of the body was not the same as their untreated counterparts. The percentage of the body that was fat was affected. Those rats that were underfed recovered by significantly increasing the synthesis and deposition of body fat. This recovery was faster than the recovery of body protein. In the overfed rats, the body protein normalized within days of cessation of the overfeeding, yet the body fat content remained elevated for weeks after the overfeeding treatment ended.

Other studies have used parabiotic rats or mice to study the consequences of overfeeding or underfeeding on body weight and composition. Parabiosis is a technique where two weanling animals are joined together surgically at the skin so that they have a common circulation. Hervey, Harris, and others have used this technique to answer the question of whether there are blood-borne factors that are involved in the regulation of feeding and body weight.[3–7] Genetically obese animals have been joined to genetically lean ones, as have normal weight partners in which one was either over- or underfed or was lesioned in either the feeding center of the hypothalamus or the satiety center. In each of these instances, the feeding behavior of both and their body weight and composition were monitored. In each instance where one partner overate and became obese, the other ate less or starved and subsequently lost body fat as well as lean body tissue. These results were interpreted as indications that there are blood-borne factors generated by the fat store that signal the feeding behavior. Indeed, some of these blood-borne factors have been identified (leptin, NPY, TNFα, etc.). Other factors have been identified that originate in the intestinal tract that also play a role in food intake. Chapter 4 describes the roles of these cytokines in the regulation of food intake.

It is apparent that although there may be controls that influence feeding and body weight, these controls may not fully regulate body fatness. That is, body weight may be set but body fat may change depending on food intake, gender, genetics, and physical activity. This may explain why aging humans may gain body fat while decreasing food intake and yet maintain their body weight. As humans age, they may decrease their physical activity. As a result, their body composition changes; they lose muscle mass and gain body fat. Their body shape changes as well. They may observe an increase in the size of their fat mass in the abdomen and on the thighs and buttocks. Again, epidemiologists have noted the differences in health risks associated with the location of the excess fat stores, the so-called apple and pear shapes. Those persons whose fat stores are distributed equally between storage sites on shoulders, arms, abdomen, hips, and thighs are said to be *apples*. Their risk of developing obesity-associated disorders is greater than that in people who have accumulated fat stores at sites below the waist, the *pears*. The depots differ in the degree of fatty acid turnover.

That is, they differ in how readily they can release their stored fat energy for use by other tissues. In humans, studies of cells isolated from the femoral, gluteal, and omental (thigh, buttocks, and abdomen) depots revealed significant differences in free fatty acid release.[3,4] On the basis of the rate of free fatty acid release and the size of the depots, the half-life of the fat depot in the femoral area was calculated to be 305 days. For the gluteal depot, it was 326 days, and for the omental depot, it was 134 days.[3] Estimates of the half-life of the fat in the other depot sites have not been made. An estimate of half-life is the estimate of time needed to exhaust one-half of the fat store. As the human uses the stored lipid, more lipid is synthesized to replace that which was used. Hence, the term fatty acid turnover means that fatty acids are both used and replaced. If they are used at a greater rate than they are replaced, a net fat loss will occur. As can be seen, however, different depots will shrink at different rates depending on their location. In addition to the aforementioned differences in depot fat use, there are also genetic and gender differences in the extent and location of the fat depots.[4] Women, for example, have larger subcutaneous fat stores than men. Men have larger omental fat depots than women of the same age and weight. The size of the fat depot determines how long the person can sustain life when food deprived.

ABNORMAL ENERGY STATES

Starvation

Starvation is the absence of sufficient food to support the body processes. The basic metabolic response to starvation of a previously healthy individual is conservation. As the gut receives less food, its emptying time is reduced. First, the stomach, then the duodenum, the jejunum, the ileum, and the large intestine lose their contents and shrink in size. Simple mono- and disaccharides are the first to disappear, followed by the products of the progressively more complex nutrients: polysaccharides, proteins, and lipids. As the sugars disappear, there is less stimulus for insulin release and basal insulin levels are approached. As glucose is less available from the gut, the body begins to mobilize its glycogen stores to provide glucose. At the same time, the body will begin to mobilize its stores of lipid (triacylglycerols) and, to a lesser extent, its body protein. It can use certain amino acids and glycerol from the triacylglycerols to synthesize glucose via gluconeogenesis and utilize the carbon skeletons of deaminated amino acids plus the fatty acids liberated from the triacylglycerols for fuel. These provide only a small percentage of the 2000–2500 kcal (8368–8577 kJ) needed per day for maintenance. Benedict[8] estimated that mobilizable body protein could provide about 15% of the body's fuel needs and that the fat stores of the adipose tissue provided the rest. Although Benedict did not have today's sophisticated technology at his disposal, his estimates were remarkably close to those of Cahill. Cahill[9] estimated that a *normal* 70 kg man required about 2000 kcal (8368 kJ) per day to maintain his body and that he had sufficient fuel stores to sustain life for about 80 days. As shown in Figure 2.1, adapted from Cahill's paper, most of the energy comes from the lipid stored in the adipose tissue. Lipids, primarily triacylglycerols, are hydrolyzed to fatty acids and glycerol through the action of hormone-sensitive lipase. This enzyme, located on the interior aspect of the fat cell membrane, is activated by the catabolic hormones, epinephrine, and the glucocorticoids. Its activity is increased when food intake is low and when glucagon is high and insulin is low. The glycerol is converted to glucose via gluconeogenesis in the liver and kidney. Most of the glucose formed in the kidney is used in situ, whereas hepatic glucose production can supply glucose to the rest of the body. The fatty acids are oxidized to ketones and then to carbon dioxide and water. Whereas the liver and some other tissues can oxidize the fatty acids completely to carbon dioxide and water, the muscle is unable to do so and thus ketones, the end products of muscle fatty acid oxidation, rise. These ketones can be used by the brain as a fuel when the supply of glucose becomes more limited. For example, after about 40 days of starvation, the brain will obtain nearly 65% of its energy from the ketones. While Cahill and others evaluated the energy losses from the whole animal, interorgan fuel fluxes have been studied as well. These fuel fluxes are

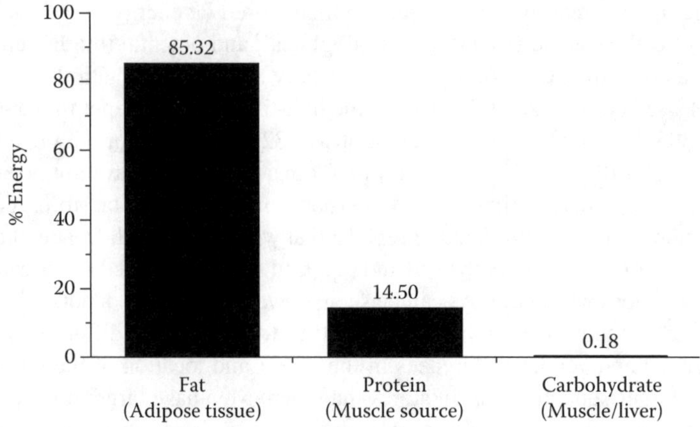

FIGURE 2.1 Sources of energy during the first 24 h of starvation.

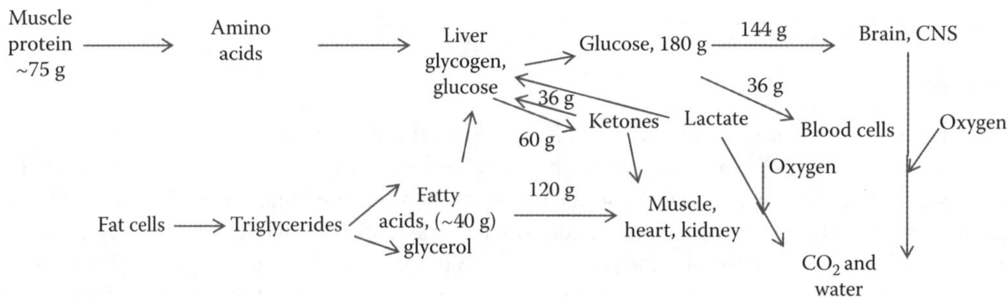

FIGURE 2.2 Intertissue fuel fluxes after 24 h of starvation. Note the central position of the liver. This organ uses glycerol, lactate, fatty acids, and amino acids to produce ketones and glucose, which serve as fuel sources for blood cells, the brain and CNS, heart, kidney, and muscle. These fuels are oxidized to carbon dioxide and water, requiring only the presence of molecular oxygen and energy from the high-energy phosphate bonds as provided by the adenine and guanine nucleotides.

diagrammed in Figure 2.2. Under normal (i.e., fed) conditions, the central nervous system (CNS) uses 115 g of glucose/day while erythrocytes, bone marrow, renal medulla, and peripheral nerves use about 36 g of glucose/day. Most of this glucose can be synthesized through gluconeogenesis from glycerol, lactate, and selected amino acids during the early phase of starvation. However, as the starvation continues, the body attempts to protect its protein component and the amino acid substrates for gluconeogenesis become less available. This, coupled with the rising ketone level (ketones can cross the blood–brain barrier), serves to induce the utilization of the ketones by the brain as a metabolic fuel.

Proteolysis, initially increased after 48 h of starvation, is suppressed by rising levels of growth hormone as the body attempts to conserve its body proteins. The initial proteolysis, however, serves to provide the needed amino acids for the synthesis of enzymes needed for survival (enzymes needed for energy mobilization and conservation). Once these mechanisms are established, body protein is conserved. The temporal relationship of fuels and the hormones that control their availability is diagrammed in Figure 2.3.

Protein–Energy Malnutrition

Starvation is the extreme state of malnutrition that occurs when the individual is provided little or no food to nourish the body. Between starvation and the state of adequate nourishment to meet

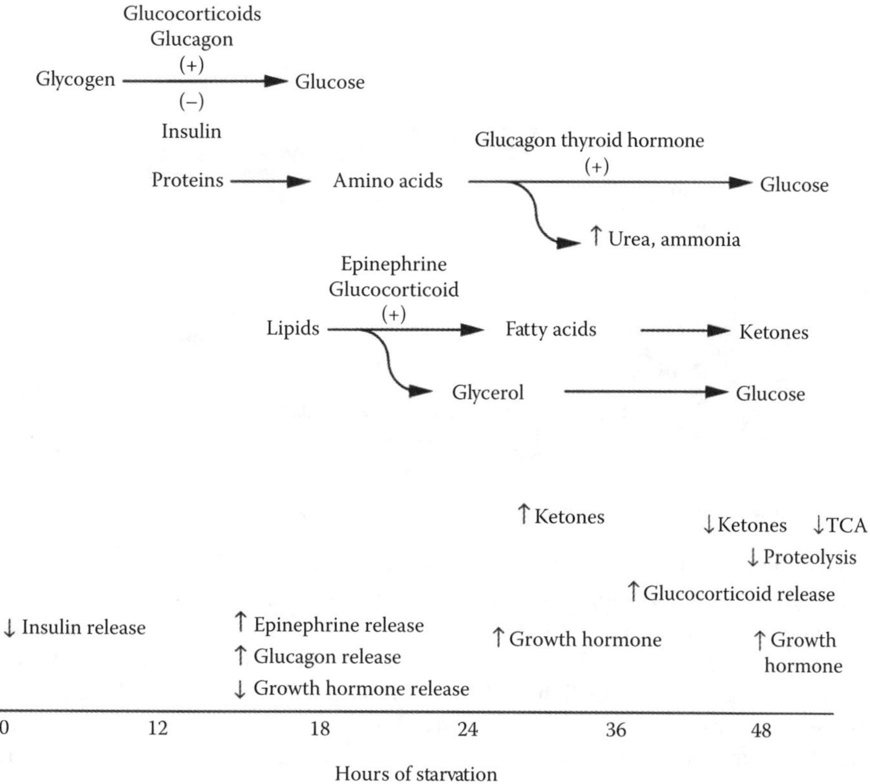

FIGURE 2.3 Temporal relations of fuels and hormones during starvation. During the first 24 h, there is a decrease in blood glucose levels and an increase in proteolysis. After 18 h, measurable increases in gluconeogenesis due to glucose production from glycerol can be observed. There is a rise in lipolysis, initially stimulated by epinephrine but then maintained by rising glucocorticoid, glucagon, and growth hormone levels. As these hormones rise, they serve to decrease peripheral tissue sensitivity to insulin and decreased glucose tolerance can be observed. With rising growth hormone levels, proteolysis is decreased and the body attempts to conserve body protein. By 48 h, ketosis, having been high, now begins to decline as the body adapts to using ketones and fatty acids as metabolic fuels.

nutrient needs, there are graded levels of inadequate nutrient intake. Although infants and children of third-world nations come to mind when malnutrition is pictured, people of all ages in all countries are vulnerable. Where the intake of macronutrients is inadequate, the syndrome is called protein–calorie malnutrition (PCM) or, more correctly, protein–energy malnutrition. Gradations in energy malnutrition are illustrated in Figure 2.4.

Chronic malnutrition is characterized not only by a negative energy balance but also by deficits in the protein intake and the intake of micronutrients. The needs for these nutrients and energy are determined by the age and health status of the individual. Rapid growth, infection, injury, and chronic debilitating disease can drive up the need for food and the nutrients it contains. Infants and young children as well as adults have been described as having PCM. Just as infection or trauma potentiates the needs for protein, energy, and micronutrients in third-world children and adults, these conditions also increase the need for nutrients in developed nations. Injury and sepsis both increase energy needs. Both adults and children may have increased nutrient needs under these circumstances, and if these needs are not met, varying degrees of malnutrition or PCM will be observed. Malnutrition has been documented in hospitalized patients in the United States, and this malnutrition may affect recovery as well as mortality. People of all ages and in all levels of society are vulnerable to nutrition deficits and these have been reported as

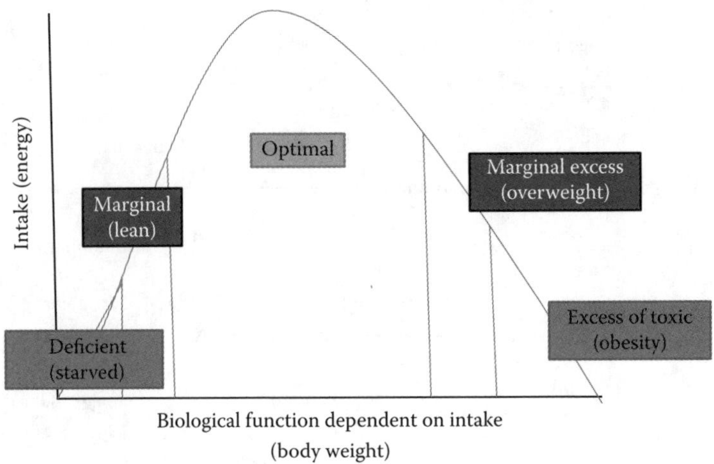

FIGURE 2.4 Body weight as a function of energy intake.

part of nutritional screening efforts by the government as well as by groups focused on specific health problems. Indeed, nutritional screening is of great value when it reliably identifies the risk factors for malnutrition, recognizes the existence of poor nutritional status, contributes to the avoidance of malnutrition, minimizes suffering, and can be reversed with appropriate dietary interventions.[10,11] Signs of malnutrition are listed in Table 2.1. These signs can be then followed by laboratory assessments that further document the presence of malnutrition. Indicators of anemia, a chief sign for malnutrition, are listed in Table 2.2. Normal values for blood and urine are shown in Tables 2.3 through 2.5. Deviations from these normal values are informative when assessing the nutritional health of a population.

Some routine laboratory tests can assist in nutrition assessment and the diagnosis of malnutrition. These include the red and white cell differential analysis, blood chemistry panels (glucose, electrolytes, minerals, lipids, indices of renal and hepatic function), and urine analysis. Tests of blood coagulation can also be informative.

Hemoglobin levels will show the presence of anemia that may be related to vitamin or mineral malnutrition and can indicate chronic disease. The red cell size and hemoglobin content can provide clues to liver disease, alcoholism, and specific nutritional deficiencies. Table 2.2 gives the measurements in blood that can indicate anemia and its nutritional cause. Anemia can arise from nonnutrient causes such as blood loss or genetic diseases, but these are not included in this table.

While serum albumin is not a sensitive indicator of protein status, it does provide a clue. Low levels may indicate a limiting amount of substrate for hepatic protein synthesis. On the other hand, nonnutritional factors may be responsible for hypoalbuminemia such as expanded extracellular fluid, accelerated protein breakdown, and impaired renal and hepatic function. Albumin levels may also be unreliable indicators of protein status in the postoperative or acutely injured patient. Some enzyme tests are indicators of nutritional cofactor status, for example, alkaline phosphatase for zinc or aminotransferase for vitamin B_6. Laboratory tests useful in clinical nutritional assessment are provided in Table 2.3. Tables 2.4 and 2.5 provide normal values for blood micronutrient and metabolite levels. The latter table gives the values in SI units.

Urine analysis (Table 2.6) can also provide information about the nutritional status of adults. The values can indicate nutrient excretion as well as the excretion of toxins such as lead. Measurements of blood and urine creatinine can be used to calculate creatinine clearance, a measure of renal function.

TABLE 2.1
Physical Signs of Malnutrition

Area of Body Examined	Common Signs of Malnutrition	Deficiency/Abnormality
Appearance in general	Significant overweight or underweight, apathetic or hyperirritable	Energy imbalance
	Loss or slowness of ankle or knee reflexes, pitting edema	Protein
Eyes	Paleness, dryness, redness, or pigmentation of membranes (conjunctiva)	Vitamin A, riboflavin
	Foamy patches or conjunctiva (Bitot's spots)	Iron, B_{12}, folate, copper
	Dullness, softness, or vascularization of the cornea	Excess, Wilson's disease
	Redness or fissures on eyelids	Hypercholesterolemia
Face	Rash, seborrhea, pallor	Riboflavin, iron, folate B_{12}
Gums	Receded, *spongy* and bleeding, swelling of the gingiva	Vitamin C
Hair	Dullness, may be brittle and easily plucked without pain	Protein
	Sometimes lighter in color than normal (depigmentation may be bandlike when hair is held up to a source of light)	
Lips	Swollen, red, corners, cracked (cheilosis)	Riboflavin
Muscles	Wasting and flabbiness of muscle, bleeding into muscle	Protein, iron, folate, B_{12}
Nails	Brittle and ridged nails, spooning	Protein, iron
Heart	Racing heartbeat (over 100 beats/min)	
	Enlargement	Selenium
	Failure	Thiamin
	Abnormal rhythm of heart	Magnesium, potassium, calcium
Organs	Palpable enlargement of liver or spleen	Alcohol abuse
	Ascites	Protein
Skeleton	Softening, swelling, or distorted shapes of bones and joints	Vitamins C and D
Skin	Roughness (follicular hyperkeratosis), dryness, or flakiness	Protein
	Irregular pigmentation, black and blue marks, lesions	Niacin
	Symmetrical, reddened lesions, rash, edema	Protein
	Looseness of skin (lack of subcutaneous fat)	Energy
	Flakiness, peeling, dry	Protein, zinc
Teeth	Caries, mottled or darkened areas of enamel	Fluoride excess
Tongue	Atrophy of papillae (the tongue is smooth) or hypertrophy of papillae	B_{12}, folate, riboflavin
	Swollen, scarlet, magenta (purple colored), or raw tongue	
	Irregularly shaped and distributed white patches	Iron

Regular assessment of the nutritional health of the population in the United States has been conducted at 10-year intervals by the Centers for Disease Control (the CDC). These surveys, called the NHANES surveys, assess the nutritional and clinical health of a cross section of the US population. The surveys include anthropometric measures (age, gender, height, weight, skinfold thickness, etc.), physical assessments as per Table 2.1, blood and urine chemistry Tables 2.3 through 2.5 (metabolites, micronutrient assessments, some hormones, etc.), food intake measures (diet recall, food frequency questionnaires, etc.), and examinations for health (blood pressure, pulse, heart rate, etc.). Subjects were also asked about their lifestyle choices, their financial status, and whether they had indoor plumbing, equipped kitchens and other

TABLE 2.2
Blood Values for Measurements Made to Assess the Presence of Anemia

Measurement	Normal Values	Iron Deficiency	B_{12} or Folic Acid Deficiency
Red blood cells (million/cu mm)	Males: 4.6–6.2		
	Females: 4.2–5.4	Low	Low
Hemoglobin (g/dL)	Males: 14–18	Low	Low
	Females: 12–16	Low	Low
Hematocrit (vol. %)	Males: 40%–54%	Low	Low
	Females: 37%–47%	Low	Low
Serum iron	60–280 μg/dL	Low	Normal
TIBC[a]	250–425 μg/dL	High	Normal
Ferritin	60	Less than 12	Normal
Percent sat.	90%–100%	Low	Normal
Hypochromia	No	Yes	None
Microcytes	Few	Many	Few
Macrocytes	Few	Few	Many
RDW (RBC size)	High	High	Very high
Red cell folate	>360 nmol/L	Normal	<315
Serum folate	>13.5 mg/mL	Normal	Low (<6.7 mg/mL)
Serum B_{12}	200–900 pg/mL	Normal	Low
MCV[b]	82–92 cu m	≤80	≥80–100

[a] Indirect measure of serum transferrin; iron-binding capacity.
[b] Mean cell volume. When volume increases, the size of the red cell has increased (↑ % of megaloblasts).

TABLE 2.3
Laboratory Tests Useful in Clinical Nutritional Assessment

Test	Index For
Hemoglobin, hematocrit, red and white cell counts, and differential (calculate total lymphocyte count)	Anemia, protein status
Urea, creatinine, glucose sodium, potassium, chloride, CO_2	Renal function, diabetes, acid–base balance
Cholesterol, triglycerides, lipoproteins	Lipid disorders
Total protein, albumin, uric acid	Renal/hepatic function
Calcium, phosphate, magnesium, bilirubin, alkaline phosphatase	Skeletal disorders
Aminotransferases, iron, ferritin	Anemia, iron status
Transferrin, transthyretin, retinol-binding protein	Iron status
Prothrombin time, partial prothrombin time, INR	Vitamin K status

features in their home that could influence their health and nutritional status. The surveys are designed to include all age groups, genders, races and ethnic background.

The NHANES surveys are not the only health and nutrition surveys that have been conducted over the years. There have been a number of others directed toward specific population groups such as the Framingham studies and the Nurses' Health Study that were directed toward understanding the etiology of cardiovascular disease and other chronic diseases. Each of these surveys provides a glimpse of factors that have relevance to the nutritional status of people in a variety of situations.

TABLE 2.4
Normal Values for Micronutrients in Blood

Nutrient	Range of Normal Values
Ascorbic acid, plasma	0.6–1.6 mg/dL
Calcium, serum	4.5–5.3 meq/L
β-Carotene, serum	40–200 μg/dL
Chloride, serum	95–103 meq/L
Lead, whole blood	0–50 μg/dL
Magnesium, serum	1.5–2.5 meq/L
Sodium, plasma	136–142 meq/L
Vitamin A, serum	15–60 μg/dL
Retinol, plasma	>20 μg/dL
Phosphorus	3.4–4.5 mg/dL
Potassium	3.5–5.0 meq/L
Riboflavin, red cell	>14.9 μg/dL cells
Folate, plasma	>6 ng/mL
Pantothenic acid, plasma	≥6 μg/dL
Pantothenic acid, whole blood	≥80 μg/dL
Biotin, whole blood	>25 ng/mL
B_{12}, plasma	>150 pg/mL
Vitamin D 25(OH)-D_3, plasma	>10 ng/mL
α-Tocopherol, plasma	>0.80 mg/dL

Notes: For more information on blood analyses, see *NHANES Manual for Nutrition Assessment*, CDC, Atlanta, GA; ICNND *Manual for Nutrition Surveys*, 2nd edn., US Government Printing Office, Washington, DC, 1963; Sauberlich et al., *Laboratory Tests for the Assessment of Nutritional Status*, CRC Press, Boca Raton, FL, 1974.

RECOVERY FROM MALNUTRITION AND STARVATION

The immediate response to the restoration of food is mediated by the stress hormones followed by the anabolic hormone, insulin. These hormones set the stage for the induction of the transporters and enzymes needed to absorb and process the influx of nutrients now available as the individual adjusts to realimentation. In rats subjected to 2 days of starvation followed by realimentation with a high-glucose diet, the adrenal corticoids serve to enhance the synthesis of the short-lived messenger RNA that carries the codes to the endoplasmic reticulum for the synthesis of the anabolic enzymes needed to process the incoming dietary glucose, protein, and fat. It takes about 18 h to see an increase in mRNA and another 12 h to see a noticeable increase in enzyme activity. The increase in enzyme activity is accompanied by an increase in liver fat. All of these responses to realimentation soon disappear as the animal then begins to return to its prestarvation metabolic characteristics.

Similarly, humans also have this short-term response to feeding after a period of starvation. The time intervals are longer than for the rat because the human is a longer-lived species. Nonetheless, upon refeeding, the human will have a short-term hyperresponse to the presence of food in the gastrointestinal tract. Depending on the duration of starvation or semistarvation, this hyperresponse can create an imbalance within the metabolic system that could be lethal if too much food is offered without realizing that humans who have withstood starvation or semistarvation for long periods of time are not as adaptable with respect to the new synthesis of transporters, enzymes, and hormones that orchestrate the recovery process. If a person is without food for only a few days, he or she will have reserves that can be used to resynthesize/reactivate his or her metabolic machinery. Preformed hormones, receptors that can be reactivated, and transporters that are in an inactive/storage form all contribute to this reserve. As mentioned

TABLE 2.5
Normal Clinical Values in SI Units for Blood Components

Component	SI Units
Ammonia	22–39 mmol/L
Calcium	8.5–10.5 mg/dL or 2.25–2.65 mmol/L
Carbon dioxide	24–30 meq/L or 24–29 mmol/L
Chloride	100–106 meq/L or mmol/L
Copper	100–200 mg/dL or 16–31 mmol/L
Iron	50–150 mg/dL or 11.6–31.3 mmol/L
Lead	50 mg/dL or less
Magnesium	1.5–2.0 meq/L or 0.75–1.25 mmol/L
pCO_2	35–40 mmHg
pH	7.35–7.45
Phosphorus	3.0–4.5 mg/dL or 1–1.5 mmol/L
pO_2	75–100 mmHg
Potassium	3.5–5.0 meq/L or 2.5–5.0 mmol/L
Sodium	135–145 meq/L or 135–145 mmol/L
Acetoacetate	<2 mmol
Ascorbic acid	0.4–15 mg/dL or 23–85 mmol/L
Bilirubin	0.4–0.6 mg/dL or 1.71–6.84 mmol/L
Carotinoids	0.8–4.0 mg/mL
Creatinine	0.6–1.5 mg/dL or 60–130 mmol/L
Lactic acid	0.6–1.8 meq/L or 0.44–1.28 mmol/L
Cholesterol	120–220 mg/dL or 3.9–7.3 mmol/L
Triglycerides	40–150 mg/dL or 6–18 mmol/L
Pyruvic acid	0–0.11 meq/L or 79.8–228.0 mmol/L
Urea nitrogen	8–25 mg/dL or 2.86–7.14 mmol/L
Uric acid	3.0–7.0 mg/dL or 0.18–0.29 mmol/L
Vitamin A	0.15–0.6 mg/dL
Albumin	3.5–5.0 g/dL
Insulin	6–20 mU/dL
Glucose	70–100 mg/dL or 4–6 mmol/L

Note: These measurements are in the blood from people who have been fasting for 8–12 h.

in the description of the metabolic response to starvation, a 70 kg man can survive without food for about 80 days. If trauma or infection or other energy-demanding tasks are imposed upon starvation, the time for survival will be much shorter. With semistarvation, survival depends on the degree of food restriction and on the fuel stores of the body before semistarvation begins. Longer periods (months, years) of semistarvation result in a gradual loss of these reserves, and when faced with the need to metabolize food once again, the individual may not be able to respond. They might have lost their ability to resynthesize components needed to use the food now presented. In this instance, the individual must be slowly realimented with small, frequent meals of simple, easy to digest, and absorbed foods. Sometimes a liquid diet is used initially because the individual may be too weak to chew and digest solid food. In any case, the individual will go through an initial period much like the rat and then gradually adjust the metabolic pathways such that a more normal substrate flux is developed.

Although survival is achieved, there may be long-lasting consequences of starvation or semistarvation. This is particularly true for infants whose mothers were starved during gestation. Several studies of the infants who are now adults have been reported. Long-term metabolic abnormalities that may affect the risk of subsequent chronic disease have been reported. For example, studies of the survivors of the Dutch famine imposed by the Germans on parts of the Netherlands during World War II have

TABLE 2.6
Normal Values for Micronutrients in Urine

Nutrient	Range of Normal Values
Calcium, mg/24 h	100–250
Chloride, meq/24 h	110–250
Copper, μg/24 h	0–100
Lead, μg/24 h	<100
Phosphorus, g/24 h	0.9–1.3
Potassium, meq/24 h	25–100
Sodium, meq/24 h	130–260
Zinc, mg/24 h	0.15–1.2
Creatinine, mg/kg body weight	15–25
Riboflavin, μg/g creatinine	>80
Niacin metabolite,[a] μg/g creatinine	>1.6
Pyridoxine, μg/g creatinine	≥20
Biotin, μg/24 h	>25
Pantothenic acid, mg/24 h	≥1
Folate, FIGLU[b] after histidine load	<5 mg/8 h
B_{12}, methylmalonic acid after valine load	≤2 mg/24 h

Notes: For more information on urine analysis, see ICNNO, *Manual for Nutrition Surveys*, 2nd edn., US Government Printing Office, Washington, DC, 1963; *NHANES Manual for Nutrition Assessment*, CDC Atlanta, GA; Gibson, R.S., *Principles of Nutrition Assessment*, Oxford University Press, New York, 1990.

[a] N^1-methylnicotinamide.

[b] Formiminoglutamic acid.

been reported. For those Dutch survivors of prenatal famine (babies born of semistarved mothers), the mortality risk for cancer particularly breast cancer and the risk for cardiovascular disease was considerably greater than in those whose mothers were not starved.[12] Female offspring of starved mothers had an abnormal blood lipid pattern.[13] Cholesterol levels were elevated and these levels were independent of body mass index, waist circumference, and midthigh circumference. Triglyceride levels were also elevated. These effects were not observed in the male progeny of starved pregnant women. Some of these gender differences could be due to the disproportionate loss of male progeny compared to female progeny of the starved or semistarved mothers. More male embryos and male fetuses were lost than female embryos and fetuses. After birth, male progeny did not survive as well as the female progeny; thus, the population of the mature survivors is skewed by the disproportionate survival of female babies. In another instance, the consequences of the 1959–1961 Chinese famine have had long-term effects on the progeny of women who were subjected to this famine. The mature progeny were smaller (shorter) and had a lower BMI than cohorts born after the famine. The famine-affected progeny had three times the risk of developing hypertension.[14] In another study of progeny of malnourished mothers in Barbados, such malnourishment was associated with persistent attention deficits in their middle-aged progeny.[15] Thus, it can be concluded that although famine can be survived as noted earlier, there can indeed be long-term consequences for the mature adult even though that adult had been well nourished during his or her subsequent childhood and adulthood.

TRAUMA AND ENERGY NEEDS

Many years ago, a disproportionate catabolic response to trauma was reported. Since that time, physicians, nutritionists, and physiologists alike have accepted this as an obligatory and necessary response to illness or injury. With the advent of parenteral and enteral feeding techniques, it has

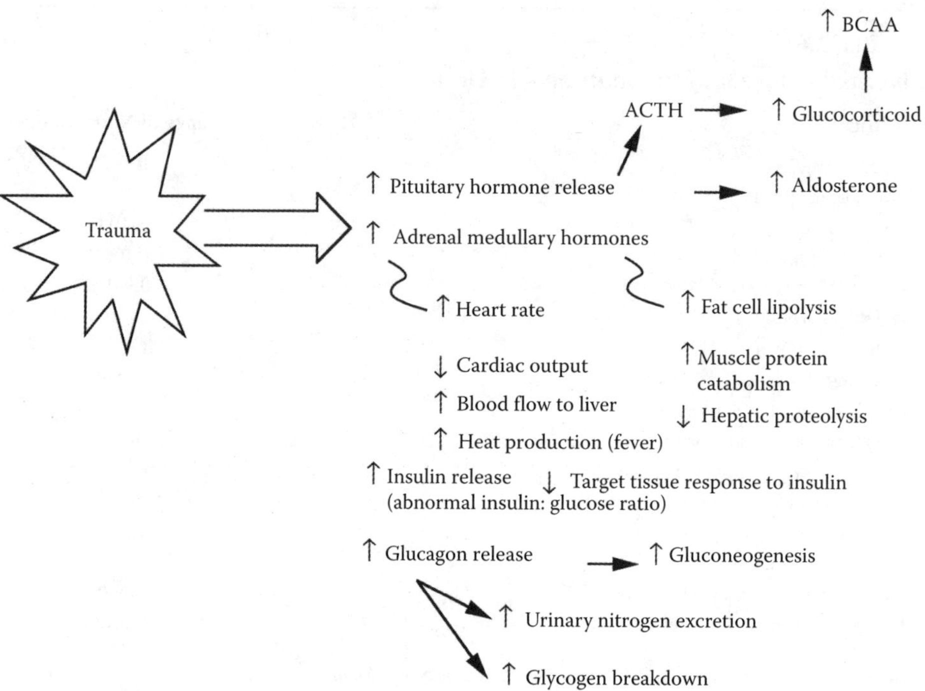

FIGURE 2.5 Trauma elicits both hormonal and metabolic responses that result in increased energy need. *Abbreviations*: ACTH, adrenocorticotropic-stimulating hormone; BCAA, branched chain amino acids.

been possible to show that this loss, formerly thought to be obligatory, is not. Indeed, losses due to surgery, infection, or burn have been shown to be minimized and even reversed (in some cases) with the provision of adequate nutritional support. This implies then that the catabolic response to trauma or illness is more a response to inadequate nutrition in the face of a greatly increased set of nutrient requirements than to the trauma or illness itself.

The endocrine and metabolic responses to injury are closely related (Figure 2.5). Increased production of some hormones and the inhibited release of others are integral parts of the body's basic defense mechanism. The primary function of this mechanism is to provide a continuous fuel supply to the CNS and the required substrates for the repair of body tissue. The body responds to trauma with an increased release of the catabolic hormones. This response, in comparison with the overall metabolic response to injury or illness, is relatively short lived. These hormonal responses to injury serve as initiators or inducers of metabolic events that must occur if recovery is to proceed. As relief from the trauma occurs, the catabolic hormonal responses recede and other metabolic control mechanisms assume command. These, in turn, give way to the normal metabolic control mechanisms as recovery proceeds. Aging patients and children likely will have a more exaggerated metabolic response to trauma than young, otherwise healthy, adults. Although the sequence of hormonal and metabolic response may be similar, the time frame and intensity of response will differ. Sometimes these differences can be life threatening if close monitoring is not practiced. The elderly may already have peripheral tissue insulin resistance, which is made worse by the trauma. The child may be more likely to quickly exhaust energy stores and have little reserve. In each instance, the difference between death and survival may rest with the provision of adequate nutrition support in terms of amounts of energy, glucose, and amino acids plus appropriate amounts of insulin to facilitate the return to normal fuel homeostasis.

The temporal changes in the choice of metabolic fuels are characterized by subtle transitions from one fuel source to another. These are orchestrated by the endocrine response to the trauma or infection. These in turn may be influenced by the preinjury nutritional status of the patient *and* the nutrients provided during the recovery period.

Basal energy requirements can increase by as much as 200% in traumatized patients. Part of this increase can be attributed to the thermogenic effects of the catecholamines released in response to the injury. In addition, increases in energy requirement may be due to the increased energy needed to support protein synthesis. Protein synthesis is highly dependent on energy intake. New proteins are needed for tissue repair and for the inflammatory and immunologic responses of the body to infection or injury or both. If the diet is inadequate, the synthesis of these proteins occurs at the expense of muscle protein. Amino acids not used for protein synthesis are deaminated and the resulting ammonia converted to urea. Urea production likewise is energetically expensive. Thus, large increases in both protein synthesis and urea genesis represent an increase in the basal energy requirement and an increase in the protein requirement in the traumatized or severely ill individual. Unless this additional energy and protein are provided, weight loss will occur.

VOLUNTARY STARVATION: ANOREXIA NERVOSA AND BULIMIA

That food intake can be consciously controlled is evident in the condition known as anorexia nervosa. This condition is frequently observed in adolescent and young adult females and is related to their inaccurate perception of their body fatness. They become obsessed with the desire to be thin and either refuse to eat and adequately nourish their bodies or they eat and then force themselves to regurgitate the food. Self-induced vomiting is called bulimia. Additional behaviors related to an obsession with body image includes the excessive use of laxatives and diuretics and the extensive participation in exercise designed to increase energy expenditure. Although the patients may be eating some food, they are not consuming enough food to meet their macro- and micronutrient requirements. Because of this, they are in negative energy and protein balance. Their serum leptin levels are low[16–18] as are serum serotonin levels.[19] These patients are characterized by little body fat. Because ovulation requires a minimal amount of fat in the body, ovulation ceases.[20] Amenorrhea, hypothermia, and hypotension also develop and, if unrecognized and untreated, anorexics may starve to death. Some people, for whatever reason, self-recognize and resume eating. Persons with anorexia have normal sensory functions; taste and smell sensory neurons are intact so if the person decides to eat once again, food becomes desirable. It tastes good and smells good.[21] In contrast, the person who has decided not to eat does not perceive food as desirable.[22] Despite an intact sensory system, patients with anorexia nervosa and/or bulima have overridden the desirable features of food and have self-starved or semistarved. In many respects, anorexic people have physiological/biochemical features that are similar to those patients described in the section on starvation. Their catabolic hormone levels are high and their body-energy stores are being raided as a result. Insulin resistance due to the catabolic hormones is observed. Liver and muscle glycogen levels are low. Fat stores are minimal. As the weight loss proceeds further, these individuals have reduced bone mass, decreased metabolic rate, decreased heart rate, hypoglycemia, hypothyroidism, electrolyte imbalance, elevated free fatty acid and cholesterol levels, peripheral edema, and finally cardiac and renal failure. When their fat stores fall below 2% of total body weight, they will die. This 2% represents the lipids essential to the structure and function of membranes as well as those complex lipids that compose the CNS. With this scenario in mind, the clinician faces the challenge of reversing the condition. Just as it is difficult to reverse starvation-induced changes in the metabolism of unintentionally starving humans (see sections on starvation, PCM, and trauma), reversing the weight loss of anorexic patients presents some special challenges. The energy requirements for weight regain in anorexic patients are highly variable and depend largely on the physiological status of the patient at the time of treatment initiation and on the pre-anorexia body weight. Those patients who had been obese prior to their self-induced anorexia regained their lost weight faster than patients who had been of normal body weight.

Successful treatment of anorexia nervosa is associated with increases in muscle mass, fat mass, and bone mineral density.[23,24] Pharmaceutical agents to stimulate appetite and reverse depression (if present) can be used. If the person is clinically depressed, treatment of the depression will frequently have a positive effect on food intake. This is not always true, however. In contrast, treatment of the anorexia with appetite-stimulating drugs, nutritional support, and counseling can reverse the condition of weight loss and, secondarily, positively affect the depression. Again, this is not always true. The outcome of the treatment depends on the time at which it is instituted. If anorexia nervosa is recognized early in the sequence of hormonal and metabolic change, then the chances of success are much greater than if treatment is initiated after irreversible tissue changes have occurred. While controversy exists as to the success of treatment as well as the accuracy of diagnosis, it is generally agreed that aggressive treatment can achieve reversal in 50% of the cases. Mortality is estimated in 6% of cases. This leaves an estimate of approximately 44% who recover spontaneously without medical intervention. Treatment success also depends on the degree of self-prescribed food intake restriction. Total food abstinence is far more threatening than mild abstinence. Included in the mortality figure of 6% are those who commit suicide. This implies a relationship between the development of depression and anorexia—two self-destructive behaviors that represent abnormalities in the CNS.

Restoring the weight loss of the anorexic patient follows a slightly different pattern from the weight regain by traumatized individuals and formerly obese individuals. In the latter groups, the fat regain precedes the protein regain.[24,25] In fact, in the genetically obese individual, fat regain takes precedence over protein regain.[26,27] In the recovering anorexic who was not genetically obese prior to anorexia, protein regain keeps pace with fat regain. As both synthetic processes utilize micronutrients, these must be provided at levels similar to those prescribed for growing children. Recovering anorexics are *growing* new tissue to replace that which was raided during the energy deficit period. They must consume sufficient nutrients to support this regrowth.

Bulimic and nonbulimic anorexics differ in their weight recovery.[26] Those who were bulimic recover their lost weight more rapidly than those who were anorexic only. This is probably due to the difference in rate of weight loss. Those anorexics who were also bulimic were more severely starved and lost weight faster than nonbulimic anorexics. Because of this, bulimics are more likely to be diagnosed and treated sooner than nonbulimic anorexics. In anorexics, as with prolonged starvation, gut absorptive capacity is compromised due to a loss of cells lining the gastrointestinal tract. In the early phase of treatment, malabsorption is likely to occur. For this reason, the diet offered during recovery must be gradually increased with respect to its energy content and with respect to the availability of the nutrients in the food. A gradual 300 kcal (1255 kJ) thrice-weekly increase from an initial 1200 kcal (5040 kJ) diet that includes about 3 g sodium is recommended. The recovery diet should also be a lactose-free diet and should be offered in six or more small meals over 24 h. A low-fat diet is sometimes recommended, but this depends on the genetic background and pre-anorexia health status of the patient. Those with diabetic tendencies might not fare as well if faced with a low-fat–high-carbohydrate diet. The medical history of the patient and family will provide clues as to the most appropriate diet design. The recovering anorexic requires more food than the recovering bulimic anorexic. The recovering anorexic has lost more absorptive cells than the bulimic anorexic. Of interest is the report that even after weight regain, the recovered anorexic has a higher than normal energy requirement and, if this is not met, will begin to lose weight once again. This suggests that not all anorexia nervosa is self-inflicted. It may begin with a conscious effort to consume less food but then may continue because of a change in the signals for food intake initiation and cessation and a change in the efficiency with which the body uses the food consumed.

ABNORMAL APPETITE: PICA

Man, as well as some lower animals, will sometimes or habitually consume items of no nutritional value. In some cases, the item in question will have a deleterious effect on the person's health. The habit is called pica, after the Latin word for magpie, a bird that will consume all manner of food and nonfood items. Pica has been observed for centuries and was described by Aetius of Amida in 1542. Many different items are consumed; however, the most common are clay (geophagia), laundry starch (amylophagia), or ice (pagophagia). A number of studies on the prevalence of pica have shown that up to 70% of some population groups may have this habit. Pregnant women as well as children are the most frequently affected, and black women are three to four times more affected than white women of the same socioeconomic group. The most common cravings were for laundry starch (as much as 8 oz a day) and clay. When both men and women were studied, few men exhibited the practice and it has been suggested that men use liquor or tobacco to meet their nonfood oral needs.

The question of why pica exists has not been satisfactorily answered. From the various epidemiological studies, age, sex, social status, and race appear to be important factors in the development of the habit. Several studies have noted that pica was associated with anemia. Pica has been reported to be accompanied by frequent nosebleeds and other spontaneous losses of blood accompanied or preceded an increased craving for certain food and nonfood items. Clay, rice, French fries, ice, green vegetables, bread, hot tea, and grapefruit were mentioned as being consumed in large quantities by these patients. The patients were treated for their anemias with iron supplements and were tested for their iron-binding capacity. Some of the patients had low uptakes of iron while others were normal.[28,29] Those with poor iron-binding capacities were usually the clay eaters; those with normal iron-binding capacities were ice eaters. Clay, even the small amount residing in the gastrointestinal tract of patients having no access to clay while hospitalized, could have adsorbed the oral iron supplements. Thus, it seems unlikely that an innate lowered iron-binding capacity was responsible for either the anemia or the pica. However, pica does appear to follow the development of anemia rather than precede it.

In addition to anemia, other conditions have been observed in pica patients. Muscular weakness and low serum potassium levels have been reported in geophagic patients. Both these conditions could be attributed to the binding of potassium in the intestine by the clay. This may also be true in patients consuming large quantities of laundry starch.

A more serious aspect of pica is the consumption of paint chips (plumbism) by young children. If the paint contains lead oxide as the pigment, lead intoxication can develop. This is characterized by anemia, low serum iron and copper values, growth depression, ataxia, kidney damage, coma, convulsions, and death. The ataxia, stupor, coma, and convulsions reflect the effect of lead on the CNS. This can be understood as the effect of lead on hemoglobin synthesis. Both copper and iron utilization are impaired and the anemia typical of lead intoxication is microcytic and hypochromic in character. In addition, lead may replace either copper, iron, or calcium in a number of tissues and, because it is metabolically inert, inhibit the functionality of that tissue. In the case of hemoglobin synthesis, it becomes obvious that the oxygen-carrying capacity of the red blood cells is decreased. Those tissues with a high oxygen requirement, that is, the neural tissue, will be the most affected. Thus, one can understand the neuromuscular response to chronic lead ingestion. If neuronal tissue suffers from prolonged oxygen deprivation, it will die and this damage is irreversible. Subjects with lead poisoning can be treated with compounds such as EDTA that will bind the circulating lead and allow the body to excrete the EDTA–lead complex. It is not possible, however, to rid the body of all of its accumulated lead nor to protect the patients from future ill effects of their lead-induced pathology. Lead will remain in its storage sites, such as bone, and, when mobilized, will have untoward effects.

In the United States today, the majority of lead-intoxication cases are young children, ages 1–6, with pica. Adults who work in lead-related industries or consume lead-contaminated illegal beverages are also affected. Increasing the levels of lead exposure generally increases the blood and tissue lead levels, yet individual variations due to age, sex, and nutritional status occur. The factors that determine the fractions of the body where lead is deposited have not been determined. It is known that well-nourished individuals are more resistant to the deleterious effects of lead than are poorly nourished individuals.

SUMMARY

1. Zero energy balance means that the energy consumed is equal to that expended; negative energy balance means that more energy is expended than is consumed.
2. The set-point theory suggests that body weight is controlled for long periods of time until or unless perturbations occur that have long-lasting effects on body weight.
3. Body fat and bodyweight are not necessarily correlated.
4. NHANES and other surveys document malnutrition.
5. Energy conservation is one of the first responses to starvation or semistarvation.
6. Recovery from starvation or semistarvation is hormonally directed and can be affected by concurrent disease, trauma, and other environmental influences. Age and gender influence recovery.
7. Anorexia nervosa and bulimia are diseases where the individual voluntarily subjects himself or herself to starvation or semistarvation. Pica also results in malnutrition due to voluntary consumption of nonfood items. Some of these are toxic.
8. Recovery must be closely monitored; there can be both short-term and long-term consequences to episodes of starvation or semistarvation.

LEARNING OPPORTUNITIES

CASE STUDY 2.1 Marcus Wants to Stop Gaining Weight

Marcus is a member of his high school wrestling team. He was 5′4″ tall, weighed 135 lb, and was 14 years old at the beginning of his sophomore year. He was just beginning his growth spurt, and in the next 6 months, he gained nearly 5 in. in height. He also gained small amounts of weight. Although at first this did not seem a very serious situation, over time, Marcus became concerned that he might have to move up to the next weight class where he thought he might be less competitive. Marcus began trying a variety of methods to keep his weight down while still preserving his hard-won muscle tissue. His methods included weight work in the gym, aerobic work such as running and swimming, taking saunas, fasting for a day before competition weigh in, and eating a high-protein diet recommend by the local diet center. Although these methods reduced his weight gain, Marcus was not satisfied. He wanted to stay in his 135–145 weight class for wrestling. He decided to try the diet pills that his mother and sister used. This seemed to work for a few weeks but Marcus found that the diet pills were not suppressing his appetite. He was still very hungry. He stopped taking them but he decided to make himself vomit the food he ate so that this food would not have an effect on his weight. He found that he could eat enough to feel satisfied, and if he then vomited all this food, he could suppress weight gain. Although he finished the season in the weight class he desired, by spring, he had gained five inches in height and he worried that through the summer he might not remain in the weight class he wanted to be in. He thought about the summer and realized that it would be a long hard slog against weight gain so Marcus continued to induce himself to vomit. He also continued his strenuous exercise program with the goal of increasing muscle strength. He stopped consuming the high-protein drink recommended by the food store. However, during the summer, a routine dental appointment revealed erosion of Marcus's tooth enamel and enlargement of his salivary glands. At the same time, Marcus complained to his dentist of constant muscle cramps at unexpected times that were hard to resolve. The dentist recognized the signs of bulimia nervosa (self-induced vomiting) and discussed this with Marcus and his father. Marcus admitted that he had been inducing vomiting to control his weight. The dentist recommended that Marcus see the family physician for a physical. The physician observed slight dehydration and esophageal inflammation and noted that Marcus's weight was only 70% of the expected weight for his height. Bulimia nervosa was confirmed but Marcus refused to see the psychologist as recommended saying instead that he would stop his self-induced vomiting.

Marcus did stop his self-induced vomiting, but then over the summer, he gained some weight. When the gain was around 10 lb, he was seriously worried about entering his junior year as a wrestler in the next weight class. He convinced himself that he did not want to do this so he decided to try laxatives as a form of weight control. He thought that this might avoid the health consequences of induced vomiting.

A few weeks into the new season, Marcus fractured his upper arm. The radiologist at the hospital noted that Marcus's bone density was low for his age and recommended a consult with his family physician. This time, a panel of tests demonstrated an electrolyte imbalance. His tissue potassium was low and the blood values likewise for chloride, potassium, sodium, magnesium, and calcium were abnormal. The blood workup showed that he was anemic, hypovolemic, and hypoproteinemic. More sophisticated bone density tests demonstrated that Marcus has osteomalacia. In addition, Marcus's EKG showed a cardiac arrhythmia. He was admitted to the local hospital for treatment and began counseling with a psychologist and a nutritionist with the goal of helping Marcus understand that his condition was induced by his forced vomiting and then his use of laxatives coupled with excess exercise. After reviewing this case, what has been happening to Marcus? What would be the best approach to take to help him understand his situation? Explain the biochemistry and physiology of this condition.

CASE STUDY 2.2 Discovering a Concentration Camp

After Germany surrendered at the end of World War II, the allied troops spread out over the territory and much to their dismay discovered numerous camps for prisoners of war and for people the Germans thought should not be citizens of their country. When the troops entered these camps, they found numerous starving people. They immediately emptied their backpacks of any food they possessed and gave it to the ex-prisoners. However, medical personnel caught up with the troops and demanded the return of the food saying that the troops were going to kill these survivors if all that food was consumed.

Analysis and resolution: What was the situation? Why would giving these people the contents of the backpacks so harmful? What homeostatic mechanisms were operative here? What would be the best treatment for these survivors?

MULTIPLE-CHOICE QUESTIONS

1. Which is a correct statement?
   a. Fatty acids can be converted to glucose.
   b. All amino acids can be converted to glucose.
   c. Starvation decreases fatty acid mobilization.
   d. During starvation, the body becomes efficient in the use of stored fuels.
2. Negative energy balance exists when
   a. Less energy is consumed than is what is needed
   b. Women are pregnant
   c. Children are growing
   d. More energy is consumed than what is needed
3. Pica is defined as
   a. The excess consumption of food
   b. The consumption of nonfood items
   c. The consumption of excess kcalories
   d. Lack of sufficient food to meet need

4. Anorexia nervosa and bulimia results in
   a. Reduced food intake
   b. Loss of body weight
   c. Loss of fat stores
   d. All of the above
5. Trauma affects energy balance because
   a. Catabolic hormones stimulate the mobilization of body fat stores and body protein
   b. Anabolic hormone release is suppressed
   c. Body temperature is increased
   d. All of the above

REFERENCES

1. Austin, G.L., Ogden, L.C., Hill, J.O. (2011) Trends in carbohydrate, fat, and protein intakes and association with energy intake in normal weight, overweight and obese individuals: 1971–2006. *Am. J. Clin. Nutr*. 93: 836–843.
2. Ford, E.S., Dietz, W.H. (2013) Trends in energy intake among adults in the United States: Findings from NHANES. *Am. J. Clin. Nutr*. 97: 848–853.
3. Prins, J.B., O'Rahilly, S. (1997) Regulation of adipose cell number in man. *Clin. Sci*. 92: 3–11.
4. Katzmarzyk, P.T., Bray, G.A., Greenway, F.L., Johnson, W.D., Newton, R.L., Rauvussin, E., Ryan, D.H., Smith, S.R., Bouchard, C. (2010) Racial differences in abdominal depot-specific adiposity in white and African American adults. *Am. J. Clin. Nutr*. 91: 7–15.
5. Hervey, G.R., Tobin, G. (1982) The part played by variation of energy expenditure in the regulation of energy balance. *Proc. Nutr. Soc*. 41: 137–153.
6. Harris, R.B.S. (1990) Role of set point theory in regulation of body weight. *FASEB J*. 4: 3310–3318.
7. Martin, R.J., White, D.B., Hulsey, M.G. (1991) The regulation of body weight. *Am. Sci*. 79: 528–541.
8. Benedict, F.G. (1915) *A Study of Prolonged Fasting*. Carnegie Institute of Washington, Washington, DC.
9. Cahill, G.F., Herrera, M.G., Morgan, A.P., Soeldner, J.S., Levy, P.L., Reichard, G.A., Kipnis, D.M. (1966) Hormone-fuel relationships during fasting. *J. Clin. Invest*. 45: 1751–1769.
10. Chernoff, R. (2013) Nutritional screen monitoring tools. In: *Handbook of Nutrition and Food* (C. Berdanier, J. Dwyer, B. Huber, eds.). CRC Press, Boca Raton, FL, pp. 505–515.
11. Kim, D.W., Khaodhiar, L., Apovian, C.M. (2013) Nutritional assessment in the clinical setting. In: *Handbook of Nutrition and Food* (C.D. Berdanier, J. Dwyer, D. Huber, eds.). CRC Press, Boca Raton, FL, pp. 755–761.
12. Van Abesian, A.F.M., Veenendaal, M.V.E., Painter, R.C., de Rooji, S.R., Dijkgraaf, M.G.W., Bossuyt, P.M.M., Elias, S.G., Grobbee, D.E., Ulterwaal, C.S.P.M., Roseboom, T.J. (2011) Survival effects of prenatal famine exposure. *Am. J. Clin. Nutr*. 95: 179–183.
13. Lumey, L.H., Stein. A.D., Kahn, H.S., Romijn, J.A. (2009) Lipid profiles in middle-aged men and women after famine exposure during gestation: The Dutch Hunger Winter Families Study. *Am. J. Clin. Nutr*. 89: 1737–1743.
14. Huang, C., Li, Z., Wang, M., Martorell, R. (2010) Early life exposure to the 1959–1961 Chinese famine has long-term health consequences. *J. Nutr*. 140: 1874–1878.
15. Galler, J.R., Bryce, C.P., Zichlin, M.L., Fitzmaurice, G., Eaglesfield, G.D., Waber, D.P. (2012) Infant malnutrition is associated with persisting attention deficits in middle adulthood. *J. Nutr*. 142: 788–794.
16. Grinspoon, G., Gulick, T., Askari, H., Landt, M., Lee, K., Anderson, E., Ma, Z., Vignati, L., Bowsher, R., Herzog, D., Klibanski, A. (1996) Serum leptin levels in women with anorexia nervosa. *J. Clin. Endocrinol. Metab*. 81: 3861–3863.
17. Herpetz, S., Wagner, R., Albers, N., Blum, W.F., Pelz, B., Langkafel, M., Kopp, W. et al. (1998) Circadian plasma leptin levels in patients with anorexia nervosa: Relation to insulin and cortisol. *Horm. Res*. 50: 197–204.
18. Eckert, E.D., Pomeroy, C., Raymond, N., Kohler, P.F., Thuras, P., Bowers, C.Y. (1998) Leptin in anorexia nervosa. *J. Clin. Endocrinol. Metab*. 83: 791–795.
19. Weltzin, T., Fernstrom, M.H., Kaye, W.H. (1994) Serotonin and bulimia nervosa. *Nutr. Rev*. 52: 399–408.
20. Frisch, R. (1991) Body weight, body fat, and ovulation. *Trends Endocrinol. Metab*. 2: 191–197.
21. Goldzak-Kunik, G., Friedman, R., Spitz, M., Sandler, L., Leshem, M. (2011) Intact sensory function in anorexia nervosa. *Am. J. Clin. Nutr*. 95: 272–282.

22. Cowdrey, F.A., Finlayson, G., Park, R.J. (2013) Liking compared with wanting for high- and low-calorie foods in anorexia nervosa: Aberrant food reward even after weight restoration. *Am. J. Clin. Nutr.* 97: 463–470.
23. Dynesen, A.W., Bardow, A., Astrup, A., Peterson, B., Holst, J.J., Nauntofte, B. (2008) Meal-induced compositional changes in blood and saliva in persons with bulimia nervosa. *Am. J. Clin. Nutr.* 87: 12–22.
24. Haas, V.K., Kohn, M.J., Clarke, S.D., Allen, J.R., Madden, S., Muller, M.J., Gaskin, K.J. (2009) Body composition changes in female adolescents with anorexia nervosa. *Am. J. Clin. Nutr.* 89: 1005–1010.
25. Mayer, L.E.S., Klein, D.A., Black, E., Attia, E., Shen, W., Mao, X., Shungu, D.C. et al. (2009) Adipose tissue distribution after weight restoration and weight maintenance in women with anorexia nervosa. *Am. J. Clin. Nutr.* 90: 1132–1137.
26. Johnston, C.A., Foreyt, J.P. (2013) Eating disorders In: *Handbook of Nutrition and Food* (C.D. Berdanier, J. Dwyer, D. Heber, eds.). CRC Press, Boca Raton, FL, pp. 793–818.
27. Johnston, C.A., Moreno, J.P., Foreyt, J.P. (2013) Psychological assessment for adults and children. In: *Handbook of Nutrition and Food* (C.D. Berdanier, J. Dwyer, D. Heber, eds.). CRC Press, Boca Raton, FL, pp. 679–691.
28. Kushner, R.F., Retelny, S. (2005) Emergence of pica (ingestion of non-food substances) accompanying iron deficiency anemia after gastric bypass surgery. *Obes Res.* 15: 1491–1495.
29. Mokhobo, K.P. (1986) Iron deficiency and anemia. *S. Afr. Med. J.* 70: 473–475.

3 Positive Energy Balance

In Chapters 1 and 2, energy need and negative energy balance were described and discussed. In this chapter, we will discuss the problems associated with chronic positive energy balance. Individuals, who continuously consume more energy than they can use, can either burn off the excess energy intake as described in the section on thermogenesis (Chapter 1) or store this excess energy intake as fat. If the stored fat is in a slight excess, the individual is *overweight*. If there is a large excess of stored fat, the individual is obese. Both humans and other species can become obese. Much of what scientists have learned about the etiology of obesity has been gained through the study of such spontaneously obese animals as the obese and lean pig, obese and lean mice, and obese and lean rats. Some of these animal models have been selectively bred to produce obesity complicated by hypertension, diabetes, or cardiovascular disease. As such, they have provided insights into the complications of obesity as observed in humans.

OBESITY

Obesity is at the other end of the spectrum of abnormal energy states. With starvation, protein-energy malnutrition, inadequate energy intake, and trauma, the body is in negative energy balance. More energy is being used than is being consumed. In contrast, excess fat stores or obesity represents that condition where more energy is consumed than is expended and the body is in positive energy balance.[1,2] Since the mid-twentieth century, the percentage of the population that is obese in the United States has risen dramatically.[1,2] More than 35% of the adult population is obese and an additional 40% are overweight (Figure 3.1). Males are more affected than are females. Excess body fat is associated with an increased risk of coronary heart disease, hypertension, stroke, heart failure, type 2 diabetes, osteoarthritis, gallstones, and many forms of cancer.[3–7] Obesity in midlife may increase the risk of mortality by two- to threefold. Excess body fat or being *overweight* is defined by a body mass index (BMI = weight/height^2) of 25–29.99, while a BMI of over 30 is the definition of obesity. As people age, there is a gradual increase in their body fat stores such that those over the age of 60 are more likely to be overweight or obese than when they were younger. More than 76% of males and 73% of females are in this category after the age of 60. More alarming is the rising numbers of obese and overweight children. Up to 17% of children from age 2 to 19 are considered overweight or obese.[8,9] This is a threefold increase in childhood obesity over that observed in the 1960s. The prevalence of obesity in children rose from about 5% before 1980 to the present ~17% in 2013. The percentage of obese children who become obese adults is 14% at 6 months of age, 41% at age 7, and about 70% at ages 10–13.[9] Obese children are also showing signs of type 2 diabetes, hypertension, and other obesity-related health problems. As with adults, there are age, race, and gender differences in the children. Youngsters of Hispanic and African-American origin are more likely to be obese than are Asian and Caucasian children. There have been intense efforts to reduce the prevalence of child obesity. Some of these efforts have been successful. Providing additional opportunities for physical activity and providing fewer energy-rich foods in the school lunch and snacks program have resulted in lessening the prevalence of obesity in school age children.

In people who are overweight or obese, their excess energy intake is stored as fat in the adipose tissue; excess fat can also be found in the internal organs and in the skeletal–muscular system. In contrast to the other body components of protein, water, and mineral matter that have a size limitation, the fat store can expand throughout life if an excess of food energy is continually provided. In some instances, both cell number and cell size are increased.[3,4] In humans, fat depots occur throughout the body.

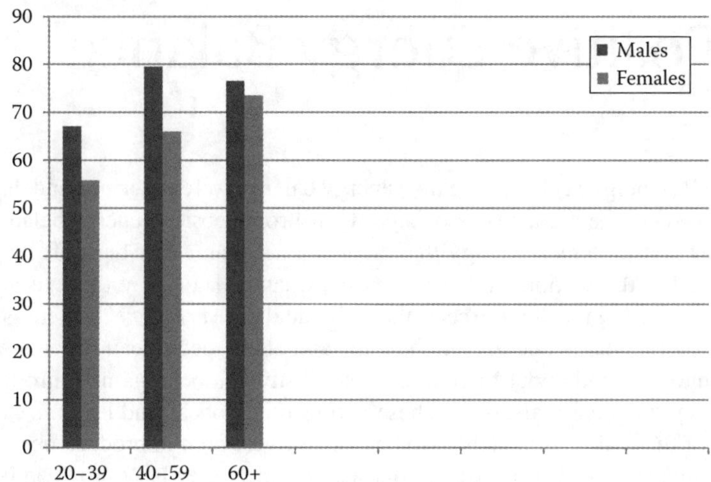

FIGURE 3.1 Percentage of the total population that are obese or overweight in three different age groups of males and females.

The major depots are in the abdomen, over the shoulders, on the hips, and on the thighs. There are differences in the distribution of fat in these depots that are due to gender, genetics, age, and lifestyle choices. Racial differences in the abdominal depot-specific adiposity in white and African-American adults have been reported.[5] While total body fatness is an important risk factor for several degenerative diseases,[6,7] the distribution of the stored fat may impact upon these disease states as well.[3,4] Males and females differ in the pattern of body fat stores. Males tend to deposit fat in the abdominal area, while females tend to deposit fat in the gluteal area. Measuring the waist and hip circumference allows computation of the waist-to-hip ratio (WHR). As this ratio increases, so does the risk for cardiovascular disease, diabetes mellitus, and hypertension.[6,7] In men, if the WHR is greater than 0.90 and in women greater than 0.80, the risk for cardiovascular disease increases significantly.

Although simple measures of body weight and waist and hip circumference can suggest that the individual is overweight or obese, there are exceptions to these measures. The body builder, for example, may develop excess muscle mass and weigh disproportionately more than the average individual, yet that individual is by no means overweight or obese. Muscle is heavier than adipose tissue, and it is the adipose fat mass that determines whether the individual is overweight or obese. The determination of the size of fat store in large animals, particularly humans, is difficult. In small animals such as mouse and rat, direct measurement is possible. The total fat in the body can be determined using a fat extraction method. Fat solvents (usually a chloroform–methanol mixture) will remove the fat, and the percentage body fat is calculated as the difference in body weight before and after extraction. In large animals, the direct determination of body fat is neither practical nor feasible especially if one wishes to determine how the body fat store might change in response to a given treatment. This is particularly a challenge when studying humans. Indirect methods are available and are described subsequently.[10–21]

Indirect Methods Used to Determine Body Fat

The determination of lean body mass (LBM) will provide an estimate of the fat mass. LBM can be calculated if one assumes that the fat-free body has constant water content (72%) and that the neutral fat is stored dry. Thus, the formula

$$\text{LBM}\left(\text{kg}\right) = \frac{\text{Total body water}\left(\text{TBW, kg}\right)}{0.72}$$

can be used. The figure 72% is an average figure derived from careful direct measurements of the water content of lean tissue.[10] Body water content varies with age. Young children, for example, have about 70% body water, while aged individuals have about 60% body water. Total body water (TBW) can be measured by infusing heavy water (deuterium), allowing this to equilibrate within the body and then withdrawing a sample of blood. This method is called the water dilution method. Knowing the concentration of the labeled water, the volume that was infused, and the concentration in the blood sample withdrawn, one can calculate the volume of dilution of the infused labeled water. This will provide a value for TBW. The calculation of TBW is as follows: $C_1V_1 = C_2V_2$ where V_2 is the volume in which the solute is distributed. Dividing TBW by 0.72 (as per the preceding equation) gives an estimate of the LBM. LBM is also equal to the total body mass minus its fat content. These methods may not be applicable to all situations and in fact may be impractical for studies using large number of subjects or subjects unwilling to provide a small sample of lean tissue for the determination of its water content or may be unwilling to have deuterium infused.

LBM can also be predicted from skeletal measurements and from bone weight. Sophisticated techniques using ultrasound, neutron activation analysis, infrared interactance, dual-energy x-ray absorptiometry (DEXA), computer-assisted tomography, magnetic resonance imaging (MRI), or bioelectrical impedance are available, and as the instrumentation improves, these methods may become practical in the clinical setting.[11–21] Presently, considerable effort is being expended to validate these methods because they are noninvasive and allow for the sequential determination of changes in one or more of the major body components as a result of a change in diet, activity, age, or endocrine status. In addition, these noninvasive methods could be useful in assessing population groups in relation to fat mass, bone density, or adipose tissue distribution. For example, Sohlström et al.[15] used MRI to estimate body fat content. They compared these estimates with those obtained from underwater weighing and from body water dilution studies. The three methods gave similar results with MRI and body weight dilution providing 1.4% ± 2.9% less and 4.7% ± 4.0% more, respectively, than underwater weighing for total body fat. However, because MRI can provide information about where this fat is found, this method is superior to the others. In MRI, images are created by a combination of electromagnetic radiation and a magnetic field. Individual body segments such as shoulders, chest, hips, and thighs can be examined as discrete entities. Thus, the amount and distribution of fat can be detailed.

DEXA is another of the newer methods used to estimate bone density and soft-tissue composition.[11–13] The advantage of this method is that it eliminates the need to use the assumption that the body exists as a two-pool system. The one pool is the fat and the other is the fat-free mass (or LBM). Bone density as a fraction of the fat-free mass can be distinguished and quantitated using DEXA. The result is that bone mass and density can be quantitated, as can the fat mass, and the remaining tissue is more legitimately the LBM. One can then distinguish and quantitate the muscle mass using its creatine content. If the major component of the lean is assumed to be the muscle, muscle mass can be determined using the dilution of radioactive creatine or creatine labeled with a heavy nonradioactive isotope.[14] This has been used successfully in rats and may be applicable to humans because creatine is almost exclusively located in the muscle. Labeled creatine is infused and after a set interval, a muscle biopsy obtained. The total muscle mass can be calculated using the following equation:

$$\frac{\text{Total}\,^{14}\text{C creatine infused}}{[^{14}\text{C creatine] in sample}} = \frac{\text{Muscle sample size}}{\text{Total muscle mass}}$$

On the assumption that LBM has a constant potassium content and that neutral fat does not bind the electrolyte, LBM can be estimated by measuring the body content of the heavy potassium isotope ^{40}K or by measuring the dilution of ^{42}K (the radioactive isotope) in the body cells.[16] The former requires a whole-body scintillation counter, whereas the latter can be determined in a small tissue (muscle biopsy) sample. The formula for calculating LBM is as follows:

$$\text{LBM} = \frac{\text{Total K content}}{\text{Concentration of K / kg tissue}}$$

Either of these methods may underestimate the LBM because of the lack of correction for the small amounts of potassium in the extracellular fluids.

LBM and percent fat can be estimated using measures of body density or specific gravity of the individual. The fat-free body will have a specific gravity of 1.1000. This will decrease as the body increases its fat content since fat has a lower (~0.92) specific gravity than the fat-free body mass. Thus, the fatter the subject, the lower the specific gravity or density. The body density can be determined in the adult using Archimedes' principle. The subject is weighed in air and again in water when immersed. The difference in the two body weights is the weight of the body that is water. Since water has a density of 1 (1 mL of water weighs 1 g), the volume of the water displaced represents both the volume of the body immersed and its density. The immersion weight/unit volume of water displaced then is diluted by the air weight/unit volume of water displaced, which in turn is the specific gravity of the subject. Corrections for the residual air in the lungs and intestines must be made. There are a number of reports on body density and body fat using this technique.[18–21] Age affects body density and percent body fat. In one study of women of different ages, Young et al.[18] reported that young (16–40 years of age) women had body densities of 1.0342–1.0343 g/mL and percent body fats of 28.69–28.75. Older women (50–70 years of age) had body densities that ranged from 1.0095 to 1.0050 g/mL and percent body fats of 41.88%–44.56%. Using the weight in air and that of underwater, body fat can be estimated using the Siri[19] equation:

$$\%\text{ Body fat} = \frac{2.118 - 1.354 - 0.78}{\text{density}} \times \%\text{TBW / body weight}$$

where 2.118, 1.354, and 0.78 are the constants and the density (g/cc), body weight (kg), and TBW (kg) are determined.

Other prediction equations for percent fat from specific gravity are available. The Pace–Rathbun[21] method calculates % fat = 100 − TBW/0.732. The Pace–Rathbun method is based on TBW only and compensates for the structural lipids (those in cell membranes, CNS, brain, and bone marrow, as contrasted to the depot lipids) by adding 3%. This gives a LBM that is somewhat different from that of Siri.[19] Underwater weighing as described earlier is based on the difference in density of the different body components. Estimating fat stores in this way is cumbersome or not feasible in many clinical settings or under conditions of field surveys. Researchers using this method have made some correlations between this estimate and estimates of body fatness using the measurements of skinfold thicknesses at key locations, that is, places where subcutaneous fat can be assessed using calipers to estimate the skinfold thickness. The fold below the upper arm (triceps fold) and the fold at the iliac crest are frequently used locations. Other locations include the abdominal fold and the thigh fold. Equations (Table 3.1) have been derived to calculate body fatness using these measurements.

For population surveys where close estimates of body fat, protein, LBM, etc., are not critical, simpler estimates of body fatness are frequently used. Using the patient's body weight and height, one can compare these values with those considered desirable for men and women. The first such tables were developed by the Metropolitan Life Insurance Company, which made the assumption that young (age 20–30) people applying for life insurance (and found insurable) were healthy. They then took the body weights of these people and arranged them according to height for both males

TABLE 3.1
General Formulas for Calculating Body Fatness from Skinfold Measurements

Males	% Body Fat = $29.288 \times 10^{-2}(x) - 5 \times 10^{-4}(x)^2 + 15.845 \times 10^{-2}(\text{Age})$
Females	% Body Fat = $29.699 \times 10^{-2}(X) - 43 \times 10^{-5}(x)^2 + 29.63 \times 10^{-3}(\text{Age}) + 1.4072$

Notes: X is the sum of abdomen, suprailiac, triceps, and thigh skinfolds. Age is in years.

and females. They called these weights *desirable* weights because they were associated with the lowest mortality due to disease. Because the weight range for each height was so large, they later subdivided each weight-for-height range into thirds and presented these thirds as being representatives of small, medium, and large frame sizes. This table has been found useful by many in estimating desirable body weight, but the user must remember that this table was not based on actual measurements of skeletal size. The table is based only on heights and weights of individuals in the third decade of life who wanted (and could afford) life insurance. In this respect, there is a bias in the table. Minority groups were largely underrepresented in the database used for these tables.

A broader database using subjects of all ages, economic status, and both sexes and from minority and majority cultural/ethnic groups has been obtained by the National Health and Nutrition Examination Survey (NHANES). The surveys by NHANES are conducted at intervals by the Centers for Disease Control of the U.S. Department of Health and Human Services. The surveys have collected data from males and females from childhood to old age. The weight and height measurements were used to create tables giving weight ranges for males and females at different ages. In addition, NHANES made more detailed measurements of skinfold thickness, skeletal size, and density and a variety of biochemical and physiological features using a representative subset of the population assessed. The NHANES tables therefore have a broader database than the Metropolitan Life Insurance tables. Despite the difference in databases used to construct the tables, both are useful in evaluating humans in terms of desirable body weight.

Perhaps more popular now is the use of BMI. This is a simple tool that is useful in assessing obesity. Body weight and height are easily measured. BMI is an index of the body weight (kg) divided by the height (m) squared ($\text{weight}/\text{height}^2$). BMI correlates with body fatness and with the risk of obesity-related disease or diseases for which obesity is a compounding factor.[6,7,20] Overweight is defined as a BMI between 25 and 30 and obesity is a BMI over 30. The BMI varies with age. A desirable BMI for people aged 19–24 is between 19 and 24, while that for people aged 55–64 is between 23 and 28. While simple in concept, this term does not assess body composition per se. It provides a basis only for assessing the health risks associated with or presumed to be associated with excess body fatness. BMI applies only to normal individuals, not the super athlete or the body builder, who may be quite heavy yet have little body fat.

Origins of Obesity

Obesity develops for a variety of reasons. Listed in Table 3.2 are some of the reasons why excess body fatness develops. Many of these reasons are genetic in origin. They consist of mutations in genes that encode components of the system that regulates food intake and energy balance. In some instances, the development of obesity is the prime phenotype of the genotype. In other instances, the phenotype is the result of an interaction between genetics and the environment. An individual may have inherited one or more mutated genes that influence the efficiency with which that individual uses the intake energy and converts it to stored energy. When provided with an ample food supply, these individuals may become fat. However, if the food supply is limited and/or if the individual leads a very active life, the excess fat store might not develop.

TABLE 3.2
Suggested Causes of Obesity

Mutations in genes for

a. Leptin, leptin receptor
b. Cholecystokinin
c. Adipsin, adiponectin
d. Ghrelin
e. Tumor necrosis factor (TNFα)
f. NPY, NPY receptor
g. CRH, CRH receptor
h. Adipocyte-specific transcription factor C/EBPα
i. Agouti protein
j. Carboxypeptidase E
k. Phosphodiesterase
l. β-Adrenergic receptor
m. Growth hormone receptor
n. Glucocorticoid receptor
o. Insulin receptor
p. Uncoupling proteins
q. Melanocortin 3 receptor

Hormone imbalance

a. Excess glucocorticoid
b. Excess insulin (hyperinsulinemia)
c. Hypothyroidism
d. Polycystic ovary disease

Other causes

a. Injury to the brain stem or hypothalamus
b. Chronic inflammatory state in adipose tissue and other tissues
c. Changes in the population of bacteria in the gastrointestinal tract
d. Social/cultural feeding behaviors

Genetics of Obesity

Research on the genetic basis for excess body fatness is very active.[22–45] Many genes have been identified as being associated with excessive body fat in humans. Listed in Table 3.3 are some of the genes reported to be associated with obesity.[31] This is not a complete list. Shown are the locations, a brief description of the phenotype, and the gene or locus of the defect. The location is in code: The first is a number that indicates the chromosome on which the base sequence is located. Next is the letter location (the structural gene is divided into segments with each segment given a letter designation), and the last is the location in the gene where a base substitution or deletion or addition can be found. The gene or locus is given an abbreviation. One can look up these associations online using the Online Mendelian Inheritance in Man (OMIM) web address (www.ncbi.nlm.nih.gov). The reader can then indicate which of the many genetic problems are of interest. The website not only gives the aberrant base sequences for a given condition but also provides some background with respect to the key citations relevant to the condition of interest. In some instances, the location of where genetic testing is available is given.

Several investigators have shown that the familial trait for body fatness has a much stronger influence on body composition than environmental influences such as culture, socioeconomic status, or food intake patterns. Stunkard and associates[27,28] as well as Bouchard and Despres[23,24] have published extensively on the responses of twins to dietary manipulation and exercise.

TABLE 3.3
Some of the Genes Associated with Obesity

Location	Phenotype	Gene/Locus
1p36.11	Mild, early-onset obesity	NR0B2
1p35.2	Obesity in association with other problems	SDC3
2p23.3	Early-onset obesity, adrenal insufficiency	POMC
3p25.3	Susceptibility to obesity	GHRL
3p25.2	Severe obesity	PPARG
3q27	Abdominal obesity, metabolic syndrome, ↑TG	GRCH37
4q31.1	Susceptibility to obesity	UCP1
4p15–p14	—	BMIQ7
5q13.2	—	CART
5q15	Obesity with impaired prohormone processing	PCSK1
5q32	—	ADBR2
5q32	Variant	PPARGC1B
6q16.3	Severe obesity	SIM1
6q23.2	Susceptibility to obesity	ENPP1
7q32.1	Morbid obesity	LEP
8q11.23	—	ADRB3
8q22.2	Cohen syndrome (hypotonia, obesity, etc.)	COH1
10q	Susceptibility to obesity	BMIQ10 and BMIQ8
11q13.4	Severe obesity and type 2 diabetes	UPC3
11p13–p12	Wilms' tumor, aniridia, mental retardation, (deletion) obesity	WAGRO
16p11.2	Severe, early-onset obesity (deletion of nine genes including that for leptin)	BMIQ16
16q22.1	Late-onset obesity	AGRP
17q21.31	Obesity	PYY
18q21.32	Obesity, autosomal dominant, (melanocortin receptor)	MC4R
20q13.2	Severe obesity	MC3R
Xq23	Susceptibility to obesity	SLC6A14

Source: http://www.ncbi.rlm.nih.gov.

They found that identical (monozygotic) twins are more nearly alike in these responses than are siblings or nonidentical (dizygotic) twins. These and other workers[22,30,32,35] have also examined the home environment with respect to body fatness. This work attempted to answer the question of whether people become overly fat because of environmental influences such as the daily coaching by the parents to eat or not eat. Most revealing in this respect are the studies of monozygotic and dizygotic twins reared by their biological parents or by adoptive parents. In one study, adopted children and their biological and adoptive parents were compared with respect to body weight and body fatness, while in other studies, twins reared together or apart were compared. Allison and colleagues[22] have calculated that the heritability of the BMI is between 0.50 and 0.70, depending on the definition of obesity and BMI used. Overfeeding studies of twins have been conducted by Bouchard and associates.[23,24] These studies showed that identical twins will gain a similar amount of weight, whereas siblings or unrelated subjects may not. After the overfeeding period, there were also genetic differences in weight loss patterns. Some people can lose weight far more easily than others. All the studies showed that the genetic influence on body fatness far outweighed the environmental influence. In some individuals, diet-induced weight loss is accompanied by a reduction in resting metabolic rate (RMR).[36,37]

There is a distinct adipose tissue response to energy restriction that predicts whether a weight loss by the obese person is maintained.[38] Those subjects who did not regain their lost weight had a significant reduction in the insulin response to glucose and also had a significant reduction in the expression of genes that encode some of the enzymes of intermediary metabolism.

A number of genetic diseases are characterized by obesity.[32] The Prader–Willi, Bardet–Biedl, Laurence–Moon, Cohen, Boyesen, and Wilson–Turner syndromes are all characterized by obesity as well as by other abnormalities. All of these syndromes are rare.[39] The Prader–Willi syndrome occurs as a result of a partial deletion of the long arm of chromosome 15. It occurs in 1/5,000–1/10,000 live births. Individuals with this syndrome are developmentally delayed, have poor muscle tone, and are growth retarded. Once the child with the Prader–Willi syndrome reaches the age of 2 or 3, other behavioral features develop. The child has a persistent food-seeking behavior that can be self-destructive. Patients with the Bardet–Biedl syndrome, although obese, have a different set of characteristics. Most are mentally retarded with polydactyly (extra fingers/toes) and hypogonadism. The prevalence of this condition is about 1/17,500 live births. These patients do not have the aggressive, persistent food-seeking characteristic like that of the patient with the Prader–Willi syndrome. Patients with the Laurence–Moon syndrome are similar to those with the Bardet–Biedl syndrome except that they are frequently diabetic and paraplegic. They do not have the polydactyly feature. The prevalence of this disorder is of the order of 1/20,000. The Cohen syndrome, also rare, is overrepresented in the Finnish population. It consists of nonprogressive mild to severe psychomotor retardation, clumsiness, microcephaly, progressive retinochoroidal dystrophy, myopia, intermittent neutropenia, and a cheerful disposition. As might be anticipated, all of these disorders are characterized by a shortened life span.

A number of spontaneous genetic errors in the animal kingdom have obesity as one of their characteristics.[25,26,29,30,40] Genetically obese rats, mice, dogs, and desert animals have been described. In rodent species, the mode of inheritance and, in some instances, the chromosomal location of genes for obesity have been found. Obesity can be inherited via an autosomal recessive or dominant or sex-linked mode. This is probably true for humans as well. In each of these mutations, an error occurs that affects energy balance. Errors in the perception of hunger and/or satiety by the brain can explain the excess food intake (hyperphagia) that characterizes several of these mutants. Inappropriate hunger signals, satiety signals, and their receptors have all been implicated (see Chapter 4).

An important cytokine that regulates energy balance is leptin.[41–45] Leptin is produced by the adipocyte and transported to the hypothalamus, where it serves to signal satiety. Leptin gene mutation is uncommon in humans. Mutations in either the gene for leptin or its receptor result in obesity. In addition, mutations in either leptin or its receptor augment the risk of insulin resistance and metabolic syndrome in humans.[41] Leptin stimulates adipocyte apoptosis as does TNFα, and so it affects both food intake and energy store through an effect on the number of fat cells available for fat storage. Leptin upregulates muscle fatty acid oxidation and muscle uncoupling protein 3 (UCP_3).[42,43] Leptin thus increases heat production via an uncoupling effect on oxidative phosphorylation (OXPHOS). In addition, leptin regulates fatty acid homeostasis. It suppresses fatty acid deposition in nonadipocytes and induces nitric oxide-mediated inhibition of lipolysis and glyceroneogenesis in white adipose tissue. Counteracting TNFα and leptin is neuropeptide Y (NPY), which stimulates appetite. While present in most neural tissues, the NPY that is closely associated with feeding is synthesized by cells of the arcuate nucleus. It is released primarily in the paraventricular nucleus, whereupon it stimulates feeding. NPY has the opposite effect of corticotropin-releasing hormone (CRH) within the hypothalamus with respect to signaling feeding. Leptin regulates both of these compounds. It downregulates NPY and upregulates CRH.

Greater than normal food intake may also characterize the genetically obese human (see Chapter 4). Yet, there are many overfat people who are not hyperphagic. There are those who cannot dissipate their surplus intake energy as heat, that is, thermogenesis, and who do not tolerate cold as well.[46–55] The common thread to these two conditions is the apparent inability of tissues to stimulate uncoupling protein (UCP) synthesis that in turn stimulates OXPHOS uncoupling that in turn results in heat production that keeps the body warm. Thus, ATP is continuously synthesized, in turn transferring its energy to the synthesis of fat. Obesity has thus been attributed to a failure of the heat producing brown adipose cells to respond to the stimulatory effects of norepinephrine and is associated with an anomalous central regulation of the sympathetic input to this tissue.

It has been hypothesized further that genetically obese animals develop subcutaneous fat pads as insulation against heat loss or gain, thereby circumventing their relative inability to thermoregulate. To increase their insulation layer, they must overeat to provide the requisite substrates for lipogenesis. Such a hypothesis has some elements of validity. The ob/ob mouse, for example, is unusually sensitive to cold and is incapable of increasing its heat production when suddenly exposed to cold or injected with norepinephrine. If gradually exposed to cold, these mice can slowly adapt to the gradual change in environmental temperature. These features of the ob/ob mouse precede the development of both hyperphagia and obesity and have been attributed to a mutation in the gene for leptin.[29,30,40] These mice do not produce normal leptin and this deficiency means that there is no leptin to travel to the brain to suppress feeding. Hence, these mice are hyperphagic. These mice also do not turn on thermogenesis very well when exposed to cold. This is because leptin has another role—that of stimulating the production of UCPs. Since the mobilization of body fuel (induction of lipolysis and glycogenolysis) is not abnormal in ob/ob mouse, it would appear that only the release of heat when these fuels are oxidized is defective. In other words, more energy is trapped in the chemical bonds of high-energy compounds than is released as heat. This, of course, is related to the increased energetic efficiency of these animals as well, since they also gain more fat per unit food consumed (and release less heat) than do lean animals.

Impaired thermoregulation has also been reported in genetically obese Zucker rats.[54] These rats produce ample amounts of leptin but they have a mutation in the gene that encodes the leptin receptor. Thus, although they produce the cytokine, it is without effect because its receptor is aberrant. It cannot bind the leptin and signal the cell accordingly. Zucker rats, like ob/ob mice, are hyperphagic and obese.[29] Similarly, they do not respond well to sudden cold exposure. Again, the missing link is not leptin but its leptin receptor that in turn affects satiety signaling and UCP production. Zucker obese rats and ob/ob mice are not the only animals affected. Lower body temperatures in neonates and an impaired ability to increase thermogenesis in response to overeating, cold exposure, or norepinephrine have been reported in a variety of genetically obese animal models. Perhaps obese humans may also have this defect. A few humans have been described with leptin defects,[34] but whether leptin or its receptor can explain all the cases of obesity is doubtful.

Normal-weight humans appear to regulate their body fat mass by increasing their heat production when overfed or exposed to cold. When stimulated by cold or infusions of norepinephrine, normal-weight subjects increased their heat production, while obese subjects did not. Several investigators developed an animal model that showed that when overfed, thermogenesis was stimulated.[46–55] They showed that when offered a variety of energy-rich snack foods, normal animals increased their heat production to maintain a normal weight. However, this mechanism is far from perfect in that, over time, these overfed animals did become fatter than their control-fed littermates. Nonetheless, the observation that heat production will increase in response to fluctuations in energy intake is a very interesting facet of energy balance. The mechanism whereby heat production is increased above basal involves the synthesis and release of UCPs. These proteins are not always present and active. In the starved animal, for example, they cannot be found.[52,55] This means that extra heat production induced by UCPs can be switched on and off. The synthesis of UCPs is rapid. Exposure to cold or hyperthyroidism or birth or starvation refeeding triggers a rapid and marked increase of messenger RNA for these proteins as well as a marked increase in the level of protein. In most animals, the increase in the level of UCPs parallels an increase in nonshivering thermogenesis. In lean animals, surplus food intake seems to signal UCP synthesis. The regulation of this synthesis occurs at the level of messenger RNA transcription.[52] The genes that encode these proteins have been isolated and sequenced. The protein completely traverses the inner mitochondrial membrane and has a C-terminal region that projects from the outer surface of the membrane. It works by dissipating the proton gradient that is developed when pairs of reducing equivalents are passed down the respiratory chain to make water. The energy that is developed by the respiratory chain is not captured in the high-energy bond of ATP but is, instead, released as heat. The control of its uncoupling function is through the external C-terminal region that contains the nucleotide (ADP)-binding site. If UCP binds the nucleotide, it is not available to the F_0F_1 ATP synthase for ATP synthesis. Fatty acids can interact with the nucleotide binding site with the result of increasing ADP binding. These fatty acids are released from the stored triacylglycerols via a hormone-stimulated cyclic AMP mechanism. This explains how norepinephrine can stimulate brown fat thermogenesis (BAT). Norepinephrine works by increasing the cAMP levels in the cytosol. This, in turn, stimulates the activity of the cytosolic lipoprotein lipase, which serves to release the fatty acids from the stored lipid. Norepinephrine is particularly effective with respect to intracellular fatty acid release in the brown fat. Other lipolytic hormones that work through increasing adenylate cyclase activity and cAMP levels also work to increase heat production. Diets rich in polyunsaturated fatty acids potentiate these hormone effects on this process.

While insulin is not thought of as a lipolytic hormone, it too has a role in regulating the synthesis and activity of the UCPs and heat production.[49] Both the synthesis of the uncoupling protein and the ability of various tissues to assist in the regulation of body temperature via the UCPs that help to dissipate the energy provided by excess food intake are impaired in the insulin-deficient animal. Once insulin is restored, the impairment is corrected. Of interest is the observation that many genetically obese rats and mice are hyperinsulinemic. This hyperinsulinemia is probably due to insulin resistance of the target tissues.

As mentioned in Chapter 2 in the description of starvation and anorexia, hormone status is important to the regulation of energy balance and normal body weight. The glucocorticoids and insulin play reciprocal roles as signals influencing energy balance. Hypercortisolism and hyperinsulinism are associated with obesity.[56] Cortisol and its related compounds, corticosterone and cortisone, play an important role in the regulation of lipogenesis as well as in the signaling of apoptosis. While these hormones are usually catabolic hormones, there are circumstances when they stimulate anabolic processes, such as fat synthesis and deposition. Other instances of the influence of hormones on body fat stores include injury to the hypothalamus, which in turn results in an increased food intake and an increase in body fat stores. Excess thyroid production results in low-fat stores, while the reverse, hypothyroidism, is characterized by an increase in fat stores together with a decrease in protein synthesis and muscle mass.

A chronic inflammatory state has been observed in obese rodents and humans.[57–64] Signs of both adipose tissue and muscle inflammation have been reported. These signs include an increase in macrophage infiltration, an increase in inflammatory cytokine production, increased TNFα production, and increases in the level of C-reactive protein. It involves the NFκB pathway resulting in a persistent elevation of the noncanonical IκB kinases IKK_e and TBK_1. These kinases attenuate β-adrenergic signaling in the adipose tissue. Treatment of 3T3-L1 adipocytes with inhibitors of these kinases restored normal β-adrenergic signaling and lipolysis attenuated by TNFα and Poly (I:C). Conversely, overexpression of the kinases reduced the induction of cAMP levels and lipolysis. Interestingly, the consumption of a high-fat diet seems to induce or potentiate the development of the chronic inflammatory state associated with obesity.[62,65] Hypocaloric low-fat diets do the reverse.

Recently, reports of the influence of specific gastrointestinal flora have appeared that indicate that microflora differences could explain obesity.[66–70] Several reports have shown a relationship between the intestinal contents of obese and lean mice and endotoxin-induced inflammation when the obesity was induced by high-fat feeding.[60,62,65,70] Studies of the different types of intestinal microflora have indicated that some (but not all) affect the production of inflammation signals generated in the gastrointestinal tract.[66–70] As the aforementioned, some of the different organisms in the colon could produce antigens that, when absorbed, would elicit signals that in turn would generate or elicit the characteristics of the inflammatory state associated with excess fat stores.

Finally, there are social and cultural influences that can ensure or potentiate genetic tendencies to develop obesity. Anthropologists and medical historians have identified examples of cultural groups that consider excess body fat a mark of beauty as well as an indication of economic status within their society. Examples of this are the various statuaries of different ages all the way from the upper Paleolithic period through the Renaissance to the eighteenth and nineteenth centuries. Women have been represented with large bellies and breasts that, to the eye of the contemporary observer, are overfat. Men, too, are of ample proportions. In fact, there is an old Pennsylvanish (Pennsylvania Dutch) expression that indicates the desire of men to have overweight women as wives: "A fat wife and a full barn never did a man harm." Even today, there are cultures, notably in Africa, that have customs that include preparing girls for marriage by fattening them. Malcom, for example, described this practice for elite Efik girls in traditional Nigeria, as well as the custom in Kenya of demanding high bride prices for fat brides. In these cultures, female fatness may not only be a testament to the families' wealth, it may also be a symbol of maternity and nurturance. This is important to the woman if the only way she gains status is through motherhood. A fat woman is thus assumed to be very maternal and nurturing.

With respect to societal determined fatness and the values of fatness, it can be assumed that the fatter a person is in a society that values fatness, the more likely that person will be to marry and produce children carrying genetic tendencies to be fat and who will be similarly taught to eat enough to be fat also. Lean people will be less likely to contribute to the gene pool because they will be considered less-desirable mates. While people in the United States, as well as other developed nations, may not have these values, there is no doubt that eating behaviors can be taught. If young children are constantly reminded and coached to overeat, there may be a continuing stimulus to overconsume food. Cultural and social dictates with respect to physical activity may be added to this. A decrease in energy expenditure ensures a positive energy balance that may well result in excess body fatness. Changes in the activity levels of adolescents change their energy balance. Chaput et al. reported on the increase in energy intake and consequent change in energy balance of adolescent boys when these boys engaged in extensive video game playing.[71]

Obesity has become a stigmatizing factor in the lives of both children and adults.[72] Antiobesity campaigns appear to embrace the thought that obesity is under the control of the individual and that if obesity is stigmatized, the obese person will be motivated to lose weight. The empirical evidence does not support this concept. Frequently, those who are overfat are told that they could become lean if they would reduce their energy intake. However, simply restricting one's food intake does not cure the problem; it merely treats the result of the positive energy balance—excess body fat. Once this fat is lost, the formerly obese person frequently abandons the restricted diet, returns to previous eating habits, and, as a result, returns to the prior weight. In some, there may also be an increase in body fatness, not just a return to the prior body weight. In part, this may be due to the action of leptin. Leptin has been shown to reverse the decline in satiation in weight-reduced obese humans.[73]

Morbidity of Severely Obese People

Health-care professionals have observed countless instances of the codevelopment of excess body fat with diabetes mellitus, hypertension, and cardiovascular disease.[1,2] Some have termed this codevelopment as metabolic syndrome. Epidemiologists have reported that obesity and overweight are risk factors in the development of these diseases. However, there are some inconsistencies with respect to the relationship of obesity to cardiovascular disease and total mortality.[6,74–79] Studies by the CDC[75] and those by Sjostrom[6] and Shea et al.[74] suggest that weight loss by the obese does not positively affect life span. The CDC report indicated an increase in mortality in people who have consciously reduced their body fat and remained lean. This report has raised serious questions about the efficacy of weight loss with respect to life-span extension. In some instances, weight loss is reversed with time and can be attributed to changes in hormonal status. This is apparent in females as they transition to menopause. With menopause, there is a change in body composition.[75]

Treatment of Obesity

Diet Strategies

In almost no other area of medicine have there been so many failures as have occurred in the treatment of obesity. Fully 90% of all those who lose weight regain it within 5 years. Data from the Chicago Gas and Electric Study suggest that one cycle of loss and regain is a risk factor for death from coronary heart disease independent of body fatness.[77] The loss–regain group, when compared with subjects who neither gained nor lost weight, had 1.8 times the risk of death from heart disease. This suggests that weight cycling is not a healthy behavior. Weight cycling is also associated with an increase in mortality and cancer incidence.[79] If weight is to be lost, it must stay lost if health benefits are to be gained. Often, this does not occur. Weight cycling consists of intermittent periods of food restriction followed by periods of *normal* eating patterns. These patterns may include periods of gorging or binge eating. One of the major effects of energy restriction on metabolism is a reduction in RMR. This lowers the overall energy requirement and increases energy efficiency, thus allowing a greater percentage of dietary energy to be partitioned into fat synthesis upon refeeding.

The effects of weight cycling on energy efficiency may be due to the composition of the weight loss during calorie restriction. One of the consequences of rapid weight loss, especially when induced by very low-energy, low-carbohydrate diets, is the loss of body protein or LBM. This is especially true when the individuals are physically inactive. Maintenance of LBM is an energy-expensive process. LBM is the most metabolically active tissue in the body with respect to energy demands, accounting for the majority of energy to support the basal energy requirement (i.e., 60%–70% of daily basal energy requirements for adults). Therefore, the less the body protein, the lower the energy requirement. If weight loss consists of significant amounts of body protein, then the formerly overfat person will have a lower basal energetic requirement and an increased energy efficiency in terms of the weight regain as fat. Attention thus must be paid to the inclusion of sufficient protein in the weight loss diet. The tendency is to reduce the amount of protein in the diet because it frequently carries with it fat. A low-energy diet could actually be an insufficient protein diet that could have negative effects on the health of the dieter. This should be avoided.[79] A weight loss diet should contain the normal amount of good-quality protein so as to sustain LBM. When a good exercise program is incorporated into the diet restriction of the energy intake, the resting energy requirement and the fat-free body mass are preserved. In addition to preserving the protein intake, attention to the calcium intake will facilitate body fat loss while preserving LBM.[80–87] Calcium plays a critical role in fat turnover and in the oxidation of stored fat. In addition, calcium plays an important role in food intake control. If the diet is designed to include calcium-rich dairy foods as contributors to the protein component of the diet, both the need for protein and calcium will be satisfied.

One of the responses of cycled humans is the tendency to overeat during the initial few days of the refeeding period. This suggests that the regulation of food intake is affected by the weight loss. The regulation of food intake is discussed in Chapter 4. Signals sent to the brain by the starved body seem to set the stage for hyperphagia (increased food intake above normal) once food is no longer restricted. These signals must be fairly enduring because this hyperphagia is of about the same duration as the duration of the restriction period. The origin of these signals is not known, but no doubt they exist because food intake is an event regulated by the central nervous system. Studies of starved and refed rats showed that these rats had a preference for dietary fat if given a choice of several energy sources. As a result of this selection, cycled rats regained more body fat than if the food offered was rich in carbohydrate and/or protein. Again, this suggests the involvement of signals to/from the brain directing the individual to select energetically rich food. This signal, coupled with the increased efficiency of the body in retaining the ingested energy, helps to explain why fat regain occurs in people who have restricted their energy intake to lose weight. Food restriction puts into place a metabolic machinery geared to save as much energy as possible and to stimulate the brain to signal the body to consume energy-rich foods. Thus, even though the patient tries to control eating and food intake, the body seeks to return to its prior overfat state. Constant vigilance is required of the patient to override these biological signals that direct the body to be fat. However, even when the patient carefully monitors food energy intake and consciously decides to regulate it, weight regain may occur due to the body's increased energetic efficiency and its tendency to synthesize and store fat in preference to protein. Here is where a good exercise program might be useful. Exercise, on a regular basis, stimulates muscle protein development and increases energy expenditure. Exercise can be a useful adjunct to energy intake restriction because it redirects energy loss from the LBM. In addition, mild and moderate exercise serves to reduce appetite and augments the desire to reduce food intake. In the sedentary individual, weight loss occurs at the expense of both fat and protein components of the body. In the exercising food-restricted individual, the weight loss is primarily fat loss. Further, mild to moderate exercise seems to suppress food intake. Thus, food restriction together with exercise is additive in a beneficial way with respect to the loss and regain of body fat.

Pharmaceutical Strategies

Pharmacologic approaches to the treatment of obesity have captured the interest of numerous pharmaceutical companies worldwide.[88–91] Table 3.4 lists some of these drugs. Drugs that target those mechanisms involved in hunger and satiety as well as drugs that target feed efficiency have been developed. The latter category includes compounds that interfere with normal digestion

TABLE 3.4
Antiobesity Drugs

Drug Class[a]	Example	Effect
Antinutrition drugs		
Gastric emptying inhibitors	(--) Threochlorocitric acid[a]	Delays gastric emptying, induces satiety
Glucosidase inhibitors	Acarbose, miglitol	Inhibits carbohydrate digestion
Inhibitors of lipid uptake	Cholestyramine	Binds bile acids, disrupts micelle formation
Pseudonutrients	Olestra	Fat substitute with less energy
	Artificial sweeteners	Sugar substitute, no energy
	Bulking agents, fibers	Induce satiety at lower energy intake
	Sugar alcohols	Reduces carbohydrate intake
Lipase inhibitor	Xenical, Alli	Inhibits hydrolysis of triacylglycerides
Compounds that affect nutrient partitioning		
Growth hormone[a]		Stimulates protein synthesis
Testosterone[a]		Stimulates protein synthesis in males
Anabolic steroids[a]		Stimulates gain of LBM suppresses fat deposition
α2-Adrenergic antagonists[a]		Enhances lipolysis
Thermogenic drugs		Reduces metabolic efficiency; increases heat production
Dinitrophenol[a]		Metabolic poison; not on market
β2- and β3-adrenergic agonists	Terbutaline[a]	Stimulates protein synthesis and lipolysis; can have serious side effects
Appetite suppressors		
β-Phenethylamine derivatives	Fastin, dexatrim	Interferes with hunger signaling via norepinephrine
Serotonergic agents	Fenfluramine,[a] fluoxetine[a]	Increases serotonin release and signals satiety
Belviq	Lorcaserin	Activates serotonin receptor and suppresses appetite
Qsymia	Phentermine + topiramate	A stimulant and an antiseizure drug combo; has severe side effects on embryos and fetuses
Amine reuptake inhibitor	Sibutramine[a]	Blocks reuptake of norepinephrine and 5-HT and suppresses appetite

[a] Not available as a weight loss drug. The FDA has determined that this drug could have adverse effects on the patient.

and absorption. Unfortunately, none of these compounds have a significant antiobesity effect. Glucosidase inhibitors as well as lipase inhibitors have been developed. The glucosidase inhibitors, for example, acarbose and miglitol, inhibit the action of amylase and thus reduce its activity. This means that the long-chain (straight and branched) starches found in many plant products are not digested as quickly as usual. In theory, this retardation of digestion should result in a retardation of absorption of the end products of starch hydrolysis. Unfortunately, this may not result in a reduction in intake energy. If starch digestion is not completed by the enzymes of the small intestine, flora of the large intestine take over and produce fatty acids that are then absorbed and used for energy.

Lipase inhibitors (Xenical) or fat absorption inhibitors (cholestyramine, neomycin, perfluorooctyl bromide) also serve to reduce energy intake. Cholestyramine binds bile acids and disrupts micelle formation. This results in an inhibition of fat absorption and increased fecal fat loss. An over-the-counter drug has recently been released: Alli. This is a weight loss drug sold in a lower dose than its parent drug, orlistat. It was originally approved in 1999 as Xenical. The drug interferes with fat absorption and can help with weight loss if used as part of an overall weight loss program that includes exercise and the use of a low-fat diet. Because it inhibits fat absorption, very uncomfortable side effects are experienced if the food plan is not low fat. Gastrointestinal discomfort (bloating, gas, loose to runny stools) occurs and some individuals may have more problems with this discomfort than others.

Neomycin, an antibiotic, reduces fat absorption as well. However, it has the side effect of reducing the intestinal mucosa. This can result in diarrhea. Perfluorooctyl bromide, a product used as a contrast medium for gastrointestinal x-ray studies, also blocks fat absorption as well as amino acid and glucose absorption. While useful in studying the functional state of the gastrointestinal tract, because it interferes with the absorption of all the macronutrients, its usefulness as an antiobesity drug cannot be considered.

Listed in Table 3.4 are some hormones that affect protein synthesis as well as fat storage. None of these should be used therapeutically to stimulate weight loss. However, they are included in the table because fat weight loss may be a secondary effect when these hormones are used for other reasons. For example, growth-hormone supplements may be given to the growth-deficient child who may be very short and fat. The supplemented child will then grow and as this growth occurs, the fat depots shrink.

The sex hormones (estrogen, testosterone) can affect body fat. In males, the percent body fat is inversely related to circulating testosterone levels. In females, increased upper abdominal and visceral fatness is associated with rising levels of testosterone. In postmenopausal females, abdominal fat stores increase due to the loss of estrogen.

Glucocorticoid excess (Cushing's disease) usually results in an accumulation of abdominal fat, whereas glucocorticoid deficiency (Addison's disease) is characterized by a depletion of fat stores. Thyroid hormone excess likewise is characterized by a reduction in fat stores, while thyroid hormone deficiency has the reverse feature. Hypothyroid individuals have enlarged fat depots. Among the pharmaceutical products, we have drugs that are thermogenic. In other words, these are drugs that stimulate energy wastage as heat. None of the known thermogenic drugs are without risk, and none of them can be used as weight loss drugs. β-Adrenergic compounds frequently have serious side effects such as tremors. One of these, terbutaline, is useful in asthma treatment. When used for this purpose, weight loss has been reported.

One group of drugs acts through the central nervous system in the regulation of hunger and satiety. The first of these is the β-phenethylamine derivatives, which work through affecting either the release or reuptake of norepinephrine. These drugs suppress appetite but they have undesirable side effects on the cardiopulmonary system and may induce insomnia. In addition, with long-term use, they lose effectiveness. Most of these drugs have been removed from the marketplace by the FDA. The second group of drugs is the serotonergic drugs. These suppress appetite by increasing serotonin levels in that part of the brain (the hypothalamus) that controls food intake. Dry mouth and insomnia are side effects and, in some instances, pulmonary hypertension has been reported. These drugs have been removed from the marketplace by the FDA. Fenfluramine is an example of this group of drugs. Fluoxetine, another of the serotonergic drugs, blocks serotonin reuptake. It too is an appetite suppressant. This drug is mainly used as an antidepressant, not as an antiobesity drug. Sibutramine, an amine uptake inhibitor, blocks the reuptake of norepinephrine, thereby suppressing food intake. All of the drugs described earlier have a measure of risk associated with their use and many have been *pulled* off the market.[90,91] Some are not available at all because they are too risky to use. Others are available by prescription only and should be used only under the close supervision of a physician. Even when used appropriately, they may not result in significant and lasting weight loss. Physicians have realized that a few weight loss drugs that are available are not long-lasting solutions to the obesity problems. While the obese patient may lose weight during the first 6 months of use, the drugs lose their effectiveness and, as mentioned, may not be safe over the long term. Indeed, the patients prescribed with these drugs often regain the lost weight if the drug is continued beyond 6 months. The FDA has removed most of the systemic weight loss drugs because of their adverse effects. Today, there are only three FDA-approved prescription drugs available to help patients lose weight: Xenical (orlistat), Belviq (lorcaserin), and Qsymia. Only one of these is approved as an over-the-counter drug for weight loss. This is Alli (orlistat).

Food companies have expanded into the *antiobesity business* by developing noncaloric sweeteners, reduced-calorie sweeteners, fat substitutes, and bulking agents. All of these products are designed to reduce the energy value of food products. Aspartame, cyclamate, saccharin, acesulfame K, and Truvia are sweeteners without energy value. Theoretically, aspartame could have an energy value since it is a dipeptide of phenylalanine and aspartic acid, but because it is 180 times sweeter than sucrose and is unstable in water and to heat, it is unlikely that significant amounts of this product will be consumed. So, for practical purposes, this sweetener would not contribute energy in any significant amount to the daily intake. The noncaloric sweeteners are used in soft drinks as well as a number of snack foods. Canned fruit and frozen desserts are also prepared with these noncaloric sweeteners. Some of the sugar alcohols, that is, mannitol, are used in prepared foods to reduce their energy content. Likewise, fat substitutes such as the sucrose polyester, olestra, are used to reduce the energy value of some foods. Table 3.5 lists some of the ingredients used in foods that reduce the energy value of the food by substituting these ingredient for the fat or sugar content usually used in the food. Bulking agents such as guar, pectin, and fiber are used as energy diluents in processed foods. All of these pseudonutrients can effectively reduce the energy intake when incorporated into a well-balanced diet that is energy restricted. This will help the overweight individual lose excess fat.

TABLE 3.5
Fat Replacers

Ingredient Name	Foods Using These Ingredients
Made from carbohydrate	
Carrageenan, cellulose gel, cellulose gum, corn syrup solids, dextrin, guar gum, salad dressing, frozen desserts, gelatin, hydrolyzed corn starch, maltodextrin, pectin, polydextrose, xanthan gum	Baked goods, candy, cheese, chewing gum pudding, sauces, sour cream, yogurt, meat-based products
Made from protein	
Microparticulated egg white and milk protein, whey protein concentrate	Butter, cheese, sour cream, mayonnaise spreads, baked goods, salad dressings
Made from fat	
Caprenin, olestra, salatrim	Soft candy, candy coatings, chips, crackers

Surgical Strategies

Over the years, as physicians have become concerned about the increasing incidence of obesity, a number of surgical interventions have been developed.[92–94] Current surgical interventions include gastric banding and gastric bypass surgery. The former is less invasive than the latter. In the latter, the procedure is called the Roux-en-Y gastric bypass. In this surgery, the size of the stomach and small intestine is radically reduced. The neck of the stomach is joined to the middle part of the intestine, thus reducing the storage capacity of the stomach and shortening the passage length of the intestine. Bypassing the small intestinal duodenal segment reduces the absorptive capacity of this organ. The patient is able to consume only very small amounts of food at each meal although with time the gastrointestinal tract adjusts such that larger meals can be consumed. With this surgery, patients can lose up to 80% of their fat mass. However, it is not without consequences. Some patients lose the weight with the surgery but then, over time, slowly regain some of the lost weight. Many patients become anemic due to a loss in iron-absorptive capacity.[95] Other effects on nutritional status have been reported. Most can be remedied by nutritional supplements.

Gastric banding is another surgical strategy that can result in moderate weight loss.[92–94] This procedure is less invasive than the gastric bypass procedure. In principle, the procedure reduces the storage capacity of the stomach forcing the patient to reduce his/her food intake. This reduction results in negative energy balance and the patient loses weight. If the patient continues to reduce the energy intake such that some body weight is lost, then the stomach banding will be efficacious. However, should the patient overrides the band, success in weight loss probably will not occur. If this procedure is combined with increased physical activity, then positive results will surely follow.

SUMMARY

1. Obesity is defined as an excess in body fat stores. It is the result of long-term positive energy balance.
2. Body fatness can be determined directly in small animals but not in large animals or humans. Indirect methods must be used. These include the use of MRI and DEXA. The measurement of creatine dilution and potassium dilution can be used to determine muscle mass.
3. The BMI = weight/height^2 is a simple estimate of body fatness. It does not apply to everyone.
4. Obesity may be due to one or more gene mutations. It can also develop secondary to head injury, hormone imbalance, chronic inflammation, abnormal array of gut flora, and/or social/cultural feeding behaviors.
5. An inability to turn on thermogenesis in response to cold or excess food intake may explain obesity in some individuals.
6. Abnormal leptin or leptin receptor may explain obesity in some individuals.
7. The treatment of obesity is fraught with difficulty. For some, simple food restriction results in body fat loss. Few drugs are available to help with this weight loss. Surgical strategies have been developed but these are very risky.

LEARNING OPPORTUNITIES

Self-Study

1. Calculate your BMI (remember to convert your weight and height to kilograms and meters, respectively).
2. Keep a 3-day record of your food intake, and using the USDA website, calculate your daily energy intake. Using the values you acquired from Chapter 1, determine whether you are in energy balance, negative energy balance, or positive energy balance.
3. Develop a strategy to normalize your energy balance.

CASE STUDY 3.1

Helen has worked in a factory painting the dials of alarm clocks with glow-in-the-dark paint. The brush she used was very fine and in order to keep a clean point on the brush, Helen has developed a technique of licking the brush every few strokes. Helen has begun to lose weight. She also has begun complaining of feeling cold when everyone else is telling her that they are quite warm. Helen visited the doctor and suspecting thyroid difficulties, he measured her oxygen consumption as well as levels of her thyroid hormones. Her thyroid hormones are well within the normal range, but Helen is cold and feeling tired all the time and she continues to lose weight. Analyze this situation. What do you think is going on? What remedy would you suggest?

MULTIPLE-CHOICE QUESTIONS

1. Which of the following is a characteristic of the Prader–Willi syndrome?
   a. Overdevelopment of bones
   b. Broad forehead and wide set eyes
   c. Lack of a satiety signal
   d. Lean body type
2. A pregnant woman seeks dietary advice to avoid the development of obesity and diabetes that is part of her family medical history. Which of the following might be useful?
   a. Consume a balanced diet.
   b. Consume a diet that helps her maintain a very modest pregnancy weight gain, and include exercise in her daily routine.
   c. Reduce stress by enrolling in a yoga class.
   d. Don't worry about diet; just monitor blood glucose levels throughout the pregnancy.
3. Obesity is a prevalent health problem in developed nations. Why?
   a. Developed nations have too much money to spend on food.
   b. Developed nations are lazy and do not do enough physical work to compensate for their increased food intake.
   c. There is an increased prevalence of genetic mutations that phenotype as obesity in developed nations.
   d. Few people recognize the health consequences of having too large a fat store.
4. Children are at an increasing risk for the development of obesity. Why?
   a. Children are not as active as they used to be.
   b. Children are encouraged to clean their plates.
   c. Children are encouraged to develop sedentary lifestyle.
   d. All of the above.
5. People who are obese are at greater risk for developing the consequences of diabetes, heart disease, and other health problems. What should be done?
   a. Encourage regular checkups with physicians.
   b. Regularly test blood glucose.
   c. Encourage the incorporation of exercise and smaller food portions in the lifestyles of these people.
   d. All of the above.

REFERENCES

1. Adler, T. (2004) Obesity sheds its mysteries. NCRR Reporter, fall, pp. 10–12.
2. Austin, G.L., Ogden, L.G., Hill, J.O. (2011) Trends in carbohydrate, fat and protein intakes and association with energy intake in normal-weight, overweight and obese individuals: 1971–2006. *Am. J. Clin. Nutr.* 95: 836–841.

3. Bjorntorp, P. (1983) The role of adipose tissue in human obesity. In: *Obesity* (M.R.C. Greenwood, ed.), Churchill Livingstone, New York, pp. 17–24.
4. Prins, J.B., O'Rahilly, S. (1997) Regulation of adipose cell number in man. *Clin. Sci.* 92: 3–11.
5. Katzmarzyk, P.T., Bray, G.A., Greenway, F.L., Johnson, W.D., Newton, R.L., Rauvussin, E., Ryan, D.H., Smith, S.R., Bouchard, C. (2010) Racial differences in abdominal depot-specific adiposity in white and African American adults. *Am. J. Clin. Nutr.* 91: 7–15.
6. Sjostrom, L.V. (1992) Morbidity of severely obese subjects. *Am. J. Clin. Nutr.* 55: 508S–515S.
7. Flegal, K.M., Graubard, B.I. (2009) Estimates of excess deaths associated with body mass index and other anthropometric variables. *Am. J. Clin. Nutr.* 89: 1213–1219.
8. Owens, S., Gutin, B., Barbeau, P. (2008) Childhood obesity and exercise. In: *Handbook of Nutrition and Food* (C.D. Berdanier, J. Dwyer, E. Feldman, eds.), CRC Press, Boca Raton, FL, pp. 889–902.
9. Suskind, D.L., Corniola, R.S., Suskind, R.M. (2013) Childhood obesity. In: *Handbook of Nutrition and Food* (C.D. Berdanier, J. Dwyer, D. Heber, eds.), CRC Press, Boca Raton, FL, pp. 783–791.
10. Berlin, N.I., Watkin, D.M., Gevirtz, N.R. (1962) Measurement of changes in gross body composition during controlled weight reduction in obesity and body density—Body water techniques. *Metabolism* 11: 302–314.
11. Clark, R.R., Kuta, J.M., Sullivan, J.C. (1993) Prediction of percent body fat in adult males using dual energy x-ray absorptiometry, skinfolds and hydrostatic weighing. *Med. Sci. Sports Exerc.* 25: 528–535.
12. Fuller, M.F., Fowler, P.A., McNeille, G., Foster, M.A. (1990) Body composition: The precision and accuracy of new methods and their suitability for longitudinal studies. *Proc. Nutr. Soc.* 49: 423–426.
13. Malina, R.M. (1999) Progress in human body composition research. *Am. J. Human Biol.* 11: 141–200.
14. Meador, C.K., Kreisberg, R.A., Friday, J.P. Jr., Bowdoin, B., Coan, P., Armstrong, J., Hazelrig, J.B. (1968) Muscle mass determination by isotopic dilution of creatinine[14]. *Metabolism* 17: 1104–1108.
15. Sohlström, A., Wahlund, L.-O., Forsum, E. (1993) Adipose tissue distribution as assessed by magnetic resonance imaging and total body fat by magnetic resonance imaging, underwater weighing and body water dilution in healthy women. *Am. J. Clin. Nutr.* 58: 830–838.
16. Christian, J.E., Combs, L.W., Kessler, W.V. (1963) Body composition: Relative in vivo determinations from potassium-40 measurements. *Science* 140: 480–490.
17. Cote, K.D., Adams, W.C. (1993) Effect of bone density on body composition estimates in young adult black and white women. *Med. Sci. Sports Exerc.* 25: 290–296.
18. Young, C.M., Martin, M.E.K., Chihan, M., McCarthy, M., Manniello, M.J., Harmuth, E.H., Fryer, J.H. (1961) Body composition of young women. Some preliminary findings. *J. Am. Diet. Assoc.* 38: 332–344.
19. Siri, W.E. (1956) The gross composition of the body. *Adv. Biol. Med. Phys.* 4: 239–280.
20. Smalley, K.J., Kneer, A.N., Kendric, Z.V., Colliver, J.A., Owen, O.E. (1990) Reassessment of body mass indices. *Am. J. Clin. Nutr.* 52: 402–408.
21. Pace, N., Rathbun, E.N. (1945) Studies on body composition; body water and chemically combined nitrogen content in relation to fat content. *J. Biol. Chem.* 158: 685–691.
22. Allison, D.B., Kaprio, J., Korkeila, M., Koskenvuo, M., Neale, M.C., Hayakawa, K. (1996) The heritability of body mass index among an international sample of monozygotic twins reared apart. *Int. J. Obes.* 20: 501–506.
23. Bouchard, C. (1989) Genetic factors in obesity. *Med. Clin. North Am.* 73: 67–81.
24. Bouchard, C., Savard, R., Despres, J.P. (1985) Body composition in adopted and biological siblings. *Hum. Biol.* 57: 61–75.
25. Bernier, J.F., Calvert, C.C., Famula, T.R., Baldwin, R.L. (1986) Maintenance energy requirement and net energetic efficiency in mice with a major gene for post weaning gain. *J. Nutr.* 116: 416–428.
26. Kasser, T.G., Mabry, J.W., Martin R.J. (1980) Heterotic and maternal effects in L and S growth strain rats: II Body weight gains, feed consumption and feed efficiency. *Growth* 50: 109–117.
27. Stunkard, A.J., Harris, J.R., Pedersen, N.L., McClearn, G.E. (1990) The body mass index of twins who have been reared apart. *N. Eng. J. Med.* 322: 1483–1487.
28. Stunkard, A.J., Sorensen, T.I.A., Harris, C., Teasdale, T.W., Chakraborty, R., Schull, W.J., Schulsinger, F. (1986) An adoption study of human obesity. *N. Eng. J. Med.* 314: 193–198.
29. Leibel, R. (1997) Single gene obesities in rodents: Possible relevance to human obesity. *J. Nutr.* 127: 1908S.
30. Fisler, J.S., Warden, C.H. (2007) The current and future search for obesity genes. *Am. J. Clin. Nutr.* 85: 1–2.
31. NIH. http://www.ncbi.nlm.nih.gov, accessed February 13, 2013.
32. Wang, C., Baumgartner, R.N., Allison, D.B. (2008) Genetics of human obesity. In: *Handbook of Nutrition and Food* (C.D. Berdanier, E. Feldman, J. Dwyer, eds.), CRC Press, Boca Raton, FL, pp. 833–846.

33. Norio, R. (2003) The Finnish disease heritage. *Hum. Genet.* 112: 441–456.
34. Montague, C.T., Faroogi, I.S., Whitehead, J.P., Soos, M.A., Rau, H., Wareham, N.J., Sewter, C.P. et al. (1997) Congenital leptin deficiency is associated with severe early-onset obesity in humans. *Nature* 387: 903–908.
35. Loos, R.J.F., Ruchat, S., Rankinen, T., Tremblay, A., Perusse, L., Bouchard, C. (2007) Adiponectin and adiponectin receptor gene variants in relation to resting metabolic rate, respiratory quotient, and adiposity-related phenotypes in the Quebec Family Study. *Am. J. Clin. Nutr.* 85: 26–34.
36. Camps, S.G.J.A., Verhoef, S.P.M., Westerterp, K.R. (2013) Weight loss, weight maintenance, and adaptive thermogenesis. *Am. J. Clin. Nutr.* 97: 990–994.
37. Stice, E., Durant, S., Burger, K.S., Schoelier, D.A. (2011) Weight suppression and risk of future increases in body mass: Effects of suppressed resting metabolic rate and energy expenditure. *Am. J. Clin. Nutr.* 94: 7–11.
38. Mutch, D.M., Pers, T.H., Ramzi Temanni, M., Pelloux, V., Marquez-Quiñones, A., Holst, C., Martinez, J.A. et al. (2011) A distinct adipose tissue gene expression response to caloric restriction predicts 6-mo weight maintenance in obese subjects. *Am. J. Clin.* 94: 1399–1409.
39. Chua, S.C., Leibel, R.L. (1994) Molecular genetic approaches to obesity. In: *The Genetics of Obesity* (C. Bouchard, ed.), CRC Press, Boca Raton, FL, pp. 213–222.
40. Leiter, E.H., Schile, A.J. (2013) Finding mouse models of human disease for use in nutrition research. In: *Handbook of Nutrition and Food*, 3rd edn. (C.D. Berdanier, J. Dwyer, D. Heber, eds.), CRC Press, Boca Raton, FL, pp. 249–256.
41. Phillips, C.M., Goumidi, L., Bertrais, S., Field, M.R., Ordovas, J.M., Cupples, L.A., Defoort, C. et al. (2010) Leptin receptor polymorphisms interact with polyunsaturated fatty acids to augment risk for insulin resistance and metabolic syndrome in adults. *J. Nutr.* 140: 238–244.
42. Gullickson, P.S., Flatt, W.P., Dean, R.G., Hartzell, D.L., Baile, C.A. (2002) Energy metabolism and expression of UCP1,2, and 3 after 21 days of recovery from intracerebroventricular mouse leptin in rats. *Physiol. Behav.* 75: 473–482.
43. Zhou, Y.T., Shimabukuro, M., Koyama, K., Lee, Y., Wang, M.Y., Trieu, F., Newgard, C.B., Unger, R.H. (1997) Induction by leptin of UCP2 and fatty acid oxidation. *Proc. Natl. Acad. Sci. USA* 94: 6386–6390.
44. Woisk, E., Mygind, H., Grendahl, T.S., Pedersen, B.K., van Hall, G. (2011) The role of leptin in human lipid and glucose metabolism: The effects of acute recombinant human leptin infusion in young healthy males. *Am. J. Clin. Nutr.* 94: 1533–1544.
45. Niang, F., Benelli, C., Ribiere, C., Collonet, M., Mehebik-Mojaat, N., Penot, G., Forest, C., Jaubert, A.-M. (2011) Leptin induces nitric oxide-mediated inhibition of lipolysis and glyceroneogenesis in rat white adipose tissue. *J. Nutr.* 141: 4–9.
46. Himms-Hagen, J. (1995) Brown adipose tissue thermogenesis in the control of thermoregulatory feeding in rats: A new hypothesis that links thermostatic and glucostatic hypothesis for control of food intake. *Proc. Soc. Exp. Biol. Med.* 208: 159–169.
47. Samec, S., Seydoux, J., Dulloo, A.G. (1998) Role of UCP homologues in skeletal muscles and brown adipose tissue: Mediations of thermogenesis or regulators of lipids as fuel substrate? *FASEB J.* 12: 715–724.
48. Simoneau, J.-A., Kelly, D.E., Neverova, M., Warden, C.H. (1998) Overexpression of muscle uncoupling protein 2 content in human obesity associates with reduced skeletal muscle lipid utilization. *FASEB J.* 12: 1739–1745.
49. Geloen, A., Trayhurn, P. (1990) Regulation of the level of uncoupling protein in brown adipose tissue by insulin requires mediation of the sympathetic nervous system. *FEBS* 267: 265–267.
50. Recquier, D., Casteilla, L., Bouillaud, F. (1991) Molecular studies of the uncoupling protein. *FASEB J.* 5: 2237–2242.
51. Negre-Salvayre, A., Hirtz, C., Cabbera, G., Cazenave, R., Troly, M, Salvayre, R., Penicaud, L., Casteilla, L. (1997) A role for uncoupling protein-2 as a regulator of mitochondrial hydrogen peroxide generation. *FASEB J.* 11: 809–815.
52. Champigny, O., Recquier, D. (1990) Effects of fasting and refeeding on the level of uncoupling protein mRNA in brown adipose tissue: Evidence for diet induced and cold induced responses. *J. Nutr.* 120: 1730–1736.
53. Rothwell, N.J., Stock, M.J. (1983) Diet-induced thermogenesis. In: *Mammalian Thermogenesis* (L. Girardier, M.J. Stock, eds.), Chapman & Hall, London, U.K., pp. 208–233.
54. Kaul, R., Heldmaier, G., Schmidt, I. (1990) Defective thermoregulatory thermogenesis does not cause onset of obesity in Zucker rats. *Am. J. Physiol.* 259: E11–E18.
55. Trayhurn, P., Jennings, G. (1986) Evidence that fasting can induce a selective loss of uncoupling protein from brown adipose tissue mitochondria of mice. *Biosci. Rep.* 6: 805–810.

56. Strack, A.M., Sebastian, R.J., Schwartz, M.W., Dallman, M.F. (1995) Glucocorticoids and insulin: Reciprocal signals for energy balance. *Am. J. Physiol.* 268: R142–R149.
57. Mowers, J., Uhm, M., Reilly, S.M., Simon, J., Chiang, S.-H., Chang, L., Saltiel, A.R. (2013) Inflammation produces catecholamine resistance in obesity via activation of PDE3B by the protein kinases IKKε and TBK1. *eLife* 2: e01119.
58. Le, N.H., Kim, C.-S., Tu, T.H., Choi, H.-S., Kim, B.-S., Kawada, T., Goto, T., Park, T., Park, J.H.Y., Yu, R. (2013) Blockade of 4-1BB and 4-1BBL interaction reduces obesity-induced skeletal muscle inflammation. *Mediat. Inflamm.* 2013: 665159–665169.
59. Sell, H., Habich, C., Eckel, J. (2012) Adaptive immunity in obesity and insulin resistance. *Nat. Rev. Endocrinol.* 8: 709–716.
60. Cani, P.D., Bibiloni, R., Knauf, C., Waget, A., Neyrinck, A.M., Delzenne, N.M., Burcelen, R. (2008) Changes in gut microbiota control metabolic endotoxemia-induced inflammation in high fat diet-induced obesity and diabetes in mice. *Diabetes* 57: 1470–1481.
61. Makki, K., Frogel, P., Wolowczuk, I. (2013) Adipose tissue in obesity-related inflammation and insulin resistance: Cells, cytokines and chemokines. *ISRN Inflamm.* 10: 139239 (ePub).
62. Teng, K.-T, Chang, C.-Y., Chang, L.F., Nesaretnam, K. (2014) Modulation of obesity-induced inflammation by dietary fats: Mechanisms and clinical evidence. *J. Nutr.* 13: 12–22.
63. Kim, C., Lee, H., Cho, Y.M., Kwon, O.J., Kim, W., Lee, E.K. (2013) TNFα-induced miR-130 resulted in adipocytes dysfunction during obesity-related inflammation. *FEBS Lett.* 587: 3853–3858.
64. Lopez-Legarrea, P., de la Iglesia, R., Navas-Carretero, S., Marinez, J.A., Zulet, M.A. (2014) The protein type within a hypocaloric diet affects obesity-related inflammation: The RESMENA project. *Nutrition* 30: 424–429.
65. Puglisi, M.J., Fernandez, M.L. (2008) Modulation of C-reactive protein, tumor necrosis factor-α and adiponectin by diet, exercise and weight loss. *J. Nutr.* 108: 2293–2296.
66. Yazigi, A., Gaborit, B., Noqueira, J.P., Butiler, M.E., Andreelii, F. (2008) Role of intestinal flora in insulin resistance and obesity. *Presse Med.* 37: 1427–1430.
67. Frazier, T.H., DiBaise, J.K., McClain, C.J. (2011) Gut microbiota, intestinal permeability, obesity-induced inflammation and liver injury. *J. Parenter. Enteral Nutr.* 35: 14S–20S.
68. Cani, P.D., Delzenne, N.M. (2009) The role of the gut microbiota in energy metabolism and metabolic disease. *Curr. Pharm. Dis.* 15: 1546–1558.
69. Cani, P.D., Detzenne, N.M. (2007) Gut microflora as a target for energy and metabolic homeostasis. *Curr. Opin. Clin. Nutr. Metabolic Care* 10: 729–734.
70. Cani, P.D., Detzenne, N.M., Amar, J., Burcelin, R. (2008) Role of gut microflora in the development of obesity and insulin resistance following high fat feeding. *Pathol. Biol. (Paris)* 56: 305–309.
71. Chaput, J.-P., Visby, T., Nyby, S., Klingenberg, L., Gregersen, N.T., Tremblay, A., Astrup, A., Sjodin, A. (2011) Video game playing increases food intake in adolescent boys: A randomized crossover study. *Am. J. Clin. Nutr.* 93: 1196–1203.
72. Vartanian, L.R., Smyth, J.M. (2013) Primum non nocere: Obesity stigma and public health. *J. Bioeth. Inq.* 10: 49–57.
73. Kissileff, H.R., Thornton, J.C., Torres, M.I., Pavlovich, K., Mayer, L.S., Kalari, V., Leibel, R.L., Rosenbaum, M. (2012) Leptin reverses decline in satiation in weight reduced obese humans. *Am. J. Clin. Nutr.* 95: 309–317.
74. Shea, M.K., Nicklas, B.J., Houston, D.K., Miller, M.E., Davis, C.C., Kitzman, D.W., Espeland, M.A., Appel, L.J., Kritchevsky, S.B. (2011) The effect of intentional weight loss on all cause mortality in older adults: Results of a randomized controlled weight loss trial. *Am. J. Clin. Nutr.* 94: 939–848.
75. Beavers, K.M., Lyles, M.F., Davius, C.C., Wang, X., Beavers, D.P., Nicklas, B.J. (2011) Is lost lean mass from intentional weight loss recovered during weight regain in postmenopausal women? *Am. J. Clin. Nutr.* 94: 767–774.
76. Dyer, A.R., Stamler, J., Greenland, P. (2000) Association of weight change and weight variability with cardiovascular and all-cause mortality. *Am. J. Epidemiol.* 152: 324–333.
77. Kroke, A., Liese, A.D., Schutz, M., Bergmann, M.M., Klipstein-Grobusch, K., Boeing, H. (2002) Recent weight changes and weight cycling as predictors of subsequent two year weight change in a middle aged cohort. *Int. J. Obes.* 26: 403–409.
78. Elliott, A.M., Aucott, L.S., Hannaford, P.C., Smith, W.C. (2005) Weight change in adult life and health outcomes. *Obesity* 13: 1784–1792.
79. Soenen, S., Martens, E.A.P., Hochstenbach-Waslen, A., Lemmens, S.G.T., Westerperp-Plantenga, S. (2013) Normal protein intake is required for body weight loss and weight maintenance, and elevated protein intake for additional preservation of resting energy expenditure and fat free mass. *J. Nutr.* 143: 591–596.

80. Weaver, C.M., Campbell, W.W., Teagarden, D., Craig, B.A., Martin, B.R., Singh, R., Braun, M.M. et al. (2011) Calcium, dairy products, and energy balance in overweight adolescents: A controlled trial. *Am. J. Clin. Nutr.* 94: 1163–1170.
81. Bortolotti, M., Rudelle, S., Schneiter, P., Vidal, H., Loizon, E., Tappy, L., Acheson, K.J. (2008) Dairy calcium supplementation in overweight or obese persons: Its effect on markers of fat metabolism. *Am. J. Clin. Nutr.* 88: 877–885.
82. Astrup, A. (1988) The role of calcium in energy balance and obesity: The search for mechanisms. *Am. J. Clin. Nutr.* 88: 873–874.
83. Zemel, M.B., Richards, J., Milstead, A., Campbell, P. (2005) Effects of calcium and dairy on body composition and weight loss in African-American adults. *Obes. Res.* 13: 1218–1225.
84. Zemel, M.B., Thompson, W., Milstead, A., Morris, K., Campbell, P. (2004) Calcium and dairy acceleration of weight and fat loss during energy restriction in obese adults. *Obes. Res.* 12: 582–590.
85. Zemel, M.B., Miller, S.L. (2004) Dietary calcium and dairy modulation of adiposity and obesity risk. *Nutr. Rev.* 62: 125–131.
86. Zemel, M.B., Richards, J., Mathis, S., Milstead, A., Gebhardt, L., Silva, E. (2005) Dairy augmentation of total and central fat loss in obese subjects. *Int. J. Obes.* 29: 391–397.
87. Tylavsky, F.A., Cowan, P.A., Terrell, S., Hutson, M., Velasquez-Mieyer, P. (2010) Calcium intake and body composition in African-American children and adolescents at risk for overweight and obesity. *Nutrients* 2: 950–964.
88. Bray, G. (1992) Drug treatment of obesity. *Am. J. Clin. Nutr.* 55: 5385–5445.
89. Bray, G., Ryan, D. (1997) Drugs used in the treatment of obesity. *Diabetes Rev.* 5: 83–103.
90. Bendich, A. (2013) Prescription and over the counter options for weight loss. *Nutr. Today* 48: 76–78.
91. Stokowski, L.A. (2010) Weight loss drugs: What works? Medscape Diabetes & Endocrinology. WebMD at http://www.medscape.com, accessed December 22, 2010.
92. Lemmon, C.R., Barbeau, P. (2005) Bariatric surgery for the obese diabetic patient: The effect on type 2 diabetes and important psychological considerations. *Pract. Diab. Int.* 22: 3–6.
93. Stanczyk, M., Martindale, R.G., Deveney, C. (2007) Bariatric surgery overview. In: *Handbook of Nutrition and Food*, 2nd edn. (C.D. Berdanier, E. Feldman, J. Dwyer, eds.), CRC Press, Boca Raton, FL, pp. 915–928.
94. Pham, T., Li, H.C., Livingston, E.H., Huerta, S. (2013) Nutritional management of the bariatric surgery patient. In: *Handbook of Nutrition and Food*, 3rd edn. (C.D. Berdanier, J. Dwyer, D. Heber, eds.), CRC Press, Boca Raton, FL, pp. 951–960.
95. Ruz, M., Carrasco, F., Rojas, P., Inostroza, J., Rebolledo, A., Basfi-fer, K., Csendes, A. et al. (2009) Iron absorption and iron status are reduced after Roux-en-Y gastric bypass. *Am. J. Clin. Nutr.* 90: 527–532.

4 Regulation of Food Intake

In Chapter 3, the health concerns of obesity were discussed as well as the observation that it is sometimes characterized by hyperphagia (overeating). In this chapter, food intake and its regulation will be discussed not only from the physiological point of view but also from the sociocultural angle. It is important for those who study the processes by which humans consume and utilize food to realize how complex the subject is. An individual does not ingest thiamine, vitamin A, protein, and selenium, those nutrients necessary for his well-being; he ingests food, be it sirloin steak, fresh juicy peaches, or chocolate-covered ants. He does not choose to eat a green salad because it is nutritionally sound to do so, but because of complex conscious and subconscious motivation peculiar to himself. This chapter is designed to explore the psychological and physiological roots of the regulation of food intake. This has relevance to our understanding of not only the development of obesity but also our understanding of the reverse problem, anorexia nervosa. Understanding the motivation for eating or not eating underpins our understanding of the whole gamut of nutrition-related problems.

PSYCHOLOGICAL ASPECTS OF FOOD INTAKE

Humans consume food, not nutrients. Although specific nutrients are necessary for the growth and maintenance of the human organism, it would be shortsighted to attempt to study human's basic nutritional needs without an appreciation of those factors that influence his intake of a sufficient variety of foods to obtain them. Most animals other than humans eat primarily to satisfy this nutritional need; human's motivation for eating (or not eating) frequently satisfies nonnutritional needs. Although his desire to eat (or not eat) may have physiological origins, his selection of the foods he consumes is based on a combination of forces arising from his culture, his family, his educational level, his economic circumstances, and his individual needs and idiosyncrasies.[1,2]

Culture is the integrated pattern of human behavior that is transmitted to succeeding generations. It dictates the role each person plays in society, as well as his responsibilities to himself, his peer group, and his family. Food habits are largely determined by one's culture. Many habits have existed for centuries and have been maintained as an integral part of a cultural heritage. The Judaic dietary law, based on passages in Leviticus and Deuteronomy in the Old Testament, has very specific regulations about meat consumption. The prohibitions include the flesh of birds and animals of prey, reptiles, creeping insects, animal blood, any animal that does not chew its cud and has a cloven hoof, and any species from the water that does not have fins and scales. This eliminates eagles, ostriches, snakes, lizards, grasshoppers, camels, pigs, rabbits, sharks, oysters, clams, shrimp, and mussels. A large portion of the world's population has its dietary habits controlled by the teachings found in Buddhism, Hinduism, and Jainism (a subset of believers in Hinduism). These philosophies support the belief that all life is sacred. This precludes killing animals for food. Such a prohibition does vary from religion to religion, and even within a religion, from cultural group to group. For example, the Hindu reveres the cow and will not kill it for food. However, when a cow or oxen dies, the untouchables (the lowest class in Hindu society) take the animal, skin it for leather, and eat the meat. Since this population ordinarily is the poorest in India, this distribution of energy and protein serves to ensure their survival.

Not only do cultural/religious practices prohibit the eating of certain foods, cultural practices also influence the foods that are eaten. The Jamaican enjoys plantain, ackee (a native food, poisonous when ripe, that looks and tastes like scrambled eggs), eggplant, papaya, mangoes, fish, lobster, naseberries, and Otaheite apples. The Otomi Indians of the Mezquital Valley in Mexico make their meals from tortillas and from local plants such as malva, hediondilla, nopal, maguey, garambullo, yucca, purslane, pigweed, sorrel, wild mustard flowers, lengua de vaca, sow thistle, and cactus fruit. They drink an intoxicating beverage, pulque, made from the century plant. A North American raised in a different culture would look askance at this diet and view it as unpalatable and perhaps nutritionally unacceptable. However, nutritional analyses of the Otomi Indians' diet showed it to be better balanced than that of an urban group from the United States. Persons from large sections of east and south Asia and tropical Africa refuse to drink milk; other African groups, on the contrary, prize milk as a precious food and serve it only to adult men. The Maasai, an African tribal group, not only drink the milk from their cattle but draw blood from the jugular vein and drink that also. Entomophagy, the eating of insects, is accepted in many cultures; the Australian bushmen consume sugar ants and witchetty grubs; local inhabitants from Central Africa eat fresh and fried termites; some Japanese groups eat dytiscid beetles (fried and made into a sauce with sugar), grasshoppers, maggots, pupae of the wasp, and the larvae of silkworms.

Within a given culture, the family has a significant influence on food acceptance.[2] This happens not because there is an active effort by elders to teach the children but because the children see the same daily ritual of food preparation. Unconsciously, they assimilate it. In primitive societies, meals are important daily social events; females prepare the food and it is distributed on the basis of sex and age. In these societies as well as in our own, important family social events (christenings, weddings, funerals, etc.) are celebrated with food. These family practices become part of the cultural heritage and influence food choice.

Similarly, in progressive industrial societies, food customs are assimilated by children through the practices of their parents. As technological advances increase the complexity of a society, food as an element in its culture becomes less important. Sociologists who study contemporary society have observed that mealtimes have become less relevant as a time for family social interaction. In the United States, many meals are consumed outside the family environment; convenience foods, sandwiches, fast foods, soft drinks, and prepared fresh or frozen foods from restaurants and grocery stores are consumed by individuals on a regular basis.

Forces outside the family influence food choices. Advertising, peer pressure, lifestyle, and age may well be more-important determinants of food choices than family food practices. There has also been a change in the roles of food in festive occasions. Whereas 100 years ago a large meal might have been served to celebrate an important life event, such as a wedding or a christening, today these events might be celebrated with a cocktail party that includes light finger foods and beverages, both alcoholic and nonalcoholic. As in less-industrialized societies, children observe these practices and apply them.

The impact that the family has on food choices is often a reflection of the educational level of the one who selects and prepares the food. If this person is limited in education, the diet may consist of a very limited number of ingredients. In turn, this could mean that the family may be poorly nourished.

In more recent times in the United States, a definite correlation has been shown between the education of a homemaker and the nutritional intake of her family. The data for this correlation came from surveys conducted to examine the extent of malnutrition in the United States. Initially, the ten-state survey mandated by the federal government conducted from 1968 to 1970 was used for this correlation. Then, on a regular basis, the Centers for Disease Control conducted the Health and Nutrition Examination Survey (HANES). For the most recent information on these surveys, visit the NHANES website http://www.cdc.gov/nchs/r&d/nchs_datalinkage/nhefs_data_htm. At this website, there are various subcategories to access. Food intake (food recalls), clinical tests, physical examinations, anthropometric examinations, medical histories, and educational and financial status have been evaluated. The surveys showed that the fewer the years of education the homemaker had, the greater the number of nutritional deficiencies in the diet of the family.

Economic circumstances also exert considerable influence on food choices. The Australian aborigine, living in an arid barren land, is very poor. He hunts for the food he consumes. To increase his food supply, his culture has evolved to include a host of insects as part of the daily diet. At the other extreme, in a more-affluent society, considerable amounts of money are spent on foods of no outstanding nutritional value. Caviar is a prime example. In 2007, Beluga caviar costs over $1300 per pound. Caviar is considered a prestigious food by many Americans and Europeans, and they delight in both serving it to guests and eating it themselves. It has no greater nutritional value than cheese, eggs, or hamburger but does impart a certain social status to the consumer.

Additionally, there are a host of other interrelated factors that influence food choices: geography, climate, methods of distribution, and storage facilities. Although the New Zealanders and the Danes live many miles apart, both their diets include an abundance of dairy products. This is a function of, in part, the similarities in their geography and climate. Citrus fruits are easily grown in Egypt. However, the food distribution system in Egypt is inadequate. As a result, many people in the country do not enjoy these fruits because they spoil in the process of being shipped. In contrast, in the United States, because of rapid transportation systems, both native grown foods and imported foods are frequently enjoyed, and foods produced in one segment of the country are available throughout the nation and in all seasons. It is not unusual to see fresh strawberries in the market year-round. These berries may be local in the appropriate season or may be from South America or from some distant point in the country when the local crop is no longer available.

Finally, among the factors that influence food choices are an individual's physiological and psychological idiosyncrasies. An example of the former is the situation in which individuals lack the intestinal enzyme, lactase, which is necessary to digest the milk sugar, lactose. When they drink milk, they experience abdominal bloating, cramps, and diarrhea. Needless to say, they elect to exclude fresh milk from their diet. Countless food allergies have been observed: allergies to wheat, corn, peanuts, chocolate, eggs, strawberries, tomatoes, and soy products, to name a few. If an allergy can be identified, frequently a very difficult task, the item is eliminated from one's diet. Sometimes, a food item is eliminated instinctively without medical documentation simply because an individual senses a relationship between his food intake and his sense of well-being.

Throughout history, there have been individuals who possessed bizarre appetites.[3] During the nineteenth century, Jeremiah Johnson, a mountain man, wandered the unexplored west, living off the land and the livers of Crow Indians. According to folklore, during the course of his travels, he devoured the livers of 247 Indians. In Hungary in the early 1600s, the Countess Elizabeth de Bathory had a penchant for the blood of young, buxomy virgins, for through their blood, she hoped to regain her youth. In her efforts to do so, she is reported to have killed 650 girls, drinking their blood and using it as a fluid in which to bathe.

All in all, man's reasons for selecting the foods he eats are a very complex issue with apparently little consideration given to his nutritional requirements. The foods one person might consider an elegant repast, another would not deign to touch. Human behavior added to the study of nutrition makes a difficult subject even more complex.

PHYSIOLOGICAL ASPECTS OF FOOD INTAKE

Sensory Perception of Food

In addition to the social, cultural, and economic influences on food intake, the selection of foods involves a complex interaction among the special senses: reactions of the eye, ear, nose, and mouth and the sensations of pain and touch are all involved. The sensations of hunger, coupled with the appearance, texture, smell, and taste of food, which, in many ways, are inextricably bound to one's cultural heritage, determine whether the hand will reach out and grasp the food, transport it to the mouth, and consume it. The appearance of the food, its color, its consistency, and its temperature are perceived by the sensory system, which includes the sense of sight, the sense of touch, the sense of temperature, and the sense of smell, and reconciled with that person's acceptance or rejection of the food based on his social/cultural background. If the mashed potatoes are green or lumpy or burned, the individual will likely reject them. The food product simply does not conform to the expectation of the consumer for the characteristics of that food.

Temperature, taste, texture, and smell are perceived via sensory receptor systems located in the nose and mouth. A receptor is a defined organization of molecules, usually a protein, within a membrane or cellular organelle that recognizes and binds compounds or elements needed by the cell. Receptors serve to translate or transmit or initiate the sending of a message to other parts of the cell or to other parts of the body. For example, the sensory receptors in the oral cavity perceive food attributes such as texture and taste. The taste/texture translates the stimulus into an electrochemical message that is relayed to the brain. Currently, far more is known about the anatomy of the area in which these events take place than about the physiology of the events themselves.

Appearance

Part of the social/cultural force that influences one's acceptance of food is the defined expectation of an acceptable food. In part, this expectation is based on the appearance of that food. Does it have the desired size and shape, and most importantly, is it the expected color?[4] Work done on the relationship between food acceptance and color has shown a striking dependence of one on the other. One study showed that when jellies were colored in an atypical manner, the fruit flavors were incorrectly identified. In another study, the flavoring of colorless syrups was incorrectly identified by most of a group of 200 pharmacy students; they were even less able to identify the correct flavor if the solutions were given unusual colors. In a third study, a trained panel of wine tasters showed a dependence on color in their evaluation of wine. Food coloring was added to dry white table wine to simulate the appearance of sauterne, sherry, rosé, claret, and Burgundy. The panel judged the rosé-colored wine to be the sweetest and the claret-colored wine to be the least sweet. Interestingly, subjects who seldom drank wine and participated in the same experiment did not relate color to sweetness.

So important are these visual aspects of food that the USDA food quality grading standards are based on the appearance of food. For example, color is an important characteristic for the grading standards of beef and of fruits. Other visual characteristics, such as the presence or absence of blemishes and bruises, are also important.

Food scientists have spent considerable time trying to relate visual characteristics to measurable physical parameters that determine the acceptance or rejection of a given food. Appearance may provide a clue about the juiciness of an apple or the tenderness of a steak; these properties, of course, are also determined in the mouth and perceived there as differences in texture.

Texture

The texture of food plays an important role in food acceptance because the sense of touch is highly developed in the mouth. Texture, traditionally defined in terms of how a food *feels* in the mouth, is perceived by four different sets of receptors: the pain, tactile, pressor, and sound receptors. The pain receptors may be activated if foods are extremely hot or cold or rich in such seasonings as cayenne pepper. The active ingredient in cayenne pepper is capsicum that acts through chemically burning the surfaces of the mouth and/or tongue.

The tactile receptor receives messages about the geometrical characteristics of the food. The size, shape, and frequency of food particles will be ascertained, and if these characteristics are expected, the food will be accepted. If, however, the ice cream is gritty, the tactile receptors will perceive this, and the food may be rejected. These tactile receptors are located in the skin of the tongue, oral cavity, and throat. Not only do they perceive characteristics such as *grittiness* or *lumpiness*, they also detect differences in moisture and fat content. These latter characteristics may describe the richness, moistness, or slipperiness of a given food.

Texture is also perceived by pressor receptors located in the muscles, tendons, and joints of the mouth, jaws, and throat. These receptors are elements of the kinesthetic sense. The characteristic resistance to chewing, as in a tough piece of meat, is an example of the perception of texture by the kinesthetic sense. *Hard or tough to chew* means extreme physical resistance to the actions of the teeth and jaws. Strenuous exertion by the voluntary muscles is required; this, in turn, is perceived as changes in the position, movement, and tension of the teeth and jaws. The kinesthetic sense is difficult to study because it is not easily located and identifiable. However, through the use of such drugs as cocaine, which blocks the muscle receptors, it has been learned that the oral kinesthetic sense originates as much from the joints as from the muscles. Four sets of receptors are involved: two in the muscles, one in the tendon, and one in the fascia associated with the muscle. There are free nerve endings (also called pressor receptors) in the muscles that are activated by the chewing of such hard items as nuts, crackers, or bones and that stimulate a sense of motion.

Some textural characteristics are sensed by sound receptors. The sound a food makes when chewed contributes to the acceptability of the item. The crunch of crisp celery or the snap of a fresh potato chip contributes to the enjoyment of that food. The stimulation of tactile and kinesthetic receptors and of the auditory receptors plays important roles in the evaluation of textural characteristics of the food. Individuals will vary in their preferences for smooth, chewy, crisp, hot, cold, or crunchy textures; all of these attributes, however, are based not on taste, smell, or appearance but on mouth *feel* and *food sounds*. In addition, cultural influences will contribute to the textural expectations of individuals. For example, a soft, smooth, bland-textured food may be associated with the food needs of infants or invalids and may not be accepted by the young male with a strong *macho* self-image. Juicy, chewy textures requiring exertion of the jaw muscles may be very acceptable to the young adult but are much less acceptable to the school-age child.

Smell (Olfaction) and Gustation (Taste)

Olfaction and gustation are intimately related. Persons who have lost their sense of smell, as frequently happens with a cold, complain that food is not as tasty as when they are well. This is because part of their appreciation of food has decreased through a temporary impairment of their ability to smell.

Among the special senses, the sense of smell is the most sensitive. The average person can detect one part in a trillion parts of air for some high-potency odorants. For example, ethyl mercaptan (ethanethiol) can be detected at 4.0×10^{-11} mg/mL air. However, the perception of a particular aroma quickly diminishes if the aroma persists. This process is called olfactory adaptation and begins the first second after an aroma is perceived.

The perception of smell is a subjective phenomenon. Depending upon a person's expectations, an item can have an intrinsically pleasant or unpleasant aroma. One example of such subjectivity is the scent of a gardenia: many people enjoy it but some find the aroma too strong or overpowering. Because the perception of smell is so highly subjective, it is difficult to study it either qualitatively or quantitatively. Some physiologists contend that whereas taste perception involves the differentiation of four primary tastes, the perception of smell involves a multitude of aromas.

The perception of taste is, as is the perception of smell, highly subjective.[4,5] Despite this, physiologists have established that humans perceive four primary tastes: sour, salty, sweet, and bitter. Chemicals that can elicit any one of these tastes are called tastants. The tastants must be in solution in order to be perceived. Both water-soluble and lipid-soluble compounds can serve as tastants.

Different substances evoke each of the primary tastes. The chemicals that elicit a sour taste are acidic compounds; the hydrogen ion, rather than the associated anion, actually stimulates the receptor. Generally, the sourness is proportional to the concentration of the hydrogen ion. A more acidic compound will trigger a stronger response than a neutral compound. An anion of an inorganic salt produces a salty taste. The halides, chloride, fluoride, bromide, and iodide are usually associated with a salty taste.

A variety of chemicals, mostly organic, trigger the sensation of a sweet taste. These include a wide variety of sugars, glycols, alcohols, aldehydes, ketones, amides, esters, amino acids, sulfonic acids, halogenated acids, and the inorganic salts of lead and beryllium. The sweetest compound known is the n-propyl derivative of 4-alkoxy-e-aminonitrobenzene. Such organic compounds as the glycosides amygdalin (found in almond kernels) and naringin (found in citrus fruit) and the alkaloids caffeine, quinine, strychnine, and nicotine taste bitter.

The average person is more receptive to a bitter taste than to a sour, salty, or sweet taste. For example, a 0.000008 M quinine solution tastes bitter, but a much higher concentration (0.0009 M) of hydrochloric acid is required to taste sour, and an even higher concentration (0.01 M) of sodium chloride to taste salty, or of sucrose to taste sweet.

Additionally, the pleasantness of a given taste relates to the concentration of the tastant. For example, as the concentration of sucrose in a solution is increased, its taste changes from unpleasant to pleasant; the pleasant sensation of sweet arises only at higher concentrations. In contrast, a bitter taste can be pleasant at low concentrations but become unpleasant at high ones. In small quantities, the white membrane of orange or grapefruit sections enhances the flavors of these fruits; however, they are seldom eaten alone because of their bitter taste.

Within a given taste modality, some chemicals can be tasted at a lower concentration than others. This can be expressed quantitatively by measuring the detection threshold and, from this, calculating the relative taste indices. Table 4.1 gives the relative taste indices of several substances with the intensities of each of the four primary sensations referred to a reference compound: the acidic substances to hydrochloric acid, the sweet substances to sucrose, the bitter ones to quinine, and the salty ones to sodium chloride. Each of these reference compounds is assigned an index value of 1.

Each of these primary tastes is perceived through the organ of taste, the taste bud. The gustatory receptor structure is about 1/30 mm in diameter and 1/16 mm in length. It contains two kinds of cells: the receptor cell and the supporting cell. The gustatory receptor cells, also called the taste buds, are barrel-shaped, modified epithelial cells. Taste buds are found in several places within the oral cavity—on the surface of the tongue, palate, pharynx, and larynx and sometimes on the cheeks. From one end of each taste cell protrudes several microvilli or taste hairs. These microvilli extend through a taste pore within the tongue's surface to contact the fluids of the mouth. The other end of each taste cell is innervated with gustatory nerve fibers. One cell may be innervated

TABLE 4.1
Relative Taste Indices of Different Substances

Sour Substances	Index	Bitter Substances	Index	Sweet Substances	Index	Salty Substances	Index
Hydrochloric acid	1	Quinine	1	Sucrose	1	NaCl	1
Formic acid	1.1	Strychnine	3.1	4-propoxy-3-amino nitrobenzene	5000	NaF	2
Chloroacetic acid	0.9	Nicotine	1.3	Saccharin	675	$CaCl_2$	1
Lactic acid	0.85	Phenylthiourea	0.9	Chloroform	40	NaBr	0.5
Tartaric acid	0.7	Caffeine	0.4	Fructose	1.7	NaI	0.35
Malic acid	0.6	Pilocarpine	0.16	Alanine	1.3	LiCl	0.4
Potassium H tartrate	0.58	Atropine	0.13	Glucose	0.8	NH_4Cl	2.5
Acetic acid	0.55	Cocaine	0.02	Maltose	0.45	KC1	0.6
Citric acid	0.46	Morphine	0.02	Galactose	0.32		
Carbonic acid	0.06			Lactose	0.3		

Source: Adapted from Guyton, A.C., *Textbook of Medical Physiology*, 7th edn., W.B. Saunders, Philadelphia, PA, 1971, p. 636.

with several fibers; there is no one-on-one line of communication between the individual taste cell and the central nervous system (CNS).

Although the tongue perceives all four of the taste modalities, it is the most sensitive to the salty and sweet tastes. The palate, on the other hand, is more sensitive to the sour and bitter tastes than to the salty and sweet tastes. The pharynx also detects all four tastes but not to the same extent as the tongue and palate. Scattered over the entire oral cavity of an adult are approximately 10,000 taste buds. The taste cells within the taste buds are short-lived cells with a rapid turnover rate. In humans, the taste cell has an approximate lifetime of 250 h. The ability to quickly regenerate is in marked contrast to most other elements of the nervous system. As one grows older, the rate at which taste cells are regenerated is decreased, and as a consequence, there is a concomitant decrease in quantity. With a decrease in number of taste cells, taste acuity declines. Very young children are more sensitive to the different tastants than are more mature people.

The anatomical features involved with gustation have been well studied, as have the tastants that elicit the sensation. Organic chemists have long known that small structural changes can alter tastes. For instance, the sugars listed in Table 4.1 are structurally similar. The taste response they elicit, however, varies from very sweet (β-d-fructose) to bitter (β-d-mannose). The most remarkable feature of these compounds is that mutarotation about the anomeric carbon of α-d-mannose makes β-d-mannose and this change elicits a bitter taste rather than a sweet one.

Saccharin is sweet, but its *N*-alkylated derivatives are tasteless. The alkali metal salts of cyclamate (cyclohexyl amine sulfate) are sweet, yet the amine salt is nearly tasteless. It has been found that the dipeptide l-aspartyl-l-phenylalanine methyl ester (aspartame) and certain related compounds are nearly 200 times sweeter than sucrose. Since this compound is composed of natural amino acids and is quite low in energy, it serves as a noncaloric sweetener. If any other amino acids are substituted for the l-aspartate (even the closely related compound l-glutamate), the resulting product is tasteless. However, sweetness is maintained if phenylalanine is replaced by methionine or tyrosine. The dipeptide free acid of the methyl ester is not sweet, nor is the ethyl ester as sweet as the methyl ester.

As with smell, the taste process includes both preneural and neural phases. The preneural event involves an interaction between the tastant and the receptor cell. It is generally believed that this is a steric interaction between these two sites, possibly involving conformational changes.[4] Then, in some incompletely understood manner, this triggers the neural phase, which is the depolarization of specific taste nerves and the passage of impulses to the brain.

For the auditory and visual senses, medical specialties have evolved to diagnose and treat, where possible, deviations from normal. Similar specialties have not been developed to solve problems of taste and smell, nor have great strides been made in the diagnosis and treatment of disorders of these senses. However, abnormalities in taste perception have provided a means for verifying and enlarging the understanding of the mechanism of the taste sensation.

Anatomic abnormalities of both the palate and the tongue have been associated with a decrease in taste sensitivity. Patients with abnormal palate structures have significantly elevated thresholds for sour and bitter tastes but not for sweet and salty ones. An increase in threshold means that a greater concentration of the tastant is required for detection and recognition of that tastant by a subject. However, not all patients with anatomic abnormalities of the hard or soft palate exhibit taste disturbances. For example, those with gross clefts of the back part of the hard palate detect and recognize all four modalities of taste.

People who wear an upper denture report an increase in the detection and recognition thresholds for sour and bitter tastes, but no change in their response to sweet and salty tastes. The upper denture fits close to the palate and covers part of the mouth area containing taste receptors. As a result, there may be an artificial masking of the taste receptor sites in these parts of the mouth, and taste perception may be affected.

Abnormalities on the surface of the tongue, such as lichen planus and tumors, cause a decrease in taste acuity. Diseases that affect the nerve supply to the tongue (such as post diphtheritic neuritis, sarcoidosis, and Bell's palsy), severe trauma, and irradiation of the oral cavity as part of treatment for a malignancy will result in a decrease in taste sensitivity. In all of these abnormal states, there is a reduction or omission in the number of taste receptor cells, which has been given as the reason for the decrease in taste acuity. Interestingly, however, congenital underdevelopment or absence of the tongue is not accompanied by a decrease in taste acuity.

Speculation about the specific functions of the taste bud in taste perception has resulted from studies of patients with type 1 familial dysautonomia (Riley–Day syndrome). In this syndrome, the tongue's surface is smooth; the sulcus terminalis, taste buds, and fungiform and circumvallate papillae are missing, and the number of unmyelinated free nerve endings is greatly diminished. Patients demonstrate significantly raised detection and recognition thresholds; some cannot consistently distinguish between water and saturated solutions of sodium chloride, sugar, urea, and 0.03 M hydrochloric acid. However, when treated with methacholine (an α-adrenergic drug), these patients have normal taste perception, while the drug remains in their system. This has led to the suggestion that the taste buds function as a chemical sieve. It is proposed that taste buds have pores of a small, controlled size through which chemical stimuli may reach the nerves. Numerous factors, not yet identified, may control this pore size. In patients with familial dysautonomia, treatment with methacholine causes an increase in membrane permeability, including that of the lingual surface, which, in turn, allows a tastant to reach the unmyelinated, free nerve endings in the tongue. Thus, the taste threshold is lowered and the patient is more responsive to the tastant.

The divalent cations, particularly copper, zinc, and nickel, have been reported to affect taste sensitivity. When given to patients with hypogeusia (low sensitivities to tastants), some improvement occurs. Observations of serum and tissue levels of copper in patients with rheumatoid arthritis and Wilson's disease (abnormal copper absorption) have led to conjectures about copper's role in the regulation of taste acuity. Patients with either of these diseases are often treated with D-penicillamine. With this therapy, patients having Wilson's disease experience no change in their taste acuity; however, patients with rheumatoid arthritis frequently report a decrease. D-penicillamine therapy is associated with a decrease in serum and tissue copper levels. For arthritic patients, treatment with penicillamine results in a change (decrease) in taste sensitivity. The taste acuity of arthritic patients, if given oral copper sulfate, returns to normal. Patients with Wilson's disease are characterized by abnormally high levels of serum copper. Penicillamine treatment reduces this high level to a normal level, yet there are no effects of this treatment on taste acuity. Recent reports indicate that taste dysfunction may be associated with impaired zinc absorption and decreased levels of zinc in the saliva. Oral therapy of zinc or nickel returns the taste acuity to normal. Thus, it would appear that copper, zinc, and nickel are involved in taste acuity and depletion may lead to hypogeusia.

Steroid hormones have also been implicated in the taste mechanism through studies of diseases of the endocrine system. Patients with Addison's disease (decreased adrenal cortical function) or panhypopituitarism have lowered detection thresholds. Patients with Addison's disease are sometimes able to detect concentrations of tastants as low as 0.01% of that perceived by normal subjects. In both cases, the heightened taste sensitivity returns to normal when the missing steroid is given. The mechanism by which the steroids influence taste perception is not known. Indeed, a comprehensive, unified theory of taste perception has not yet been realized. But the taste of food, as well as its appearance, texture, and smell, is intimately involved in man's desire to eat.

NEURONAL SIGNALS FOR HUNGER AND SATIETY

Internal cues regulate food intake through a number of signals and responses that ultimately result in the initiation or cessation of feeding. These cues are in addition to those described earlier, which involve the cerebrum. Both short-term and long-term controls are exerted that, over time, serve to regulate the food intake of normal individuals so that they neither gain nor lose weight. Food intake control rests, in part, with the integration of a variety of hormonal and nonhormonal signals that are generated both peripherally and centrally. The hypothalamus is thought to be the main integrator of these signals. Other discrete areas are also involved. The hypothalamus is located beneath the thalamus, a part of the diencephalon forebrain, close to the pituitary and directly linked to the pituitary via the hypothalamus portal system. The hypothalamus is involved in both the initiation and cessation of food and water intake. It serves as an endocrine organ that produces the hormones that, in turn, modulate the release of hormones from the posterior pituitary. It also releases other hormones, called releasing factors or tropins, which control the activity of the anterior pituitary. The area of the brain that includes the thalamus, hypothalamus, and pituitary has been called the center of existence, because it controls much of what is known as instinctive behavior. In addition to its regulatory effect on appetite, satiety, and thirst, the hypothalamus serves, through its effect on the pituitary, as the main subcortical control center for the regulation of the parasympathetic and sympathetic systems, for the regulation of heart rate, and for the regulation of vasodilation and vasoconstriction, two important processes for the maintenance of body temperature. If the body temperature rises, vasodilation (increased blood flow through skin capillaries), along with increased respiration and increased sweat loss, occurs, thus increasing body heat loss. Conversely, if the body is in a cold environment, vasoconstriction (decreased blood flow) occurs and body heat is conserved. Vasoconstriction, vasodilation, and heart rate are also important to the regulation of blood pressure. Indirectly, the hypothalamus regulates the activity of the gastrointestinal system, the emotions, and spontaneous behavior.

The role of the hypothalamus in the control of eating behavior has been well studied. As early as 1840, extreme obesity in humans was reported to occur in patients with hypothalamic tumors. Recognition of the involvement of the ventromedial hypothalamus in the regulation of food intake did not come until it was shown that if the ventromedial hypothalamic area was destroyed or lesioned in animals, these animals overate, with a resulting increase in body fat. If the lateral hypothalamus was lesioned, animals became both adipsic (had no thirst response) and aphagic (did not eat). This relationship of feeding behavior to drinking behavior can be understood when the consequences of dehydration due to absence of fluid intake are realized. In adipsic animals, saliva production is significantly reduced; thus, laterally lesioned animals have difficulty, initially, in swallowing dry food. As the lesioned animal recovers or adapts to the lesion, he drinks when he eats dry food but does not eat when water deprived. In addition, the lesioned rat does not drink in response to serum hyperosmolarity (increased levels of solutes in the blood), hyperthermia (increased body temperature), or hypovolemia (decreased blood volume). Animals with lesions in the lateral hypothalamus do not respond to reductions in blood sugar levels (via insulin injections) and will die in severe hypoglycemia rather than eat readily available food. This observation suggested that both the lateral and ventromedial nuclei in the hypothalamus interact via chemical signals to control eating and drinking. Since eating and the cessation of eating are under hypothalamic control, it is reasonable to assume that this behavior is initiated or stopped by a series of signals emitted from and/or received by this tissue. The nature of this signal system is rather complex. As research continued in this area, it was learned that other areas of the brain are involved. The paraventricular nucleus (PVN) located slightly in front of the dorsomedial nucleus appeared to be involved in the regulation of glucose intake as it relates to the maintenance of glucose homeostasis. The dorsomedial nucleus, found on either side of the third ventricle, seems to be involved in the control of body size but not body fat and, because of this involvement, is likely to play a role in food intake. In addition, the area postrema of the brain stem and the caudal medial nucleus have been implicated in food intake regulation. All of these studies implicating various portions of the brain in the regulation of food intake were conducted using brain lesioning experimental protocols. These protocols, however crude, provided the basis for the concept that feeding behavior was coordinated by the CNS in response to factors in the blood and that likely this was a neuroendocrine system.[6,7]

Studies of energy balance in relation to brown fat thermogenesis (BAT) supported this concept since BAT could be stimulated by infusions of norepinephrine. Stimulation of BAT was energy wasting and led to body weight loss if that stimulation persisted over a period of time. Again this was a gross measurement, not one likely to occur on a regular basis in normal individuals. Nonetheless, it gave a hint of the involvement of the CNS in the regulation of energy balance. Since energy intake

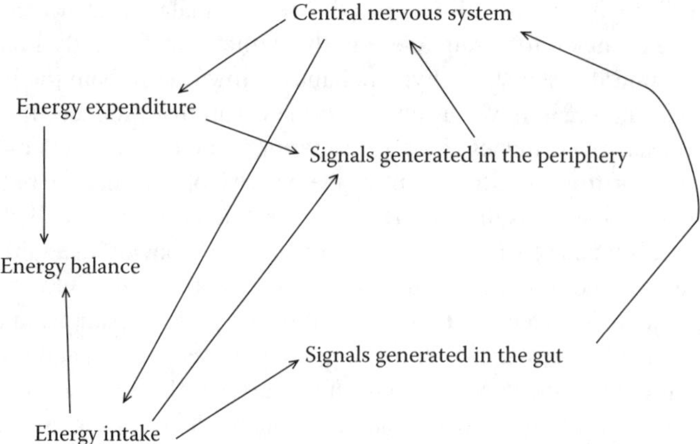

FIGURE 4.1 A general scheme for integrating the various signals for food intake with the regulation of energy balance. In this scheme, energy balance is central to determining energy intake. Food, when consumed, stimulates the production and release of signals that travel to the brain that in turn elicit signals that regulate energy expenditure and also serve to reduce subsequent food intake.

is an integral part of energy balance, it suggested that neuroendocrine factors are indeed involved in the regulation of feeding behavior.

That energy balance was related to food intake was not a novel concept, yet it was one that investigators in a wide variety of fields had to study together in order to make sense of it all. There had to be an integration of the peripheral and central signaling systems that could then explain why animals (and humans) increased or decreased their food consumption.[8,9] Models such as that shown in Figure 4.1 were devised to allow for the further investigation of these systems that then contributed to our understanding of how food intake is controlled. The nature and identity of the signals were not known, but using a variety of techniques, they were presumed to occur.

Several different approaches were used to elucidate these signals. Among these were the use of the parabiotic technique as mentioned in Chapter 2 in the discussion of set point theory.[10–14] Parabiosis involves the surgical pairing (skins of each animal were sutured together so that the animals shared their interstitial fluids but nothing else) of two animals. After recovery from the surgery, one was force fed an overabundance of food.[11,12] The second member of the pair was allowed to eat ad libitum. The first member became fat. This animal stored the excess energy intake as fat. The second member of the pair ate very little and became very thin. The thin member of the pair had decreased adipocyte lipogenic activity.[11] In another paradigm, the members of the pairs were siblings that differed in their genetic background: one carried the homozygous recessive fatty gene, while the other did not.[10,13,14] Both were allowed ad libitum access to food. The fatty member of the pair was hyperphagic. Hyperphagia is one of the traits of the genetic obesity. The other member ate very little. In both paradigms, there clearly was a signal circulating from the obese animal to the lean partner influencing its appetite since its food intake was significantly less than control parabiosed animal without the obesity gene.

That there was a blood-borne factor(s) was now clearly evident, but the identity of this factor(s) and its mechanism of action was not known until some investigators interested in genetic obesity began looking at possible genes that if mutated could phenotype as obesity.[15–17] Truett et al. mapped the rat fatty (fa) gene to chromosome 5 and showed that it was homologous to the db gene in the mouse.[15,16] Later Zhang et al. showed that the ob gene in mice mapped to chromosome 6, not chromosome 5, as found in rats.[17] Chromosome 6 had been identified years ago as the location of the ob gene in mice. Chromosome 4 was identified as the location for the diabetic (db) trait by scientists at the Jackson Laboratory in Bar Harbor, Maine. The phenotype of all three mutations included hyperphagia and obesity and type 2 diabetes. Although the mutations were mapped to different locations on different chromosomes, the common phenotype of hyperphagia suggested a possible linkage. That linkage turned out to be the cytokine, leptin and its receptor. Leptin is a cytokine produced and released by the adipose tissue. A cytokine is a soluble polypeptide or glycoprotein. It travels in the blood to the brain where it signals satiety. In this instance, the adipose tissue is an endocrine organ and the brain the target tissue. The brain has multiple receptors for leptin. The hypothalamus in particular has an abundance of the long form of the receptor on its surface with an intracellular domain of 303 amino acid residues.[21] This intracellular domain probably has signaling properties. When leptin is bound to the extracellular domains, cell signaling occurs that results in the perception of satiety by the individual.[27–30]

The mutation in the ob/ob mouse was a mutation in the gene that encoded leptin, while the mutation in the fa/fa rat and the db/db mouse was in the gene for the leptin receptor.[18–21] A number of leptin gene polymorphisms have been reported in humans that associate with excess body fat, type 2 diabetes mellitus, prostate cancer, and non-Hodgkin's lymphoma.[22–24] Adipocyte-selective reduction of leptin receptors in knockout mice resulted in adiposity, lipemia, and insulin resistence.[25] Leptin deficiency in humans is rare yet it has been reported.[26] Leptin receptor defects in humans are more likely. Mutations in both leptin and its receptor associate with obesity.[26,27] Leptin receptors are found in many tissue types. In particular, they can be found in the PVN that contains neurons that stimulate thyrotropin-releasing hormone (TRH) released by the anterior pituitary. TRH stimulates the release of thyroid-stimulating hormone (TSH) that, in turn, stimulates the synthesis and release of the thyroid hormones. The thyroid hormones regulate metabolic rate, lipolysis, oxidative phosphorylation, and energetic efficiency. Leptin has been shown to elicit these same changes in metabolism.[29–42]

As research in leptin developed, it was discovered that it had other functions in addition to signaling satiety. It signals apoptosis of adipocytes[31] and serves as the link between adipose tissue mass and the central neural network.[32] With age, leptin receptor sensitivity falls, while serum leptin levels rise;[33–35] this may explain the change in energy balance that occurs as people (and animals) age. Leptin is also a potent stimulator of growth hormone release.[43] This hormone has effects on metabolic efficiency and in particular on protein homeostasis associated with growth.[43,44] Glucocorticoid-mediated lipolysis is responsive to leptin,[44] and conversely, leptin gene expression is activated by glucocorticoids.[45] Central leptin administration increases glucocorticoid release.[46] Leptin has been shown to modulate glucose homeostasis as well by affecting insulin action.[46,47] Thus, it should come as no surprise that leptin directly alters lipid synthesis, deposition, mobilization, and oxidation. It also plays an important role in the management of glucose homeostasis as well as protein homeostasis.[42,48,49]

Leptin, as mentioned, is a major player in the regulation of food intake, yet food or food components can have effects on leptin production and release. For example, zinc deficiency regulates leptin production and release.[50,51] No doubt other nutrients will be shown to have this effect as well when a deficiency of their intake is characterized by a decrease in food intake.[52–57]

Lastly, leptin has a role in oxidative stress.[58–60] Leptin stimulates angiogenesis and exerts an atherogenic effect through the generation of oxidative stress in endothelial cells. Leptin appears to regulate peroxisome proliferator–activated receptor γ (PPARγ), tumor necrosis factor α (TNFα), and uncoupling protein 2 (UCP2) in adipose tissue. These are proinflammatory responses and are typical of the pathophysiology of degenerative disease. This action of leptin might explain the association of diabetes, atherosclerosis, and obesity that commonly occurs if in fact, the obesity is due to an abnormality in the leptin system. If there is too much circulating leptin produced because of receptor insensitivity due to either age or perhaps some polymorphism in the leptin receptor, this leptin could then be available to stimulate chronic disease development.

In addition to leptin, other neuropeptides or cytokines have been identified that affect satiety and hunger. Neuropeptide Y has been shown to stimulate feeding.[33,52,53] Ghrelin stimulates satiety and is responsive to protein intake as well as physical activity.[54,55] In humans with metabolic syndrome, a carbohydrate-restricted diet that induced weight (fat) loss resulted in increases in ghrelin levels as well as increases in another of the satiety signaling compounds, cholecystokinin.[56] Cholecystokinin is released by cells in the intestine. There are many cytokines and not all of them are involved in the regulation of food intake; some are involved in the function of the immune system. Listed in Table 4.2 are the cytokines of importance to signaling hunger and satiety.

TABLE 4.2
Cytokines, Their Receptors, and Their Signaling Mechanisms

Cytokine	Receptor Distribution	Signaling Mechanism
Ghrelin	Synthesized in stomach. Receptors are in hypothalamus.	Transfers information from stomach to hypothalamus and influences growth hormone release in response to changes in energy homeostasis
Cholecystokinin	Receptors are in brain, gall bladder, and endocrine pancreas.	Stimulates bile release and pancreatic exocrine enzyme release; signals satiety
Adiponectin	Released by adipose tissue; receptors in insulin target tissues.	Increases insulin sensitivity
TGFα, TGFβ	Several related cytokines and receptors. Found in most cells.	Involves the tyrosine kinase system
NPY	Found in most neural cells.	Involves the tyrosine kinase system
Leptin	Found in brain cells as well as other cell types.	?

Although the literature is rapidly expanding with respect to the neurological signals that regulate satiety and hunger, there still needs to be an overall understanding of feeding and satiety that not only includes the signals for hunger and those for satiety but also signals the continuation of feeding once feeding has commenced. One theory suggests that eating is a response to variations in the level of circulating glucose.[61] This theory, called the glucostatic theory, proposes that cellular energy requirements determine feeding behavior. In particular, it suggests that brain cells, which use glucose almost exclusively as their metabolic fuel, are exquisitely sensitive to fluctuations in blood glucose levels and, as such, will activate the *feeding center* to initiate feeding when blood glucose levels dip below normal or activate the *satiety center* to stop feeding when blood glucose levels are high.[62] Support for this theory comes from the observation that feeding is initiated by animals injected with insulin and from the observation that gold thioglucose (which destroys the satiety center of the hypothalamus) is ineffective in diabetic animals. In the latter case, eating continues because gold thioglucose does not get into the hypothalamic cells of diabetic animals to destroy the satiety center. This occurs because the penetration of gold thioglucose into the hypothalamic cells is insulin dependent. This is a very simplistic approach to food intake regulation, but it has provided a framework for the building of a more cohesive explanation of the systems that operate to ensure energy balance. More recently, Pannacciulli et al.[62] showed that carbohydrate oxidation and balance predicts subsequent ad libitum food intake and can influence short-term weight change. They concluded that carbohydrate balance is a contributing metabolic factor affecting food intake.

Another school of thought is that eating behavior is controlled by the fat cell size and number.[63] This is called the lipostatic theory. It speculates that there is a set point for each animal in terms of the number of fat cells and their fat content. When this set point is reached, the animal ceases to eat. In the absence of eating, these fat stores are mobilized and used until a lower set point is reached and feeding again commences. This theory is supported by observations that starved animals eat large amounts of food when provided with food after starvation until they regain their prestarvation weight; then, they resume their prestarvation eating behavior. In other words, they overate to fill their fat depots, then ate only enough to maintain these depots. Modulation of food intake by signals arising in adipose tissue is an important component of our understanding of energy balance as discussed in Chapters 1 through 3 and the preceding discussion.[64]

It is possible that the theories described earlier (as well as some others) may be integrated into a comprehensive set of pathways that readily allow for the understanding of the signals needed to initiate, maintain, and stop feeding. Most of the hormonal signals have short-term effects on feeding, but do not affect overall long-term food consumption. These signals may truly be hunger or satiety signals, but one must not confuse a satiety signal with a food intake–inhibition signal or confuse a hunger signal with a food intake–initiation signal. The initiation may occur but not be sustained sufficiently to result in significant food consumption. Similarly, inhibition may occur but may not significantly alter overall food intake. Therefore, not only the stop and start signals need to be examined, but so too does the overall control of food intake that has a long-term effect on energy balance. Sustaining feeding or food abstinence may involve not only the factors discussed earlier but may also include those listed in Table 4.3. Initiation may be hormonally induced but feeding may be sustained because the food is found to be pleasing as per the discussion on the hedonistic qualities of food—its taste, smell, texture, etc. Similarly, cessation of feeding even though hormones have signaled initiation may occur if the food is not palatable or culturally acceptable. Hormones that can enhance food intake at one

TABLE 4.3
Factors That Affect Food Intake

Enhance	Suppress
Insulin	Leptin
Testosterone	Estrogen
Glucocorticoids	Mazindol
Thyroxine	Phenylethylamines[a]
Low serotonin levels	Substance P
Galanin	Glucagon
Neuropeptide Y	Neurotensin
TRH	Bombesin
Dynorphin	Cyclo-his-pro
β-Endorphin	High-protein diets
Opioid peptides	Fluoxetine
Histidine (precursor of histamine)	TNFα
Desacetyl-melanocyte-stimulating hormone	Amylin
Tryptophan (precursor of serotonin)	Melanocortin
Somatostatin	Glucagon-like peptide-1
TSH	α-Melanocyte-stimulating hormone
Growth-hormone-releasing hormone	Anorectin
Melanin-concentrating hormone	Corticotropin-releasing
Orexin-A	Hormone
Ghrelin	Satietin[b]
Agouti-related peptide	High blood glucose
	Enterostatin
	Calcitonin
	Amino acid imbalance
	Pain
	Antidepressants[c]

[a] These are drugs and except for phenylpropanolamine are controlled substances. Many have serious side effects. They are structurally related to the catecholamines. Most are active as short-term appetite suppressants and act through their effects on the CNS, particularly through the β-adrenergic and/or dopaminergic receptors. This group includes amphetamine, methamphetamine, phenmetrazine, phentermine, diethylpropion, fenfluramine, and phenylpropanolamine. Phenylpropanolamine-induced anorexia is not reversed by the dopamine antagonist haloperidol.

[b] This is a blood-borne factor.

[c] All of these drugs are controlled substances and their use as antidepressants must be carefully monitored. This group includes amitriptyline, buspirone, chlordiazepoxide, chlorpromazine, cisplatin, clozapine, ergotamine, fluphenazine, imipramine, iprindole, and others that block 5-HT receptors.

level can suppress it at another. Insulin is a prime example. Thyroxine is another. Normal individuals given a low dose of insulin will experience hunger. However, large doses of insulin can provoke a serious hypoglycemia that will have the opposite effect. Other hormones are involved as well. In hypothyroidism, hunger signals are poorly perceived. The patient, although not anorexic, does not have a strong drive to eat. In contrast, hyperthyroidism is characterized by strong, almost unremitting hunger. Within this framework are a number of afferent and efferent systems that influence food intake by providing information to the brain and relaying instructions via neuronal signals from the brain to the rest of the body.[61–69] Food intake can be increased or decreased with reciprocal effects on the CNS when these peptides are administered. Galanin, neuropeptide Y, the opioid peptides, growth-hormone-releasing hormone, and desacetyl-melanocyte-stimulating hormone increase food intake, whereas insulin excess, glucagon, leptin, cholecystokinin, anorectin, corticotropin-releasing hormone, neurotensin, bombesin, cyclo-his-pro, and TRH reduce food intake. Several of these hormones or peptides have specific actions with respect to the intake of specific food components. For example, increases in neuropeptide Y result in increased carbohydrate intake, while increases in the level of galanin and opioid peptides increase fat intake. Fat intake is suppressed when the blood level of enterostatin rises. Rising blood levels of glucagon suppress protein intake. All of the aforementioned are short-term signals that appear to regulate food selection as well as the amount of food consumed. Although most of these studies have been done in carefully prepared experimental animals (usually rats), there is sufficient indirect evidence to suggest that short-term food intake is similarly regulated in humans. In humans, serotoninergic agents have been used as treatments for mental disorders.

These agents either block the binding of serotonin (5-hydroxytryptamine, 5-HT) to its receptor or upregulate the receptors' binding affinity. 5-HT receptors are widespread throughout the cerebral cortex, the limbic system, the striatum, the brain stem, the choroid plexus, and almost every other region of the CNS. These drugs have a side effect of affecting food intake. Because serotonin suppresses feeding if the receptor is blocked, feeding is enhanced. Thus, drugs that block these receptors are useful in treating anorexia (decreased desire to eat) especially the anorexia that accompanies anxiety, depression, obsessive–compulsive disorders, panic disorders, migraine, and chemotherapy emesis. In contrast, drugs that potentiate the binding of 5-HT to its receptor will result in a suppression of appetite and may be useful in treating the hyperphagia of Prader–Willi syndrome and other conditions associated with genetic obesity. As the database on various cytokines and their receptors expands, doubtless there will be drugs that either interfere with cytokine action or potentiate it. Perhaps these drugs might be useful in the treatment of obesity, while other drugs might be helpful in treating anorexia.

Drugs, particularly those used in cancer chemotherapy, frequently have appetite suppression as a side effect. In part, this reduction in food intake may be due to disease- or drug-induced changes in taste and aroma perception and, in part, due to the effects of the disease or drugs on the CNS, particularly the adrenergic and serotonergic receptors. Several of the compounds listed in Table 4.3 are appetite suppressants and are chemically related to the catecholamines. These drugs can be addictive and have deleterious side effects.

Some steroids affect food intake. Adrenalectomized animals or humans with Addison's disease, both glucocorticoid-deficient states, do not perceive normal hunger signals. If there is no food for extended periods of time, these individuals are difficult to realiment. However, once eating commences, a normal feeding pattern will be maintained. In excess, glucocorticoid stimulates feeding, and patients with Cushing's disease (excess glucocorticoid production) or patients who are receiving long-term glucocorticoid treatment will report increased hunger and food intake. Patients with Cushing's disease are often characterized by large fat depots across the shoulders and in the abdomen. In addition, obese patients are frequently characterized by excess blood levels of both glucocorticoids and insulin. As noted earlier, these hormones stimulate appetite and feeding.

Within the normal range, doses of testosterone and estrogen, although also steroids, have opposite effects with respect to food intake. In experimental animals, day-to-day variations in food intake by females will follow the same pattern as their day-to-day variation in estrogen level. When estrogen is high, food intake is suppressed and vice versa. Women who are anestrus due to ovariectomy or who are postmenopausal frequently lose their day-to-day estrogen-mediated food intake pattern.[70] With this loss is a more even (and somewhat increased) food intake and subsequent body fat gain. This has been found as well in castrated female rats, dogs, and cats.

The gain in body weight as fat may be explained by the loss in food intake control exerted by the estrogens rather than by an estrogen-inhibiting effect on lipogenesis. Testosterone increases food intake marginally but also stimulates protein synthesis and spontaneous physical activity. As a result, body fat does not increase. As testosterone levels decline in males with age, protein synthesis declines and the body tends to sustain its fat synthetic activity. This results in a change in body composition with an increase in body fat stores. The age-related decline in testosterone production may not be accompanied by a decline in food intake.

Although food intake can vary from day to day in response to minor day-to-day variations in food supply, activity, and hormonal status, body weight is relatively constant.[65–69] The mechanisms that control body weight are very complex, and the fine details of this regulation are far from clear. However, suffice it to say, major long-term deviations in either food intake or physiological state can affect body weight or energy balance. If food intake (energy intake) is curtailed for days to months, body weight will fall; similarly, if food intake is dramatically increased, body weight will increase. This relationship assumes no change in body energy demand. As described in Chapter 2 in the section on trauma, the energy requirement can be increased up to 10-fold by major illness or trauma despite the fact that the patient may be recumbent and perhaps sedated. Similarly, individuals who have markedly changed their activity levels will affect their energy balance.

If strenuous exercise is added without an increase in food intake, this will increase energy expenditure and negative energy balance, or weight loss will occur. In most individuals, therefore, long-term changes in energy balance, through changes in either intake or expenditure, will result in a body weight change.

SUMMARY

1. Food intake is regulated by physiological cues and genetically dictated signals and by social and cultural factors.
2. The sensory perception of the various characteristics of a food determines food acceptance/rejection and may also influence how much of the food is consumed.
3. Neuronal signals influence initiation of food intake and its cessation. The cytokines function as signals for hunger and satiety.
4. The hypothalamus is the central integrator of signals for hunger, thirst, and satiety.
5. Hormonal status affects food intake and subsequent body composition.

LEARNING OPPORTUNITIES

CASE STUDY 4.1

Andrew is a catcher for the local baseball team. One day as he was squatting behind the hitter, the pitcher threw a wild pitch and the ball came in at 90 miles/h and struck Andrew on the side of his head just behind his left ear right where his protective hat did not cover his skull. It was such a strong hit that it knocked him out. He went to the hospital where x-rays showed a severe bruise to his skull. Further NMR studies showed a concussion and injury area that extended deep into his brain. A neurosurgeon was called in and was able to reduce the brain swelling and fluid accumulation. With an extended period of rest and recovery, Andrew was able to resume his normal activities. All was well until Andrew began to notice that he was gaining weight and that he was always looking for something to eat. What's going on here? Describe and analyze the situation.

MULTIPLE-CHOICE QUESTIONS

1. The desire to eat comes from
   a. Availability of food
   b. Knowledge of food preparation technique
   c. Observation of others
   d. Activity of the CNS
2. Separation of meat preparation areas and dishes from those used for the preparation of dairy foods is an example of
   a. Cultural control of food intake
   b. Requirement by state and federal law
   c. Proper sanitary procedure
   d. Saving money for food purchases
3. An undiagnosed lesion in the brain results in abnormal fluid and food intake. Appropriate studies showed the location of the lesion. Where is it?
   a. Amygdala
   b. Hippocampus
   c. Thalamus
   d. Hypothalamus
4. Marmite is well liked by Australians but rejected by Americans. Why?
   a. Marmite is culturally accepted by Australians.
   b. Marmite is a cheap vitamin supplement.
   c. Marmite helps to get rid of the waste products for beer manufacture.
   d. Americans and Australians differ in their taste detectors.
5. Signals for satiety include
   a. Leptin
   b. NPY
   c. TNFα
   d. Cholecystokinin

REFERENCES

1. Sanjur, D. (1982) *Social and Cultural Perspectives in Nutrition*. Prentice Hall Englewood Cliffs, NJ, 336pp.
2. Bryant, C.A., Courtney, A., Markebury, B.A., DeWalt, K.M. (1985) *The Cultural Feast*. West Publishing Co., New York, 481pp.
3. Booth, D.A. (1992) Integration of internal and external signals in intake control. *Proc. Nutr. Soc.* 51: 21–28.
4. Palmer, R.K. (2007) The pharmacology and signaling of bitter, sweet, and umami taste sensing. *Mol. Interv*. 7: 87–98.
5. Guyton, A.C. (1971) *Textbook of Medical Physiology*, 7th edn. W. B. Saunders, Philadelphia, PA, p. 639.
6. Bray, G.A. (1986) Autonomic and endocrine factors in the regulation of energy balance. *Fed. Proc.* 45: 1404–1410.
7. Girardier, L., Seydoux, J. (1981) Is there a sympathetic regulation of the efficiency of energy utilization? *Diabetologia* 20: 362–365.
8. Martin, R.J., Beverly, J.L., Truett, G.E. (1989) Energy balance regulation. In: *Animal Growth Regulation* (D.R. Campion, G.J. Hausman, R.J. Martin, eds.). Plenum Publishing, New York, pp. 211–235.
9. Sukhaime, P.V., Margen, S. (1982) Autoregulatory homeostatic nature of energy balance. *Am. J. Clin. Nutr*. 35: 355–365.
10. Harris, R.B., Hervey, G.R., Tobin, G. (1987) Body composition of lean and obese Zucker rats in parabiosis. *Int. J. Obes*. 11: 275–283.
11. Harris, R.B., Martin, R.J. (1990) Site of action of putative lipostatic factor: Food intake and peripheral pentose shunt activity. *Am. J. Physiol*. 259: R45–R52.

12. Harris, R.B., Martin R.J., Bruch, R.C. (1995) Dissociation between food intake, diet composition, and metabolism in parabiotic partners of obese rats. *Am. J. Physiol.* 268: R4874–R4883.
13. Harris, R.B. (1997) Loss of body fat in lean parabiotic partners of ob/ob mice. *Am. J. Physiol.* 272: R1809–R1815.
14. Harris, R.B. (1999) Parabiosis between db/db and ob/ob or db/+ mice. *Endocrinology* 140: 138–145.
15. Truett, G.E., Bahary, N., Friedman, J.M., Leibel, R.L. (1991) Rat obesity gene fatty (fa) maps to chromosome 5: Evidence for homology with the mouse gene diabetes (db). *Proc. Natl. Acad. Sci.* 88: 7806–7809.
16. Truett, G.E., Jacob, H.J., Miller, J., Drouin, G., Smoller, J.W., Lander, E.S., Leibel, R.L. (1995) Genetic map of rat chromosome 5 including the fatty (fa) locus. *Mammalian Genome* 6: 25–30.
17. Zhang, Y., Proenca, R., Maffei, M, Barone, M., Leopold, L., Friedman, J.M. (1994) Positional cloning of the mouse obese gene and its human homologue. *Nature* 372: 425–432.
18. Caro, J.F., Sinha, M.K., Kolaczynski, J.W., Zhang, P.L., Considine, R.V. (1996) Leptin: The tale of an obesity gene. *Diabetes* 45: 1455–1462.
19. Bray, G.A., York, D.A. (1997) Leptin and clinical medicine: A new piece in the puzzle of obesity. *J. Clin. Endocrinol. Metab.* 82: 2771–2776.
20. Kline, A.D., Becker, G.W., Churgay, L.M., Landen, B.E., Martin, D.K., Muth, W.L., Rathnachalam, R. et al. (1997) Leptin is a four helix bundle: Secondary structure by NMR. *FEBS Lett.* 407: 239–242.
21. Tartaglia, L.A. (1997) The leptin receptor. *J. Biol. Chem.* 272: 6093–6096.
22. Van der Lende, T., Te Pass, M.F., Veerkamp, R.F., Liefer, S.C. (2005) Leptin gene polymorphisms and their phenotypic associations. *Vitam. Horm.* 71: 373–404.
23. Han, H.R., Ryu, H.J., Cha, H.S., Go, M.J., Ahn, Y., Cho, Y.M, Lee, H.K. et al. (2008) Genetic variations in the leptin and leptin receptor genes are associated with type 2 diabetes mellitus and metabolic traits in the Korean female population. *Clin. Genet.* 74: 105–115.
24. Jeon, J.P., Shim, S.M., Nam, H.Y., Ryu, G.M., Hong, E.J., Kim, H.L., Han, B.G. (2010) Copy number variation at leptin receptor gene locus associated with metabolic traits and the risk of type 2 diabetes mellitus. *BMC Genomics* 11: 426–430.
25. Huan, J.N., Li, J., Han, Y., Chen, K., Wu, N., Zhao, A.Z. (2003) Adipocyte-selective reduction of the leptin receptors induced by antisense RNA leads to increased adiposity, dyslipidemia, and insulin resistance. *J. Biol. Chem.* 278: 45638–45650.
26. Montague, C.T., Farooql, S., Whitehead, J.P., Soos, M.A., Rau, H., Wareham, N.J., Sewtwe, C.P. et al. (1997) Congenital leptin deficiency is associated with severe early onset obesity in humans. *Nature* 387: 903–908.
27. Dagogo-Jack, S. (1999) Regulation and possible significance of leptin in humans: Leptin in health and disease. *Diabetes Rev.* 7: 23–38.
28. White, D.W., Kuropatwinski, K.K., Devos, R., Baumann, H., Tartaglia, L.A. (1997) Leptin receptor signaling. *J. Biol. Chem.* 272: 4065–4071.
29. Mistry, A.M., Swick, A.G., Romsos, D.R. (1997) Leptin rapidly lowers food intake and elevates metabolic rates in lean and ob/ob mice. *J. Nutr.* 127: 2065–2072.
30. Harris, R.B. (2013) Direct and indirect effects of leptin on adipocytes metabolism. *Biochim. Biophys. Acta* S0925–4439: 163–164.
31. Qian, H., Azain, M.J., Compton, M., Hartzell, D.L., Hausman, G.A., Baile, C.A. (1998) Brain administration of leptin causes deletion of adipocytes by apoptosis. *Endocrinology* 139: 791–794.
32. Campfield, L.A., Smith, F.J., Burn, P. (1996) The ob protein (leptin) pathway—A link between adipose tissue mass and central neural networks. *Horm. Metab. Res.* 28: 619–632.
33. Li, H., Matheny, M., Tumer, N., Scarpace, P.J. (1998) Aging and fasting regulation of leptin and hypothalamic neuropeptide Y gene expression. *Am J. Physiol.* 275: E405–E411.
34. Scarpace, P.J., Matheny, M., Moore, R.L., Tumer, N. (2000) Impaired leptin responsiveness in aged rats. *Diabetes* 49: 431–435.
35. Orban, Z., Bornstein, S.R., Chrousos, G.P. (1998) The interaction between leptin and the hypothalamic-pituitary–thyroid axis. *Horm. Metab. Res.* 30: 231–235.
36. Havel, P.J. (2004) Update on adipocytes hormones: Regulation of energy balance and carbohydrate/lipid metabolism. *Diabetes* 53 (Suppl. 1): S143–S151.
37. Havel, P.J. (2002) Control of energy homeostasis and insulin action by adipocytes hormones: Leptin, acylation stimulating protein and adiponectin. *Curr. Opin. Lipidol.* 13: 51–59.
38. Jequier, E. (2002) Leptin signaling, adiposity and energy balance. *Ann. NY Acad. Sci.* 967: 379–388.
39. Korbonits, M. (1998) Leptin and the thyroid—A puzzle with missing pieces. *Clin. Endocrinol.* 49: 569–572.

40. Breslow, M.J., Lee, K.M., Brown, D.R., Chacko, V.P., Palmer, D., Berkowitz, D.E. (1999) Effect of leptin deficiency on metabolic rate in ob/ob mice. *Am. J. Physiol.* 276: E443–E449.
41. Unger, R. H., Zhou, Y-T, Orci, L. (1999) Regulation of fatty acid homeostasis in cells: Novel role of leptin. *Proc. Natl. Acad. Sci. USA* 96: 2327–2332.
42. Brown, L.M., Clegg, D.J. (2013) Food intake regulation. In: *Handbook of Nutrition and Food* (C.D. Berdanier, J. Dwyer, D. Heber, eds.). CRC Press, Boca Raton, FL, pp. 125–131.
43. Tannenbaum, G.S., Gurd, W., Lapointe, M. (1998) Leptin is a potent stimulator of spontaneous pulsatile growth hormone (GH) secretion and the GH response to GH-releasing hormone. *Endocrinology* 139: 3871–3875.
44. Heiman, M.L., Chen, Y., Caro, J.F. (1998) Leptin participates in the regulation of glucocorticoid and growth hormone axes. *J. Nutr. Biochem.* 9: 553–559.
45. DeVos, P., Lefebvre, A-M., Shrivo, I., Fruchart, J.-C., Auwerx, J. (1998) Glucocorticoids induce the expression of the leptin gene through a non-classical mechanism of transcriptional activation. *Eur. J. Biochem.* 253: 619–626.
46. Van Dijk, G., Donahey, J.C.K., Thiele, T.E., Scheurink, A.J.W., Steffens, A.B., Wilkinson, C.W., Tenenbaum, R. et al. (1997) Central leptin stimulates corticosterone secretion at the onset of the dark phase. *Diabetes* 46: 1911–1914.
47. Cohen, B., Novick, D., Rubinstein, M. (1996) Modulation of insulin activities by leptin. *Science* 274: 1185–1186.
48. Muoio, D.M., Dohm, G.L., Fiedorek, F.T., Tapscott, E.B., Coleman, R.A. (1997) Leptin directly alter lipid partitioning in skeletal muscle. *Diabetes* 46: 1360–1363.
49. Butler, A.A., Kozak, L.P. (2010) A recurring problem with the analysis of energy expenditure in genetic models expressing lean and obese phenotypes. *Diabetes* 59: 323–329.
50. Mantzoros, C.S., Prasad, A.S., Beck, F.W.J., Grabowski, S., Kaplan, J., Adair, C., Brewer, G.J. (1998) Zinc may regulate serum leptin concentrations in humans. *J. Am. Coll. Nutr.* 17: 270–275.
51. Ott, E.S., Shay, N.F. (2001) Zinc deficiency reduces leptin expression and leptin secretion in rat adipocytes. *Exp. Biol. Med.* 226: 841–846.
52. Plata-Salaman, C.R. (1996) Leptin (OB protein), neuropeptide Y, and interleukin-1 as interface mechanisms for the regulation of feeding in health and disease. *Nutrition* 12: 718–723.
53. White, B.D., Martin, R.J. (1997) Evidence for a central mechanism of obesity in the Zucker rat: Role of neuropeptide Y and leptin. *Proc. Exp. Biol. Med.* 183: 1–10.
54. Lejeune, H.P., Westerterp, K.R., Adam, T.C., Luscombe-Marcsh, N.D., Westerterp-Plantenga, M.S. (2006) Ghrelin and glucagon-like peptide 1 concentrations, 24 h satiety, and energy and substrate metabolism during a high-protein diet and measured in a respiration chamber. *Am. J. Clin. Nutr.* 83: 89–94.
55. Jurimae, J., Jurimae, T., Purge, P. (2007) Plasma ghrelin is altered after maximal exercise in elite male exercise. *Exp. Biol. Med.* 232: 904–909.
56. Hayes, M.R., Miller, C.K., Ulbrecht, J.S., Mauger, J.L., Parker-Klees, L., Gutschall, M.D., Mitchell, D.C., Smiciklas-Wright, H., Covasa, M. (2007) A carbohydrate-restricted diet alters gut peptides and adiposity signals in men and women with metabolic syndrome. *J. Nutr.* 137: 1944–1950.
57. Leidy, H.J., Campbell, W.W. (2011) The effect of eating frequency on appetite control and food intake: Brief synopsis of controlled feeding studies. *J. Nutr.* 141: 154–157.
58. Bouloumie, A., Marumo, T., Lafontan, M., Busse, R. (1999) Leptin induces oxidative stress in human endothelial cells. *FASEB J.* 13: 1231–1238.
59. Qian, H., Hausman, G.J., Compton, M.M., Azain, M.J., Hartzell, D.L., Baile, C.A. (1998) Leptin regulation of peroxisome proliferator-activated receptor-g, tumor necrosis factor, and uncoupling protein expression in adipose tissues. *B.B.R.C.* 246: 660–667.
60. Loffreda, S., Yanag, S.Q., Lin, H.Z., Karp, C.L., Brengman, M.L., Wang, D.J., Klein, A.S. et al. (1998) Leptin regulates proinflammatory immune responses. *FASEB J.* 12: 57–65.
61. Langhans, J. (1996) Metabolic and glucostatic control of feeding. *Proc. Nutr. Soc.* 55: 497–515.
62. Pannacciulli, N., Salbe, A.D., Ortega, E., Venti, C.A., Bogardus, C., Krakoff, J. (2007) The 24-hour carbohydrate oxidation rate in human respiratory chamber predicts ad libitum food intake. *Am. J. Clin. Nutr.* 86: 625–632.
63. Harris, R.B.S., Martin R.J. (1984) Lipostatic theory of energy balance. *Nutr. Behav.* 1: 253–275.
64. Martens, M.J.I., Born, J.M., Lemmens, S.G.T., Karhunen, L., Heinecke, A., Goebel, R., Adam, T.C., Westerterp-Plantenga, M.S. (2013) Increased sensitivity to food cues in the fasted state and decreased inhibitory control in the satiated state in the overweight. *Am. J. Clin. Nutr.* 97: 471–479.
65. Jeanrenaud, J. (1985) An hypothesis on the aetiology of obesity: Dysfunction of the central nervous system. *Diabetologia* 28: 502–513.

66. Hirschberg, A.L. (1998) Hormonal regulation of appetite and food intake. *Ann. Med.* 30: 7–20.
67. Fry, M., Hoyda, H.D., Ferguson, A.V. (2007) Making sense of it: Roles of the sensory circumventricular organs in feeding and regulation of energy homeostasis. *Exp. Biol. Med.* 232: 14–26.
68. Bray, G.A. (2000) Reciprocal relation of food intake and sympathetic activity: Experimental observations and clinical implications. *Int. J. Obes. Relat. Disorders* 24 (Suppl. 2): S8–S17.
69. Lam, C.K.L., Chari, M., Lam, T.K.T. (2009) CNS regulation of glucose homeostasis. *Physiology* 24: 159–170.
70. Frisch, R. (1991) Body weight, body fat, and ovulation. *Trends Endocrinol. Metab.* 2: 191–197.

5 Exercise

Physical activity is an important component of the energy balance equation. The energy associated with exercise apart from the activities of daily living including work is an additive to that needed to support basal metabolism, growth, pregnancy, lactation, work, and the recovery from trauma and/or disease. By definition, exercise is a physical activity that is apart from that associated with daily living. It is designed to improve fitness and health. In the extreme, it is designed to prepare one to compete in athletic events. The elite athlete is in a class by himself or herself with respect to energy output and nutrient needs.

DEFINITIONS

Physical activity (exercise) is defined as bodily movements produced by the contraction of skeletal muscles resulting in an increase in energy expenditure above that required to sustain the other functions of the body. Exercise is a physical activity that is planned, structured, repetitive, and purposive. When well designed, it improves physical fitness. The degree to which energy expenditure is increased depends on the activities selected for the exercise period, the intensity of the exercise, and the duration of the exercise.

To some extent, energy expenditure associated with daily living can be significant when the individual leads a very active life. The individual may work as a day laborer and have an employment digging ditches or building houses or working in a manufacturing setting. These occupations call for an energy expenditure that falls into the domain of occupational energy expenditure (work). Individuals with these occupations may not engage in exercise given that their daily living includes so much physical activity. Individuals in this category expend energy outside of the definition of a planned, purposeful activity called exercise.

There are quantitative dimensions of physical activity that include frequency (how often the activity is repeated), intensity (how much effort is required to perform the activity), and duration (how long the activity is sustained). The energy expended varies with the type of activity and on the body weight, body composition, and efficiency of performance of the individual. Table 5.1 shows the effects of exercise intensity on energy expenditure by untrained adult men and women.[1] The gender difference is primarily due to the difference in body size and aerobic muscle mass, although there are also differences in hormonal status that can affect energy expenditure. Age can modify these figures. Children and adolescents have less muscle mass as a percent of their total body mass and smaller bodies that in turn affect their energy expenditure while exercising. The elderly may have diminished muscle mass as a percentage of their total body mass due to sarcopenia (muscle loss with aging). Some of the loss in their percent muscle mass is due to an increase in the percent of the body mass that is the fat mass.[2] Aging muscle is characterized by an infiltration of fat into the muscle. In Table 5.1, light exercise is defined as an exercise that raises the energy expenditure up to three times that of the resting energy expenditure. Heavy exercise raises the expenditure six to eight times that of the resting energy expenditure. Moderate exercise falls in between light and heavy energy expenditure. Energy expenditure can be expressed as kcal per minute, or liters of oxygen consumed per minute, or milliliters of oxygen consumed per kilogram body weight per minute or METS.

The term, MET, is a multiple of the resting metabolic rate. One MET is equivalent to the resting oxygen consumption that ranges from 200 to 250 mL/min. Two METs require twice as much oxygen, and three METs require three times as much oxygen as that used during rest. The MET can

TABLE 5.1
Average Energy Expenditure by Men and Women in Terms of Exercise Intensity[a]

	Energy Expenditure			
Level	**kcal/min**	**L O_2/min**	**mL/kg/min**	**METS**
Men (65 kg Body Weight)				
Light	2.0–4.9	0.40–0.99	6.1–15.2	1.6–3.9
Moderate	5.0–7.4	1.00–1.49	15.3–22.9	4.0–5.9
Heavy	7.5–9.9	1.50–1.99	23.0–30.6	6.0–7.9
Women (55 kg Body Weight)				
Light	1.5–3.4	0.30–0.69	5.4–12.5	1.2–2.7
Moderate	3.5–5.4	0.70–1.09	12.6–19.8	2.8–4.3
Heavy	5.5–7.4	1.10–1.49	19.9–27.1	4.4–5.9

Source: Adapted from Durnin, J.V.G.A. and Passmore, R., *Energy Work and Leisure*, Heinmann, London, U.K., 1967.

[a] L/min is based on 5 kcal/L O_2; mL/kg/min is based on body weight; one MET (a multiple of resting metabolic rate) is equivalent to the average resting oxygen consumption.

be expressed in terms of body mass: one MET is the oxygen consumed per unit of body mass or approximately 3.6 mL O_2/kg min.

The average physically active male or female may expend up to 2 h/day on recreational sport or exercise. This amount of purposeful activity added to the energy costs of daily living ensures that the individual can maintain a healthy weight as well as maintain a useful muscle mass. Table 5.2 gives some examples of exercise-induced energy expenditure (kcal/min kg) and gives examples showing how body weight can influence energy expenditure.

As shown in the examples in Table 5.2, body mass is an important factor in determining the energy expended by exercise. As body mass increases, the energy expended for a particular exercise increases. This is particularly evident in weight-bearing exercises such as walking, jogging, and running. In exercises where the body is supported such as biking or swimming, the influence of body mass on energy expenditure is reduced, yet the total energy expended by the heavier person is greater than that expended by the lighter person. If the energy cost is expressed in relation to body mass, the difference in energy expenditure due to differences in body mass is almost eliminated. However, the total energy expended by a particular exercise by the heavier person is still greater than that expended by the lighter one simply because the body mass must be transported in the activity and this requires proportionately more total energy.

The assessment of physical activity is not precise.[4] There are individual variations in the conduct of an activity as well as individual differences in the reporting of same. To one individual, playing baseball is a vigorous event that includes running, catching, ball throwing, and batting. For another, it is keeping the score card and keeping the bats in order. Both people are *playing baseball but* the energy expenditure by the former is greater than that of the latter. Monitoring the actual energy expenditure is a challenge under these circumstances. As noted in Chapter 1, early energy investigators compiled lists of activities and calculated the energy expenditure associated with each activity through measuring the oxygen consumption of the subject(s). However, it is not always possible to measure the energy expenditure using oxygen consumption. The investigator or subject burden might be too high. An approximation of oxygen consumption can be achieved by using heart rate. Small detectors can be worn by the subject that measure heart rate. Within limits, heart rate and oxygen consumption tend to be linearly related throughout a large portion of the aerobic work range. Heart rate can thus be used as a measure of activity and as an indirect estimate of energy expenditure. However,

TABLE 5.2
Energy Expenditure for Various Sports and Exercises

		Body Weight (kg)							
Activity	**kcal/min/kg**	**50**	**56**	**62**	**68**	**74**	**80**	**89**	**98**
Archery	0.065	3.3[a]	3.6	4.0	4.4	4.8	5.2	5.8	6.4
Badminton	0.097	4.9	5.4	6.0	6.6	7.2	7.8	8.6	9.5
Basketball	0.183	6.9	7.7	8.6	9.4	10.2	11.0	12.3	13.5
Boxing (in ring)	0.222	6.9	7.7	8.6	9.4	10.2	11.0	12.3	13.5
Canoeing (leisure)	0.044	2.2	2.5	2.7	3.0	3.3	3.5	3.9	4.3
Circuit training									
Hydra-fitness	0.132	6.6	7.4	8.2	9.0	9.7	10.5	11.7	12.9
Nautilus	0.092	4.6	5.2	5.8	6.3	6.8	7.4	8.2	9.1
Free weights	0.086	4.3	4.8	5.3	5.8	6.3	6.8	7.6	8.4
Hill climbing	0.121	6.1	6.8	7.5	8.2	9.0	9.7	10.8	11.9
Cycling									
5.5 miles/h	0.064	3.2	3.6	4.0	4.4	4.7	5.1	5.7	6.3
9.4 miles/h	0.100	5.0	5.6	6.2	6.8	7.4	8.0	8.9	9.8
Field hockey	0.134	6.7	7.5	8.3	9.1	9.9	10.7	11.9	13.1
Football	0.132	6.6	7.4	8.2	9.0	9.8	10.6	11.7	12.9
Golf	0.085	4.3	4.8	5.3	5.8	6.3	6.8	7.6	8.3
Gymnastics	0.066	3.3	3.7	4.1	4.5	4.9	5.3	5.9	6.5
Jumping rope									
70/min	0.162	8.1	9.1	10.0	11.0	12.0	13.0	14.4	15.9
125/min	0.177	8.9	9.9	11.0	12.0	13.1	14.2	15.2	17.3
Running, cross country	0.163	8.2	9.1	10.1	11.1	12.1	13.0	14.0	16.9
Skiing level									
Moderate speed	0.119	6.0	6.7	7.4	8.1	8.8	9.5	10.2	11.7
Squash	0.212	10.6	11.9	13.1	14.4	15.7	17.0	18.2	20.8
Swimming									
Backstroke	0.169	8.5	9.5	10.5	11.5	12.5	13.5	14.5	16.6
Table tennis	0.068	3.4	3.8	4.2	4.6	5.0	5.4	5.8	6.7
Walking									
Hard surface	0.080	4.0	4.5	5.0	5.4	5.9	6.4	6.9	7.8

Source: Adapted from McArdle, W.D. et al., *Exercise Physiology, Energy, Nutrition, and Human Performance*, 3rd edn., Appendix D, Lea & Febiger, Philadelphia, PA, 1991, pp. 804–811.

[a] kcal/min; 1 kg = 2.2 lb.

heart rate and oxygen consumption are not always parallel. The type of activity can determine whether heart rate and oxygen consumption are linearly related. For example, the oxygen consumption of an individual participating in aerobic dance will increase heart rate to a much higher level than that of an individual consuming the same amount of oxygen but running on a treadmill.[5,6] In arm exercise where the arm muscles are contracting statically as in a straining type exercise, heart rates are significantly higher than when leg muscles are being similarly exercised. Just as energy expenditure measurements can be influenced by environmental factors, so too can heart rate. These factors include environmental temperature, emotional state, food intake, body position, the muscle groups being exercised, and whether the exercise is continuous or intermittent. Whether the muscles are working rhythmically or contracting isometrically also influences heart rate.

The total energy expended through physical activity is additive to the basal energy needed to sustain the body in the resting state. Hence, the net energy expended by an individual equals the total energy expended minus the resting energy expenditure for the equivalent period of time. As individuals repeat these activities on a regular basis, there is a measure of efficiency of movement that develops over time. This means that with time and repetition, there is an increase in mechanical efficiency such that more work can be accomplished per unit of energy expended. Whether the work is defined as miles walked or laps in a swimming pool or jumps per minute using a jumping rope, the energy expended per unit of time will decrease as the individual becomes more proficient in this activity. The increase in proficiency is interpreted to mean that a training effect has developed. Trained persons consume less oxygen and use less energy over a given period of time than untrained individuals. Training improves the mechanical efficiency of the whole body, not just the particular muscle groups used for the exercise. Training improves heart action and lung function as well as muscle metabolism.

With exercise, oxygen consumption increases until a steady state is achieved where the oxygen consumed equals the target tissue oxygen uptake. With training, this steady state is achieved sooner than without training. Oxygen consumption does not increase instantly at the start of exercise. In the beginning stage of exercise, the oxygen uptake is considerably below the steady state even though the energy need remains unchanged. The lag in oxygen consumption is compensated for by the use of immediate energy-producing reactions in the muscle, primarily those reactions involving the high-energy bonds of creatine phosphate and ATP. Oxygen becomes important for the subsequent reactions of energy transfer via oxidative phosphorylation and the aerobic reactions of the citric acid cycle, fatty acid oxidation, and amino acid oxidation. Until the steady state is achieved, there is an oxygen debt. This deficit can be viewed quantitatively as the difference between the total oxygen consumed during the exercise and the total that would have been consumed had a steady rate of aerobic metabolism been reached immediately at the initiation of the exercise. Until aerobic metabolism is fully engaged, anaerobic metabolism takes place (see review, nutritional biochemistry). Primarily, this involves the use of the glycolytic pathway. Glucose and glucose released from glycogen serve as fuels for this pathway. As aerobic metabolism is lagging, the glycolytic pathway produces lactic acid. Normally, the end product of glycolysis is pyruvate, which then enters the mitochondrial citric acid cycle. However, this is impaired when there is an oxygen debt. As the debt increases, so too does the level of lactate, not only in the muscle but also in the blood. With the establishment of the steady state, the oxygen debt is resolved, and a balance between aerobic and anaerobic metabolism is reestablished. Although there is an accumulation of lactate initially, this dissipates as the steady state is achieved. Training facilitates this transition (reestablishment of the balance between aerobic and anaerobic metabolism). Furthermore, training facilitates an efficient use of available fuels for muscle metabolism. Glycogen stores can be made more available within the muscle, and there is an adaptation in metabolism with respect to the use of alternate fuel sources such as free fatty acids. Although training assists in establishing a steady state with respect to oxygen use and consumption, there is a limit to the steady state. When this limit is achieved, fatigue is sensed, and the willingness of the person to exercise actively is reduced. The individual will then need a period of recovery. If fatigue is ignored, exhaustion will set in and the individual will no longer be able to exercise. With fatigue, lactate levels are higher than during the preexercise period and the acidity of muscle and blood increases. This has a dramatic effect on the intracellular environment. The alkaline reserve is called into play in order to buffer the acidity of the muscle and blood. Trained individuals appear to tolerate higher levels of blood and muscle lactate levels than untrained individuals.

In addition to the aforementioned metabolic changes in muscle, there are pulmonary and cardiovascular responses to exercise that are part of the whole body response to physical activity. Respiration and heart rate increase immediately with the initiation of exercise. The extent of these increases depends on the work load and its intensity. The respiratory response is fully integrated with the cardiovascular response such that the exercise-induced increase in heat and CO_2 production can be removed. With an increase in heart rate, there is an increase in circulation to the muscle where there are increases in the extraction of oxygen from the blood in exchange for CO_2 and in the lungs where there are increases in the reverse direction: increased extraction of CO_2 from the blood in exchange for oxygen. The increase in respiratory exchange carries with it an increase in the elimination of heat via the expired air. Heat is also dissipated through sweat and through radiation from the body surface.

MINIMUM PHYSICAL ACTIVITY RECOMMENDATIONS

In order to achieve the health benefits of an active lifestyle, the individual should include at least 150–500 min/week of moderately intense exercise.[7–9] If the exercise is very intense, then the time can be reduced to 75–150 min/week. Regardless of the intensity of the exercise, the exercise period should include muscle strengthening exercises. Including both aerobic and anaerobic activities will result in an increase in body fitness with its accompanying health benefit. According to the most recent (2008) Physical Activity Guidelines for Americans,[8] adults should include the following activities:

- Two hours, 30 min/week of moderate intensity or 1 h and 15 min of vigorous intensity/week of aerobic physical activity. It need not be a single type of activity but can vary according to the wishes of the individual. The activity should be performed in episodes of at least 10 min spread out through the week.
- Additional health benefits are provided when the activity period is increased to 5 h/week of moderate intensity or 2 h and 30 min of vigorous intensity activity.
- The activity period should include muscle strengthening exercises that involve all the major muscle groups, and this set of exercises should be performed at least twice a week.

The benefits as described earlier associated with regular physical activity/exercise are listed in Table 5.3.

The American College of Sports Medicine (ACSM) has prepared guidelines for exercise testing and prescription.[10] These are very useful in developing plans to increase the physical activity of sedentary people. The guidelines include pretest clinical evaluation, physical fitness testing and interpretation, and clinical exercise testing and interpretation. The pretest clinical evaluation should

TABLE 5.3
Benefits of Regular Physical Activity/Exercise

Increased maximal oxygen uptake due to both central and peripheral adaptations
Lower minute ventilation at a given submaximal intensity
Lower myocardial oxygen cost for a given absolute submaximal intensity
Lower heart rate and blood pressure at a given submaximal intensity
Increased capillary density in skeletal muscle
Increased exercise threshold for the accumulation of lactate in the blood
Increased exercise threshold for the onset of disease signs/symptom: reduction in coronary artery disease risk factors (reduced resting systolic/diastolic pressures, reduced blood triglycerides, reduced body fat), improvements in glucose homeostasis (reduced insulin needs, improved_target tissue sensitivity to insulin, improved glucose tolerance), and reduction in intra-abdominal fat.

Sources: U.S. Department of Health and Human Services, 2008. Physical activity guidelines for Americans, http://www.health.gov/PAGuidelines/guidelines/default.aspx, Accessed October 7, 2013; U.S. Department of health and Human Services, 2010. Healthy people 2020, http://www. healthypeople.gov, Accessed October 8, 2013; *ACSM's Guidelines for Exercise T and Prescription*, 6th edn., American College of Sports Medicine, Lippincott Williams & Wilkins, Philadelphia, PA, 2000, 368pp.

include a medical history and physical examination that includes measuring blood pressure; blood analysis for glucose, lipids, and lipoproteins; alternative stress testing; and pulmonary function testing. Medical screening is important if the exercise program is to have therapeutic benefits. There are risks associated with exercise particularly by previously sedentary individuals.[11] Indications for increased risk include blood pressure abnormalities, history of cardiac problems, respiratory problems (abnormal pulmonary function), history of diabetes, history of disordered blood lipids, and other medical problems. Those with concurrent infectious disease or with metabolic diseases such as those associated with mitochondrial malfunction should be regarded as at risk of an untoward outcome with exercise.[12] Individuals at risk for medical problems associated with exercise should be closely monitored and intervention strategies developed to prevent these problems. Often, patients recovering from cardiac problems or other disabilities will benefit from medically supervised exercise programs that are geared to improving the recovery from such problems. Cardiac rehabilitation, for example, is a significant and important adjunctive exercise therapy that has benefits for the patient recovering from heart surgery or cardiovascular events.

EXERCISE AND NUTRIENT NEEDS

There is no doubt that nutrition supports physical activity and vice versa. Without good nutrient intakes, physical activity is limited. Regardless of whether the goal is to attain peak competitive status or to optimize one's health and fitness, at the heart of each of these is the provision of appropriate fluid and food intakes that support normal metabolism.[13–17] The appropriate selection of foods and fluids that meet nutritional needs is essential to the optimal response to exercise. It is the key to achieving optimal physical performance.

According to the most recent (2009) Nutrition and Athletic Performance position paper[15] issued by the Academy of Nutrition and Dietetics (formerly the American Dietetics Association), Dieticians of Canada, and the ACSM, "physical activity, athletic performance and recovery from exercise are enhanced by optimal nutrition." The energy intake recommendation categorized by physical activity level (PAL) is shown in Table 5.4, while the recommendations for the intakes for the macronutrients are shown in Tables 5.5. The recommendations for the intakes of the vitamins and minerals are those of the Food and Nutrition Board of the National Academy of Sciences. The daily dietary recommended intakes (DRIs) for males and females who exercise and who are not in the category of the elite athlete are usually not different from those of sedentary people. The DRIs[16] for the vitamins and minerals for adult males and females (age 19 to <70) are shown in Table 5.6. Strenuous exercise as performed by the elite athlete *may* increase the needs for the micronutrients, but there is little research to document this possibility.[14] It is generally accepted that if the athlete (elite or otherwise) meets his/her macronutrient needs and consumes enough food energy to maintain a healthy body weight, then that athlete will consume sufficient amounts of the micronutrients. Table 5.6 also includes the recommendations for micronutrient intake as outlined in the Position on Nutrition and Athletic Performance.[15] Not all of the micronutrients are addressed by the Position statement. Hence, there are a number of blank entries in this table with respect to the Position statement on the micronutrients.

In addition to meeting the nutrient needs to support physical activity, attention to the fluid intake is essential. Hydration must be maintained to support optimal performance. Water balance can be disturbed if the exercise is of high intensity for long periods of time. Individuals sweating profusely will lose considerable amounts of water (and electrolytes) that must be replaced if the individual is to continue the exercise. Electrolyte solutions may be of benefit to the physically active individual. The heat and humidity of the environment will influence water loss. Loss is greater in warm environments than in cool environments. The perception of water loss is greater in humid environments than in dry ones because the dry environment facilitates evaporative water loss from the skin. Losing water in this way (without the perception of water loss) can be dangerous if the water loss is not replaced continuously. Dehydration in dry environments can occur quickly.

TABLE 5.4
Energy Intake Recommendations Based on DRIs and the Dietary Guidelines for Americans

DRI[16] for Energy (EER)[a–c]			Dietary Guidelines for Americans[7] (kcal)[d–f]		
Height (in meters)/ Activity level	**EER Males (BMI 18.5–24.99)**	**EER Females (BMI 18.5–24.99)**	**Age (in years)/ Activity level avg.**	**Males (BMI, 22.1 avg.)**	**Females (BMI, 21.6)**
1.50 M			*19–30 years*		
Sedentary	1848–2080	1625–1762	Sedentary	2400–2600	1800–2000
Low active	2009–2267	1803–1956	Moderate active	2600–2800	2000–2200
Active	2215–2506	2025–2198	Active	3000	2400
Very active	2554–2898	2291–2489			
1.65 M			*31–50 years*		
Sedentary	2068–2349	1816–1982	Sedentary	2200–2400	1800
Low active	2254–2566	2016–2202	Moderate active	2400–2600	2000
Active	2490–2842	2267–2477	Active	2800–3000	2200
Very active	2880–3296	2567–2807			
1.80 M			*51 + Years*		
Sedentary	2301–2635	2015–2211	Sedentary	2000–2200	1600
Low active	2513–2884	2239–2459	Moderate active	2200–2400	1800
Active	2882–3200	2519–2769	Active	2400–2800	2000–2200
Very active	3225–3720	2855–3141			

[a] DRIs represent recommendations for males and females 30 years of age; for each year below/above 30, add/subtract 7 kcal/day for females and 10 kcal/day for males.

[b] EER is the average energy intake that is predicted to maintain energy balance in healthy normal-weight individuals of a defined age, sex, weight, height, and level of activity consistent with good health (based on a BMI value between 18.5 and 24.99).

[c] Regression equations based on doubly labeled water data: female EER = 354–691 × age (years) + PA × [9.36 weight (kg) + height (m)]; male EER = 662–9.53 × age (years) + PA × [15.91 × weight (kg) + 539.6 × height (m)]. PA represents physical activity, which differs depending on PAL (the ratio of total energy expenditure/basal energy expenditure): PA = 1.0 for both males and females if PAL is 1.0–1.39; PA = 1.11 (males) or 1.12 (females) if PAL is 1.4–1.59, low active (typically daily activities + 30–60 min of daily moderate activity). PA = 1.25 (males) and 1.27 (females) if PAL is 1.6–1.89, active (typical daily living activity plus at least 60 min of daily moderate activity). PA is 1.48 (males) or 1.45 (females) if PAL is 1.9–2.5, very active (typical daily living activities plus at least 60 min of moderate activity plus 60 min of vigorous activity or at least 120 min of moderate activity).

[d] Dietary guideline recommendations are used when no quantitative DRI value is available and are applied to ages 2 and older.

[e] Values are rounded to the nearest 200 kcal; an individual's energy needs may be higher or lower than these average estimates.

[f] Values are based on EER and the reference size of median height and weight; for adults, the reference man is 5 ft 10 in. tall and weighs 154 lb. The reference woman is 5 ft 4 in. tall and weighs 126 lb. Sedentary is a lifestyle that includes only light physical activity. Moderately active is a lifestyle that includes physical activity equivalent to walking 1.5–3 miles/day at 3–4 miles/h in addition to activities associated with daily living. Active is a lifestyle that includes physical activity equivalent to walking 3 miles/day at 3–4 miles/h in addition to the light physical activity associated with daily living. The kcal ranges shown are to accommodate the needs of different ages within the group; fewer kcal are needed at older ages. Estimates for females do not include women who are pregnant or who are breast feeding.

TABLE 5.5
Carbohydrate, Fat, and Protein Intake Recommendations Based on the DRIs and the Position on Nutrition and Athletic Performance

DRI[16] Recommendations for the Macronutrients	Position on Nutrition and Athletic Performance[15]
AMDR (carbohydrate as a % of total energy)*	
Adults, 19 to >70 yrs: 45%–65%	Range for exercising adults: 6–10 g/kg body weight/day.
Carbohydrates: males: 130; females 130	
Total fiber, AI: males 19–50: 38; females 19–50: 25; males 51 to >70: 30; females 51 to >70: 21	Caution is recommended in using specific percentages, for example, 60% of energy from added sugars. Limit to no more than 25% of energy carbohydrates as a basis for meal planning.
ADMA (protein as a % of energy intake)	
Adults, age 19–70: 10%–35%	Most individuals should include 0.8 g/kg/day.
RDA, g/day: Males: 56, females 46	Range for endurance athletes is ~1.2–1.4 g/kg/day.
Essential Amino acids RDAs (mg/kg/day)	Range for strength-trained athlete: 1.2–1.7 g/kg/day.
Adult males and females	
Histidine: 14	The amount of protein needed to maintain muscle mass may be lower for resistance training due to more efficient protein utilization.
Isoleucine:19	
Leucine: 42	
Lysine: 38	
Methionine + cysteine: 19	The amount of protein needed to maintain muscle mass may be higher in the initial phase of training.
Phenylalanine + tyrosine: 33	
Threonine: 20	
Tryptophan: 5	Protein intake recommendations can usually be met through diet without the need for supplements. Vegetarian athletes may need dietetic advice to ensure adequacy of intake.
Valine: 24	
AMDR (percent of energy from fat)	
Adults, 19 to >70: 20%–35%	Recommendation: 20%–30% of energy.
AMDR (% of energy), n-6 polyunsaturated fatty acids	Fat composition should be equal portions of saturated, monounsaturated, and polyunsaturated fat.
Adults, age 19 to >70: 5%–10%	
AMDR (% energy), n-3 polyunsaturated fatty acids	
Adults, 19 to >70 years: 0.6–1.2	A trained individual uses a greater % of fat as fuel than an untrained person.
Linoleic acid AI (g/day)	There is no benefit in consuming a low fat or fat free diet (diets having < than 15% fat).
Males, age 19–50: 17; Females, age 19–50: 12	
Males, age 51 to >70: 14; Females, age 51 to >70: 11	High fat (>70% of energy) diets are not recommended.
α-Linolenic acid AI (g/day)	
Males, age 19 to >70: 1.6; Females, age 19 to >70: 1.1	

* Abbreviations used: DRI; acceptable macronutrient distribution range (AMDR); recommended dietary allowances per day (RDA); adequate intake (AI).

ELITE ATHLETES

The highly competitive professional athlete is in a special group of physically active individuals. The elite athlete differs from the recreational athlete in the time spent in training for competition. These athletes may spend many hours a day preparing for competitive events, whether they are involved in team sports such as football or in individual sports such as running or gymnastics. The elite athlete usually trains at high intensity for long periods of time to hone their skills to perform in competitions.

TABLE 5.6
Daily Vitamin and Mineral Intake Recommendations for Adult Males and Females

	DRI[16]	
Nutrient	**Gender/amount**	**Position on Nutrition and Athletic Performance[15]**
Thiamin (mg)	Male, 1.0; female, 0.9	0.5 mg/1000 kcal is recommended.
Riboflavin (mg)	Male, 1.3; female, 1.1	0.6 mg/1000 kcal is recommended.
Niacin (mg)	Male, 16; female, 14	Same as DRIs.
Vitamin B_6 (mg)	Male, 1.3–1.7; female, 1.3–1.5	Exercise *may* increase needs.
Folacin (μg)	Male, 400; female, 400	
Pantothenic acid (mg)[a]	Male, 5; female, 5	
Vitamin B_{12} (μg)[a]	Male, 2.4; female, 2.4	
Biotin (μg)[a]	Male, 30; female, 30	
Choline (mg)[a]	Male, 550; female, 425	
Ascorbic acid (mg)	Male, 75; female, 60	
Vitamin A (μg)	Male, 625; female, 500	
Vitamin D (μg)	Male, 5–10; female, 5–10	
Vitamin E (mg)	Male, 12; female, 12	
Vitamin K (μg)	Male, 120; female, 90	
Sodium (g)[a]	Male, 1.5; female, 1.5	
Potassium (g)[a]	Male, 4.7; female, 4.7	
Chloride (g)[a]	Male, 2.3; female, 2.3	
Calcium (mg)[a]	Male, 1000; female, 1000	Attention to calcium intake is important to prevent osteopenia, stress fractures, and loss of bone mineral.
Phosphorus (mg)	Male, 700; female, 700	
Magnesium (mg)	Male, 400–420; females, 310–320	Calcium, iron, zinc, and magnesium intakes may be inadequate if diets are restricted.
Iron (mg)	Male, 8; female, 15–18[b]	Iron deficiency can develop if athletes do not consume sufficient amounts of iron-rich foods.
Zinc (mg)	Male, 11; female, 8	Vegetarian athletes are at risk for zinc deficiency.
Iodide (pg)	Male, 150; female, 150	
Selenium (pg)	Male, 55; female, 55	
Chromium (μg)[a]	Male, 30–35; female, 20–25	
Copper (μg)	Male, 900; female, 900	
Fluoride (mg)[a]	Male, 4; female, 3	
Manganese (mg)[a]	Male, 2.3; female, 1.8	
Molybdenum (μg)	Male, 45; female, 45	

Source: www.nap.edu. Accessed October 2013.

[a] Acceptable intake; not enough data to determine DRI for this nutrient.

[b] Applies to menstruating females.

Although the sports may differ in the details of their performance, training will involve both strength and conditioning workouts that are specific to that particular sport. The nutrient needs of the elite athlete are similar to the recreational athlete with respect to the qualitative dimensions of the diet but the quantitative dimension differs.[14] The diet must provide sufficient energy from carbohydrates, proteins, and fats to maintain the body in peak physical condition and to support the activity. This broad statement lacks the detail needed for concrete recommendations for nutrient intakes. Research is lacking with respect to the particular nutrient needs. That is, we do not know how much of each of the essential nutrients should be consumed by the elite athlete to maximize his/her physical health. Many athletes follow bizarre dietary regimens that they believe will maximize their athletic performance. In many instances, these dietary routines are not based on rigorously tested scientific concepts.

Carbohydrates are important to athletic performance and have received research attention.[14] Carbohydrate intake or carbohydrate availability should be maximized for optimal performance. The 2010 International Olympic Committee (IOC) Consensus Statement on Sports Nutrition[19] advises elite athletes to begin competition with adequate carbohydrate reserves, that is, maximal glycogen reserve and maximal blood glucose levels consistent with good health. The rationale for this statement resides with the concept that the carbohydrate needs are not static but change daily based on training schedules and competition dates. Carbohydrate needs also are affected by injuries, recovery from same, and intensity of the competition. Aside from these are the adjustments needed to accommodate differing competition types: individual performance versus team performance, skill sports versus endurance competitions, and sports for persons of low body weight versus sports where large body weight is important. All of these factors need to be considered with respect to the carbohydrate intake. Carbohydrate ingestion during endurance exercise has been shown to improve performance.[20]

In those sports where muscle breakdown and resynthesis are characteristic of the competition (power and strength athletes, i.e., weight lifters and wrestlers), the need for protein intake might be higher than for sports where muscle turnover is normal. For the elite athlete trying to alter body composition to increase lean body mass while decreasing fat mass, an intake of 1.7 g/kg protein may be warranted. Mettler et al.[21] studied weight lifters who reduced their energy intake by 40%. One group consumed 2.3 g protein/kg/body weight (35% energy as protein), while a control group consumed 0.7 g protein/kg/body weight. Both groups consumed the same amount of carbohydrate. When protein was increased, fat intake was decreased. Both groups lost weight as fat, but the group consuming the higher amount of protein lost very little lean body mass, whereas the control group lost about 1.5 kg of muscle mass. Many athletes believe that dietary protein is the key to athletic success. However, it is not the quantity of protein consumed but the quality and the timing of the food consumed. Resistance training leads to changes in muscle tissue in the hours following the training stimulus. The postworkout period is the preferred time to consume protein/amino acids to encourage muscle protein synthesis and accretion. The amount of protein/amino acids needed for this effect is very small: ~6 g of essential amino acids or ~20 g of high-quality protein will elicit this effect. This is less than the protein found in a quarter-pound hamburger at the local fast-food shop. Excessive protein intakes (above that recommended for protein maintenance) mean that the excess protein consumed is deaminated and the amino acids used for metabolic fuel. This is a costly process and places a burden on the kidneys to excrete the excess nitrogen from the deaminated amino acids. There is very little storage of dietary protein consumed in excess of need (see Chapter 8). Little is known about the needs for the micronutrients by the elite athlete. As with the recreational athlete, the assumption is that if the elite athlete is consuming sufficient carbohydrate, protein, and fat to maintain body weight and achieve optimal athletic performance, then the micronutrient needs are met.

AGING AND EXERCISE

Aging impacts both the quality of life and longevity through reduced musculoskeletal function (sarcopenia). This loss in function represents molecular aging. It is not known whether the process can be reversed. One 20-week study examined the impact of exercise on the phenotypic expression of aging and then attempted to identify unique gene pathways associated with age-related muscle change.[22] The investigators generated genome-wide transcript profiles from 44 subjects who had supervised resistance training. There was a wide range of responses from these subjects with respect to hypertrophy of the skeletal muscle. The range was from 3% to 28%. Those who gained the most had inhibited mTOR activation of muscle growth as characterized by inhibited activation of the muscle growth genes. There were inconsistent molecular responses to the exercise treatment that were independent of age.

Despite the inconsistent results in this study, there are a number of reports showing that exercise has a beneficial effect on a number of measures in elderly people. For example, Shibata and Levine[23] reported on the effects of progressive exercise training of people over the age of 65. The exercise was progressively increased over a 1-year period to 200 min/week. After 1 year, the effective arterial elastance, peripheral vascular resistance, and systemic arterial compliance were improved even though there was no change in aortic age nor was there any improvement in aortic stiffening. Vaughan et al. reported that exercise improved cognition and physical functioning of elderly women.[24] Swift et al. reported that exercise improved blood pressure of elderly women.[25] Other investigators have also reported similar results yet none have reported a reversal of the age-induced changes in the musculoskeletal system, the cardiovascular system, the neural system, or any other critical system. Exercise improves the quality of life but does not reverse age degenerative change.

SUMMARY

1. Physical activity (exercise) is defined as body movement that is planned, structured, repetitive, and purposive. Its purpose is to increase energy expenditure.
2. The impact of exercise on energy expenditure is dependent on body size, age, gender, aerobic muscle mass, and the frequency and intensity of the activity.
3. Energy expenditure is expressed as kcal/min or L O_2/min or mL O_2 consumed/kg body weight/min.
4. Measuring heart rate can approximate oxygen consumption.
5. Training increases the efficiency of muscular activity with respect to oxygen use.
6. Fatigue is associated with increased muscle and blood lactate levels, increased muscle and blood acidity, and an increased use of the alkaline reserve.
7. Nutrient needs are not usually affected by the recreational athlete.
8. The elite athlete may have an increase in energy need, an increase in protein need, and small increases in micronutrient needs.
9. The minimum physical activity of an adult should be 150–200 min/week.

LEARNING OPPORTUNITIES

There are several over-the-counter drink mixtures. They promise to keep the drinker awake and functional to party, study, work, and generally live life in top gear. These drinks contain varying amounts of caffeine and sugar and few or no electrolytes.

Depending on the brand, caffeine content of these drinks ranges from about 50 to 500 mg/8 oz serving. In addition, again depending on the brand, these drinks may contain a range of additional ingredients such as many of the B complex vitamins, ginseng, guarana, and taurine.

Based on this information, answer the following questions:

1. Suggest a purpose for each of the listed ingredients.
2. What are the positive and negative aspects of caffeine consumption?
3. Is there such a thing as too much caffeine? What are some of the physiologic consequences of too much caffeine consumption over an extended period of time?
4. In 2002, many energy drink companies began offering a product that was both an energy drink and an alcoholic drink with higher alcohol percentage than many beers. Suggest why the complicated effects of such drinks were widely concerning to many college administrators across the country. What would happen if a 5′2″ female weighing 110 lb consumed a can and a half of one of these drinks?
5. Using your knowledge of energy production and body energy stores, explain why, during exercise, cells rely more on glucose and fat for energy than on protein.
6. Do a risk–benefit analysis of three ergogenic aids. List the risks and benefits of each. Focus on both cellular level and tissue level effects of such aids. Write a conclusion as to whether each is really helpful.

REFERENCES

1. Durnin, J.V.G.A., Passmore, R. (1967) *Energy, Work and Leisure*. Heinmann, London, U.K., pp. 1–340.
2. Delmonico, M.J., Harris, T., Visser, M., Park, S.W., Conroy, M.B., Velasquez-Mieyer, P., Boudreau, R. et al. (2009) Longitudinal study of muscle strength, quality, and adipose tissue infiltration. *Am. J. Clin Nutr.* 90: 1579–1585.
3. McArdle, W.D., Katch, F.I., Katch, V.L. (1991) *Exercise Physiology: Energy, Nutrition, and Human Performance*, 3d edn. Lea & Febiger, Malvern, PA, 853pp.
4. Keim, N., Jahns, L. (2013) Energy assessment: Physical activity. In: *Handbook of Nutrition and Food* (C.D. Berdanier, J. Dwyer, D. Heber, eds.), 3rd edn. CRC Press, Boca Raton, FL, pp. 693–702.
5. Mass, S. (1989) The validity of the use of heart rate in estimating oxygen consumption in static and in combined static/dynamic exercise. *Ergonomics* 32: 141–149.
6. Parker, S.B. et al. (1989) Failure of target heart rate to accurately monitor intensity during aerobic dance. *Med. Sci. Sport Exerc.* 21: 230–236.
7. U.S. Department of Agriculture and the U.S. Department of Health and Human Services. (2010) Dietary guidelines for Americans. http://www.cnpp.usda.gov/dietaryguidelines.htm. Accessed October 7, 2013.
8. U.S. Department of Health and Human Services. (2008) Physical activity guidelines for Americans. http://www.health.gov/PAGuidelines/guidelines/default.aspx. Accessed October 7, 2013.
9. U.S. Department of health and Human Services. (2010) Healthy people 2020. http://www. healthypeople.gov. Accessed October 8, 2013.
10. (2000) *ACSM's Guidelines for Exercise T and Prescription*, 6th edn. American College of Sports Medicine, Lippincott Williams & Wilkins, Philadelphia, PA, 368pp.
11. Bouchard, C, Blair, S.N., Church, T.S., Earnest, C.P., Hagberg, J.M., Hakkinen, K., Jenkins, N.T. et al. (2012) Adverse metabolic response to regular exercise: Is it a rare or common occurrence? *PLoS One* 7: e37887–e37894.
12. Mancuso, M., Angelini, C., Bertini, E., Carelli, V., Cmoi, G.P., Minetti, C., Moggio, M. et al. (2012) Fatigue and exercise intolerance in mitochondrial diseases. Literature revision and experience of the Italian Network of mitochondrial diseases. *Neuromuscul. Disord.* 22: S226–S229.
13. Laing, E.M. (2013) Exercise and nutrient needs. In: *Handbook of Nutrition and Food* (C.D. Berdanier, J. Dwyer, D. Heber, eds.), 3rd edn. CRC Press, Boca Raton, FL, pp. 359–371.
14. Rosenbloom, C. (2013) Nutrient needs of the elite athlete (2013) In: *Handbook of Nutrition and Food*, 3rd edn. (C.D. Berdanier, J. Dwyer, D. Heber, eds.). CRC Press, Boca Raton, FL, pp. 373–379.
15. Rodriguez, N.R., DiMarco, N.M., Langley, S. (2009) Position of the American dietetic association, dietitians of Canada and the American college of medicine: Nutrition and athletic performance. *J. Am. Diet Assoc.* 109: 509–527.
16. Institute of Medicine. (2005) *Dietary Reference Intakes for Energy, Carbohydrate, Fiber, Fatty Acids, Cholesterol, Protein, and Amino acids* (*Macronutrients*). National Academy Press, Washington, DC.
17. Steen, S.N., Butterfield, G. (1998) Diet and nutrition. In: *ACSM's Resource Manual for Guidelines for Exercise Testing and Prescription* (J. Roitman, M. Williams, eds.), 3rd edn. Williams and Wilkins, Baltimore, MA, pp. 27–35.
18. www.nap.edu. Accessed October 2013.
19. IOC consensus statement on sports nutrition 2012. www.olympic.org/Documents/Reports/EN/CONSENSUS-FINAL-v8-en-pdf. Accessed October 2013.
20. Temesi, J., Johnson, N.A., Raymond, J., Burdon, C.A., O'Connor, H.T. (2011) Carbohydrate ingestion during endurance exercise improves performance in adults. *J. Nutr.* 141: 890–896.
21. Mettler, S., Mitchell, N., Tipton, K.D. (2010) Increased protein intake reduces lean body mass loss during weight loss in athletes. *Med. Sci. Sports Exerc.* 42: 326.
22. Phillips, B.E., Williams, J.P., Gustagsson, T., Bouchard, C., Rankinen, T., Knudsen, S., Smith, K., Timmons, J.A., Atherton, P.J. (2013) Molecular networks of human muscle adaptation to exercise and age. *PLoS Genet.* 9: e1003369.
23. Shibata, S., Levine, B.D. (2012) Effects of exercise training on biologic vascular age in healthy seniors. *Am. J. Physiol. Heart Circ. Physiol.* 302: H1340–H1346.
24. Vaugh, S., Morris, N., Shum, D., O'Dwyer, S., Polit, D. (2012) Study protocol: A randomized controlled trial of the effects of a multi-modal exercise program on cognition and physical functioning in older women. *BMC Geriatr.* 12: 60–66.
25. Swift, D.L., Earnest, C.P., Katzmarzk, P.T., Rankinen, T., Blair, S.N., Church, T.S. (2012) The effect of different doses of aerobic exercise training on exercise blood pressure in overweight and obese post-menopausal women. *Menopause* 19: 503–509.

6 Cell Cycle, Life Cycle

Living creatures consist of one or more cells. The more complex the organism, the more cells and cell types are found in that organism. Higher-order mammals contain a variety of cell types that are organized anatomically into specific tissues, organs, and systems. These tissues, organs, and systems have specific functions that are integrated into the whole functioning animal. Nutrition can affect these functions, so it is the purpose of this chapter to describe the functions of cells and their integration into the tissues, organs, and systems that function in the cycle of life.

CELL STRUCTURE AND FUNCTION

The typical eukaryotic cell (Figure 6.1) consists of a nucleus, mitochondria, lysosomes, endoplasmic reticulum, Golgi apparatus, and microsomes surrounded by the cell sap or cytosol. Membranes surround the organelles within the cytosol as well as the cell itself. Each segment or organelle has a particular function and is characterized by specific reactions and metabolic pathways. These are listed in Table 6.1. Both the macronutrients and the micronutrients affect these functions. For example, an inadequate intake of folacin (see Chapter 12) will affect the synthesis of the bases that are used for DNA and RNA synthesis; this will affect cell division. Amino acid deficiency will compromise protein synthesis as will an inadequate intake of energy (see Chapters 1, 2, and 8). As a result, growth of the young will be compromised. An inadequate supply of active vitamin D will compromise bone mineralization and result in bone malformations (see Chapter 11). The kind and amount of carbohydrate in the diet will affect the cytosolic metabolic pathways with subsequent effects on intermediary metabolism (see review and Chapter 9). The types and amounts of dietary fat will affect the composition and function of the membranes in and around the cell (see Chapter 10). Altogether, nutrient intake affects the function of the various cells in the body. Some of these effects are long term, while others are short term. Some are direct, while others are indirect via nutrient effects on cell signaling systems.

RECEPTORS

Among the components of the cell are a group of proteins called receptors. There are both plasma and intracellular membrane receptors. Plasma membrane receptors typically bind peptides or proteins. These are called ligands. In many instances, these compounds are hormones, or growth factors. Upon binding, one of two processes occurs. In one, the binding of a peptide or protein (ligand) to its cognate receptor is followed by an internalization of this ligand–receptor complex. In the other, the receptor is not internalized, but when the ligand is bound to its receptor, it generates a signal that alters cell metabolism and function. Internalization of the ligand allows for its entry into the cell. It can enter either as the intact ligand or as an activated fragment that may target specific intracellular components. If it enters as an intact ligand, it can either transfer to another receptor or move to its target site in the cell by itself as it dissociates from its plasma membrane receptor. The receptor in turn is either recycled back to the plasma membrane or it is degraded. Figure 6.2 illustrates this plasma membrane–hormone binding.

There are actually four types of membrane-spanning receptors: (1) simple receptors that have a single membrane-spanning unit, (2) receptors with a single membrane-spanning unit that also involves a tyrosine kinase component on the interior aspect of the plasma membrane, (3) receptors with several membrane-spanning helical segments of their protein structures that are coupled to a

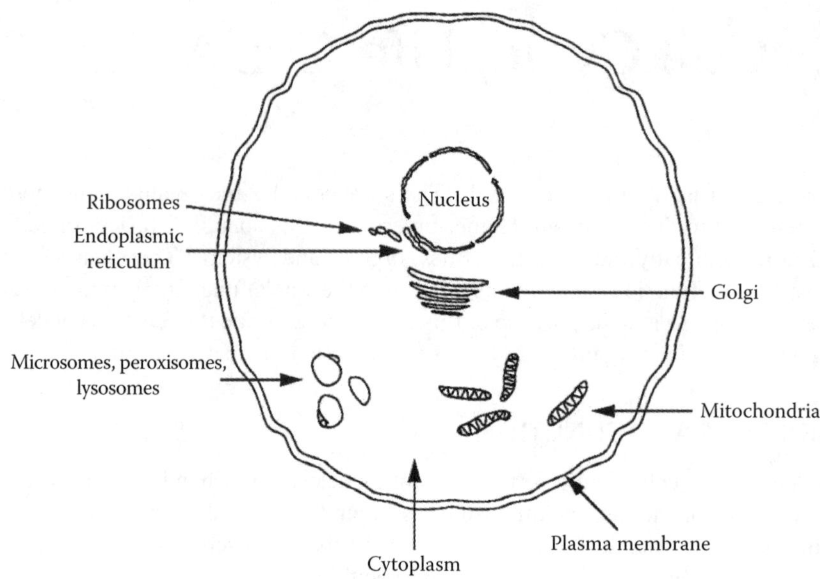

FIGURE 6.1 Typical eukaryotic cell showing representative subcellular structures.

TABLE 6.1
Functions of the Organelles/Cell Fractions of a Typical Eukaryotic Cell

Organelle/Cell Fraction	Function
Plasma membrane	Cell boundary; holds receptors for a variety of hormones; signal systems begin here; processes, exports, and imports substrates, ions, etc.; binds hormones to their respective receptors.
Cytosol	Medium for a variety of enzymes, substrates, products, ions, transporters, and signal systems; glycolysis, glycogenesis, glycogenolysis, lipogenesis, pentose shunt, part of urea synthesis, and part of protein synthesis occur in the cytosol.
Nucleus	Contains DNA, RNA, and many proteins that influence gene expression; protein synthesis starts here with DNA transcription.
Endoplasmic reticulum	Ca^{++} stored here for use in signal transduction; glucose transporters accumulate here until needed; has role in many synthetic processes.
Golgi apparatus	Sequesters, processes, and releases proteins; export mechanism for release of macromolecules.
Mitochondria	Powerhouse of cell; contains DNA that encodes 13 components of oxidative phosphorylation; Krebs cycle, respiratory chain, ATP synthesis, fatty acid oxidation, and the first step of urea synthesis occur here.
Ribosomes	Site for completion of protein synthesis.
Lysosomes	Intracellular digestion; protein and macromolecule degradation.
Peroxisomes	Suppression of oxygen free radicals; contain antioxidant enzymes.
Microsomes	Drug detoxification; detoxification and fatty acid elongation can occur here.

separate G protein (G proteins are proteins that bind guanosine triphosphate [GTP] or guanosine diphosphate [GDP]) on the interior aspect of the plasma membrane, and (4) receptors that not only have membrane-spanning units but also have a membrane-spanning ion channel. Examples of each of these are shown in Table 6.2.

Immunoglobulins typically are moved into the cell via the single membrane-spanning receptor, as are nerve growth factor (NGF) and several other growth factors. The receptors for these proteins are usually rich in cysteine. The cysteine-rich region projects out from the plasma membrane and

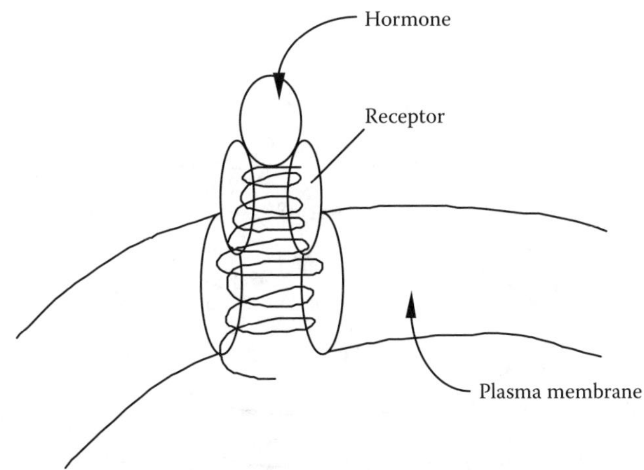

FIGURE 6.2 Schematic representation of a hormone bound to its cognate receptor in the plasma membrane.

TABLE 6.2
Types of Plasma Membrane Receptors and Examples of Ligands

Single membrane-spanning unit, no tyrosine kinase	
Ligands	Immunoglobulins
	T-cell antibodies
	Insulin-like growth factor (IGF)
	NGF
	GH
Single membrane-spanning unit with tyrosine kinase activity	
Ligands	TSH
	Insulin
	Platelet-derived growth factor (PDGF)
Multiple membrane-spanning units coupled with G protein	
Ligands	Calcitonin
	Parathyroid hormone (PTH)
	Luteinizing hormone
	Rhodopsin
	Acetylcholine
	Thyrotropin releasing hormone
Multiple membrane-spanning units coupled with G protein and an ion channel	
Ligand	γ-Aminobutyric acid (GABA)

is important for the binding of the ligand through disulfide bonds. Insulin and thyroid-stimulating hormone (TSH) are moved into the cell via a single membrane-spanning unit that has a tyrosine kinase activity. There is a considerable homology between the first type of receptor and this type of receptor in the portion of the receptor that binds the ligand. Where the receptors differ is in the portion that extends into and projects through the interior aspect of the plasma membrane. On the interior aspect of these single membrane-spanning receptors is a tyrosine kinase domain. The tyrosine kinase portion of the receptor is involved in the intracellular signaling systems. These can be very complex cascades, as illustrated in Figure 6.3. In this illustration, an ion (Ca^+) channel is also depicted, as are the two major intracellular signaling systems, the phosphatidylinositol (PIP) and the adenylate cyclase signaling systems.

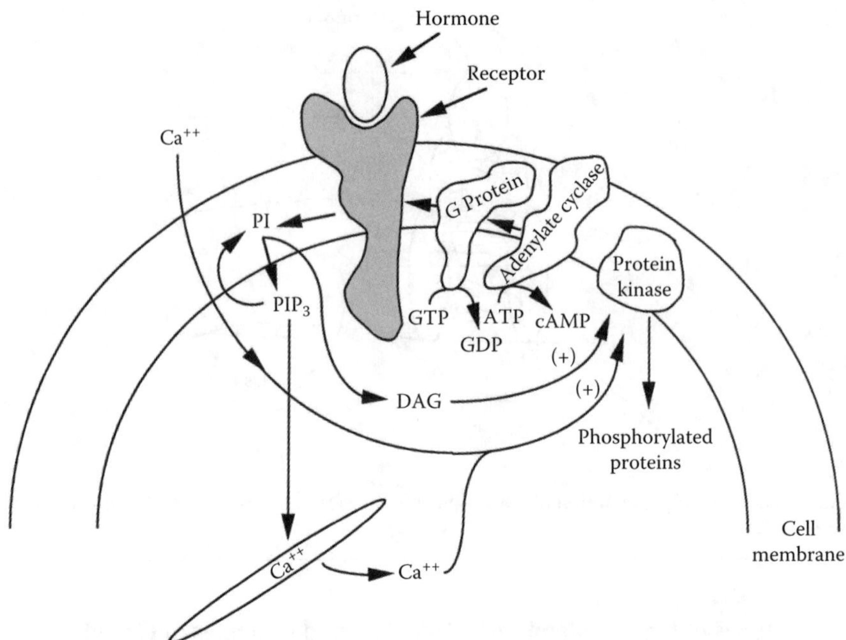

FIGURE 6.3 Hormone–receptor reaction that involves G proteins, adenylate cyclase, proteins, the PIP cycle, and cAMP. When the hormone binds to the receptor, a cascade of events follows. The G protein moves over to the receptor protein and binds GTP. Adenylate cyclase moves over and binds to the G protein and, in the process, energy is released. The cAMP level then rises and through the action of phosphodiesterase is converted to 5′ AMP. ATP is regenerated by the mitochondrial oxidative phosphorylation system or through substrate phosphorylation. The ATP furnishes the phosphate group and the energy for the subsequent phosphorylation of intracellular proteins via the membrane-bound protein.

Once the ligand has entered the cell, one of two events occurs. If the ligand is a hormone that has its primary effect at the plasma membrane, then its *job* is done. It will then be taken into the cell and degraded via the enzymes of the lysosomes. If the ligand has an intracellular function, it will move to its target within the cell. One of these targets may be DNA. The ligand may be transferred to an intracellular transport protein and/or to another receptor protein that has a DNA-binding capacity or may bind directly to the DNA affecting its transcription. These binding proteins make up another group of receptor proteins, the intracellular receptors. These intracellular receptors function in the movement of ligands from the plasma membrane to their respective targets. In this instance, the ligands may be lipid-soluble materials, or minerals or vitamins, or carbohydrates, peptides, or proteins. There is no evidence that these receptors participate in the intracellular signaling cascades except as recipients of their ligands. Intracellular receptors bind such compounds as the retinoids, vitamin D, certain minerals, steroid hormones, thyroid hormone, and some of the small amino acid derivatives that regulate metabolism.[1] As such, they serve to move these materials from their site of entry to their site of action. Sometimes, more than one receptor is involved in the action of a specific nutrient. For example, vitamin A is carried into the cell via cellular binding proteins (vitamin A binding proteins). These proteins carry the DNA active form of the vitamin (retinoic acid) to the nucleus or mitochondrion whereupon it is then bound to a nuclear or mitochondrial receptor that in turn binds to specific base sequences of the DNA. With some of the nutrient ligands, the intracellular receptor binds not only DNA but other cell components as well. The retinoic acid receptor is a member of a family of receptors known as the steroid super family of DNA-binding receptors. Each of these receptors binds a specific steroid. One of these receptors binds the thyroid hormone.

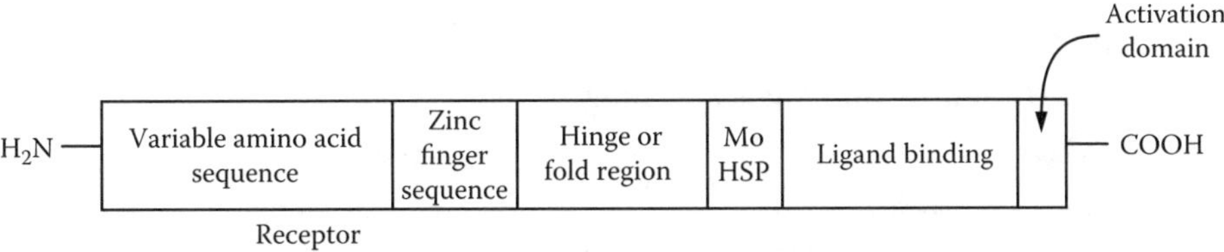

FIGURE 6.4 Generic structure of a receptor having a single polypeptide chain with six segments. The first is a variable amino acid sequence that confers immunologic identity to the receptor. The second is the zinc finger domain, which is rich in histidine and cysteine. Next is the hinge or fold region, which provides flexibility to the polypeptide chain. This is followed by the ligand-binding domain and the activation domain.

The family name is something of a misnomer, because not all of the ring-structured compounds they bind are steroids or steroid hormones nor do all of them bind DNA.

In this family of receptors, there are six basic domains (Figure 6.4) that have functional importance with respect to transcription. There are both homologous and nonhomologous domains. Homology exists in 60%–95% of the amino acid sequence of the zinc finger domain, in 65%–75% of the heat shock domain (HSP), and in 30%–60% of the ligand-binding domain. The regions where nonhomology exists determine which of the many ligands will be bound. The first hypervariable region provides the identity of the receptor based on its immunoreactivity. This has a use in the study of gene expression, especially in the area where investigators are trying to understand how specific nutrients affect the expression of specific genes. Other members of this receptor class of cellular components bind specific ligands and proteins that bind copper or zinc or one or more of the vitamins or one of the many amino acids, fatty acids, carbohydrates, or metabolites. In addition, there are intracellular receptors that bind one or more of these substances but do not bind to DNA. Instead, these binding proteins serve as transporters of their ligands from their point of entry to their point of use. Altogether, the proteins called receptors are important structural components of living cells.

SIGNAL SYSTEMS

Once hormones or nutrients are bound to their cognate receptors, changes in cell function occur. How are these changes brought about? As mentioned in the section on plasma membrane receptors, a number of hormones, particularly the protein and peptide hormones, affect cellular metabolism via a signaling system. There are several of these. Some couple to adenylate cyclase and others to guanylate cyclase, and still others are involved in the PIP pathway. Some use the calcium ion as a second messenger and others use ion channels. Some hormones use elements of all of these in signaling the cell to respond appropriately. Table 6.3 lists some of the hormones and the signaling systems they use. A hormone that uses the G protein as part of its signaling system does so when bound to its cognate receptor. G proteins are proteins that bind the nucleotide GDP or GTP. When the hormone binds to the receptor, a conformational change occurs that causes the G protein to exchange GTP for GDP. This activates the G protein. The activated G protein modulates the catalytic subunit of the membrane-bound adenylate cyclase, which in turn catalyzes the conversion of ATP to cyclic AMP. Cyclic AMP stimulates protein kinase A, which phosphorylates a number of proteins, thereby amplifying the original signal elicited by the binding of the hormone to the receptor.[2–11]

Some G proteins are coupled to the PIP_3 phospholipase C pathway. Phospholipase C catalyzes the hydrolysis of the membrane phospholipid, PIP releasing two second messengers, diacylglycerol (DAG) and phosphatidylinositol 4,5 phosphate (PIP_2), which is phosphorylated to the 1,4,5 phosphate form (PIP_3). Each of these second messengers has its own target. PIP_3 migrates to the

TABLE 6.3
Some Hormones and Their Signaling Systems

Hormone	System
Atrial natriuretic hormone (ANH)	Cyclic GMP
Bradykinin, α2-adrenergic norepinephrine, somatostatin	Cyclic AMP
Adrenocortical-stimulating hormone (ACTH)	Cyclic AMP and PIP pathway
Acetylcholine	Ion channel
Calcitonin, follicle stimulating hormone (FSH)	Cyclic AMP
Glucagon, PTH	Cyclic AMP
Vasopressin, β-adrenergic norepinephrine	Cyclic AMP

endoplasmic reticulum and, when bound to its receptor on this organelle, opens up a calcium channel. The calcium ions sequestered in the endoplasmic reticulum are then free to migrate out into the cytoplasm, whereupon they serve as cofactors in several reactions or are bound to calmodulin or they stimulate exocytosis. Exocytosis is important to the insulin-producing β cell of the pancreatic islets.[12,13] Insulin is exocytosed and this exocytosis is calcium stimulated and energy dependent.

DAG, the other second messenger released through the action of phospholipase C, binds to an allosteric binding site on protein kinase C that, in the presence of phosphatidylserine and the calcium ion, becomes activated so that still another group of proteins become phosphorylated.

G proteins also regulate the ion channels in both the plasma membrane and the sarcoplasmic reticulum.[14] There are two types of channels, one that is voltage gated (depolarization/repolarization) and the other that is coupled to specific membrane receptors via G proteins. Altogether then, hormones that bind to membrane-bound receptor proteins elicit their effects on cell functions via an integrated set of intracellular signals. These signal cascades are both simple and complex and involve a number of different proteins, each having a specific role in this signal transduction.

CELL DIFFERENTIATION

Although all nucleated cells possess the same DNA, some of the specific DNA regions (genes) are not transcribed or translated in all cell types. If translated, some gene products are not very active. Thus, not all cells have the same processes with the same degree of activity. Cellular differentiation has taken place so that muscle cells differ from fat cells, which differ from brain cells, and so forth. In each cell type, there are processes and metabolic pathways that may be unique to that cell type. An example is the great lipid storage capacity of the adipocyte, a feature not found in a bone or brain or muscle cell, although each of these cells does contain some lipids. Similarly, the capacity to form and retain a mineral apatite (a mixture of different minerals) is characteristic of a bone cell; the synthesis of contractile proteins by muscle cells is also an example of cell uniqueness.

Cells differ in their choice of metabolic fuel. Hepatic and muscle cells make, store, and use significant amounts of glycogen. Adipocytes and hepatocytes make, store, and sometimes use triacylglycerols. All of these special features have an impact on the composition of specific organs and tissues in the body that collectively contribute to the whole-body composition. The analysis of the composition of specific organs and tissues does not necessarily reflect the whole-body composition. One must consider the function of each organ and tissue in the context of the whole body. Similarly, the determination of the activity of a single process in a single cell type or organ may not necessarily predict the activity (and cumulative result) of that process in the whole body. However, some processes are unique to certain tissues so some exceptions to the aforementioned role are possible. For example, one can measure glycogenesis and glycogenolysis in samples of liver and muscle and be fairly confident that these measures will represent whole-body glycogen synthesis and breakdown. Other cell types may make, store, and use glycogen but not to the extent found in the liver or muscles.

TABLE 6.4
Life Span (Days) of Epithelial Cells from Different Organs in Man and Rat

Cell Type	Man	Rat
Cells lining the gastrointestinal tract	2–8	1.4–1.6
Cells lining the cervix	5.7	5.5
Skin cells	13–100	19.1
Corneal epithelial cells	7	6.9

With respect to cell function and its contribution to the body's metabolic processes, a mention should be made of the differing rates of cell renewal or cell half-life. Cells differ in their life span depending on their location and function.[15] Skin cells (epithelial cells) are short lived compared with brain cells. The turnover time for an epithelial cell in man is of the order of 7 days. Brain cells are not extensively regenerated and renewal of neural tissue is fragmented. That is, there is a turnover of individual cellular components such as the lipid component, but the cell once formed is not replaced as an entity to the same extent, as are the epithelial cells. Epithelial cells, especially those of the skin and the lining of the intestinal tract, are shed on a daily basis. Shown in Table 6.4 are some estimates of the life span of several sources of epithelial cells in man and in rats. While the average life span of man is on the order of 70 years, that of the rat is between 2 and 3 years. Despite this species difference in whole-body life span, the life span of epithelial cells is surprisingly similar.

Another short-lived cell is the erythrocyte, the red blood cell.[16] It has a half-life of about 60 days in the human. Replacement cells must be made constantly through the process of hematopoiesis. Hematopoiesis is responsible for all of the blood cells (white cells, platelets, and red cells) and takes place in the pluripotent stem cells of the bone marrow. Erythropoiesis is solely responsible for the red cell proliferation through a process of proliferation and differentiation. It is dependent on an intact bone marrow environment and on a cascade or network of cytokines, growth factors, and nutrients. The main function of the red cell is to carry oxygen to all cells of the body and exchange it for carbon dioxide. A shortfall in the number of red cells or in its oxygen-carrying capacity is called anemia. Table 6.5 lists the nutrients important to normal red cell production.

There are a number of nonnutritional reasons for anemia. These include excessive blood loss, drug-induced red cell destruction, and the genetic diseases: thalassemia and hemolytic anemia. Some toxic conditions, that is, lead intoxication, can also cause anemia. It is of interest to note that many of the symptoms of malnutrition include lesions of the skin and anemia (see Chapter 2). This is because skin cells and red blood cells are among the shortest-lived cells in the body and abnormalities in them are readily apparent. As noted, cell types differ in their life span. We do not know all the details of how cells reproduce themselves either in part or whole. Doubtless, there are signaling systems in place that control this process. A number of systems have been described that include not only cell multiplication (growth) but also cell death (necrosis or apoptosis). Many of

TABLE 6.5
Nutrients Needed for Red Cell Production

Protein
Energy
Vitamins E, A, B_6, B_{12}
Folacin
Iron, copper, zinc
Riboflavin
Niacin

these systems are hormonally controlled. Growth factors including growth hormone (GH) play key roles in new cell production. These factors have been elucidated through the study of conception, embryogenesis, and fetal development. Studies of the growth of animals and man after birth have also provided information about this process.[17,18] When growth begins, its velocity is high and then it gradually slows down. When growth ceases, that is, when the number of new cells appears to equal the number of cells that have died, a steady state is achieved (maturity). When a steady state has developed, the half-life of the cell can be determined or calculated. By definition, the half-life of the cell (or of any biologically active material) is defined as the amount of time required for half of the number of cells or amount of active material to disappear or be eliminated. Careful measurements of both time and the number of labeled cells or biologic material must be made.[19] The half-life of a cell can be calculated using measurements of the appearance and/or disappearance of a labeled material such as thymidine. Thymidine is taken up by the nuclear DNA as the cell prepares to divide or renew itself. It then disappears as the cell dies. The fractional elimination constant (which is the same as the fractional appearance rate) can then be calculated and the half-life of the item in question derived.[20] Suppose the number of cells initially equals *Co*. Over a period of time (*t*), this number is reduced to half (the half-life).

The equation can be written and solved as follows:

$$C = Coe - kt$$

$$\ln C = \ln Co - ket$$

$$\text{Rearranging gives us } \ln\left(Co/C\right) = ket$$

$$\text{At one half-life, } C = 0.5Co$$

$$\text{Therefore, } \ln\left(2.0\right) = ket_{1/2}$$

$$0.693 = ket_{1/2}$$

$$t_{1/2} = 0.693/ke$$

Note that 0.693 is always equal to the natural log of 2. This concept of half-life is part of the overall concept of steady state. Steady state, a feature of living systems, is that state where no net change occurs yet there is a steady flow of materials through the system. There are no net losses or gains, merely maintenance of the status quo. This probably characterizes the steady ebbs and flows of the nonpregnant, nongrowing adult. In this individual, there is no body weight gain or loss, no change in skeletal or muscle mass, and no measurable changes in body function. Perturbation of steady state occurs from birth to death under well-defined conditions but in the adult, the steady state is the maintenance state.

APOPTOSIS

Cell growth has been studied and a number of growth factors have been identified that have relevance to our understanding of how mammalian growth and development occurs. The half-life of cells varies throughout the body and is dependent on cell types. It depends on a variety of factors including age, nutritional status, health status, and genetics, as well as factors not yet identified. Age is important. Growing individuals are in a phase of life in which cell number is increasing exponentially.[18] Once growth and development is complete, this increase in cell number slows down. In contrast, senescence is characterized by a gradual loss in total cell number as well as losses in discrete cell types. In part, these changes in cell number are analogous to the observations of cell biologists, who have reported on the growth of cells in culture. Cultured cells go through a rapid growth phase doubling in number for 50–100 generations. Eventually, the cells reach a *turning point* and grow poorly or not at all, despite the continual provision of new media. Finally, the culture ceases to thrive and the number of cells begins to decline. At this time, the cells begin to die off slowly through a process called apoptosis or programmed cell death.[21–24] Cell cultures that do not become apoptotic are called immortal; that is, they do not have the mechanism for programmed cell death. Immortal cells have been genetically altered so that they can sustain themselves indefinitely provided that they have their culture medium replenished in a timely fashion. The alteration in the genetic control of the life of a cell is called transformation. Transformed cells are powerful research tools and the study of these cells allows for learning about their metabolism.

Cell turnover has two parts: cell replacement and cell death. Cell death is either a concerted, all-at-once event or a programmed, gradual process. If the former, cell death is called necrosis. This occurs if a tissue sustains an injury, small or large. A small cut in the skin results in necrosis of the injured cells in and around the cut. A ruptured coronary vessel results in the death of the heart muscle supplied by that vessel. If only a small capillary ruptures, the necrosis of the myocardium will be small. If a larger vessel ruptures, damage to the heart can be quite large and indeed may be a mortal event. Necrotic cell death is preceded by cell enlargement and a swelling of all the organelles within the cell. The DNA disintegrates and its nucleotides are degraded.

In contrast, programmed cell death or apoptosis involves a shrinkage of the cell and enzyme-catalyzed DNA fragmentation. This fragmentation can be detected as a laddering when the DNA is extracted from the cell and separated by electrophoresis. Apoptosis is a process that is an integral part of living systems. It is part of the growth process as well as part of the maintenance of cell and tissue functions. It is also part of wound healing and recovery from traumatic injury. Adipose tissue remodeling, immune function, epithelial cell turnover, and the periodic shedding of the uterine lining are but a few examples of this process. Apoptosis is viewed as a defense mechanism to remove unwanted and potentially dangerous cells such as virally infected cells or tumor cells. The process involves the mitochondria as the *central executioner*.[25,26] The mitochondria produce reactive oxygen (free radicals) as well as other materials that participate in apoptosis. Alterations in mitochondrial function have been observed to occur prior to any other feature of apoptosis. A decrease in mitochondrial membrane potential that, in turn, affects membrane permeability is an early event. The increase in permeability is followed by a release of cytochrome c that in turn regulates the caspases, which are cysteine proteases.[27] These caspases stimulate the proteolysis of key cell proteins in various parts of the cell. Altogether, the fragmentation of the DNA and the destruction of cell proteins result in the death of the cell via a very orderly process.

Apoptosis is the mechanism used in the thymus to eliminate thymocytes that are self-reactive. By doing so, the development of an autoimmune disease is suppressed. Indeed, this mechanism is being examined as an explanation of autoimmune insulin-dependent diabetes mellitus. Apoptosis is being carefully studied to learn about the signals that initiate or suppress it. Figure 6.5 illustrates the process of apoptosis and Table 6.6 lists some of the signals and regulatory compounds that influence this process.

Many cells can be stimulated to become apoptotic.[28,29] The p53 protein, for example, can induce apoptosis as one of its modes of protecting the body against tumor cells. The p53 protein is a DNA-binding protein. Mutations in tumor cells that cause an inactivation of p53 have been found.[30] The result of such a mutation is that tumor cells grow and multiply. The gene for p53 likewise can mutate, and this mutation has been associated with tumor development and growth. Apparently, this gene has several *hot spots* (likely places for mutation to occur), which explains its role in carcinogenesis and its loss in normal function. The Bcl-2 protein, a membrane-bound cytoplasmic protein, is another player in this regulation of apoptosis.[28] It is a member of the family of proteins called protooncogenes. Its normal function is to protect valuable cells against apoptosis. It is downregulated when cells are stimulated to die. Inappropriately high Bcl-2 protein levels can provoke cell overgrowth. The cell regulates Bcl-2

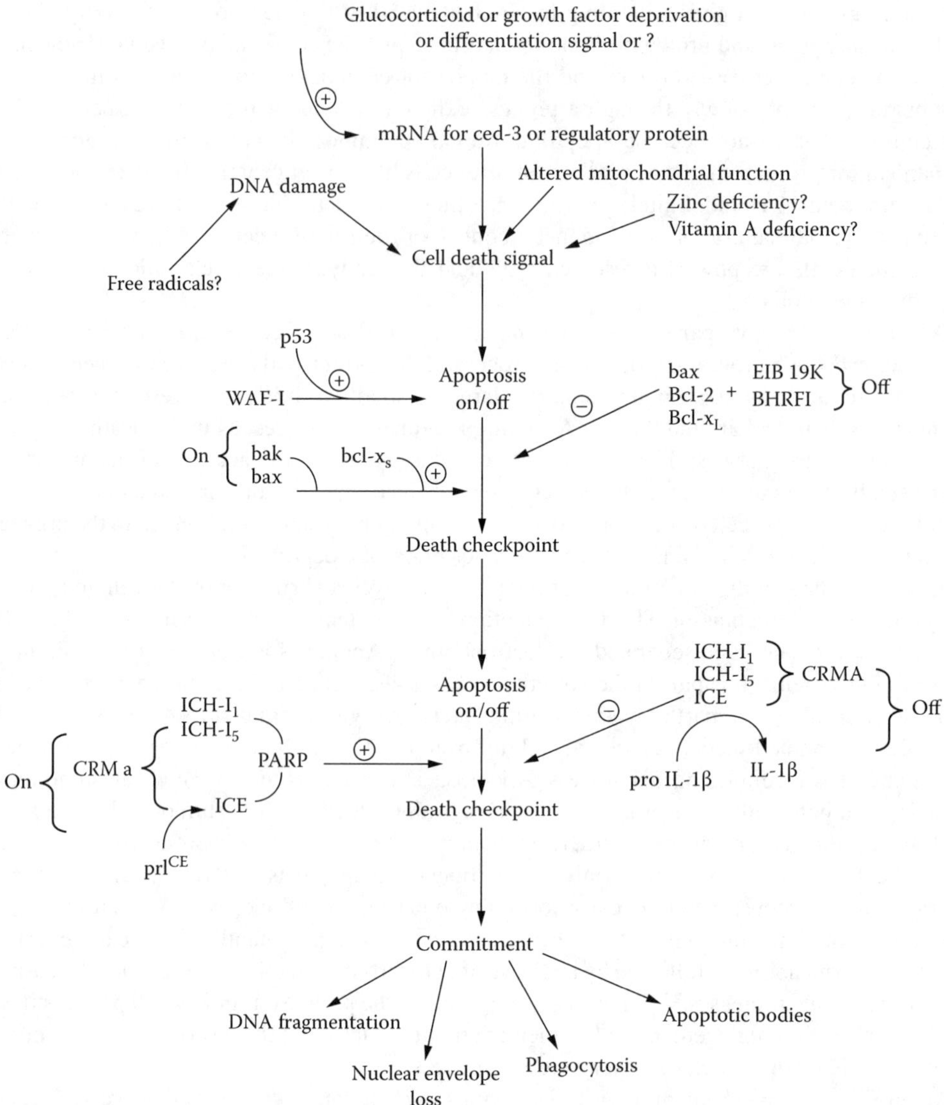

FIGURE 6.5 Flow chart for apoptosis. Note the many question marks, indicating that there are as many unknown factors in this process as there are known.

protein so as to maintain a normal homeostatic state. Bcl-2 and its homologue, Bcl-xL, block apoptosis. Both Bcl-2 and Bcl-xL can heterodimerize with Bax or Bcl-xs and, when Bcl-2 or Bcl-xL is overexpressed, an enhancement of oxidative stress mutagenesis can be observed. This occurs because these proteins suppress the apoptotic process, allowing more exposure of the cell to DNA damage by mutagens.

Nutrients play a role in apoptosis. High levels of zinc (500 μm) have been found to block apoptosis in cultured thymocytes.[31] The zinc blocks the action of the glucocorticoids in stimulating apoptosis. Zinc also interferes with tumor necrosis factor (TNF)-induced apoptosis as well as heat-induced cell death. In contrast, low levels of zinc (0.3–200 μm) have the reverse effect. That is, at low levels of zinc, apoptosis is stimulated by TNF, glucocorticoid, and heat exposure. The mechanism whereby zinc has these effects must be multifaceted. Zinc has an important role in transcription control as part of the zinc fingers, but it is not known how this relates to apoptosis.

TABLE 6.6
Contributory Factors[a] in the Regulation of Apoptosis

	Effect	
Factor	**Suppress**	**Stimulate**
Age	✓	
Apaf-1 protein		✓
p53 protein		✓
Bcl 2 protein	✓	
Bcl-x3 protein		✓
Bcl-xL protein	✓	
Bax protein		✓
Bak protein		✓
WAF-1	✓	
ced 3 and 4		✓
Glucocorticoids		✓
ced 9		✓
High zinc		✓
Low zinc		✓
Low retinoic acid	✓	
High retinoic acid		✓
Interleukin 1β		✓
Leptin		✓
TNFα		✓
Insulin		✓
Low manganese		✓
IGF_1	✓	
Low SOD activity	✓	
Peroxidized lipid	✓	

[a] It may appear that the names of these factors are in *code*. Actually, their names were given by the investigators working with them and are somewhat arcane. Some are abbreviations: TNFα is tumor necrosis factor α; IGF_1 is insulin-like growth $factor_1$; SOD is superoxide dismutase.

Manganese, another essential nutrient, also is involved as a cofactor for superoxide dismutase (SOD).[32] In instances where SOD is less active than normal, apoptosis is stimulated coincident with an increase in C2-ceramide, TNFα, and hydrogen peroxide. Peroxides form from unsaturated fatty acids as well as certain of the amino acids. There may be a link, therefore, between the fatty acid intake of the individual and apoptosis of certain cell types. In one study of genetically obese diabetic rats, an increase in fatty acid intake was associated with an increase in β cell apoptosis.

Retinoic acid (and dietary vitamin A) deficiency stimulates apoptosis.[33,34] The well-known feature of vitamin A deficiency (suppressed immune function) suggests that vitamin A and its metabolite, retinoic acid, serve to influence the sequence of events leading to cell death. This link is made because it is known that T-cell apoptosis is an important defense mechanism and T cells are part of the immune system. Vitamin A is also an antiproliferative agent, so its effect on abnormal cell growth is two pronged—it stimulates apoptosis and suppresses proliferation.

Genetic regulation of apoptosis involves not only the transcription factors mentioned earlier but also specific genes. Already described are the p53 and Bcl-2 DNA-binding proteins that, like zinc, retinoic acid, and fatty acids, affect gene expression. Add to this list the mitogen-activated protein kinases (p42/44) Erk1 and Erk2. When phosphorylated, these proteins suppress apoptosis in brown adipocytes.[35] Apoptosis is also suppressed by certain of the cytokines (IL6, IL3, interferon [γ]) and stimulated by others (leptin).[36,37] Finally, the gene Nedd 2 encodes a protein similar to the nematode cell death gene ced 3 and the mammalian interleukin 1b-converting enzyme.[38] Overexpression of this gene induces apoptosis.

With the understanding of apoptosis comes the understanding of how and why the body changes in its composition as it ages from conception to death. We have also begun to understand the role of apoptosis (and its control) in the pathophysiology of such degenerative diseases as diabetes.[39,40] All of the factors described earlier play roles in the gradual changes that occur not only in the pancreas but also in other tissues: muscle, adipose tissue, neural tissue, and so forth. All of these systems are coordinately regulated in the healthy young animal, but as animals (including man) age, subtle small modulations occur that then cumulatively result in cell, tissue, and lastly organ dysfunction.

Looking at just the age-related changes in body fat, one can observe small but incremental differences in body fat with age. For example, the young animal has little stored fat, while the older one has gained fat sometimes at the expense of body protein. Clearly, the body is continually being remodeled, and quite clearly, this remodeling is the result of a combination of many factors including the apoptotic process.

LIFE CYCLE

Just as cells have a finite existence, so too do whole bodies. Like the cell with its cycle of formation, maintenance, and death, whole bodies have a life cycle that includes the stage from conception to birth, from birth to growth and development, to adulthood (maintenance), and then to senescence. For the human, the time frame for these stages is long, while that for the rat or mouse is relatively short. Scientists have learned much from these shorter-lived species about the processes involved and how nutrition can affect the time frame for these stages of the life cycle. The reader is reminded of the different nutrition needs for these stages. The National Research Council Food and Nutrition Board (www.nap.edu) has set out recommendations for the intakes of each of the essential nutrients that are appropriate for each of the life stages. The recommendations are for daily intakes, yet there can be some variations from day to day as the food choices vary from day to day. In the chapters on the specific nutrients, these recommended intakes are stipulated (see Chapters 8 through 14). Bear in mind that these are recommendations, not requirements; the intake recommendations are greater than the nutrient requirement, which is an individual intake need. Thus, the daily recommendation has a safety factor such that the needs of about 90% of the population should be met if this intake recommendation is followed. Above and beyond these recommendations designed to optimize the health and well-being of the individual, we have a large body of information related to the effects of reduced food energy intake on development and longevity gleaned from hundreds of studies using rats and mice.

When well-balanced but energy-restricted diets are provided to rats and mice, the life span is extended.[41–45] Some of these reported effects are listed in Table 6.7. The design of these experiments is critical. If just the amount of food is reduced without accounting for the need for adequate intakes (AIs) of protein, essential fatty acids, and the micronutrients, nutrient insufficiency will develop. It is critical that the diet be low only in its energy content and nothing else. Care must also be exercised as to when the diets are offered to the experimental animals. If they are offered all at once, then a phenomenon of meal feeding occurs with unexpected results vis-a-vis fuel flux. If the *meal* is offered during the daylight hours to a nocturnal feeding rat, then there will be a 12 h time shift in lipogenic capacity and glucose flux. A carefully designed restricted feeding experiment will provide food throughout the 24 h period so that the animals do not receive (and consume) all their food at once. There are automatic feeding devices that can deliver at hourly intervals the food such that the restricted animal receives 1/24th of its daily ration each hour. Another aspect of this feeding paradigm for rats and mice is the tight control of their environment. Usually, the environment is carefully controlled with respect to temperature, humidity,

TABLE 6.7
Energy Restriction Effects in Rodents

Increased life span
Decrease in PTH release
Longer maintenance of serum vitamin D levels
Lower blood levels of calcium and phosphorus
Smaller excursions in blood glucose levels throughout the 24 h light cycle
Greater spontaneous activity
Reduced weight gain
Delay in the development of chronic nephropathy
Smaller fat cells
Fat cells more responsive to epinephrine, ACTH, glucagon, and fluoride
No difference in hepatic protein DNA or RNA content or protein synthetic rates
Less serum calcitonin
Decreased serum lipid levels
Greater bone mass
Delay in onset of puberty

light, and pathogen contamination. These rodents are reared in a stress-free environment with respect to cage space and other environmental considerations.

How do these findings relate to humans? Obviously, humans are not kept in a controlled environment free of stress. Furthermore, humans eat a variety of foods on an ad libitum basis. Obviously, surfeit feeding with subsequent excess fat gain has been recognized as a detrimental characteristic in humans. However, there are some humans who seem to regulate their food intake (and energy expenditure) so as to avoid gaining excess fat stores (see Chapter 4). Is there a lifetime benefit to this eating pattern similar to what was reported to occur in rats? We cannot do the critical experiment in humans to answer this question. Yet, it is a tantalizing one.

GROWTH AND DEVELOPMENT

From the single fertilized cell to maturity, the human (as well as other species) passes through several important stages. From conception to birth is one of these followed by infanthood and childhood followed by adolescence. Each of these stages is characterized by both an increase in cell number and a concerted and coordinated change in cell/tissue/organ characteristics and function. Longitudinal growth of the skeleton is the most obvious feature accompanied by the growth and maturation of the muscles, the internal organs, the reproductive system, and the central nervous system.[17–19] Physical activity as well as the consumption of a well-balanced diet adequate in all the needed nutrients ensures this coordinated growth pattern. Should one or more of the essential nutrients be inadequate, growth abnormalities will be observed. Familiar images of poorly nourished infants and children throughout the world document these nutritional effects on growth and development. Further, malnourished females have more pregnancy complications and greater numbers of miscarriages and fetal malformations than well-nourished females.[46] Their babies likewise have more postnatal difficulties than babies of well-nourished mothers. Lactation is compromised such that the babies of malnourished mothers are malnourished as well.

As described in Chapter 2, there may be some long-lasting effects of maternal malnutrition on the health and well-being of the progeny. Birth complications for both mother and child, birth weight, postbirth development, growth of children and adolescents, mental development, and physical development have been shown to be affected by the nutritional status of the pregnant female.[47] Some of these maternal effects on the progeny have been demonstrated in rats and mice. Some of the effects are long lasting, while other effects disappear with time. Some of these are listed in Table 6.8.

TABLE 6.8
Maternal Diet Effects on Rodent Progeny

Maternal dietary fat affects fat stores in progeny but this effect disappears with time.
Maternal carbohydrate intake affects glucose metabolism in young pups but not mature ones.
Maternal dietary protein affects fetal development: low protein → poorly developed pups.
Maternal essential fatty acid diet results in fetal resorptions.
Maternal food restriction results in smaller litters.

Whether all the findings in rodents are applicable to humans is unclear. Rodents differ appreciably from humans with respect to gestation, birth, and growth of the progeny. Rodent progeny come in litters; humans usually give birth to single infants. Twins and multiple births occur but not as frequently. Rodent progenies are born 21 days after conception in a very undeveloped state. They are blind, have mere stubs for limbs, and have no fur and their heads and central nervous systems are in a primitive state. Within a few days, fur appears, legs and feet appear, eyes develop and open, and the typical movement and responses of the rodent are apparent. In 3 weeks, they are ready to be weaned from the mother who, under the usual colony conditions, is already pregnant with another litter. These species differences are important if we are to understand whether the maternal diet affects progeny outcome independent of the postnatal environment and whether the findings from rats and mice are applicable to humans.

CONCEPTION TO BIRTH

The fertilization of the egg by a sperm results in conception. The fertilized egg (zygote) rapidly undergoes cell division forming an embryo. The DNA of the egg and sperm are mixed and half of it is discarded leaving the embryo with 46 chromosomes, approximately half from the mother and half from the father. The embryo also inherits mitochondrial DNA that encodes 13 components of the mitochondrial oxidative phosphorylation system. All of this is inherited from the mother; the paternal mitochondrial DNA is somehow lost during the conception process.[48] The embryonic/fetal DNA dictates the amino acid sequence of all of the peptides and proteins in the body. Some of the early peptides and proteins play a role in the ordered sequence of events that characterize the growth and development of the embryo/fetus. The initial DNA molecules are duplicated time and again so that as each new cell is formed it contains its requisite DNA. The formation or synthesis of this DNA is nutritionally dependent. During pregnancy, the nutrients needed for DNA synthesis are provided by the mother. If the mother is inadequately nourished prior to conception, the nutrient stores needed for this synthesis may be inadequate. Of particular interest is the maternal supply of folacin. It is essential to DNA synthesis as well as for cell replication, division, and specialization. Population surveys have shown that mothers who are folacin deficient have a greater risk of maldevelopment of the spinal cord and brain. Neural tube defects can be reduced by 70% in babies whose mothers consumed at least 400 μg folacin/day prior to conception and 600 μg/day during pregnancy.[49] Iron adequacy is another concern for pregnancy. Iron supplementation results in a substantial reduction of anemia in both the mothers and the newborns.[47]

Calcium, magnesium, and vitamin D are important for bone formation in the fetus. If the maternal diet is lacking in any of these nutrients, the developing fetus will raid the maternal supply. Maternal bone turnover is increased during pregnancy and if the fetus raids the maternal supply, it does so resulting in a loss of bone mineral by the mother. Calcium and magnesium supplementation improves fetal outcome and also prevents the bone loss observed in the malnourished mother. Some pregnant females develop hypertension during pregnancy that can be partially reversed with supplementation. Vitamin D deficiency during pregnancy has been linked to preeclampsia, low-birth-weight babies, and other complications such as neonatal rickets and asthma. There are racial differences in the rates of vitamin D deficiency with African-American and Hispanic women having more problems with vitamin D deficiency than Caucasian women.

The brain and the rudiments of the central nervous system are among the first systems to develop. As the brain develops, so too does the reproductive system, the cardiovascular system, and other systems vital to the development of the embryo/fetus. By 8 weeks, embryonic male genitalia develop and release testosterone that sets the stage for subsequent behavioral patterns typical of males. Similarly, by 8 weeks of embryonic development, female embryos develop uterine tubes (oviducts) and a uterus. These and other systems develop as well under the influence of maternal hormones such as the human chorionic gonadotropin (hCG), relaxin, human chorionic somatomammotropin (hCS), estradiol, estriol, progesterone, and prolactin. The placenta produces hormones that influence growth and development. These include proopiomelanocortin, β-endorphin, corticotropin-releasing hormone, α-melanocyte-stimulating hormone and dynorphin, and GnRH and inhibin (two hormones that interact with respect to hCG secretion). The embryo produces prorenin and this has effects on renal development and function. The fetus and the placenta interact in the formation of the steroid hormones that in turn have effects on growth and metabolic development.

Growth of the fetus has been estimated but true measurements cannot/have not been made. Some measurements have been inferred from the sizes of premature infants. However, prematurely born babies may not represent a fetus that has a few more weeks or months of gestation before birth. Zeigler et al.[50] have constructed a model for the gain in weight of the fetus from week 24 of gestation to week 40 of gestation. Over this period of time, the fetus gains protein (from 7.8 to 19.8 g/day), mineral matter, and fat (from 10.8 to 13.9 g/day) and loses water as a percentage of the body mass. This model indicates that the growth of the fetus involves all compartments of the body. Muscle mass, bone mass, organ mass, and fat mass are all coordinately affected and normal growth is accomplished. Over the 42 weeks of pregnancy, the embryo/fetus will grow from almost nothing to 7–8.5 lb. At birth, the length of the newborn will vary from 46 to 53 cm. The genetic background of the parents will affect the weight and length of the fetus. Parents who are quite small will have small babies and in contrast, parents who are very large (tall and muscular but not obese) will have large babies. Women who develop gestational diabetes (diabetes diagnosed during pregnancy) often give birth to babies who are much heavier (some have weighed up to 16 lb) when allowed to give birth at term.[47,51,52] These babies have gained excessive amounts of fat during gestation. Often, an obstetrician will induce the birth of the baby if it is apparent that the fetal weight gain is excessive. When the baby becomes too large to pass through the birth canal, it may be necessary to perform a cesarean birth.

BIRTH TO CHILDHOOD

The first 2 years of an infant's life is marked by rapid growth. GH is essentially unimportant for fetal development in utero but is primary to growth after birth. The rate of growth of males and females from birth to age 20 is shown in Figure 6.6. Postnatal growth is a complex process orchestrated not only by GH and the somatomedins but also by the thyroid hormones, the glucocorticoids, and insulin. It is also affected by the genetic background of the individual and by the supply of the essential nutrients.

Growth is an orderly sequence of maturational changes that involves the accretion of body protein and an increase in the length and size of the individual not just an increase in weight. The food supply is the most important extrinsic factor in determining this growth and development. From birth to weaning, the infant's main source of nutrients is from milk. Some mothers will elect to bottle-feed their infants from birth until weaning, while other mothers will elect to breastfeed. The breastfed infant will gain passive immunity from the breast milk, while the bottle-fed infant will not. Both feeding styles will adequately nourish the infant.

The well-nourished lactating mother will supply her infant with the nutrients he or she needs to support good growth. During lactation, the requirements for carbohydrates; dietary fiber; water;

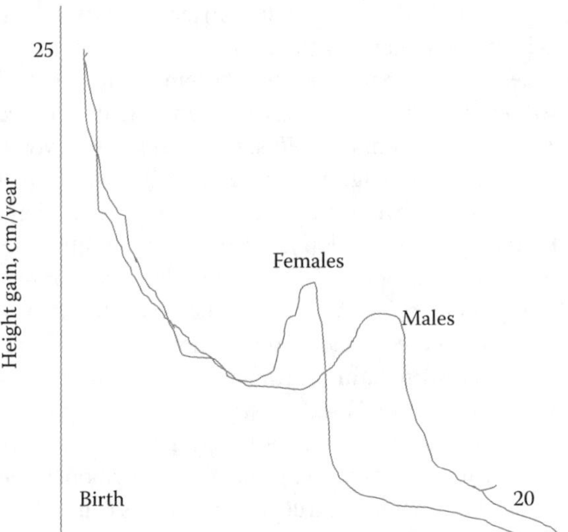

FIGURE 6.6 Rate of growth in males and female from birth to age 20.

biotin; chlorine; chromium; copper; manganese; pantothenic acid; riboflavin; selenium; zinc; vitamins A, B_6, B_{12}, E, and C; iodine; and potassium are increased over that needed to support pregnancy (www.nap.edu). In lactation, the iron requirements are slightly reduced. The lactating woman must consume enough energy to support adequate milk production to meet the needs of her infant. She must balance that need against her desire to lose the weight she gained during pregnancy that was not directly related to the growth of the fetus and supporting maternal tissue. Sometimes, the pregnant woman will gain 20–30 lb of nonrelated gestation tissue, and this poses a problem for the mother who now wishes to lose that excess body weight. She can increase her physical activity and thus her energy expenditure, and she can reduce her energy intake but not her intake of the essential nutrients.

Lactating mothers release significant amounts of ghrelin and peptide YY.[53] These two cytokines are involved in appetite regulation and energy homeostasis. As lactation continues, the level of ghrelin diminishes but peptide YY remains elevated. It is thought that the intentional loss of body weight following parturition might be helped by these changes in neuroendocrine signals. Lactation thus is a useful adjunct to the mother desiring to attain her prepregnancy body weight.

CHILDHOOD AND ADOLESCENCE

Just as GH is the primary regulator of growth in infants, it plays an important role in the growth of young children and adolescents. There are many stimuli that affect GH secretion in humans. Some of these are listed in Table 6.9.

The basal GH concentration ranges from 0 to 3 ng/mL in normal adults. Secretion rates are variable as can be assumed by perusal of the factors that affect GH release. Most of the enhancers of hormone release are those that are important to the regulation of energy homeostasis. Hence, the reader will observe that hypoglycemia, exercise, and fasting stimulate GH release and that high blood glucose will have the reverse effect. Note in Figure 6.6 that there are growth spurts (probably due to spurts in GH release) in both males and females during the adolescent period. Peak GH release occurs just prior to the onset of puberty. Growth is also dependent on other hormones as well. The thyroid hormones, if insufficient, will result in stunting.

As can be anticipated, normal growth demands that the diet consumed during this period contains all of the essential nutrients in the appropriate amounts.[54,55] Growth is very sensitive to the need for energy. Protein synthesis is highly dependent on the provision of sufficient energy

TABLE 6.9
Factors That Increase and Decrease GH Release

Increase	Decrease
Low blood sugar	REM sleep
2-deoxyglucose	Glucose
Exercise	Glucocorticoids
Protein meal	Free fatty acids
Glucagon	Medroxyprogesterone
Stress	Circulating GH
Glucagon	IGF-1
Thyroid hormones	
Lysine vasopressin	
L-dopa	
Estrogens and androgens	

as well as a balanced amino acid supply. Hence, the rapidly growing child and very rapidly growing adolescent will need both an increase in the amount of dietary protein and an increase in dietary energy to support this growth. In addition, growth demands the provision of essential vitamins and minerals. Should there be a temporary deficit in the intake of essential nutrients, there will be an effect on growth. This has been observed under a variety of circumstances including a temporary food shortage or a period of acute or chronic illness. Following such circumstances, there will be a period of *catch-up* growth during which the child or adolescent grows faster than expected. The accelerated growth continues until the prestarvation or preillness growth curve resumes. If the food shortage is chronic, this catch-up growth may not resume, and the child does not achieve his or her potential adult size. Stunting has been observed in populations that are chronically undernourished. In contrast, when people move from areas that are chronically subjected to food shortages, there is a generational effect on the progeny. Stunted adults produce children who mature at greater heights than their parents. It may take several generations for the achievement of the optimal height and body mass to occur when people migrate from an area of chronic food shortage to one where food is plentiful.

MATURITY

After the human has attained his or her adult height and the body has acquired sufficient bone and muscle mass, the individual is said to be mature. The period of maturity is a long one in the human. Depending on gender and genetic heritage, maturity is attained somewhere between age 20 and 22. The maturity period lasts until senescence sets in. The time interval is highly variable and depends on a variety of factors. Certainly, appropriate nutrient intake is a key determinant as is one's genetic heritage, exposure to noxious elements, degree of physical activity, and other environmental factors. Body mass can continue to accrue if the individual gains fat mass (see Chapter 3) and/or the individual develops an interest in body building where, through exercise, muscle mass is increased. In both of these instances, specific cell types are expanding. In obesity, both the fat cell size and fat cell number can increase. With body builders, it is the muscle cell that increases both in size and number.

Dietary and nutrient recommendations for healthy adults are designed not only to meet basic nutrient needs and prevent nutrient deficiencies but also to prevent or delay the appearance of chronic diseases that can shorten the length and quality of life. The dietary reference intakes (DRIs) are recommendations for nutrient intakes by healthy people. They are based on the results of current and past research designed to determine the optimal nutrient intakes for people of different age groups. Not all of the essential nutrients have an associated DRI. This is because there are insufficient data to base a DRI recommendation. Thus, some of the essential nutrients have recommendations that are called AIs and others have, in addition, a tolerable upper limit (UL) where there is some suspicion that an excess intake might be deleterious to the individual. Many of the nutrients with the UL designation are minerals. Too high an intake results in a toxic situation and care must be taken to avoid such toxicities.

The DRIs include the recommended intakes for nutrients or the recommended daily dietary allowance (RDA). RDAs are intended to guide the intakes of 97%–99% of the population. Intake guidelines have been developed that will help consumers select the amounts and kinds of foods that will provide the needed nutrients in the needed amounts. The current terminology is less inclusive in that the DRIs are intended to cover the needs of 90% of the population. This reduction in coverage was thought to narrow the possibility of adverse responses to excess intakes.

One of the current health problems associated with excess intake is that of excess dietary energy intake (see Chapter 3). It is difficult to make a recommendation for energy intake since there is so much individual variation in energy need. What would be appropriate for one individual might be excessive in another and too little for a third. The needs for some of the other nutrients are certainly less variable.

AGING (SENESCENCE)

The very nature of life is that one begins aging at conception and stops at death. However, for the purposes of this section on the life cycle, the period of interest is the period of life that occurs after the attainment of maturity and its conclusion. Senescence occurs when the individual loses the steady state and lasts until the individual dies. It is characterized by a steady and inevitable loss of function of cells, tissues, and organs.

The elderly are the fastest growing segment in our population today.[56–59] Citizens of western, technologically advanced nations are living longer than their ancestors. In the United States, the segment of the population over the age of 65 has grown rapidly. For example, between 1960 and 1990, the total US population increased by 39%. The segment of that population over the age of 65 grew by 89%. In 2010, the number of people over 65 was 40 million. It is expected that this number will increase to 55 million in 2020 and to be more than 88 million by 2050. The number of people over the age of 85 was approximately 5.4 million in 2010 and is expected to grow to 19 million by 2050. The segment of the population over the age of 85 will grow by 232%.[58,60] Those who are 65 today can expect to live more than 18 years, and those who are 85 can expect to live an additional 6 years.

Due to the increase in the over-65 segment, scientists are beginning to pay much more attention to the nutrition-related health problems facing these people. Firm recommendations for nutrient intakes by the senescent population are lacking. There are no DRIs for this population group. Obviously, the health-care system will need to be expanded as the elderly segment of the population expands. The costs of elder care and its delivery will need continual reexamination.

As people age, many aspects of their lives change. Upon retirement, their income may be reduced and their health-care expenses may increase. Age-related changes in the muscular–skeletal systems of the elderly will probably mean less mobility. Older sensory systems may be less acute. Diminished senses of balance, hearing, smell, sight, and the overall perception of self in society have an impact on health and well-being, as well as on aging individuals' ability to care for themselves. The development of senile dementia of the Alzheimer's type (SDAT) with subsequent losses in both mental and physical function occurs more frequently as the population ages. Shown in Table 6.10 are the predicted age-specific prevalence rates for SDAT. With the significant gain in average life expectancy, a parallel rise in these age-related failures in brain function must be anticipated.

However, as the studies by Johnson and colleagues[59] have shown, some deteriorated mental function might not be strictly age related. It might be due to malnutrition. Older adults may show signs

TABLE 6.10
Predicted Age-Specific Prevalence Rates (%) for DSM-III Senile Dementia and SDAT

Age	DSM-III Dementia	SDAT
62.5	0.9	0.2
67.5	1.6	0.4
72.5	2.8	0.9
77.5	4.9	2.1
82.5	8.7	4.7
87.5	15.5	10.8
91.5	24.5	21.0
95.0	36.7	37.4

Source: Ritchie, K., *Facts Res. Gerontol.*, 4(2), 1994.
Note: SDAT: epidemiology and public health issues.

of inadequate protein, mineral, and vitamin nutriture that impact on mental function. The lack of vitamin B_{12}, folacin, and protein, as well as other nutrient inadequacies, has been identified. If these inadequacies can be addressed and nutritional status improved, some of the so-called age-related impaired mental functions can be reversed. Some malnutrition can also be attributed to the loss of ability to purchase the needed food—either for economic reasons or because elders may not be able to get to the grocery store to select the foods they need. Their diminished sensory faculties may mean that they can no longer drive and thus must depend on their families and communities for their food supply. They may also be unable to prepare the food or store it appropriately, due to their diminished sensory function. If dentition is poor, the choice of foods might be limited to those items that are easy to swallow with minimal mastication. The absence of dentures or the presence of poorly fitted dentures can be a major impediment to the consumption of the wide variety of foods needed to assure good nutritional status.

How can these problems be identified and corrected? This is not an easy question to answer. The nutrition screening of people over the age of 65 can present some special problems and hurdles. For a variety of reasons, many elders may not be able to read. Thus, acquiring information about their usual food intake has this additional complication. Short-term memory loss may cause some elderly to be unable to recall the food they consumed yesterday or the day before. If elders are blind or have failing vision, they may not be able to complete a diet-recall form or to compile a food intake diary. Innovative techniques must be developed to address this problem. Some researchers have used a picture-sort approach where the subject selects pictures of foods and recalls to the interviewer how frequently that food is consumed. Other researchers have used interview techniques that involve the use of food group patterns as well as individual food-recall methods. Having an observer record the actual food consumed is a possibility, but this method is labor intensive and time consuming unless the elderly are in a group setting such as in an assisted-care facility. Individual observation may not be practical if the elderly person is living independently. In addition, the line between screening and diagnostic testing is blurred. In areas where there is good, widely available geriatric care, the need for such testing is reduced. In other words, where the elderly are well served by the medical community, the need for screening is much less than where they are poorly served. Early indications of health being impacted by malnutrition are usually observed in the former situation and ignored in the latter. Thus, anemia due to mineral or vitamin deficiency might be corrected as elderly people are routinely cared for by their physicians. Osteoporosis, arthritis, and other degenerative diseases that have a nutrition component likewise can be identified and effectively treated.

Good geriatric care also includes the recognition that some of the medications used in managing such chronic diseases as hypertension or diabetes mellitus may interact with certain nutrients, thus placing the patient at risk for malnutrition. Thiazide diuretics, for example, are widely prescribed for the management of hypertension. They are excellent medications for this purpose; however, they increase the loss of potassium. Frequently, the elderly need to supplement their diets with potassium-rich foods (citrus fruits, bananas, etc.) or take a potassium supplement. The elderly may develop chemical imbalances in the brain that affect their emotional state. It is not unusual for physicians to prescribe antidepressants. Those drugs that are anticholinergics can have the side effects of dry mouth, altered taste perception, nausea, vomiting, constipation, and reduced appetite. All of these side effects can affect nutritional status because of their influence on food consumption. Similarly, nutritional status can be affected by the use of antacids and laxatives. Some of the elderly believe that a daily large bowel movement is essential. Despite day-to-day variation in the kinds and amounts of foods consumed, there is this belief that a daily movement is a feature of good health. Thus, many elderly are chronic laxative users. This use may disturb gastrointestinal function and promote diarrhea as well as the possibility of an electrolyte imbalance. In turn, this will reduce gut passage time and thus absorptive cell exposure time for nutrients. Again, this can result in impaired nutritional status.

Diseases of the joints and connective tissue are frequently managed with the use of anti-inflammatories. Both steroids and nonsteroids are used to reduce the inflammation and associated pain. Aspirin and indomethacin are among the nonsteroidal, over-the-counter medications frequently used. If used daily in large doses, both can result in iron-deficiency anemia. High aspirin intake can deplete the hepatic iron stores because it interferes with normal blood coagulation. The elderly can have bruises and small *bleeds* that result in blood loss and anemia. A number of other drugs can influence nutritional status. However, many drugs have not been studied at all with respect to their effect on nutritional status especially in the elderly. Nonetheless, interest in drug–nutrient interactions is building as we learn more about the gradual losses in body function that characterize aging.[61]

Aging in itself has effects on the pathways of intermediary metabolism as well as on the endocrine system. Some of these effects are listed in Table 6.11.

Insulin resistance may be a feature of aging. With age, the pancreas becomes less responsive to signals for insulin release, and the target tissues become less responsive to its action. In part, this may be due to age-related increased plasma membrane phospholipid saturation, but it is also due to age-related increases in fat cell size. As fat cells accumulate stored fat, they become less sensitive to the action of insulin in promoting glucose uptake and use. Muscle cells likewise may have age-related changes in membrane fluidity that impair their response to insulin. As well, there is an age-related decrease in muscle use. Working muscles have little need for insulin bound to its receptor to facilitate glucose use. Altogether then, this decrease in muscle activity plus the increase in fat cell size has a negative effect on the insulin–glucose relationship. Glucose levels rise and the β cells of the pancreatic Islets of Langerhans increase their output of insulin to meet the glucose challenge. However, this excess output does little good in reducing the blood glucose in the aging overly fat inactive individual, and it is not uncommon to have type 2 diabetes develop as a consequence. Age-related impaired glucose tolerance can be mitigated by food restriction and increased physical activity, which reverses the aforementioned physiological state. Because insulin is one of the main regulators of intermediary metabolism and because its action is counterbalanced by the glucocorticoids, the catecholamines, the thyroid hormones, glucagon, and several other hormones, it should be no surprise that age changes in these hormones occur as well. Again, some of these changes can be attributed to age changes in membrane lipids, but some can be attributed to changes in hormone production and in the synthesis and activity of the receptors that mediate their action. Table 6.12 lists some hormones affected by age. The blood levels of most of these hormones decrease in the aging human and laboratory animal. A few pass through a phase where they are elevated above normal then fall below normal as aging continues. All of these hormones

TABLE 6.11
Effects of Age on Intermediary Metabolism and Its Control

Pathway	Control Points	Age
Glycolysis	(a) Transport of glucose into the cell (mobile glucose transporter)	↓
	(b) Glucokinase	↓
	(c) Phosphofructokinase	↓
	(d) α-glycerophosphate shuttle	
	(e) Redox state, phosphorylation state	
Pentose phosphate shunt	(a) Glucose-6-phosphate dehydrogenase	↓
	(b) 6-phosphogluconate dehydrogenase	↓
Glycogenesis	(a) Stimulated by insulin and glucose	ND
	(b) High-phosphorylation state (ratio of ATP/ADP)	ND
Glycogenolysis	(a) Low-phosphorylation state	ND
	(b) Stimulated by catecholamines	ND
Lipogenesis	(a) Stimulated by insulin	
	(b) Acetyl-CoA carboxylase	
	(c) High-phosphorylation state	
	(d) Malate citrate shuttle	↓
Gluconeogenesis	(a) Stimulated by epinephrine	
	(b) Malate aspartate shuttle	↓
	(c) Redox state	↑
	(d) Phosphoenolpyruvate carboxykinase	↓
	(e) Pyruvate kinase	
Cholesterogenesis	(a) HMG CoA reductase	
Ureogenesis	(a) Carbamyl phosphate synthesis	↑, ↓
	(b) ATP	ND
Citric acid cycle	(a) All three shuttles	ND
	(b) Phosphorylation state	↓
Lipolysis	(a) Lipoprotein lipase	↓
Respiration	(a) ADP influx into the mitochondria	↓
	(b) Ca^{2+} flux	
	(c) Shuttle activities	↓
	(d) Substrate transporters	↓
Oxidative phosphorylation	(a) ADP/ATP exchange	↓
	(b) Ca^{2+} ion	
Protein synthesis	(a) Accuracy of gene transcription	↓
	(b) Availability of amino acids	↓
	(c) ATP	↓

Note: ↑, increased as the animal ages; ↓, decreased as the animal ages.

serve to regulate the metabolism of carbohydrates, lipids, and proteins. Age has unique effects on each of these tissues and their respective metabolic processes. Each of the pathways of intermediary metabolism has specific control points, which in turn are affected by age. Although various studies have shown age-related declines in enzyme activities, it should be remembered that these are in vitro measurements in conditions where substrates and coenzymes are in optimal amounts to assure saturation. This rarely occurs in vivo. Hence, a decline in activity may not mean a decline in in vivo function. In a number of instances, the age-related decline in activity of a pathway or reaction can be inhibited by chronic food restriction. With chronic food restriction, the elderly may lose fat mass that in turn has effects on peripheral cell responsiveness to insulin vis-á-vis glucose use.

TABLE 6.12
Hormone Changes with Age

Hormone	Age—Effects
Thyroxine (T_4)	↓
Triiodothyronine (T_3)	↓
Thyroid binding globulin	No change or ↑
TSH	↓
Insulin	↑ followed by ↓
ACTH	↓
Epinephrine	↓
Glucagon	↓
GH	↓
Estrogen	↓
Testosterone	↓
Cortisol (glucocorticoids)	↓
Pancreatic polypeptide	↓

Note: ↑, increase; ↓, decrease.

In the absence of hyperinsulinemia, there is a decreased release of the anti-insulin hormones. As described earlier, age-related alterations in hormone balance do occur, and these alterations have an impact on carbohydrate oxidation, glycogen storage and mobilization, hexose monophosphate shunt, and gluconeogenesis.

As aging proceeds, there is a rise in blood lipids coupled with a decrease in adipose tissue lipoprotein lipase. With age, adipocytes have a less competent lipid uptake system due to this decline in lipase activity. In normal aging animals, the rates of cholesterol synthesis do not change; however, the uptake of this cholesterol as well as its oxidation and excretion declines. This has the result of an age-related increase in serum cholesterol levels. Genetics plays an important role in these age-related changes in serum lipids (see Chapters 7 and 10). Some genotypes are characterized by a sharper decline with age in lipid uptake processes than other genotypes. For example, those whose lipoprotein receptors are genetically aberrant will, as a result, show a far earlier rise in serum lipids than those whose receptors are fully functional. Some may only have a decline in cholesterol uptake or triacylglyceride uptake, while others will have a decline in the uptake of both. Age-related declines in thyroid hormone production, thyroxine conversion to triiodothyronine, glucocorticoid release, and the insulin/glucagon ratio will have effects on fatty acid mobilization and oxidation, and the results of this decline in hormone-stimulated lipolysis are observed as an age-related expansion of the fat stores and perhaps increases in blood lipids. While age has effects on fatty acid synthesis in rats and mice, these effects are minimal in humans consuming the typical western diet. This is because this diet is relatively rich in fat, so the need for its synthesis is almost nonexistent. Humans tend to use the dietary carbohydrate as their primary fuel and the surplus dietary fat is transported to the adipose tissue for storage. Hence, de novo fatty acid synthesis is negligible. In the young animal, there is considerable protein synthesis and with age there is a decline in this synthetic activity. With an age-related decline in protein synthesis, there is an increased need to rid the body of amino groups as the surplus amino acids are deaminated for use in gluconeogenesis and lipogenesis. This means that if the protein intake is not reduced to accommodate the decreased need for protein, there will be an increase in the activity of the urea cycle. Studies in aging rats have shown that dietary intake excess of energy and protein is associated with an age-related increase in urinary protein and renal disease that is preceded first by an increase then a decrease in ureogenesis. Food restriction or protein restriction ameliorates these age-related changes in renal function and urea synthesis. In humans, age has effects on voluntary food intake. Whether these effects are truly age related or due to other factors (disease, drugs, loneliness, etc.) is difficult to assess.

All of the age-related changes in intermediary metabolism are linked together by age changes in mitochondrial oxidative phosphorylation that in turn are affected by mitochondrial DNA sequence.[62] Age carries with it a progressive change (increase) in mitochondrial membrane saturation, a progressive loss in ATP synthetic efficiency, and an increase in free radical damage to mitochondrial DNA and its translation products. These progressive changes mean a progressive loss in the tight control of intermediary metabolism exerted by the concentration and flux of the adenine nucleotides. In turn then, one might expect to find progressive changes as described earlier in carbohydrate, lipid, and protein metabolism in addition to and in response to the progressive changes with age in the endocrine system and those changes associated with the central nervous system.

SUMMARY

1. Cells contain organelles that have specific functions within the cell. These functions provide cell identity. Complex mammals have many different cell types that are organized into tissues, organs, and systems. The functions of this organization are nutritionally sensitive.
2. Receptors bind ligands that in turn affect cell function that in turn are regulated by one of several signal systems.
3. As organisms become more complex, their cells differentiate such that specific cell types have specific functions and these in turn contribute to the characteristics of the individual.
4. Nutritional status affects cell function and cell turnover.
5. Apoptosis (programmed cell death) contributes to cell turnover. The length of time needed to maintain cell number differs by cell type and this time is the cell's half-life.
6. Complex mammals like simple cell organisms have a life cycle. In man, this includes the period from conception to birth, the period of growth and development, the mature period, and the postmature-aging period called senescence.
7. All aspects of the life cycle are nutritionally sensitive.

LEARNING OPPORTUNITIES

Self-Study Your Nutritional Status

Using the food diary you constructed for Learning Opportunity 3.1, calculate estimates of your daily mineral and vitamin intake. Compare this value to those recommended for your age and gender. Go to the website www.nap.edu to obtain your daily recommended intakes for the essential nutrients, and then create a two-bar graph for each of the essential vitamins and minerals. One bar should be your intake and the second one (next to it) should be that recommended for you. For any of the micronutrients where there is more than a 10% difference, show how you are going to alter your food intake to erase this difference. The difference can either be on the plus side or the negative side. Do not include your intake of micronutrients via a vitamin/mineral supplement. If you take a supplement, you should look at your bar graphs to determine whether you need to take this supplement or perhaps select another type of supplement. Show this comparison and list your conclusions.

CASE STUDY 6.1 Gramma is Tired

Gramma is 70 years old. Lately, she has been complaining of feeling tired. While she used to enjoy working outside in her garden, she no longer does so and her garden is full of weeds. Her beautiful flowers are disappearing as the weeds take over. Gramma no longer wants to go shopping. She goes to the store for her groceries but minimizes the number of items she buys. She says she is too tired to carry all those groceries home but her grandson, Allan, thinks she may not be able to afford both food and the medications she needs to manage her hypertension. Gramma also complains of joint stiffness and, reluctantly, she admits to using large amounts of aspirin to control her joint pain. Allan decides that Gramma should go to her doctor for evaluation. The doctor orders x-rays to determine the cause of the joint pain and also a blood workup to determine what other factors might cause her tiredness. Analyze this situation and describe what you think is going on. What recommendations would you make to improve Gramma's situation?

MULTIPLE-CHOICE QUESTIONS

1. Aging can be speeded up by
   a. Obesity
   b. Lack of food
   c. Lack of medicines
   d. None of the above
2. Apoptosis is
   a. Programmed cell death
   b. Essential to tissue/organ renewal
   c. Nutrition dependent
   d. All of the above
3. The cycle of life
   a. Mimics cell cycle
   b. Differs between species
   c. Differs between males and females
   d. None of the above
4. All cells contain
   a. A plasma membrane
   b. Mitochondria
   c. Nucleus
   d. Endoplasmic reticulum
5. Receptors function to
   a. Move ligands from place to place
   b. Contribute to the control of cell function
   c. Are essential to gene expression
   d. All of the above

REFERENCES

1. Tsai, M.-J., O'Malley, B.W. (1994) Molecular mechanisms of action of steroid/thyroid receptor super family members. *Ann. Rev. Biochem.* 63: 451–486.
2. Kahn, R.A., Der, C.J., Bokoch, G.M. (1992) The ras superfamily of GTP-binding proteins: Guidelines on nomenclature. *FASEB J.* 6: 2512–2513.

3. Macara, I.G., Lounsbury, K.M., Richards, S.A., McKiernan, C., Bar-Sagi, D. (1996) The ras superfamily of GTPases. *FASEB J.* 10: 625–630.
4. Bygrave, F.L., Roberts, H.R. (1995) Regulation of cellular calcium through signaling cross-talk involves as intricate interplay between the actions of receptors, G-proteins, and second messengers. *FASEB J.* 9: 1297–1303.
5. Lincoln, T.M., Cornwell, T.L. (1993) Intracellular cyclic GMP receptor proteins. *FASEB J.* 7: 328–338.
6. Koesling, D., Bohme, E., Schultz, G. (1991) Guanyl cyclases, a growing family of signal transducing enzymes. *FASEB J.* 5: 2785–2791.
7. Allende, J.E. (1988) GTP-mediated macromolecular interactions: The common features of different systems. *FASEB J.* 2: 2356–2367.
8. Weiss, E.R., Kelleher, D.J., Wai-Woon, C., Soparkar, S., Osawa, S., Heasley, L.E., Johnson, G.L. (1988) Receptor activation of G proteins. *FASEB J.* 2: 2841–2848.
9. Premont, R.T., Inglese, J., Lefkowitz, R.J. (1995) Protein kinases that phosphorylate activated G protein-coupled receptors. *FASEB J.* 9: 175–182.
10. Strader, C.D., Fong, T.M., Graziano, M.P., Tota, M.R. (1995) The family of G-protein-coupled receptors. *FASEB J.* 9: 745–754.
11. Rens-Domiano, S., Hamm, H.E. (1995) Structural and functional relationships of heterotrimeric G-proteins. *FASEB J.* 9: 1059–1066.
12. Saltiel, A.R. (1994) The paradoxical regulation of protein phosphorylation in insulin action. *FASEB J.* 8: 1034–1040.
13. Knutson, V.P. (1991) Cellular trafficking and processing of the insulin receptor. *FASEB J.* 5: 2130–2138.
14. Brown, A.M. (1991) A cellular logic for G protein-coupled ion channel pathways. *FASEB J.* 5: 2175–2179.
15. Brozek, J. (1963) Body composition. *Ann. NY Acad. Sci.* 110: 1–1018.
16. Limbaugh, B.H., Hendricks, L.K., Kutlar, A. (2007) Anemia. In: *Handbook of Nutrition and Food* (C.D. Berdanier, E.B. Feldman, J. Dwyer, eds.). CRC Press, Boca Raton, FL, pp. 1093–1109.
17. Reeds, P.J., Fiorotto, M.L. (1990) Growth in perspective. *Proc. Nutr. Soc.* 49: 411–420.
18. Meisami, E., Timiras, P.S. eds. (1990) *Handbook of Human Growth and Developmental Biology*, Vol. II: Part B. CRC Press, Boca Raton, FL, 362pp.
19. Christian, J.E., Combs, L.W., Kessler, W.V. (1963) Body composition. Relative in vivo determinations from ^{40}K measurements. *Science* 140: 480–490.
20. Hargrove, J.L. (1998) *Dynamic Modeling in the Health Sciences*. Springer-Verlag, New York.
21. Fesus, L. (1993) Biochemical events in naturally occurring forms of cell death. *FEBS Lett.* 328: 1–5.
22. Hacker, G., Vaux, D.L. (1997) A chronology of cell death. *Apoptosis* 2: 247–256.
23. Krolmer, G., Petit, P., Zamzame, N., Vayasiere, J-L., and Mignotte, B. (1995) The biochemistry of cell death. *FASEB J.* 9: 1277–1287.
24. Lotem, J., Sachs, L. (1998) Different mechanisms for suppression of apoptosis by cytokines and calcium mobilizing compounds. *Proc. Natl. Acad. Sci. USA* 95: 4601–4606.
25. Mignotte, B., Vayssiere, J.-L. (1998) Mitochondria and apoptosis. *Eur. J. Biochem.* 252: 1–15.
26. Petit, P.X., Zamzami, N., Vayssiere, J.-L., Mignotte, B., Kroemer, G., Castedo, M. (1997) Implication of mitochondria in apoptosis. *Mol. Cell. Biochem.* 174: 185–188.
27. Zheng, T.S., Schlosser, S.F., Dao, T., Hingorani, R., Crispe, I.N., Boyer, J.L., Flavell, R.A. (1998) Caspase-3 controls both cytoplasmic and nuclear events associated with fas-mediated apoptosis in vivo. *Proc. Natl. Acad. Sci. USA* 95: 13618–13623.
28. Cherbonnel-Lasserre, C., Dosanjh, M.K. (1997) Suppression of apoptosis by overexpression of Bcl-2 or Bcl-X_L promotes survival and mutagenesis after oxidative damage. *Biochimie* 79: 613–617.
29. Lotoki, G., Keane, R.W. (2002) Inhibitors of apoptosis proteins in injury and disease. *IUMB Life* 54: 231–240.
30. Wright, S.C., Zhong, J., Larricck, J.W. (1994) Inhibition of apoptosis as a mechanism of tumor promotion. *FASEB J.* 8: 654–660.
31. Tubek, S. (2007) Zinc supplementation or regulation of the homeostasis: Advantages and threats. *Biol. Trace Elem. Res.* 119: 1–9.
32. Zhao, V., Chaiswing, L., Velez, J.M., Batinic-Haberie, I., Colburn, N.H., Oberley, T.D., St. Clair, D.K. (2005) p53 translocation to mitochondria precedes its nuclear translation and targets mitochondrial oxidative defense protein-manganese superoxide dismutase. *Cancer Res.* 65: 3745–3750.
33. Nagy, L., Thomazy, V.A., Heyman, R.A., and Davies, P.J.A. (1998) Retinoid induced apoptosis in normal and neoplastic tissues. *Cell Death Differ.* 5: 11–19.
34. Szondy, Z., Reichert, U., and Fesus, L. (1998) Retinoic acids regulate apoptosis of T lymphocytes through an interplay between RAR and RXR receptors. *Cell Death Differ.* 5: 4–10.

35. Lindquist, J.M., Rehnmark, S. (1998) Ambient temperature regulation of apoptosis in brown adipose tissue. *J. Biol. Chem.* 273: 30147–30156.
36. Lotem, J., Sachs, L. (1998) Different mechanisms for suppression of apoptosis by cytokines and calcium mobilizing compounds. *Proc. Natl. Acad. Sci. USA* 95: 4601–4606.
37. Desai, B., Gruber, H.E. (1999) Anti-apoptotic actions of cytokines in mammalian cells. *Proc. Soc. Exp. Biol. Med.* 221: 1–13.
38. Kumar, S., White, D.L., Takai, S., Turczynowicz, S., Juttner, C., Hughes, T.P. (1995) Apoptosis regulatory gene NEDD2 maps to human chromosome segment 7q34–35, a region frequently affected in haematological neoplasms. *Hum. Genet.* 95: 641–644.
39. Shimabukuro, M., Zhou, Y.T., Levi, M., and Unger, R.H. (1998) Fatty acid-induced ß cell apoptosis: A link between obesity and diabetes. *Proc. Natl. Acad. Sci. USA*. 95: 2498–2502.
40. Maurico, D., Mandrys-Poulsen, T. (1998) Apoptosis and the pathogenesis of IDDM. *Diabetes* 47: 1537–1543.
41. Aspnes, L.E., Lee, C.M., Weindruch, R., Chung, S.S., Roecker, E.B., Aiken, J.M. (1997) Caloric restriction reduces fiber loss and mitochondrial abnormalities in aged rat muscle. *FASEB J.* 11: 573–581.
42. Masoro, E.J. (1990) Assessment of nutritional components in prolongation of life and health by diet. *Proc. Soc. Exp. Biol. Med.* 193: 31–34.
43. Yu, B.P., Masoro, E.J., McMahan, C.A. (1985) Nutritional influences on aging of Fisher 344 rats: I Physical, metabolic, and longevity characteristics. *J. Gerontol.* 40: 657–670.
44. Little, M.E., Hahn, P. (1990) Diet and metabolic development. *FASEB J.* 4: 2605–2611.
45. Chatterjee, B., Fernandies, G., Yu, B.P., Song, C, Kim, J.M., Demyan, W., Roy, A.K. (1989) Calorie restriction delays age-dependent loss in androgen responsiveness of the rat liver. *FASEB J.* 3: 169–173.
46. Stein, Z., Susser, M., Saenger, G., Marolla, F. (1975) *Famine and Human Development*. Oxford University Press, Oxford, U.K., 350pp.
47. Kolasa, K.M., Weismiller, D.G. (2013) Nutrition during pregnancy and lactation In: *Handbook of Nutrition and Food* (C.D. Berdanier, J. Dwyer, D. Heber, eds.). CRC Press, Boca Raton, FL, pp. 261–278.
48. Giles R.E., Blanc, H., Cann, H.M., Wallace, D.C. (1980) Maternal inheritance of human mtDNA. *Proc. Natl. Acad Sci. USA* 77: 6715–6719.
49. www.nap.edu (Accessed October 18, 2013).
50. Ziegler, E.E., O'Donnell, A.M., Nelson, S.E., Fomon, S.J. (1976) Body composition of the reference fetus. *Growth* 40: 329–341.
51. Catalano, P.M., Thomas, A.J., Huston, L.P., Fung, C.M. (1989) Effect of maternal metabolism on fetal growth and body composition. *Diabetes Care* 21(Suppl. 2): B85–B90.
52. Durnwald, C., Huston-Presley, L., Amini, S., Catalano, P. (2004) Evaluation of body composition of large for gestational age infants of women with gestational diabetes mellitus compared with women with normal glucose tolerance levels. *Am. J. Obstet. Gynecol.* 191: 804–808.
53. Larson-Meyer, D.E., Ravussin, E., Heilbronn, L., DeJonge, L. (2010) Ghrelin and peptide YY in postpartum lactating and nonlactating women. *Am. J. Clin. Nutr.* 91: 366–372.
54. Demerath, E.W., Czerwinsky, S.A., Chumlea, W.C. (2013) Height, weight, and body mass index in childhood. In: *Handbook of Nutrition and Food* (C.D. Berdanier, J. Dwyer, D. Heber, eds.). CRC Press, Boca Raton, FL, pp. 641–657.
55. Baxter, S.D. (2013) Nutrition for healthy children and adolescents ages 2–18. In: *Handbook of Nutrition and Food* (C.D. Berdanier, J. Dwyer, D. Heber, eds.). CRC Press, Boca Raton, FL, pp. 292–335.
56. Rose, M.B., Nusbaum, T.J. (1994) Prospects for postponing human aging. *FASEB J.* 8: 925–928.
57. Manton, K.G., Corder, L.S., Stallard, E. (1997) Monitoring changes in the health of the US elderly population: Correlates with biomedical research and clinical innovations. *FASEB J.* 11: 923–930.
58. Ritchie, K. (1994) Facts and research in gerontology 1994. *Supplement on Dementia and Cognitive Impairment*, Vol. 4, p. 2.
59. Johnson, M.A., Haslam, A. (2013) Nutrition in the later years. In: *Handbook of Nutrition and Food* (C.D. Berdanier, J. Dwyer, D. Heber, eds.), 3rd edn. CRC Press, Boca Raton, FL, pp. 347–358.
60. US Census Bureau. (2010) Resident population by race, Hispanic origin, status, and age: 2020–2015. US Government Printing Office, Washington, DC.
61. Hargrove, J.L. (2007) Drug-nutrient Interactions In: *Handbook of Nutrition and Food* (C.D. Berdanier, E.B. Feldman, J. Dwyer, eds.), 2nd edn. CRC Press, Boca Raton, FL, pp. 1237–1240.
62. de Benedictis, G., Rose, G., Carrieri, G., DeLuca, M., Falcone, E., Passarino, G., Bonafe, M. et al. (1999) Mitochondrial DNA inherited variants are associated with successful aging and longevity in humans. *FASEB J.* 13: 1532–1536.

7 Nutrigenomics

Over the last few decades, there has been a growing interest in unraveling the mysteries surrounding the individuality of nutrient need and tolerance. Scientists have sequenced both the human nuclear[1] and mitochondrial genome.[2,3] The mitochondrial genome has been sequenced and mapped, and the far larger nuclear genome is being mapped piece by piece. We can now identify many of the genes of importance to nutrition and metabolism. Nutritionists have been interested not only in how nutrients affect gene expression but also in how small differences in the base sequence of a given gene or in the factors that influence gene expression could affect the gene product. Scientists have been especially interested in how specific nutrients function as promoters or suppressors of specific genes. This area of research is quite active.

Biochemical individuality has been known to exist for decades, and nutrition scientists have realized that the recommendations of nutrient intakes must allow for this. Hence, the early intake recommendations were made such that nearly all people could avoid the consequences of malnutrition if they followed these intake recommendations. Now, however, scientists have come to realize that some intake recommendations are inappropriate for some people. As mentioned in the chapter on energy, a single recommendation of energy intake might be too little for one individual, while for another, it would be too much. This is perhaps the most interesting example of how nutrients and genetic heritage interact to determine the nutrient status of an individual. Other instances can be cited as well. However, before these instances are listed, it is important to consider how genes are expressed and how nutrients affect this expression.

GENES

The sequence of amino acids in each protein synthesized by the body is determined from a subunit of the DNA molecule known as the gene. It consists of several thousands of bases (abbreviated as kb, 1000 bases = 1 kb). Each protein has a unique base sequence in its cognate gene. While only four bases are used in the DNA, the combinations and sequences of the combinations provide a specific code for the messenger RNA (mRNA) that in turns encodes the amino acid sequence of each and every protein and peptide. DNA also functions to transmit genetic information from one generation to the next in a given species. Thus, DNA has a broad spectrum of function—it ensures the identity of both specific cell types and specific species.

GENE EXPRESSION

The characteristics of a body within a species are determined by the base sequence of its genetic material, DNA. Most of this DNA is found in the nucleus, while a small amount is found in the mitochondria. Through its sequence of bases, it dictates the sequence of amino acids in each of the peptides and proteins it encodes. Each amino acid has one or more codons that specify it in a chain of amino acids that constitutes the gene product. These codons are listed in Table 7.1.

Note that for every amino acid except tryptophan, there is more than one codon. This serves as a fail-safe mechanism in that if a base substitution should occur and the substitution produces a codon that also encodes the same amino acid, then the base substitution is without effect on the gene product. Note too that there are stop codons and a start codon. These codons signal the start and stop of a given structural gene. These codons (start and stop) dictate the length of the transcription product (mRNA) and in turn signal the length of the amino acid chain.

TABLE 7.1
Codons for the Amino Acids

	First Base							
Second Base	**U**		**C**		**A**		**G**	
U	UUU	Phe	CUU		AUU		GUU	
	UUC		CUC	Leu	AUC	Ile	GUC	Val
	UUA	Leu	CUA		AUA		GUA	
	UUG		CUG		AUG[a]	MET	GUG	
C	UCU		CCU		ACU		GCU	
	UCC	Ser	CCC	Pro	ACC	Thr	GCC	Ala
	UCA		CCA		ACA		GCA	
	UCG		CCG		ACT		GCG	
A	UAU	Tyr	CAU	His	AAU	Asn	GAU	Asp
	UAC		CAC		AAC		GAC	
	UAA	STOP	CAA	Gln	AAA	Lys	GAA	Glu
	UAG	STOP	CAG		AAG		GAG	
G	UGU	Cys	CGU		AGU	Ser	GGU	
	UGC		CGC	Arg	AGC		GGC	Gly
	UGA	STOP	CGA		AGA	Arg	GGA	
	UGG	Trp	CGG		AGG		GGG	

[a] AUG also serves as a start codon.

The process of protein synthesis using the sequence of bases in the DNA provides the basis for understanding genetic differences. It is also the basis for understanding how the unique properties of each cell type are maintained, since the properties that make cells unique are usually conferred by the peptides and proteins within them. Some of these proteins are the structural elements of the cell. Others are enzymes that catalyze specific reactions and processes that characterize the cell in question. Still other proteins confer a particular biochemical function on the cell. Should there be a change in the sequence of the bases within the structural gene, the sequence of amino acids in the resultant gene product may or may not be different. As described earlier, the most innocuous change might result in a codon that will indicate the same amino acid in the gene product. In another setting, the change in base sequence of a codon could mean a substitution of one amino acid for another. If the two are similar in size and charge, this codon base change might not be a serious defect. The gene product might retain its functional properties. This is especially true if the amino acid in question is not in the active site of the protein or is far removed from the working part of the gene product. If the protein whose amino acid sequence has been changed is crucial to the normal functioning of the organism, then this change is serious indeed. If, on the other hand, the protein is of minor importance, then a change in its sequence is of little consequence. In addition, there can be base sequence changes in portions of the DNA that have control properties on transcription. Cis and trans transcription factors, if aberrant, can affect mRNA synthesis and therefore affect the synthesis of the gene product.

DNA Structure

As mentioned earlier, DNA is composed of four bases: adenine, guanine, thymine, and cytosine. These bases are condensed to form the DNA chain in a process analogous to the condensation of amino acids that serve as the primary structure of a protein. Species vary in the percentage distribution of these bases in their DNA. The chain of nucleotides that makes up the DNA is formed by joining adenine, guanine, thymine, and cytosine through phosphodiester bonds. The phosphodiester linkage is between the 5′ phosphate group of one nucleotide and the 3′ hydroxyl group of the adjacent nucleotide. This provides a direction (5′ to 3′) to the chain. A typical segment of the chain is illustrated in Figure 7.1. The hydrophobic properties of the bases plus the strong charges of the polar groups within each of the component units are responsible for the helical conformation of the DNA chain. Hydrogen bonding between the bases stabilizes this conformation, as shown in Figure 7.2. The bases themselves interact so that, in the nucleus, the two chains are intertwined. Hence, the term *double helix* applies to the structure of the nuclear DNA. In the mitochondria, the DNA is also a double strand but is arranged as a double circle with connections between the light and heavy strands. Both the base sequence of the double-stranded ring and the location of each of the genes in this DNA have been determined. This structure is illustrated in Figure 7.3.

In contrast to nuclear DNA that has a promoter region before each of the structural genes, the mitochondrial genome has a single promoter for all of the structural genes. This promoter region is

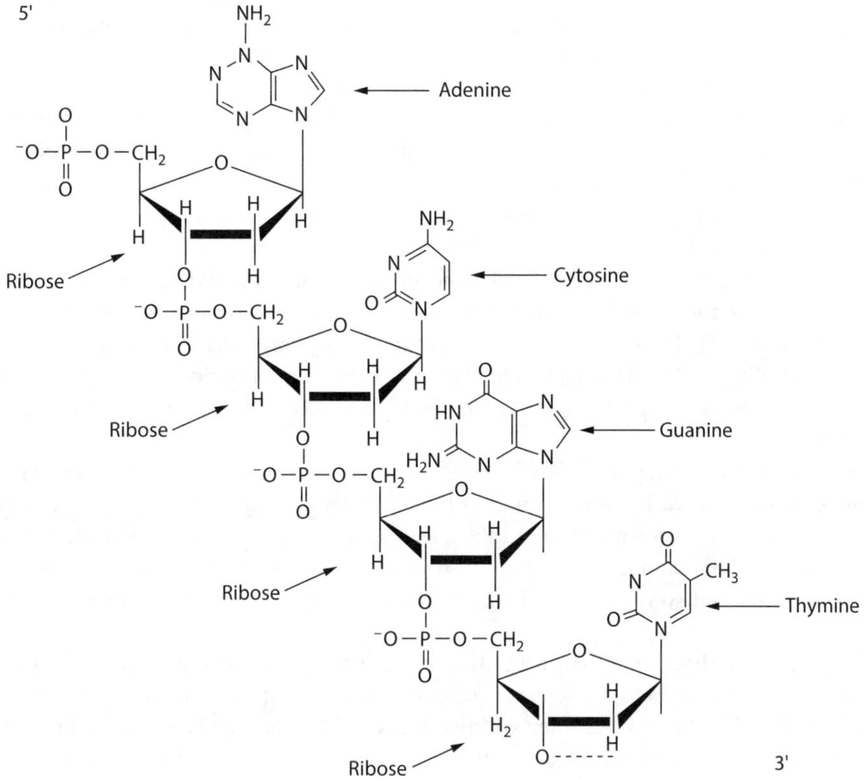

FIGURE 7.1 The bases that make up the DNA polynucleotide chain are joined together by phosphodiester bonds using ribose as the common link between the bases.

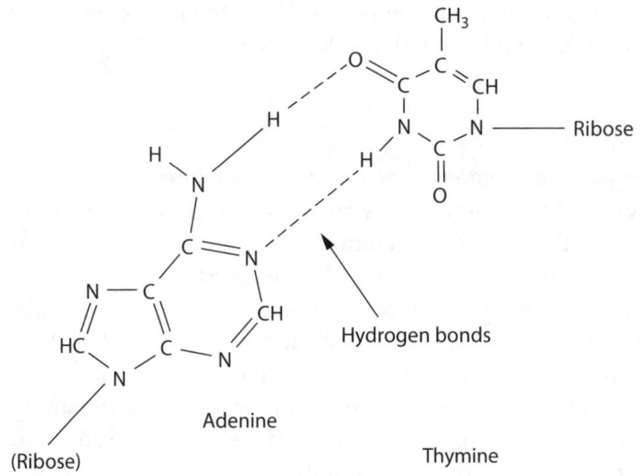

FIGURE 7.2 Hydrogen bonds form between complementary bases: adenine complements thymine; guanine complements cytosine. These bonds stabilize the double-helical array of the two DNA strands.

located in the D-loop. It has putative elements for the binding of the receptors for vitamins A and D as well as for other members of the steroid receptor family and other transcription factors.

The mitochondrial genome contains 12 structural genes that encode components of the oxidative phosphorylation (OXPHOS) system (Figure 7.3). One of these encodes a subunit of the F_1F_0 ATPase, while the rest encode subunits of the sites one and three of the respiratory chain. Mutations in this genome are passed from mother to child. The nature of the mutations is such that only heterozygotes survive when the mutation affects the active sites of the gene products. Homozygosity is lethal since such a mutation would mean that the OXPHOS system would not work. With respect to heterozygosity, if the percent mutated DNA is less than 50%, there might not be any discernible symptoms. When the mutated DNA approaches 90%, serious disease is observed. Because of the randomness of the distribution of mutated and normal DNA, siblings of an affected mother can evidence a variety of symptoms. Individuals with such mutations frequently have larger than normal requirements for vitamins A and D as well as increased needs for the antioxidant vitamin E.

In the nucleus, the DNA is found in the chromosomal chromatin shown in Figure 7.4. Chromatin contains very long double strands of DNA and a nearly equal mass of histone and nonhistone proteins.[5] The histones, H1, H2A, H2B, H3, and H4, are highly basic proteins varying in molecular weight from ~11,000 to ~21,000. As a result of their high content of basic amino acids, the histones serve to interact with the polyanionic phosphate backbone of the DNA so as to produce uncharged nucleoproteins.

Histones also serve to keep the DNA in a very compact form and, as well, serve to protect this DNA from damage by external agents such as free radicals or viruses or drugs. In mammals, the mitochondrial DNA does not have this protective histone coat. It is *naked* and much more vulnerable to damage. This damage can be quite severe yet because there are so many copies of the mitochondrial DNA and so many mitochondria in a cell, the effects of this damage might not be apparent.

The DNA and the histones form repetitive nucleoprotein units, the nucleosomal core particles. Each particle consists of 146 base pairs of DNA wrapped around an octamer of core histones (one H3–H3–H4–H4 tetramer and two H2A–H2B dimers). The DNA located between nucleosomal core particles is associated with histone H1 (Figure 7.4). This 11 nm histone fiber is then further packed into an irregular 30 nm chromatin fiber structure, which is coiled into even more complex structures to eventually assemble the chromosome. The amino terminal tails of histones protrude from the nucleosomal surface; covalent modifications of these tails affect the

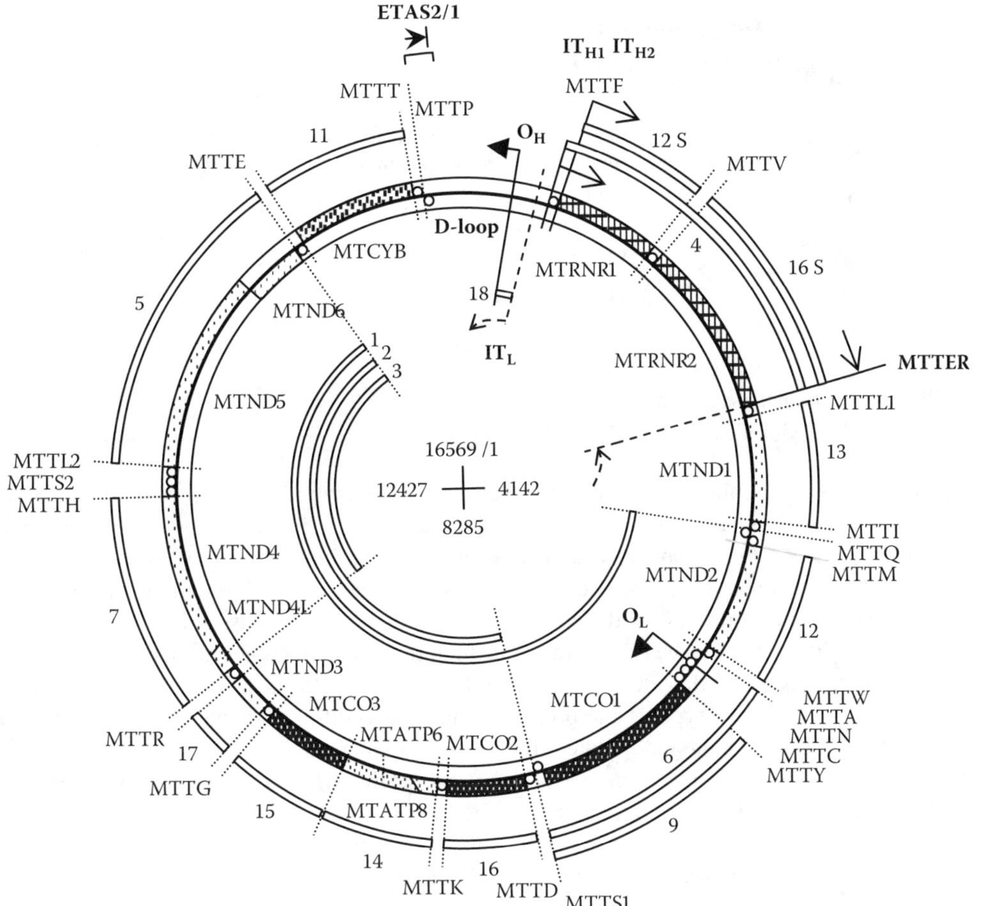

FIGURE 7.3 Genetic and transcriptional map of the human mitochondrial genome.[4] The circle represents the mtDNA duplex. Shaded areas on the outer ring represent those genes encoded on the heavy strand, while the light strand is shown as the inner circle. There are 22 tRNA genes shown as open dots. The 7S DNA species is in the control region (the D-loop or the common promoter region for this genome) shown as a broken line box within the two circles. The nucleotides in the human are numbered from 1 to 16,569. Transcripts are numbered according to size, 1–18, and include the 12 structural genes that encode subunits of the respiratory chain and the F_1F_0 ATPase. These are abbreviated: MTATP6, MTATP8 (subunits of the F_1F_0 ATPase), MTND6, MTND5, MTND4, MTND4L, MTND2, MTND1 (subunits of complex 1), MTCO3, MTCO2, and MTCO1 (subunits of complex 3). The remaining transcripts are those of the ribosomal proteins (12S and 16S) and the RNA at the R-loop. The site where transcription terminates is indicated by MTERF. This is where the nuclear-encoded mitochondrial transcription termination factor binds.

structure of chromatin and form the basis for the epigenetic regulation of chromatin structure and gene function.[6,7]

During cell division, the nuclear DNA, as soon as its replication is completed, becomes highly condensed into distinct chromosomes of characteristic shapes. These chromosomes exist as pairs and are numbered. There are 46 chromosomes in the human. Included in this number are the sex chromosomes, the X and Y chromosomes. If the individual has one X and one Y, he is a male; if two X's are present, she is a female. The chromosomes are the result of a mixing of the nuclear DNA of the egg and sperm. Approximately half of each pair comes from each parent. If identical codes

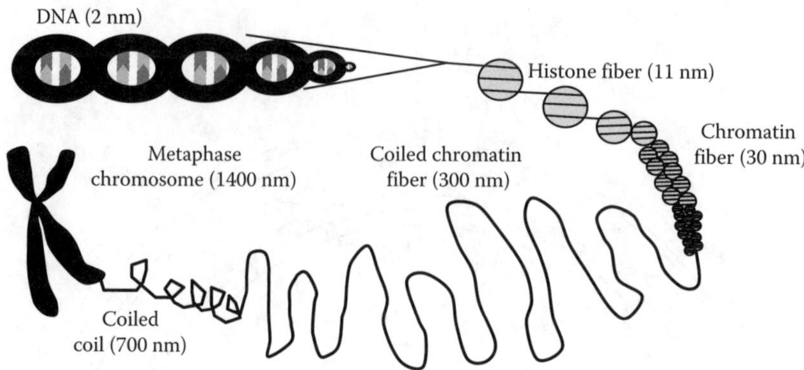

FIGURE 7.4 Chromatin structure.

for a given protein are inherited from each parent, the resultant progeny will be a homozygote for that protein. If nonidentical codes are inherited, the progeny will be a heterozygote. Within the heterozygote population, there may be certain codes that are dominant, for example, eye color or hair color. These are dominant traits and are expressed despite the fact that the individual has inherited two different codes for this trait. A difference in a code that is not expressed is a recessive trait. If, by chance, the difference in the code represents a mutation and two copies of this aberrant code are inherited, the expression of this mutated code will be observed. This is the basis for genetic diseases of the autosomal recessive type. If the progeny inherits two different copies of the aberrant code and one of these is dominant and mutated, the disease is an autosomal dominant type. Autosomal means a mutation in any of the chromosomal DNA except that which is in the X or Y chromosome. A mutation of the DNA in this chromosome is called a sex-linked mutation. If it results in a disease, it is called sex-linked genetic disease. There is another inheritance pattern based on the mitochondrial genome. Because this genome is primarily of maternal origin, certain of the characteristics of the OXPHOS system will be inherited via maternal inheritance. A number of mitochondrial mutations result in a number of degenerative diseases.

Mutation or Polymorphisms

Changes in the normal sequence of bases in the DNA can occur. If the change results in an aberrant gene product (the protein it encodes), then it is called a *mutation*. If the change has little or no effect on the gene product, then it is called a polymorphism. Sometimes, a change can occur that results in a change in the amino acid sequence of the gene product, but if this change has no effect on the functionality of the product, it too is called a *polymorphism*. DNA and protein polymorphisms can have subtle effects on how an individual responds to a nutrition variable. Examples of these responses are listed in Table 7.2.

A mutation can be spontaneous or one induced by free radicals or drugs that induce free radical damage, a virus, or any one of a number of external variants that target the genetic material of the cell. Mutations can be base substitutions, base rearrangements, base deletions, or base additions. The DNA damage is random, in most cases. That is, it does not occur in the same place in every cell. There are some places in the DNA that are more vulnerable to damage than are other places. These are the places where there are direct repeats of bases.

DNA damage whether spontaneous or caused by external agents can be repaired in the nucleus,[27] but the mitochondrial DNA has little self-repair.[4] Sometimes, repair takes place but is inaccurate. That is, the repair does not fully restore the base sequence to its predamaged state.[27] In this scenario,

TABLE 7.2
Interactions of Polymorphisms with Nutrient Variables

Gene/Protein	Polymorphism	Nutrient variable	Result
β-2-adrenoceptor Gln27Glu	Carbohydrate		↑ Insulin levels; obesity.[8]
Hepatic lipase	480C→T	Fat	↑ Lipase activity in CT and TT than CC.[9]
PPARα	162L→V	PUFA	V had lower apoC-III.[10]
MTHFR	C677T	Folate, B_{12}	TT genotypes had higher serum homocysteine levels, ↓ RBC folate, and need more dietary folate.[11–14]
MTHFR	677+/+ vs. +/–	Folate and choline	↑ Choline turnover.[15]
MTHFR	1298A→C	PUFA	↑ Homocysteine; ↑ hypertension.[16]
IL2	330A→C	Vitamin E	↓ Respiratory infection in C.[17]
IL10	819G→C	Vitamin E	↓ Respiratory infection in C.[17]
IL10	1982C→T	Vitamin E	↓ Respiratory infection in T.[17]
ANGPTL4	A→G	Fat intake	A had ↑ HDL-C and ↓ TG.[18]
TCN267	A→G vs. AA Vitamin B_{12}		↓ Holotranscarbamylase in A.[19]
GST	M1 vs. T1	Vitamin C	↑ Vitamin C, ↓ malondialdehyde, ↑ iron, ↑ total LDL cholesterol in GSTM1 than in GSTT1.[20]
GSTM and GSTT	(Deletion mutations)	Iron	GSTM mothers, responsive; GSTT mothers, not responsive—with respect to infant birth weight.[21]
TNFα	308G→A	Fat intake	G allele, more responsive to fat intake than A allele.[22]
LEPR	A→G	PUFA	G allele had ↑ insulin and insulin resistance compared to the A allele when fed PUFA.[23]
	G→A	Oral glucose	↑ Blood pressure; ↑ BMI.[24]
FTO	A→T	Food intake	AA genotypes were fatter than AT.[25]
ADIPOQ	G→A	Sat. fat	GG genotype produced more adiponectin than AG genotype.[26]

Abbreviations: PPARα, peroxisome proliferator-activated receptor alpha; MTHFR, methyltetrahydrofolate reductase; IL, interleukin; GST, glutathione S-transferase; TNFα, tumor necrosis factor alpha; LPR, leptin receptor; FTO, fat mass obesity; ADIPOQ, adiponectin; and PUFA, polyunsaturated fatty acids.

a base addition or a different base substitution or mismatch repair could occur. This mutation will then become part of the genetic information transmitted to the next generation. Polymorphisms are useful research tools, because they allow population geneticists to track mutation and evolutionary events through related family members. Polymorphisms in the amino acid structures of a given protein occur between species. Sometimes, the polymorphism is such that a protein from one species can be given to another with little chance of rejection of that protein by the recipient. Such was the case before the development of human insulin (a biotech reproduction of human insulin). Prior to this development, insulin was extracted from the pancreas of pigs and cows and prepared for use by insulin-dependent diabetics. Although there were species differences in the amino acid sequence of these insulins, these differences did not prevent their use as a hormone replacement for those who needed it. The species differences were not in the active sites of the hormone, nor were they in sites that rapidly induced an immune response to the foreign protein.

Epigenetics

Genetic change can also be due to environmental factors that affect chromatin but that do not affect the DNA base sequence. This is called epigenetic change. The amino acid residues in histone tails can be modified by covalent acetylation, biotinylation, methylation, phosphorylation, or ubiquitination (Figure 7.5), and this will have effects on gene transcription, mitotic condensation of chromatin, and DNA repair.[28–40] Many epigenetic events are due to environmental factors. For example, air pollutants or nutrient deficiencies or exposure to toxic materials can evoke an epigenetic event.

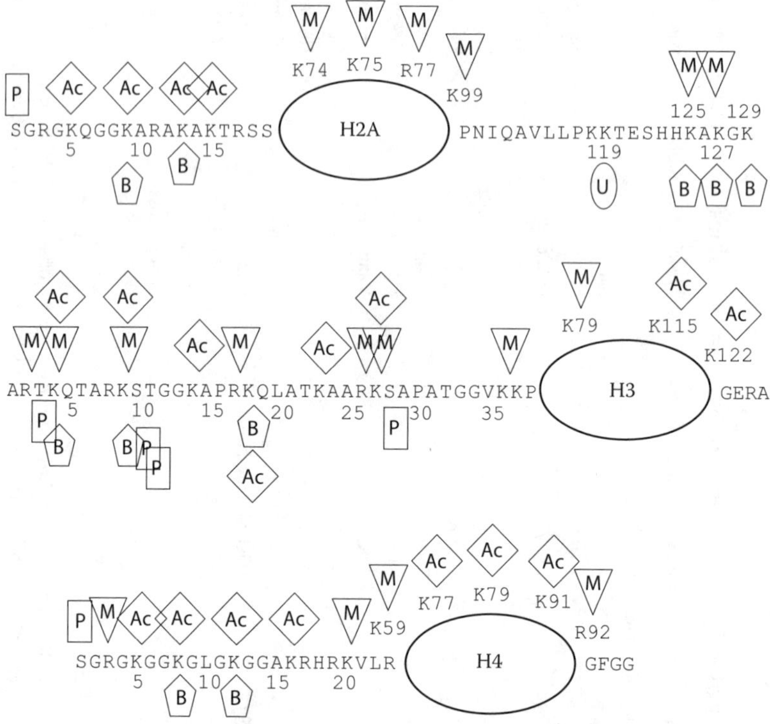

FIGURE 7.5 Modification sites in histones H2A, H3, and H4. The abbreviations used are Ac, acetate; B, biotin; M, methyl; P, phosphate; and U, ubiquitin.

The modifications due to acetylation, biotinylation, methylation, and so forth are deciphered by proteins containing motifs that target them to chromatin. For example, some transcription factors contain bromo domains that have an affinity for acetylated histones, increasing gene expression.[33] For another example, trimethylation of lysine (K)-4 in histone H3 is associated with the transcriptional activation of the surrounding DNA, whereas dimethylation of K9 is associated with transcriptional silencing.[28,29] Covalent modifications of histones can be reversed in a number of ways.[28] Several vitamin-dependent histone modifications have been identified that use biotin. Biotin can bind to the lysine residues in the histones. In one example, the sodium-dependent multivitamin transporter gene is regulated at the chromatin level by histone biotinylation.[30–32,35] In another example, transposable elements are repressed by histone biotinylation. Transposable elements serve to stabilize the genome. If the chromatin histone coat is biotinylated, there is an increase in genome instability and this, in turn, increases cancer risk.[35,36] In addition, there is folate-dependent methylation of lysine residues[37] and niacin-dependent poly-ADP-ribosylation of glutamate residues.[38] The acetylation of histones represents a vitamin-dependent form of chromatin structure regulation. This is based on the observation that pantothenate-derived coenzyme A is critical to the formation of acetyl-CoA. Acetyl-CoA, in turn, is the acetyl donor for histone acetylation. Niacin (as part of NAD and NADP) is also an important player in this process.[38] The methylation of histones can alter acetylation patterns. Finally, another folate-dependent epigenetic event is the covalent binding of methyl groups (derived from folate) to produce 5-methylcytosine in mammalian DNA.[34,37] This modification of DNA depends on a number of nutrients: S-adenosyl methionine, vitamin B_{12}, vitamin B_6, methionine, betaine, riboflavin, zinc, and choline.[34] Methylation of cytosine residues in DNA is associated with repression of transcription.

Epigenetic responsiveness to dietary manipulation such as caloric restriction has been invoked to explain why some individuals are more responsive to this treatment than others.[39] Significant DNA methylation differences in 35 loci have been reported between 2 groups of obese women who were given an energy-restricted diet. One group responded well to the treatment losing significant weight, while the other group was resistant to this treatment. Similarly, there have been reported differences in response by persons with type 2 diabetes with respect to epigenetic responses to environmental stimuli.[40] Aging, physical activity, and dietary protocols have elicited epigenetic responses such as DNA methylation at specific loci in some people but not in others. Clearly, there are individual differences in the histone coat of the chromatin that can explain the differential responses of these people. A full understanding of these differences is not in hand.

Synthesis of Purines and Pyrimidines

The synthesis of DNA and RNA depends on the synthesis of the purine and pyrimidine bases that are building blocks of the nucleic acids. Note that mRNA contains uracil in place of thymine; the latter is found only in DNA (see below). Purine and pyrimidine syntheses are nutrient dependent. When insufficient purines and pyrimidines are provided, cell replacement, growth, and tissue repair are not possible. In this respect, one can understand the many symptoms of nutrient deficiency disorders such as pellagra, scurvy, beriberi, and anemia. Short-lived cells that must replicate themselves often will show signs of deficiency far earlier than long-lived cells. Hence, skin lesions and anemia are characteristics of water-soluble vitamin deficiency as well as protein deficiency. Nutrients that can be stored, that is, the fat-soluble vitamins, will have a longer time for symptom development, yet the first signs of deficiency will likewise be seen in the short-lived cells of the epithelia and blood. Many of the micronutrients as well as energy and protein are needed for the synthesis of the purine and pyrimidine bases.

Before pyrimidines and purines can be incorporated into DNA and RNA, they must be synthesized. They are synthesized de novo and this synthesis requires, both directly and indirectly, a number of vitamins and minerals as well as energy. The purines are adenine and guanine, while the pyrimidines are cytosine, uracil, and thymine. The purines form glycosidic bonds to ribose via the N(9) atoms, whereas the pyrimidines do this using their N(a) atoms. Pyrimidine synthesis is shown in Figure 7.6, while purine synthesis is shown in Figure 7.7.

In this pathway, the addition of ribose occurs prior to ring closure and phosphorylation. Also shown in Figures 7.6 and 7.7 are the micronutrients needed for these pathways. Where ATP is involved in a reaction step, all of the vitamins that serve as coenzymes in intermediary metabolism are needed. This includes niacin, thiamin, riboflavin, lipoic acid, pantothenic acid, biotin, folacin, vitamin B_{12}, pyridoxine, choline, and inositol. Also needed are the minerals of importance to the redox reactions of OXPHOS, that is, iron, copper, and, of course, iodine as a component of the thyroid hormones (synthesized from the amino acid tyrosine) that regulate OXPHOS and the selenium-containing enzyme (5′ deiodinase) that converts thyroxine to its active form, triiodothyronine.

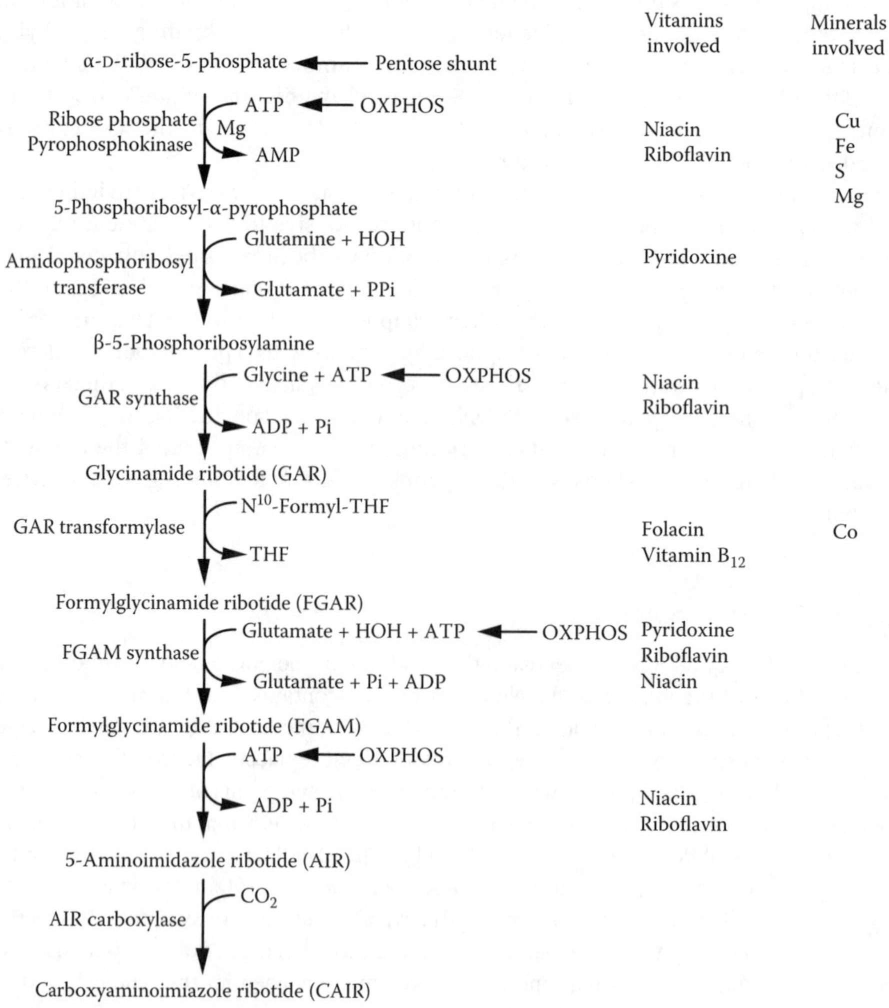

FIGURE 7.6 Purine synthesis. *(Continued)*

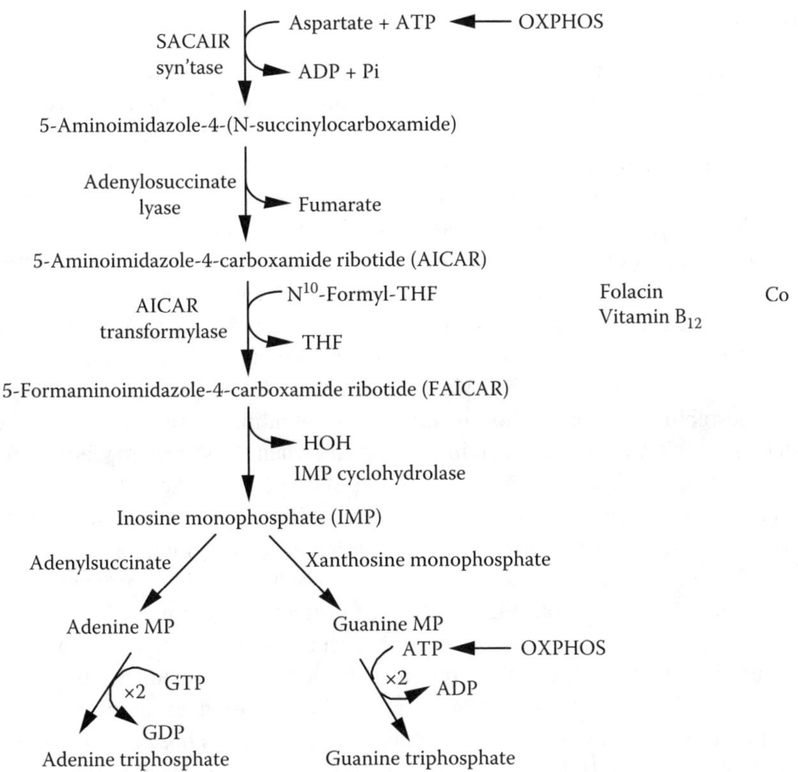

FIGURE 7.6 (CONTINUED) Purine synthesis.

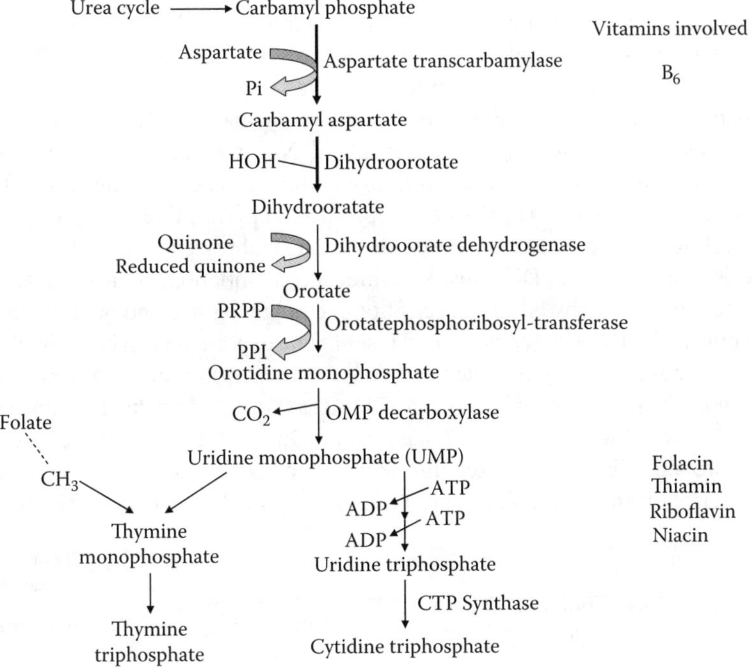

FIGURE 7.7 Pyrimidine synthesis. In this pathway, the pyrimidine ring is formed before it is attached to ribose and phosphorylated.

TRANSCRIPTION

Having the codes in the nucleus for the synthesis of protein in the cytoplasm implies a communication between the cytoplasm and the nucleus and between the nucleus and the cytoplasm. Signals are sent to the nucleus that *inform* this organelle of the need to synthesize certain proteins. Signals include substrates for the needed proteins, nutrients, hormones, and other signaling compounds, some of which have yet to be identified.[41–48] The nucleus directs protein synthesis in the cytoplasm by sending mRNA to the cytoplasmic compartment. This process is called *transcription.*

Each gene will have its own unique signals for the initiation of transcription. Some signals are very strong and will stimulate the transcription of a group of related genes. An example of this is the four genes that encode the components of fatty acid synthetase. All are stimulated to transcribe by the same set of signals. Transcription does not occur spontaneously and it follows that the DNA is quite stable unless signaled to transcribe. Many factors serve to stabilize the structure of the DNA. When DNA is destabilized, transcription is initiated. Unwinding a small portion of the DNA is a necessary step in the initiation of transcription and occurs when the stabilizing factors are perturbed and signals are sent to the nucleus that transcription of a specific gene should begin. Unwinding exposes a small (~17 kb) segment of the DNA (the gene), allowing its base sequence to be available for complementary base pairing for the synthesis of mRNA. The segment that is exposed contains not only the portion of the gene that codes for the corresponding mRNA (*coding region*) but also a sequence called the *promoter* region (Figure 7.8). The promoter region precedes the start site of the coding region, and this is said to be *upstream* of the structural gene. Sequences of bases that bind specific proteins are called *elements.* The proteins that bind to these elements are receptors that in turn bind substances that affect transcription. Some of these substances are nutrients, while others may be hormones or other gene activators, enhancers, or silencers. Those bases following the start site are *downstream.* The nucleotides that code for a specific protein may not be adjacent to each other on the DNA strand but may be located nearby.

mRNA is used to carry genetic information from the DNA of the chromosomes to the surface of the ribosomes (Figure 7.9). It is synthesized through the activity of RNA polymerase II as a single strand in the nucleus.[43–47,49–52] Chemically, RNA is similar to DNA. It is an unbranched linear polymer in which the monomeric subunits are the ribonucleoside-5′-monophosphates. The bases include the purines (adenine and guanine) and pyrimidines (uracil and cytosine). RNA is single stranded rather than double stranded. It is held together by molecular base pairing and will contract if in a solution of high ionic strength. RNA, particularly the mRNA, is a much smaller molecule than DNA and is far less stable. It has a very short half-life (from minutes to hours) compared to that of nuclear DNA (years). Because it has a short half-life, the purine and pyrimidine bases are reused whenever possible. If recycling does not occur, the bases must be resynthesized.

The synthesis of mRNA from DNA involves three steps: initiation, elongation, and termination. Initiation is the process whereby basal transcription factors recognize and bind to DNA. These factors form a complex with RNA polymerase II. Most of gene expression can be defined as transacting factors (proteins) binding to cis-acting elements (base sequences) in the promoter regions of genes. Within the promoter, approximately 25 base pairs upstream of the start site, is a consensus sequence called the TATA box, which contains A-T base pairs. One of the basal transcription factors, the TATA-binding protein (TBP), recognizes this sequence of DNA and binds there. This begins the process of transcription initiation. The transacting TBP binds to the cis-acting TATA box, and a

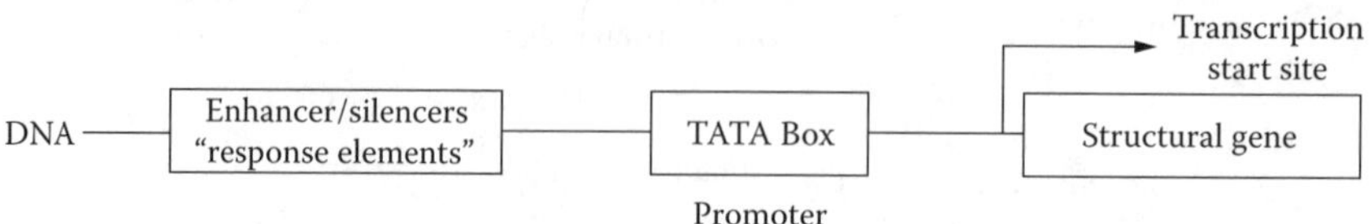

FIGURE 7.8 Detailed structure of the components of a gene that is to be transcribed.

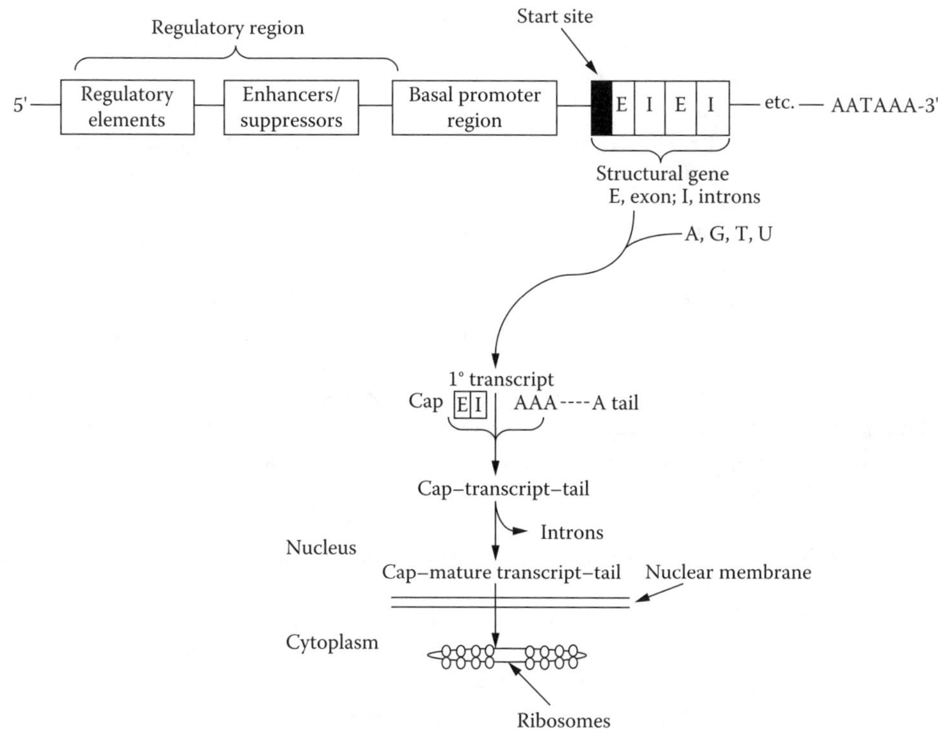

FIGURE 7.9 Synthesis of mRNA and its migration to the ribosomes in the cytoplasm.

large complex of basal transcription factors, RNA polymerase II, and DNA is formed. Elongation is the actual process of RNA formation through the use of a DNA template in the 5′-to-3′ direction. Shortly after elongation begins, the 5′ end of mRNA is capped by 7-methylguanosine triphosphate. This cap stabilizes the mRNA and is necessary for processing and translation. The third step is the termination of the chain.

Transcription control is exerted by that portion of the DNA called the promoter region plus transcription factors that bind either to this region or to an upstream region that in turn affects the activity of either cis-acting factors or the polymerase II activity. RNA polymerase II binds to the promoter region just upstream of the start codon for the gene. The promoter region is located in the 5′ flanking region upstream from the structural gene on the same strand of DNA. Cis-responsive elements are located about −40 to −200 bp from the start site. Some promoters, that is, TATA, GC, and CCAAT boxes, are common to many genes transcribed by RNA polymerase II. These sequences interact with transcription factors that in turn form preinitiation complexes. The mechanisms of such transcriptional regulation have been reviewed by Semenza[46] and Johnson et al.[47] Transacting factors are usually proteins produced by other genes that influence transcription. Transacting factors can be proteins or peptide hormones or steroid hormone–receptor protein complexes, or vitamin–receptor protein complexes, or minerals, or mineral–protein complexes. The mechanism for binding hormone receptors to specific regions of DNA has been reviewed and described by Freedman and Luisi.[42] The promoter region contains the start site for RNA synthesis. RNA polymerase II binds to this specific DNA sequence, and under the influence of the various transcription factors, RNA transcription is initiated.[41–52] The RNA polymerase II opens up a local region of the DNA double helix so that the gene to be transcribed is exposed. One of the two DNA strands acts as the template for complementary base pairing with incoming ribonucleotide triphosphate molecules. The nucleotides are joined until the polymerase encounters a special sequence in the DNA called the termination sequence. At this point, transcription is complete. Following this process, the newly formed RNA is edited and processed.

This processing removes nearly 95% of the bases. The resultant shortened RNA then migrates out of the nucleus and becomes associated with ribosomes whereupon translation takes place.

This outline of transcription has omitted a number of important details with respect to transcription control. For example, the regulation of transcription is exerted by a group of proteins that determine which region of the DNA is to be transcribed. Cells contain a variety of sequence-specific DNA-binding proteins. Nutrients can bind to these proteins and have their effect in this way. These proteins are of low abundance, and they function by binding to specific regions (elements) on the DNA. The regions are variable in size but are usually between 8 and 15 nucleotides. Depending on the binding protein and the nutrient bound to it, transcription is either enhanced or inhibited and indeed cell types may differ because of these proteins. Since all cells contain the same DNA, gene expression in discrete cell types is controlled at this point simply by the binding of these very specific DNA-binding proteins. Thus, genes for the synthesis of insulin, for example, could be turned on in the pancreatic β cell, but not in the myocyte, simply because the β cell has the needed specific DNA-binding proteins that the myocyte lacks. At some point in differentiation, the myocyte failed to acquire sufficient amounts of these regulatory factors and thus cannot synthesize and release insulin.

In many instances, specific DNA-binding proteins contain zinc and the portions on the zinc-containing protein that binds to DNA are referred to as zinc fingers.[48,53] Gene expression is regulated by the formation of these zinc fingers, yet they are only a part of this regulation. Most genes are regulated by a combination of regulatory factors. In some, a group of DNA-binding proteins interact to control the activation or inhibition of transcription. Not all of these proteins are of equal power in all instances. There may be a *master* regulatory protein that serves to coordinate the binding of several *lesser* proteins. This is important for the coordinate expression of genes in a single pathway, as happens, for example, in the expression of the genes that encode the multienzyme complex, fatty acid synthetase.

Mutations in genes that encode any one of these transcription factors could result in disease.[54–56] Mutations in genes encoding transcription factors often have pleiotropic effects because these factors regulate a number of different genes. So, too, are the effects of nutrients that are required components of these transcription factors. An example is the series of genes that encode the enzymes needed for the conversion of a fibroblast to a myocyte.[54] The mammalian skeletal muscle cell is very large and multinucleated. It is formed by the fusion of myoblasts (myocyte precursor cells) and contains characteristic structural proteins as well as a number of other proteins that function in energy metabolism and nerve–muscle signaling. When muscle is being synthesized, all of these proteins must be synthesized at the same time. In proliferating myoblasts, very few of these proteins are present, yet as these myoblasts fuse, the mRNAs for these proteins increase as does the synthesis of the proteins. This indicates that the expression of the genes for muscle protein synthesis is responding to a single regulatory DNA-binding protein. This protein (Myo D1) has been isolated and identified and occurs only in muscle cells. Should this protein be inserted in some other cell type such as a skin cell or an adipocyte, for example, the same expression will occur. That is, the skin or fat cell will look like a muscle cell. It will take on the characteristics of a myoblast and become a myocyte.

Of interest is the fact that although all of the genes needed for synthesis in the myocyte and its master controller are present, synthesis will not occur or will occur at a very limited rate if one or more of the essential amino acids needed for this synthesis are absent or deficient in the diet. Here is an example of a gene–nutrient interaction that has control properties with respect to muscle protein synthesis, and this interaction ultimately affects the overall process of growth. Turning this situation around, if the master regulator Myo D1 is aberrant or if one or more of the genes that encode the enzymes needed for protein synthesis in the myocyte have mutated such that the enzyme in question is nonfunctional or only partly functional, muscle development will cease or be retarded. In either instance, abnormal growth will result.

As mentioned, transcription is regulated by both the nearby upstream promoter region and the distant enhancer elements. The upstream enhancer element can include a TATA box and extends for about 100 bp. Enhancer fragments further upstream can bind multiple proteins which, in turn, can influence transcription. These factors are proteins and are labeled JUN, AP2, ATF, CREB,

SP1, OTF1, CTF, NF1, SRE, and others. One well-studied group of DNA-binding proteins is that which binds the steroid hormones.[57–63] These are called the steroid receptors and are members of a group of proteins called the steroid superfamily of receptor proteins. They bind to specific base sequences called steroid response elements (SREs). Included in this superfamily are receptors for vitamins A and D, the glucocorticoids, the sex hormones, and the thyroid hormones. This group of receptors is regulated by ligand binding. The ligands are the aforementioned steroids and hormones. All members of this family of DNA-binding proteins contain two zinc fingers in their DNA-binding domains. Zinc is bound to the histidine- and cysteine-rich regions of the protein that envelops the DNA in a shape that looks like a finger.[48,57] The zinc finger is shown in Figure 7.9. The zinc ion plays an enormous role in gene expression because of its central use in the zinc finger.

The action of these complexes explains how cells respond to a steroid hormone stimulus. Each receptor protein consists of about 100 amino acids and zinc. As mentioned, they recognize a specific DNA sequence. For some members of this family of proteins, the transcription-enhancing domain is localized at the amino terminus of the polypeptide chain. This is the part of the molecule that binds to the promoter region of the DNA of a specific gene. At the carboxy terminus is the binding site for the hormone. Steroid hormones have their effects through binding to their cognate receptors that in turn binds to the hormone response element on the DNA. Members of the superfamily also enhance the transcription of mitochondrial genes.[58,62] The recognition of this function of steroid hormones provides a further explanation of how these hormones function in energy balance. Enhanced mitochondrial gene expression should result in an increased mitochondrial function, that is, enhanced activity of OXPHOS. In turn, this would result in increased ATP production that is needed for cell function and tissue growth.

The regulation of transcription occurs at the initiation step. The promoter region contains many cis-acting elements, each named for the factor that controls them. An element is a particular sequence of bases in the DNA that binds with a specific binding protein. In general, these regions are called *response elements*. Examples include the retinoic acid response element (RARE), heat shock element (HSE), and cAMP response element (CRE). The transacting factors that bind these elements are in general called *transcription factors*. They are also referred to as DNA-binding receptor proteins. They are proteins with at least two domains, DNA binding and transcription activation. A number of nutrients bind to nuclear receptors that in turn bind to DNA, and together these nutrient-bound receptors have effects on transcription. Recently, it has been shown that coactivators are needed to bind transcription factors and increase transcription by both interacting with basal transcription factors and altering chromatin structure. Nutrient-dependent DNA-remodeling events (*epigenetics*) also play a critical role in the regulation of transcription.[58] Corepressors act to decrease transcription at both the level of basal transcription factors and chromatin structure. Coactivators and corepressors are proteins.

The true regulation of transcription occurs by the regulation of transcription factors.[64,65] Transcription factors can be regulated by

- Their rates of synthesis or degradation
- Phosphorylation or dephosphorylation
- Ligand binding
- Cleavage of a protranscription factor
- Release of an inhibitor

There are other examples of the effects of nutrients on gene transcription. It has been shown that supplementation with the vitamin biotin increases the synthesis of transcription factors Spl and Sp3[60] enhancing the transcriptional activity of Spl-/Sp3-dependent genes. Another mechanism of biotin-dependent gene expression is increased phosphorylation of *a NF-κB inhibitor* in the cytoplasm.[61] Phosphorylation of the inhibitor of NF-κB causes its dissociation from NF-κB in the cytoplasm. Subsequently, NF-κB is shuttled to the cell nucleus where it binds to regulatory regions in genes, mediating transcriptional activation of these genes.

Posttranscriptional regulation of gene expression is the next stage of control.[40–52] As mentioned in the "Transcription" section, newly formed mRNA is edited prior to leaving the nucleus. RNA transcription can be terminated prematurely with the result of a smaller than expected gene product. A single mRNA can be translated into several different gene products, usually peptides. These proteins or peptides may have comparable or opposing functions depending on the products in question. As described, mRNA is edited and processed such that only ~5% of this RNA leaves the nucleus. The 95% that remains is degraded and the purine and pyrimidine bases are reused or are subject to further degradation. The RNA that leaves the nucleus does so through pores in the nuclear membrane. This is an active process, the details of which are not well understood. Not all of the mRNA that exits the nucleus is immediately translated into protein.

All of the aforementioned mechanisms serve to control transcription, a vital step in controlling gene expression. Once the bases are joined together in the nucleus to form mRNA, the nucleus must edit and process it. Processing it includes capping, nucleolytic, and ligation reactions that shorten it, terminal additions of nucleosides, and nucleoside modifications (Figure 7.8). Through this processing, less than 5% of the original RNA migrates from the nucleus to the ribosomes, where it attaches prior to translation. The editing and processing are needed because immature RNA contains all those bases corresponding to the DNA introns. Introns are those groups of bases that are not part of the structural gene. Introns are intervening sequences that separate the exons or coding sequences of the structural gene. The removal of these segments is a cut-and-splice process whereby the intron is cut at its 5′ end, pulled out of the way, and cut again at its 3′ end; at the same time, the two exons are joined. This cut-and-splice routine is continued until all the introns are removed and the exons joined. Some editing of the RNA also occurs with base substitutions made as appropriate. Finally, a 3′-terminal poly(A) tail is added.

The editing and processing step is now complete. The mature mRNA now leaves the nucleus and moves to the cytoplasm for translation. The nucleotides that have been removed during editing and processing are either reused or totally degraded. Of note is the fact that editing and processing also are mechanisms used to degrade the whole message unit. This serves to control the amount and half-life of this RNA. The endonucleases and exonucleases used in the cut-and-splice processing also come into play in the regulation of mRNA stability. The mRNAs have a very short half-life when compared to DNA and the ribosomal and transfer RNAs (tRNAs). If mRNA half-life is shortened or prolonged, gene expression is affected. Many of the very unstable mRNAs have half-lives in terms of minutes—among these are those that code for short-lived regulatory proteins such as the protooncogenes fos and myc. This instability is probably due to an A- and U-rich 3′ untranslated region (UTR). Stability of mRNA can be affected by steroid hormones, nutritional state, viruses, and a variety of pharmaceuticals.

Some gene products are needed for only a short time. Hormones and cell signals must be short lived, and therefore the body needs to control or counterbalance their synthesis and action. One of the ways to do this is by regulating the amount of mRNA (number of copies of mRNA for each gene product) that leaves the nucleus. Another way is to degrade mRNA faster than it can be used for translation. As an example of the former, mRNA for some of the anabolic enzymes is greatly increased when an animal is briefly starved and then refed.[65–68] Once this animal has adjusted to the presence of food, the production of the mRNA is reduced and its degradation is increased.

Mitochondrial Gene Expression

Mitochondrial gene expression is similar to nuclear expression in several respects. Transcription is responsive to some of the same nutrients and hormones that also affect nuclear transcription.[4,62] Both genomes require binding proteins but it seems that each compartment has its preferred binding form. Unlike the nuclear genome where each gene has its own promoter region, all of the genes in the mitochondrial genome have a common promoter found in the D-loop.[4] In contrast to nuclear gene transcription and translation that involves both the nuclear and cytoplasmic compartments, mitochondrial transcription and translation occurs totally within the mitochondrial compartment. It is affected by a wide variety of nuclear-encoded transcription factors and nutrients.[4,58,62]

TRANSLATION

Once the mRNA has migrated from the nucleus to the cytoplasm and attaches to ribosomes, translation is ready to begin. Translation is the synthesis of the protein using the order of the assemblage of constituent amino acids as dictated by the mRNA. All of the amino acids needed for the protein being synthesized must be present and attached to a tRNA. These tRNA–amino acids dock on the mRNA again using base pairing, and the amino acids are joined to one another via the peptide bond. The newly synthesized protein is released as it is made on the ribosome and changes to its conformation and structure occur. These changes depend on the constituent amino acids and their sequence.

Translation is also influenced by specific nutrients. The translation of the ferritin gene, for example, is influenced by the amount of iron available in the cell.[69] In iron deficiency, the mRNA start site for ferritin translation is covered up by an iron-responsive protein. This protein binds the 3′ UTR and inhibits the movement of the 40S ribosome from the cap to the translation start site (Figure 7.10). When iron status is improved, the start site is uncovered and translation can proceed. The actual site of translation is on the ribosomes. Some ribosomes are located on the membrane of the endoplasmic reticulum, and some are free in the cytosol. Ribosomes consist almost entirely of ribosomal RNA and ribosomal protein. Ribosomal RNA is synthesized via RNA polymerase I in the cell nucleus as a large molecule; in this location, this ribosomal RNA molecule is cleaved and leaves the nucleus as two subunits, a large one and a small one. The ribosome is then reformed in the cytoplasm by the reassociation of the two subunits; the subunits, however, are not necessarily derived from the same precursor molecule.

Ribosomal RNA makes up a large fraction of total cellular RNA. A smaller fraction consists of small RNAs that bind to specific amino acids and transfer these amino acids to their site on the polysomes (clusters of ribosomes) in the synthesis of specific proteins. The ribosomal RNA serves as the *docking* point for the activated amino acids bound to the tRNA and the mRNA that dictates the amino acid polymerization sequence. Each amino acid has at least one specific tRNA. Each tRNA molecule is thought to have a cloverleaf arrangement of nucleotides. With this arrangement of nucleotides, there is the opportunity for the maximum number of hydrogen bonds to form between base pairs. A molecule that has many hydrogen bonds is very stable. tRNA also contains a triplet of bases known, in this instance, as the *anticodon*. The amino acid carried by tRNA is identified by the codon of mRNA through its anticodon. The amino acid itself is not involved in this identification.

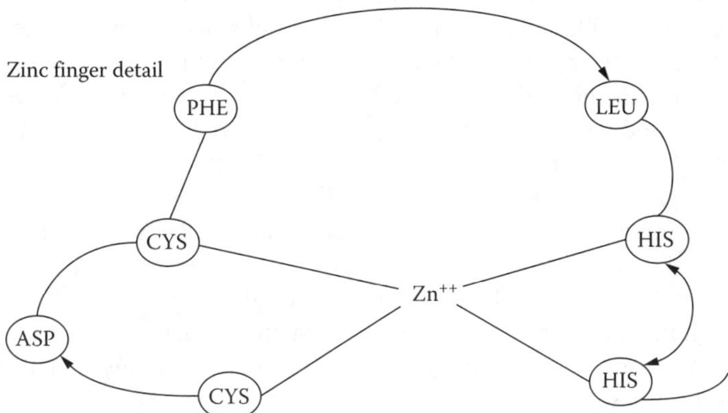

FIGURE 7.10 Detail of the bonding of the zinc ion to histidine and cystine residues of a DNA-binding protein that has zinc fingers.

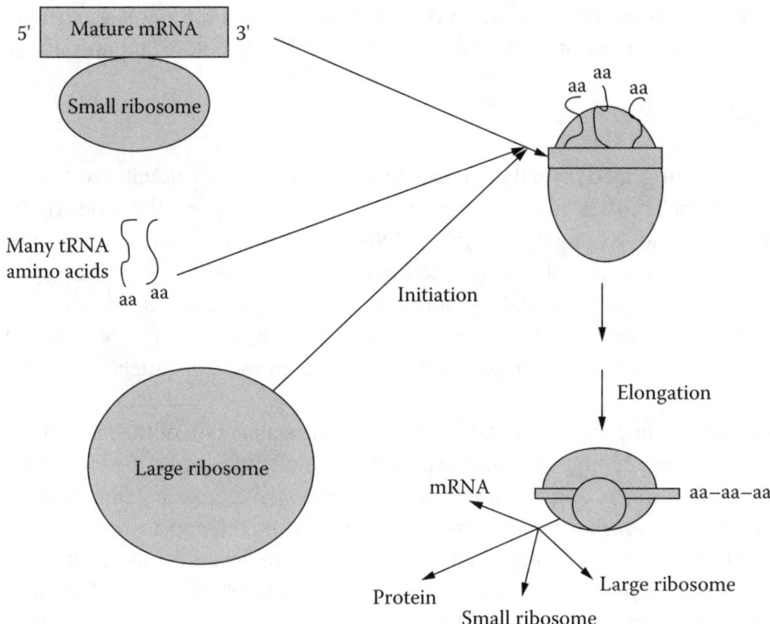

FIGURE 7.11 Overview of translation involving mRNA, tRNA–amino acids, and small and large ribosomal units.

Translation takes place in four stages, as illustrated in Figure 7.11. Each stage requires specific cofactors and enzymes. In the first stage, which occurs in the cytosol, the amino acids are activated by esterifying each one to its specific tRNA. This requires a molecule of ATP. In addition to a specific tRNA, each amino acid requires a specific enzyme for activation.

During the second stage of translation, the initiation of the synthesis of the polypeptide chain occurs. Initiation requires that mRNA binds to the ribosome. An initiation complex is formed by the binding of mRNA cap and the first activated amino acid–tRNA complex to the small ribosomal subunit. The ribosome finds the correct reading frame on the mRNA by *scanning* for an AUG codon. The large ribosomal unit then attaches, thus forming a functional ribosome. A number of specific protein initiation factors (eIFs) are involved in this step.

In the third stage of protein synthesis, the peptide chain is elongated by the sequential addition of amino acids from the tRNA complexes. The amino acid is recognized by base pairing of the codon of mRNA to the bases found in the anticodon of tRNA, and a peptide bond is formed between the peptide chain and the newly arrived amino acid. The ribosome then moves along the mRNA; this brings the next codon in the proper position for attachment of the next activated amino acyl–tRNA complex. The mRNA and nascent polypeptide appear to *track* through a groove in the ribosomal subunits. This protects them from attack by enzymes in the cytosol.

The final stage of protein synthesis is the termination of the polypeptide chain. The termination is signaled by one of three special codons (stop codons) in the mRNA. After the carboxy terminal amino acid is attached to the peptide chain, it is still covalently attached to tRNA, which is, in turn, bonded to the ribosome. A protein-release factor promotes the hydrolysis of the ester link between the tRNA and the amino acid. Once the polypeptide chain is generated and free of the ribosome, it assumes its characteristic 3D structure. At this point, some posttranslational modification can occur. These modifications can include a wide variety of changes. For example, nuclear-encoded proteins needed for mitochondrial OXPHOS are synthesized with a leader sequence that allows them to migrate into the mitochondria. This leader is then removed as the OXPHOS system is assembled. Another example is prothrombin, which is assembled with a large number of glutamic acid residues. In the presence of vitamin K, these residues are carboxylated, and this posttranslational change results in a dramatic increase in the calcium-binding capacity of the resultant protein. Unless prothrombin can bind calcium, it cannot function in the clotting process. This is an example of how a nutrient can affect gene expression at the posttranslational stage: in this instance, the expression of functional prothrombin. The site of the nutritional effect is that of posttranslational protein modification.

If, during the course of synthesis, there is any interference in the continuity of a supply of the needed amino acids, protein synthesis is stopped. Since protein biosynthesis is very costly in terms of its energy requirement, synthesis is severely inhibited by starvation or energy restriction. In experimental animals, it has been shown that starvation inhibits the polymerization of mRNA units, thus significantly reducing the activity of the transcription process. Other studies have shown that animals starved and then refed *overcompensate* for this period of reduced mRNA synthesis by markedly increasing mRNA synthesis above normal during the period of realimentation after the starvation period.[65] This *starvation–refeeding*-induced increase in mRNA is manifested as an increase in the synthesis of enzymes necessary for the metabolism of the various ingredients in the diet used for realimentation. The signal(s) for the release of the starvation-induced inhibition of mRNA and enzyme synthesis include the macronutrients in the diet as well as hormones such as glucocorticoids, thyroxine, and insulin.[65–68]

Effects of Diet on Genetic Diseases

Some genetic diseases can be treated by dietary choices. For example, mutations of the *biotinidase* gene in humans are associated with decreased recycling of the vitamin biotin in human tissues, leading to increased urinary excretion of biotin metabolites and, hence, biotin deficiency.[69] Afflicted individuals can be treated by lifelong supplementation with pharmacological doses of biotin. A similar example is lactose intolerance, which is caused by reduction in the enzyme lactase, leading to decreased tolerance to dietary lactose (*milk sugar*) in afflicted individuals. Lactose intolerance (gastrointestinal discomfort, gas, diarrhea in response to lactose feeding) can be observed in many ethnic groups that do not consume milk or milk products after weaning.[40,70] People with lactose intolerance are symptom-free as long as their diet does not contain significant amounts of milk. In fermented milk products (e.g., yogurt and cultured buttermilk), most of the lactose has been metabolized by microbe cultures, and hence, these products are tolerated reasonably well by most people with lactose intolerance.

In contrast to biotinidase deficiency and lactose intolerance, many genetic diseases cannot be influenced by diet.[71] There are a number of reasons for this. First, some gene mutations are lethal to embryos and are associated with the loss of the pregnancy. For example, there is not one reported case of a living patient with a complete absence of holocarboxylase synthetase, a gene that controls crucial steps in biotin metabolism. Second, some genes control essential steps in intermediary metabolism, and expression of these genes cannot be sufficiently modulated by diet. For example, expression of *interleukin-2 receptor gamma* is absolutely critical for immune function,[72] but the expression of this gene can be affected by diet only within narrow limits.[73,74]

Nutrient–Gene Interactions

In addition to nutrients that affect transcription via specific receptors that bind certain base sequences in the promoter region, we also have nutrients that by themselves stimulate or suppress transcription. Examples include some of the fatty acids and the glucose molecule. Long-chain PUFAs inhibit the transcription of the fatty acid synthetase gene complex, while glucose stimulates the transcription of the enzyme glucokinase by binding to a glucose-sensitive region in the promoter for this gene. Only the β cell and the hepatocyte DNA have this region exposed, and only these cell types express the glucokinase gene. Glucokinase catalyzes the phosphorylation of glucose. In the β cell, glucokinase serves as the glucose sensor of circulating blood glucose. When blood glucose is elevated, this sensor signals the β cell to release insulin. Mutation in the glucokinase gene is associated with an inadequate sensing of blood glucose and a corresponding reduction in glucose-stimulated insulin release. The particular form of diabetes associated with this defect is called maturity-onset diabetes of the young (MODY). MODY can also be found associated with a defective nuclear receptor that is in the promoter region of the glucokinase gene. It too results in defective glucose sensing and inadequate insulin release. Other cell types have the glucokinase gene but do not express it probably because their glucose promoter site is unexposed. Instead, these other cell types express a similar (but different) gene for the enzyme hexokinase that catalyzes the phosphorylation of glucose. Hexokinase also catalyzes the phosphorylation of other monosaccharides. There are a numerous examples of specific nutrient effects on transcription. Some of these effects concern the transcription of genes that encode enzymes or receptors or carriers that are important to the use of that nutrient. Examples of these are listed in Table 7.3.

Some serve more than one function with respect to gene expression. Some influence both transcription and translation, while others serve to enhance the transcription of one gene while suppressing the transcription of another. Nutrient–gene interactions can result in either an increase or a decrease in a specific mRNA, yet there may be no increase in gene product or a measurable increase in gene product function. This speaks to the complicated nature of metabolic control. Simply synthesizing more message units or more enzyme protein does not automatically mean an increase in enzyme activity or an increase in a metabolic pathway or an increase in a metabolic product.

An example of an effect of a specific nutrient on translation is that of iron in the synthesis of ferritin.[74] Iron storage in cells occurs through chelation to a protein called ferritin. This occurs at the outer aspect of the mitochondrial membrane. Ferritin synthesis is highly regulated by iron intake. In iron deficiency, the mRNA start site for ferritin translation is covered up by an iron-responsive protein. This protein binds the 3′ UTR and inhibits the movement of the 40S ribosome from the cap to the translation start site. When the diet contains sufficient iron and iron status is improved, the start site is uncovered and translation then proceeds.

TABLE 7.3
Some Examples of Nutrient Effects on Gene Expression

Nutrient	Gene/Gene Product	Effect
Manganese	Mg-superoxide dismutase	Increases both transcription and translation
Cholesterol	LDL receptor	Suppresses transcription
Vitamin D	Calcium-binding proteins	Increases transcription of genes for calcium-binding proteins in bone cells
Glucose	Glucokinase	Increases transcription in β cells and hepatocytes
Copper	Metallothionien	Increases transcription of this metal-carrying protein
Fatty acids	Fatty acid synthetase and S_{14} gene	Suppresses transcription in liver
	Fatty acid–binding protein	Increases transcription
Selenium	Glutathione peroxidase	Increases transcription
	5′ deiodinase	
Vitamin A (acid)	Many proteins	Increases transcription
Zinc	Zinc transporters, zinc-containing DNA-binding proteins	Increases transcription
Iron	Ferritin	Increases translation
Vitamin K	Prothrombin, bone gla protein, osteocalcin	Serves as cosubstrate for the posttranslational carboxylation of glutamic acid–rich regions of these proteins

The epigenetic changes in the chromatin should also be included in this listing as described in the "Epigenetics" section. Methylation, acetylation, and other reactions affect gene expression but not through a change in base sequence or in transcription, translation, or posttranslation modification.

GENETIC DISEASES OF INTEREST TO NUTRITION

If there is a mutation in the genetic code for a given protein, the amino acid sequence generated for that protein will be incorrect. In the synthesis of the important protein, hemoglobin, if the genetic code calls for the use of valine instead of the usual glutamic acid in the synthesis of the β chain in the hemoglobin molecule, the resulting protein is less able to carry oxygen. This mutation characterizes the disease sickle cell anemia. The amino acid substitution not only affects the oxygen-carrying capacity of the red blood cell but also affects the solubility of the hemoglobin in red blood cells. The decreased solubility of the hemoglobin can be understood if one remembers the relative polarity of the glutamic acid and valine molecules. The glutamic acid side chain is more ionic and thus contributes more to the solubility of the protein than the nonpolar carbon chain of valine. This change in pH decreases its solubility in water, and, of course, a change in solubility leads to an increased viscosity of the blood as the red cells rupture spilling their contents into the blood stream.

There are a number of metabolic diseases affecting nutrient metabolism that are genetically determined. Most of these are quite rare and most are recessive disorders.[71] Table 7.4 is a list of these disorders and the mutation responsible for the disorder. This is a partial list and not all of the genetic diseases are listed. For some of the disorders, there is more than one mutation associated with the disease. For example, there are a number of genetic mutations in the code for red cell glucose-6-phosphate dehydrogenase. The code is carried as a recessive trait on the X chromosome, and thus only males are affected. These mutations are usually silent. That is, the male, having a defective red cell glucose-6-phosphate dehydrogenase, does not know he has the problem unless his cells are tested or unless he is given a drug such as quinine or one of the sulfur antibiotics that increase the oxidation of $NADPH^+H^+$. When this happens, $NADPH^+H^+$ is depleted and is not available to reduce oxidized glutathione. In turn, the red cell ruptures. In almost all cases, the affected male has sufficient enzyme activity to meet the normal demands for $NADPH^+H^+$. It is only when stressed by these drugs that a problem develops.

There are other genomic defects that are silent as well. For example, people unable to metabolize the pentoses found in plums and cherries are usually unaware of their condition. It may come to light if a nonglucose-specific screening test is used for diabetes screening just after the individual has consumed these fruits. There may appear to be an elevated level of sugar in the blood and urine, and diabetes might be thought to be present. If a specific assay for glucose (glucokinase) is used for diabetes screening rather than a nonspecific test, this mistake in diabetes diagnosis will not be made. Another example of a silent genetic disease is that of McCardle's disease.[72] In this disease, the individual is intolerant of exercise. This occurs because the individual is unable to use the glycogen in their muscles for fuel. Unless forced to exercise, these people might not be aware of their metabolic defect. They may have adopted a very sedentary lifestyle by unconscious realization of their intolerance.

Unconscious food selection has been observed in children with some of the macronutrient intolerances. Children who are lactose intolerant may refuse to consume milk; those who are gluten intolerant may avoid wheat-containing products and so forth. There may be an instinctive avoidance that helps the individual enjoy their food without serious consequences.

Many of the disorders listed in Table 7.4 have no cure, and many are characterized by a shortened life span. However, for some, there are nutrition strategies that may be helpful. Diseases associated with the malabsorption of carbohydrate, that is, lactose intolerance and galactose intolerance, can be managed by the omission of these carbohydrates from the diet. Some of the amino acid disorders can be managed by the reduction of the dietary intakes of the particular amino acid in question.

TABLE 7.4
Genetic Disorders in Nutrient Metabolism

Disease	Mutated Gene	Characteristics
Amino acid diseases		
Maple Syrup Urine Disease	Branched-chain keto acid dehydrogenase	Elevated levels of α-ketoacids and their metabolites in blood and urine; mental retardation, ketoacidosis, early death.
Homocysteinemia	Cystathionine synthase	Absence of cross-linked collagen; eye malformations, osteoporosis; mental retardation, thromboembolism and vascular occlusions.
Phenylketonuria	Phenylalanine hydroxylase	Mental retardation, decreased neurotransmitter production; shortened life span; six mutations in this gene have been reported.
Tyrosinemia	Tyrosine transaminase	Eye and skin lesions, mental retardation.
	Fumarylacetoacetate hydroxylase	Normocytic anemia, leukocytosis, increased serum bilirubin, increased hepatic enzymes, prolonged prothrombin time.
Albinism	Tyrosinase	Lack of melanin production; sensitivity to sunlight.
Alkaptonuria	Homogentisate oxidase	Elevated homogentisate levels in blood, bones, and internal organs; increased susceptibility to viruses and arthritis.
Histidinemia	Histidase	Elevated blood and urine levels of histidine; decreased histamine.
Hyperprolinemia	Proline oxidase	Mental retardation; seizures; two mutations.
Hyperornithinemia	Ornithine-δ-aminotransferase	Increased levels of ornithine in blood; progression vision loss; increased urine loss of ornithine.
Urea cycle defects	Arginase Carbamyl phosphate synthase Ornithine transcarbamylase Arginisuccinate synthase Argininosuccinase	Progressive lethargy; mental retardation; urea cycle failure; symptoms of ammonia toxicity; early death.
Hyperlysinemia	α-Aminoadipic semialdehyde synthase	Elevated levels of lysine in blood and urine; condition is generally benign.
Hypermethioninemia	Methionine adenyltransferase	Benign.
Nonketotic hyperglycemia	Glycine cleavage system (three mutations)	Early death; hypoglycemia, mental retardation, seizures.
Gout	?	Excess uric acid production; renal uric acid stones; uric acid crystals accumulate in joints.
Lesch–Nyhan	Hypoxanthine phosphoribosyl transferase	Hyperuricemia, choreoathetosis, spasticity; mental retardation; self-mutilation; gouty arthritis.
Lipid diseases other than those relating to lipemia		
Tay–Sachs	Hexosaminidase A	Early death, CNS degeneration, ganglioside GM2 accumulation.
Gaucher's	Glucocerebrosidase	Hepatomegaly, splenomegaly, erosion of long bones and pelvis, mental retardation, glucocerebrosidase accumulation.
Fabry's	α-Galactosidase A	Skin rash, renal failure, pain in legs, ceramide trihexoside accumulation.
Niemann–Pick	Sphingomyelinase	Enlarged liver and spleen, mental retardation, sphingomyelin accumulation.
Krabbe's	Galactocerebroside	Mental retardation, absence of myelin.
Gangliosidosis	Ganglioside: β-galactosidase	Enlarged liver, mental retardation.
Sandhoff–Jatzkewitz	Hexosaminidases A and B	Same as Tay–Sachs but develops quicker.
Fucosidosis	α-L-Fucosidase	Cerebral degeneration, spastic muscles, thick skin.
Refsum's	α-Hydroxylating enzyme	Neurological problems: deafness, blindness, cerebellar ataxia.

(Continued)

TABLE 7.4 (*CONTINUED*)
Genetic Disorders in Nutrient Metabolism

Disease	Mutated Gene	Characteristics
Carbohydrate-related disorders		
Lactose intolerance	Lactase	Chronic or intermittent diarrhea, flatulence, nausea, vomiting, growth failure in young children.
Sucrose intolerance	Sucrase	Diarrhea, flatulence, nausea, poor growth in infants.
Galactose intolerance	Galactose carrier	Diarrhea, growth failure in infants, stools containing large amounts of glucose, galactose, and lactic acid.
Galactosemia	Three genes: galactose-1-P	Increased cellular content of galactose-1-phosphate, eye cataracts.
	Uridyl transferase	Mental retardation, cell galactitol; three mutations in this gene.
	Galactokinase	Cataracts, cellular accumulation of galactose and galactitol.
	Galactoepimerase	No severe symptoms; two mutations in this gene.
Fructosemia	Fructokinase	Fructosuria, fructosemia.
	Fructose-1-P-aldolase	Hypoglycemia, vomiting after a fructose load, fructosemia, fructosuria. In children, poor growth, jaundice, hyperbilirubinemia, albuminuria, amino aciduria.
	Fructose-1,6-diphosphatase	Hypoglycemia, hepatomegaly, poor muscle tone, increased blood lactate.
Pentosuria	NADP-linked xylitol dehydrogenase	Elevated levels of pentose in urine.
Hemolytic anemia	Red cell glucose-6-phosphate dehydrogenase	Low red cell NADPH, hemolysis of red cell especially with quinine treatment.
	Pyruvate kinase	Nonspherocytic anemia, accumulation of glucose metabolites in red cells; jaundice in the newborn.
Type VII glycogen storage disease	Phosphofructokinase	Intolerance to exercise, elevated muscle glycogen levels, accumulation of hexose monophosphates in muscle.
Von Gierke's (type I glycogen storage)	Glucose-6-phosphatase	Hypoglycemia, hyperlipidemia, brain damage in some pts, excess liver glycogen, shortened life span, increased glycerol utilization.
Amylopectinosis (type IV glycogenosis)	Branching enzyme, hepatic amylo-(1,4→1,6)-transglucosidase	Tissue accumulation of long-chain glycogen that is poorly branched; intolerance to exercise.
Pompe's (type II glycogenosis)	Lysosomal α-1,4-glucosidase (acid maltase)	Generalized glycogen excess in viscera, muscles, nervous system muscle weakness, hepatomegaly, enlarged heart.
	Amylo-1,6-glucosidase (debranching enzyme)	Generalized glycogen excess in viscera, nervous system, muscles, hepatomegaly, enlarged heart.
Forbes (type III glycogenosis)	Muscle phosphorylase	Tissue accumulation of highly branched glycogen, hypoglycemia, acidosis muscle weakness, enlarged heart.
McArdle's (type V glycogenosis)	Liver phosphorylase	Intolerance to exercise.
Hers (type VI glycogenosis)	Phosphorylase kinase	Hepatomegaly, increased liver glycogen content, elevated serum lipids, growth retardation.
Micronutrient-related disorders		
Porphyria	Uroporphyrinogen III cosynthase	Increased red cell porphyrin, excess excretion of δ-aminolevulinic acid (urine) and porphobilinogen (stool); photosensitivity.
	Ferrochelatase	Excess protoporphyrin in stool; photosensitivity.
	ALA dehydratase	Neurovisceral symptoms; excess δ-aminolevulinic acid in urine.

(*Continued*)

TABLE 7.4 (*CONTINUED*)
Genetic Disorders in Nutrient Metabolism

Disease	Mutated Gene	Characteristics
	Porphobilinogen deaminase	Neurovisceral symptoms; excess δ-aminolevulinic acid and porphobilinogen in urine.
	Coproporphyrinogen oxidase	Photosensitivity; neurovisceral symptoms; excess δ-aminolevulinic acid, porphobilinogen, and coproporphyrin in urine.
	Protoporphyrinogen oxidase	Photosensitivity; neurovisceral symptoms; excess δ-aminolevulinic acid, porphobilinogen, and coproporphyrin in urine; coproporphyrin and protoporphyrin in feces.
	Uroporphyrinogen decarboxylate (two mutations)	Photosensitivity; uroporphyrin and 7-carboxylate porphyrin in urine; isocoproporphyrin in feces.
Wilson's	?	Reduction in the rate of the incorporation of copper into ceruloplasmin; reduction in the biliary excretion of copper; increased urinary copper; excess hepatic copper; liver disease.
Menkes	Intestinal copper	Symptoms of copper deficiency; deficient copper-dependent enzyme carrier.
Hemochromatosis	?	Excess serum iron; excess liver iron; excess serum ferritin.
Molybdenum cofactor deficiency	?	Mental retardation; deficient sulfite oxidase and xanthine dehydrogenase activity; neuronal loss and demyelination; early death.
Rickets	$25(OH)_2$ D hydroxylase	Vitamin D–deficient rickets.
	D receptor resistance (five mutations)	Vitamin D–deficient rickets.

Source: Scriver, C.R. et al., eds., *The Metabolic Basis of Inherited Disease*, 6th edn., McGraw-Hill, New York, 1989, p. 3000.

For example, phenylketonuria can be managed by a reduction in the phenylalanine content of the diet. This is rather tricky since enough of this essential amino acid must be provided but not too much so that there is a surplus that cannot be appropriately metabolized. In addition, since phenylalanine is used to make tyrosine, this amino acid must then be provided in the diet in sufficient amounts to meet the need.

There are two genetic disorders that have assisted scientists in understanding the function and metabolism of copper. In one disorder, that is, the Menkes syndrome, copper absorption is faulty. Intestinal cells absorb the copper but cannot release it into the circulation. Parenteral copper corrects most of the characteristics of the condition that resembles copper deficiency, but care must be exercised in its administration. Too much can be toxic. In addition, parenterally administered copper does not reach the brain and cannot prevent the cerebral degeneration and premature death characteristic of patients with the Menkes disease.

Another genetic disorder in copper status is Wilson's disease. This condition is also associated with premature death and is due to an impaired incorporation of copper into ceruloplasmin and decreased biliary excretion of copper. This results in an accumulation of copper in the liver and brain. Early signs of Wilson's disease include liver dysfunction, neurological disease, and deposits of copper in the cornea manifested as a ring that looks like a halo around the pupil. This lesion is called the Kayser–Fleischer ring. Renal stones, renal aciduria, neurological deficits, and osteoporosis also characterize Wilson's disease. Periodic bleeding that removes some of the excess copper can be helpful in managing Wilson's disease as can treatment with copper-chelating agents such as D-penicillamine and by increasing the intake of zinc that interferes with copper absorption.

Iron is an essential mineral for hemoglobin formation. However, there are a number of genetic reasons why excess iron in the blood can be encountered. These are the porphyrias and hemochromatosis. In the latter, excess iron accumulates and in the former, there are abnormalities in porphyrin metabolism. Some of these disorders are devastating, while others are less so. Vitamin D and the uptake of calcium and phosphate are linked. In the absence of active vitamin D, rickets develops. Some individuals are unable to activate the vitamin. That is, they do not have a normal activity of the renal enzyme $25(OH)_2D$ hydroxylase. As a result, these individuals develop vitamin D rickets. The bones are not appropriately mineralized because there is a deficiency of the active vitamin. This can be managed by providing the active form of the vitamin in the diet. In addition, there is also a disease characterized by resistance to the activity of active vitamin D. The genetic problem here is a deficiency in the receptor for the vitamin. Five different mutations have been reported, which accounts for this problem. Patients with these genetic problems also develop rickets and collectively are referred to as having vitamin D–resistant rickets. Lastly, there are a couple of complex disorders that affect more pathways in addition to those of vitamin D. These include the Fanconi syndrome, X-linked hypophosphatemia, and pseudohypoparathyroidism. In each of these, there is a disturbed mineralization of the skeletal system as well as disturbed regulation of calcium status, phosphorus status, and soft tissue mineralization.

SUMMARY

1. The genetic heritage of an individual is vested in the sequence of bases that make up the DNA. The DNA consists of specific regions called genes.
2. Genes hold the codes for the proteins and peptides in the body. Their expression is often influenced by specific nutrients.
3. Nutrients can function in the transcription, translation, or posttranslation of the gene product.
4. The DNA in the nucleus is protected by a histone layer. The DNA in the mitochondria is naked and has no protective coat.
5. Changes in the base sequence of a gene can be either a mutation or a polymorphism. In either situation, the function of the gene product might be altered.
6. Epigenetic change occurs when there is a change in gene expression without a change in the base sequence of the gene.
7. The syntheses of the bases that make up the DNA are dependent on the presence of a number of micronutrients. If one or more are lacking, DNA synthesis is impaired.
8. Mutation in either the structural gene or its promoter(s) can result in disease.
9. There are numerous examples of nutrient–gene interactions.

LEARNING OPPORTUNITIES

LEARNING ACTIVITY: Your Family Tree

Prepare a four-generation family tree showing all of your biological relatives. You will need to ask your family members to provide this information. When you make the tree, do not give names to your family members to protect their privacy. Give them a number. Begin numbering either with your generation or with your great grandparents' generation. It does not matter where you begin numbering with respect to the generations. However, each generation should have its own first number. For example, you might start with your generation. You would be #1, your sister would be #2, and your brothers would be #3 and #4. Your parents would be #10 and #11;

their brothers and sisters likewise, double digits. Be sure to keep the family lines separate. That is, do not put all your father's sisters and your mother's sisters together but separate them by families. Your grandparents' numbers would be triple digits and your great grandparents would have four digits. If you are adopted, this might not apply to you but you should go through the activity anyway. Do not include step relatives, that is, step sisters and step parents. Show yourself; your siblings; your parents, aunts, and uncles; your grandparents, grandaunts, and granduncles; and your great grandparents, great grandaunts, and great granduncles. With each individual, show whether they are alive or dead by providing their birth dates and death dates (if applicable). If dead, indicate cause of death as well as any chronic conditions they might have had before they died. If alive, indicate the presence of all of their medical problems. There may be many. List them all. Indicate any congenital problems and any genetic problems. Once you have put this tree together, you will then look at it to determine whether there might be any trends that could have significance with respect to your medical future. For example, you might note whether there is a lot of type 2 diabetes mellitus or a lot of colon cancer. These are diseases that have strong genetic linkages, yet they are diseases that can be avoided or postponed with appropriate intervention.

After you have considered and completed your family tree, think about the following case studies. They have been written to help you understand situations where inheritance as well as lifestyle choices can impact the health and well-being of the individual.

CASE STUDY 7.1 African Adventure

John and Mary are excited by their upcoming trip to Africa. In preparation for their trip, they visit their doctor who pronounces them fit and healthy enough for their adventure. Their doctor prescribes prophylactic doses of quinine since they will be visiting an area of Africa where malaria is endemic. Mary tolerates the quinine very well but after a week, John begins to complain of feeling tired. Two weeks after beginning to take the quinine, John is really under the weather and is feeling poorly. The two return to the doctor who orders a full-scale clinical examination of John. His blood work comes back and the red cell count has fallen from 5.8 to 3.9 million cells/mm^3. There is evidence of extensive hemolysis. By the time the lab results are in, John is close to collapse and the doctor admits him into the hospital for care. What is the problem?

CASE STUDY 7.2 BoBo Hates Milk: It Gives Him a Tummy Ache

BoBo, his nickname, is a delightful 4-year-old. He is developing normally and is growing adequately. His mom, however, is concerned that he is not eating right. She has read that young growing children should consume milk because it is an excellent source of calcium for strong bones and teeth. It is a good source for easily digested protein and contains essential vitamins and minerals. Every time she gives BoBo a glass of milk, he avoids drinking it. He plays at the table and eventually manages to tip the glass over and spill the milk on the floor. His mom gets upset and cleans up the mess but doesn't think about BoBo's behavior as an avoidance mechanism. Finally, she forces BoBo to drink the milk. Within an hour, BoBo has a tummy ache. He cries, draws his little legs up to his tummy, and clearly is very uncomfortable. After a couple of hours, he expels some gas and has a bit of diarrhea and then is back to his sunny self. Analyze this situation; suggest causes and remedies.

PROBLEM SOLVING

Look up the amino acid sequence of bradykinin. This is an eight-amino-acid peptide. Construct the possible base sequences of the DNA that encodes this compound. Do not forget to include the stop and start codons. Provide all of the possible base sequences.

MULTIPLE-CHOICE QUESTIONS

1. Transcription means
   a. The synthesis of mRNA
   b. The synthesis of ribosomal protein
   c. The construction of new protein
   d. None of the above
2. A gene is
   a. A unit of DNA
   b. A message for transcription
   c. Controlled by ATP synthesis
   d. None of the above
3. Nutrients can affect gene expression through
   a. Providing substrates for oxidation
   b. Stimulating transcription and translation
   c. Providing the ingredients for purine and pyrimidine syntheses
   d. All of the above
4. Genetic diseases can be
   a. Treated by dietary means
   b. Transmitted to the next generation
   c. Caused by dietary factors
   d. Associated with many chronic disorders
5. The DNA in the nucleus
   a. Is fragile and subject to damage
   b. Can be damaged but repaired
   c. Is in the shape of a helix
   d. Is unstable

REFERENCES

1. Strausberg, R.L., 82 co Authors (2002) Generation and initial analysis of more than 15,000 full-length human and mouse cDNA. *Proc. Natl. Acad. Sci. USA* 99: 16899–16903.
2. Wallace, D.C. (1992) Diseases of the mitochondrial DNA. *Annu. Rev. Biochem.* 61: 1175–1212.
3. Giles, R.E., Blanc, H., Cann, H.M., Wallace, D.C. (1980) Maternal inheritance of human mitochondrial DNA. *Proc. Natl. Acad. Sci. USA* 77: 6715–6719.
4. Taanman, J.W., Williams, S.L. (2005) The human mitochondrial genome: Mechanisms of expression and maintenance. In: *Mitochondria in Health and Disease* (C.D. Berdanier, ed.). Taylor & Francis, Boca Raton, FL, pp. 95–244.
5. Wolffe, A. (1998) *Chromatin*, 3rd edn. Academic Press, San Diego, CA, p. 300.
6. Camporeale, G., Zempleni, J. (2006) Biotin. In: *Present Knowledge in Nutrition* (B.A. Bowman, R.M. Russell, eds.), 9th edn. I.L.S.I., Washington, DC, pp. 314–326.
7. Espino, P.S., Drobic, B., Dunn, K.L., Davie, J.R. (2005) Histone modifications as a platform for cancer therapy. *J. Cell. Biochem.* 94: 1088–1102.
8. Martinez, J.A., Corbalan, M.S., Sanchez-Villegas, A., Forga, L., Marti, A., Martinez-Gonzaez, M.A. (2003) Obesity risk is associated with carbohydrate intake in women carrying the Gln27Glu beta2-adrenoceptor polymorphism. *J. Nutr.* 133: 2549–2554.

9. Bos, G., Dekker, J.M., Feskens, E.J., Ocke, M.C., Nijpels, G., Stehouwer, C.D., Bouter, L.M., Heine, R.J., Jansen, H. (2005) Interactions of dietary fat intake and hepatic lipase –480C>T polymorphism in determining hepatic lipase activity: The Hoorn study. *Am. J. Clin. Nutr.* 81: 911–915.
10. Tai, E.S., Corella, D., Demissie, S., Cupples, L.A., Coltell, O., Schaefer, E.J., Tucker, K.L., Ordovas, J.M. and the Framingham Heart Study (2005) Polyunsaturated fatty acids interact with PPARA-L162V polymorphism to affect plasma triglyceride and apolipoproteins C-III concentrations in the Framingham Heart Study. *J. Nutr.* 135: 397–403.
11. Huh, H.J., Chi, H.S., Shim, E.H., Jang, S., Park, C.J. (2006) Gene-nutrition interactions in coronary artery disease: Correlations between the MTHFR C677T polymorphism and folate and homocysteine status in a Korean population. *Thromb. Res.* 117: 501–506.
12. Robitaille, J., Hamner, H.C., Cogswell, M.E., Yang, Q. (2009) Does the MTHFR 677C-T variant affect the recommended dietary allowance for folate in the US population? *Am. J. Clin. Nutr.* 89: 1269–1273.
13. Tsai, M.Y., Loria, C.M., Cao, J., Kim, V., Siscovick, D., Schreimer, P.J., Hanson, N.Q. (2009) Clinical utility of genotyping the 677C>T variant of methylenetetrahydrofolate reductase in humans is decreased in post-folic acid fortification era. *J. Nutr.* 139: 33–37.
14. Crider, K.S., Zhu, J.-H., Hao, L., Yang, Q.-H., Yang, T.P., Gindler, J., Maneval, D.R. et al. (2011) MTHFR 677C-T genotype is associated with folate and homocysteine concentrations in a large population-based, double-blind trial of folic acid supplementation. *Am. J. Clin. Nutr.* 93: 1365–1372.
15. Yan, J., Wang, W., Gregory, J.F., Malysheva, O., Brenna, J.T., Stabler, S.P., Allen, R.H., Caudill, M.A. (2011) MTHFR C677T genotype influences the isotopic enrichment of one-carbon metabolites in folate compromised men consuming d6-choline. *Am. J. Clin. Nutr.* 93: 348–356.
16. Huang, T., Tucker, K.L., Lee, Y.-C., Crott, J.W., Parnell, L.D., Shen, J., Smith, C.E., Ordovas, J.M., Li, D., Lai, C.-Q. (2011) Methylenetetrahydrofolate reductase variants associated with hypertension and cardiovascular disease interact with dietary polyunsaturated fatty acids to modulate plasma homocysteine in Puerto Rican adults. *J. Nutr.* 141: 654–660.
17. Belisle, S.E., Hamer, D.H., Leka, L.S., Dallat, G.F., Delgado-Lista, J., Fine, B.C., Jacques, P.F., Ordovas, J.M., Meydani, S.N. (2010) IL-2 and IL10 gene polymorphisms are associated with respiratory tract infection and may modulate the effect of vitamin E on lower respiratory tract infections in elderly nursing home residents. *Am. J. Clin. Nutr.* 92: 106–114.
18. Nettleton, J.A., Volcik, K.A., Hoogeveen, R.C., Boerwinkle, E. (2009) Carbohydrate intake modifies association between ANGPTL4 [E40K] genotype and HDL–cholesterol concentrations in white men from the atherosclerosis risk in communities study. *Atherosclerosis* 203: 214–220.
19. Riedel, B.M., Molloy, A.M., Meyer, K., Fredricksen, A., Ulvik, A., Schneede, J., Nexa, E., Hoff, G., Ueland, P.M. (2011) Transcobalamin polymorphism 67A>G but not 776C>G affects serum holotranscobalamin in a cohort of healthy middle-aged men and women. *J. Nutr.* 141: 1784–1790.
20. Block, G., Shaikh, N., Jensen, C.D., Volberg, V., Holland, N. (2011) Serum vitamin C and other biomarkers differ by genotype and phase 2 enzyme genes $GSTM_1$ and $GSTT_1$. *Am. J. Clin. Nutr.* 94: 929–937.
21. Hur, J., Kim, H., Ha, E.-H., Park, H., Ha, M., Kim, Y., Hong, Y.-C., Chang, N. (2013) Birth weight of Korean infants is affected by the interaction of maternal iron intake and $GSTM_1$ polymorphism. *J. Nutr.* 143: 67–73.
22. Joffe, Y.T., van der Merwe, L., Carstens, M., Collins, M., Jennings, C., Levitt, N.S., Lambert, E.V., Goedecke, J.H. (2010) Tumor necrosis factor gene-308G/A polymorphism modulates the relationship between dietary fat intake, serum lipids and obesity risk in Black South African women. *J. Nutr.* 140: 901–907.
23. Phillips, C.M., Goumidi, L., Bertrais, S., Field, M.R., Ordovas, J.M., Cupples, A., Defoort, C. et al. (2010) Leptin receptor polymorphisms interact with polyunsaturated fatty acids to augment risk of insulin resistance and metabolic syndrome in adults. *J. Nutr.* 140: 238–244.
24. Han, H.R., Ryu, H.J., Cha, H.S., Go, M.J., Ahn, Y., Koo, B.K., Cho, Y.M. et al. (2008) Genetic variations in the leptin and leptin receptor genes are associated with type 2 diabetes mellitus and metabolic traits in the Korean female population. *Clin. Genet.* 74: 105–115.
25. Tanofsky-Kraff, M., Han, J.C., Anandalingam, K., Shomaker, L.B., Coilumbo, K.M., Wolkoff, L.E., Koslosky, M. et al. (2009) The FTO gene rs9939609 obesity-risk allele and loss of control over eating. *Am. J. Clin. Nutr.* 90: 1483–1488.
26. AlSaleh, A., O'Dell, S.D., Frost, G.S., Griffin, B.A., Lovegrove, J.A., Jebb, S.A., Sanders, T.A.B. (2011) Single nucleotide polymorphisms at the ADIPOQ gene locus interact with age and dietary intake of fat to determine serum adiponectin in subjects at risk of metabolic syndrome. *Am. J. Clin. Nutr.* 94: 262–270.
27. Kunkel, T.A. (1992) DNA replication fidelity. *J. Biol. Chem.* 267: 18251–18254.
28. Jenuwein, T., Allis, C.D. (2001) Translating the histone code. *Science* 293: 1074–1080.

29. Fischle, W., Wang, Y., Allis, C.D. (2003) Histone and chromatin cross-talk. *Curr. Opin. Cell Biol.* 215: 172–183.
30. Camporeale, G., Shubert, E.E., Sarath, G., Cerny, R., Zempleni, J. (2004) K8 and K12 are biotinylated in human histone H4. *Eur. J. Biochem.* 271: 2257–2263.
31. Kobza, K., Camporeale, G., Rueckert, B. (2005) K4, K9, and K18 in human histone H3 are targets for biotinylation by biotinidase. *FEBS J.* 272: 4249–4259.
32. Chew, Y.C., Camporeale, G., Kothapalli, N., Sarath, G., Zempleni, J. (2006) Lysine residues in N- and C-terminal regions of human histone H2A are targets for biotinylation by biotinidase. *J. Nutr. Biochem.* 17: 225–233.
33. Dey, A., Chitsaz, F., Abbasi, A., Misteli, T., Ozato, K. (2003) The double bromodomain protein Brd4 binds to acetylated chromatin during interphase and mitosis. *Proc. Natl. Acad. Sci. USA* 100: 8758–8763.
34. Christman, J.K. (2003) Diet, DNA methylation and cancer. In: *Molecular Nutrition* (J. Zempleni, H. Daniel, eds.). CAB International, Wallingford, U.K., pp. 237–265.
35. Zempleni, J., Gralla, M., Camporeale, G., Hassan, Y.I. (2009) Sodium-dependent multivitamin transporter gene is regulated at the chromatin level by histone biotinylation in human Jurkat lymphoblastoma cells. *J. Nutr.* 139: 163–170.
36. Zempleni, J., Chew, Y.C., Bao, B., Pestinger, V., Wijeratne, S.S.K. (2009) Repression of transposable elements by histone biotinylation. *J. Nutr.* 139: 2389–2392.
37. Haggarty, P., Hoad, G., Campbell, D.M., Horgan, G., Plyathilake, C., McNeill, G. (2012) Folate in pregnancy and imprinted gene and repeat element methylation in the offspring. *Am. J. Clin. Nutr.* 97: 94–99.
38. Kirkland, J.B. (2009) Niacin status impacts chromatin structure. *J. Nutr.* 139: 2397–2401.
39. Bouchard, L., Rabasa-Lhoret, R., Faraj, M., Lavoie, M.-E., Mill, J., Perusse, L., Vohl, M.-C. (2010) Differential epigenomic and transcriptomic responses in subcutaneous adipose tissue between low and high responders to caloric restriction. *Am. J. Clin. Nutr.* 91: 309–320.
40. Ling, C., Groop, L. (2009) Epigenetics: A molecular link between environmental factors and type 21 diabetes. *Diabetes* 58: 2718–2724.
41. Clarke, S.D., Abraham, S. (1992) Gene expression: Nutrient control of pre and posttranscriptional events. *FASEB J.* 6: 3146–3152.
42. Freedman, L.P., Luisi, B.F. (1993) One of the mechanisms of DNA binding by nuclear hormone receptors: A structural and functional perspective. *J. Cell. Biochem.* 51: 140–150.
43. Kollmar, R., Farnham, P.J. (1993) Site specific utilization of transcription by RNA polymerase II. *P.S.E.B.M.* 203: 127–139.
44. Lea, M.A. (1993) Regulation of gene expression in hepatomas. *Int. J. Biochem.* 25: 457–469.
45. Reichel, R.R., Jacob, S.T. (1993) Control of gene expression by lipophilic hormones. *FASEB J.* 7: 427–436.
46. Semenza, G.L. (1994) Transcriptional regulation of gene expression: Mechanism and pathophysiology. *Hum. Mutat.* 3: 180–199.
47. Johnson, P.F., Sterneck, E., Williams, S.C. (1993) Activation domains of transcriptional regulatory proteins. *J. Nutr. Biochem.* 4: 3386–3398.
48. Klug, A., Rhodes, D. (1987) Zinc fingers: A novel protein motif for nucleic acid regulation. *Trends Biochem. Sci.* 12: 464–469.
49. Shilatifard, A. (1998) Factors regulating the transcriptional elongation activity of RNA polymerase II. *FASEB J.* 12: 1437–1446.
50. Aso, T., Conaway, J.W., Conaway, R.C. (1995) The RNA polymerase I elongation complex. *FASEB J.* 9: 1419–1428.
51. Ren, H., Stiles, G.L. (1994) Post transcriptional mRNA processing as a mechanism for regulation of human A1 adenosine receptor expression. *Proc. Natl. Acad. Sci. USA* 91: 4864–4866.
52. Weiss, L., Reinberg, D. (1992) Transcription by RNA polymerase II: Initiator-directed formation of transcription-competent complexes. *FASEB J.* 6: 3300–3309.
53. Bray, P., Lichter, H.J., Ward, D.C., Dawid, I.B. (1991) Characterization and mapping of human genes encoding zinc finger proteins. *Proc. Natl. Acad. Sci. USA* 88: 9563–9567.
54. Hastings, K.E.M., Emerson, C.D. (1984) Proliferation, differentiation and gene expression in skeletal muscle myogenesis; recombinant DNA approaches. In: *Recombinant DNA and Cell Proliferation* (G.S. Stein, J.L. Stein, eds.). Academic Press, Orlando, FL, pp. 219–241.
55. Coates, P.M., Tanaka, K. (1992). Molecular basis of mitochondrial fatty acid oxidation defects. *J. Lipid Res.* 33: 1099–1110.
56. Miller, S.G., DaVos, P., Guerre-Mills, M., Wong, K., Hermann, T., Staels, B., Briggs, M.R., Auwers, J. (1996) The adipocytes specific transcription factor C/EBP modulates human gene expression. *Proc. Natl. Acad. Sci. USA* 93: 5507–5511.

57. Tsai, M.-J., O'Malley, B.W. (1994) Molecular mechanisms of action of steroid/thyroid receptor super family members. *Annu. Rev. Biochem.* 63: 451–486.
58. Berdanier, C.D. (2006) Mitochondrial gene expression: Influence of nutrients and hormones. *Exp. Biol. Med.* 231: 1593–1602.
59. Robyr, D., Wolfe, A.P. (1998) Hormone action and chromatin remodeling. *CMLS Cell. Mol. Life Sci.* 54: 113–124.
60. Griffin, J.B., Rodriguez-Melendez, R., Zempleni, J. (2003) The nuclear abundance of transcription factors Sp1 and Sp3 depends on biotin in Jurkat cells. *J. Nutr.* 133: 3409–3415.
61. Rodriguez-Melendez, R., Schwab, L.D., Zempleni, J. (2004) Jurkat cells respond to biotin deficiency with increased nuclear translocation of NF-κB, mediating cell survival. *Int. J. Vitam. Nutr. Res.* 74: 209–216.
62. Everts, H.B., Classen, D.O., Hermoyian, C.L., Berdanier, C.D. (2002) Nutrient-gene interactions: Dietary vitamin A and mitochondrial gene expression. *IUBMB-Life* 53: 295–301.
63. Falvey, E., Schibler, U. (1991) How are the regulators regulated? *FASEB J.* 5: 309–314.
64. Wurdeman, R., Berdanier, C.D., Tobin, R.B. (1978) Enzyme overshoot in starved-refed rats: Role of glucocorticoid. *J. Nutr.* 108: 1457–1452.
65. Berdanier, C.D., Shubeck, D. (1979) Interaction of glucocorticoid and insulin in the responses of rats to starvation refeeding. *J. Nutr.* 109: 1766–1771.
66. Bouillon, D., Berdanier, C.D. (1980) Role of glucocorticoid in adaptive lipogenesis in the rat. *J. Nutr.* 110: 286–297.
67. Berdanier, C.D. (1981) Effects of estrogen on the responses of male and female rats to starvation refeeding. *J. Nutr.* 111: 1425–1429.
68. Wolf, B., Heard, G.S. (1991) Biotinidase deficiency. In: *Advances in Pediatrics* (L. Barness, F. Oski, eds.). Medical Book Publishers, Chicago, IL, pp. 1–21.
69. Heyman, M.B. (2006) Lactose intolerance in infants, children and adolescents. *Pediatrics* 118: 1279–1286.
70. Byers, K.G., Savaiano, D.A. (2005) The myth of increased lactose intolerance in African-Americans. *J. Am. Coll. Nutr.* 24: 569S–573S.
71. Scriver, C.R., Beaudet, A.L., Sly, W.S., Valle, D., eds. (1989) *The Metabolic Basis of Inherited Disease*, 6th edn. McGraw-Hill, New York, p. 3000.
72. Sugamura, K., Asao, H., Kondo, M. (1996) The interleukin-2 receptor g chain: Its role in the multiple cytokine receptor complexes and T cell development in XSCID. *Annu. Rev. Immunol.* 14: 179–205.
73. Rodriguez-Melendez, R., Camporeale, G., Griffin, J.B., Zempleni, J. (2003) Interleukin-2 receptor g-dependent endocytosis depends on biotin in Jurkat cells. *Am. J. Physiol. Cell Physiol.* 284: C415–C421.
74. Munro, H.N., Kikinis, Z., Eisenstein, R.S. (1993) Iron dependent regulation of ferritin synthesis. In: *Nutrition and Gene Expression* (C.D. Berdanier, J.L. Hargrove, eds.). CRC Press, Boca Raton, FL. pp. 525–546.

8 Protein

After the energy need is met, protein is the next most important macronutrient need. Food proteins provide the amino acids that are needed to synthesize proteins in the body. On the average, Americans consume about 100 g of protein per day. This is far more than what is actually needed. Protein, in its many forms, is an essential and universal constituent of all living things. As much as one-half of the dry weight of the cell is protein. The human body is, on the average, 18% protein. Besides being plentiful, proteins serve a variety of functions. They serve as structural components, as biocatalysts (in the form of enzymes), as antibodies, as lubricants, as messengers (in the form of hormones and cytokines), as receptors, and as carriers or transporters. The building blocks of all proteins are the amino acids. In this chapter, the chemistry and physiology of the proteins are discussed.

AMINO ACIDS

Chemistry

Amino acids consist of carbon, hydrogen, oxygen, nitrogen, and occasionally sulfur. All amino acids with the exception of proline have a terminal carboxyl group

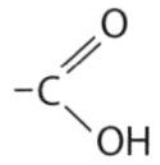

$$-C\begin{matrix}\nearrow O \\ \searrow OH\end{matrix}$$

and an unsubstituted amino ($-NH_2$) group attached to the α-carbon. Proline has a substituted amino group and a carboxyl group. Also attached to the α-carbon is a functional group identified as R; R differs for each amino acid (Table 8.1). The general structure of amino acids can be represented as

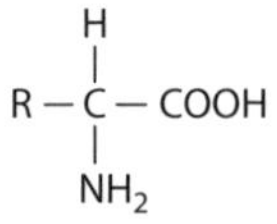

$$\begin{array}{c} H \\ | \\ R-C-COOH \\ | \\ NH_2 \end{array}$$

While it is convenient to represent amino acids in this manner, in reality, amino acids exist as the dipolar ion

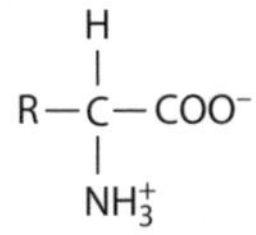

$$\begin{array}{c} H \\ | \\ R-C-COO^- \\ | \\ NH_3^+ \end{array}$$

in the range of pH values (5.0–8.0) found within the body. In learning the structures of the essential amino acids, the student will find it useful to remember the basic structure of alanine. All of the other amino acids have R groups that replace the terminal methyl group in alanine. For example, in valine, the methyl group is replaced with an isopropyl group; in phenylalanine, it is replaced with a phenyl group. The exception to this structure is the amino acids proline and hydroxyproline. These two are ring structures.

There are several ways to classify amino acids. Protein chemists use the polarity of the R group as the basis for their classification of the amino acids. This classification system divides the amino acids into four groups: (1) nonpolar, (2) polar but not charged, (3) positively charged at pH 6.0–7.0, and (4) negatively charged at pH 6.0–7.0. The distribution of the amino acids into these groups is shown in Table 8.2. This classification system is considered more useful than others

TABLE 8.1
Structures and Abbreviations of the Amino Acids (the Single-Letter Abbreviations Are Used as Shorthand in Delineating Large Protein Sequences)

Name	Abbreviation	Structure
Glycine	Gly, G	$H-CH(NH_2)-COOH$
Alanine	Ala, A	$CH_3-CH(NH_2)-COOH$
Valine	Val, V	$(CH_3)(H_3C)CH-CH(NH_2)-COOH$
Leucine	Leu, L	$(CH_3)(H_3C)CH-CH_2-CH(NH_2)-COOH$
Isoleucine	Ile, I	$CH_3-CH_2-CH(H_3C)-CH(NH_2)-COOH$
Serine	Ser, S	$CH_2(OH)-CH(NH_2)-COOH$
Threonine	Thr, T	$CH_3-CH(OH)-CH(NH_2)-COOH$
Cysteine (Cystein)	Cys, C	$CH_2(SH)-CH(NH_2)-COOH$
Methionine	Met, M	$CH_2(S-CH_3)-CH_2-CH(NH_2)-COOH$
Aspartic acid	Asp, D	$HOOC-CH_2-CH(NH_2)-COOH$
Asparagine	Asn, N	$H_2N-C(=O)-CH_2-CH(NH_2)-COOH$
Glutamic acid	Glu, E	$HOOC-CH_2-CH_2-CH(NH_2)-COOH$
Glutamine	Gln, Q	$H_2N-C(=O)-CH_2-CH_2-CH(NH_2)-COOH$
Arginine	Arg, R	$H_2N-C(=NH)-N(H)-CH_2-CH_2-CH_2-CH(NH_2)-COOH$

(*Continued*)

TABLE 8.1 (*CONTINUED*)
Structures and Abbreviations of the Amino Acids (the Single-Letter Abbreviations Are Used as Shorthand in Delineating Large Protein Sequences)

Name	Abbreviation	Structure
Lysine	Lys, K	$CH_2-CH_2-CH_2-CH_2-CH-COOH$ NH_2 NH_2
Hydroxylysine	Hyl	$CH-CH-CH_2-CH_2-CH-COOH$ NH_2 OH NH_2
Histidine	His, H	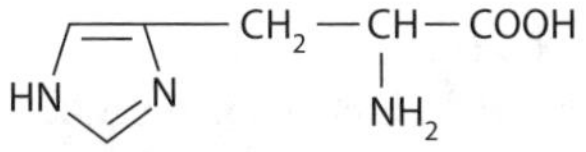 $CH_2-CH-COOH$ HN N NH_2
Phenylalanine	Phe, F	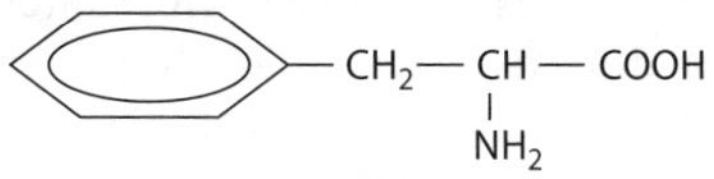 $CH_2-CH-COOH$ NH_2
Tyrosine	Tyr, Y	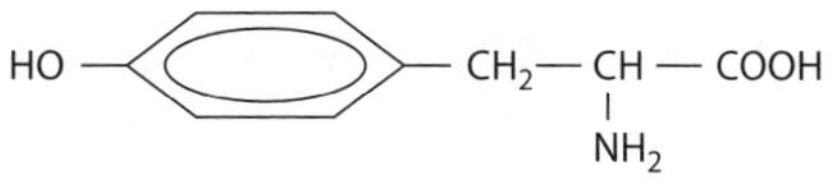 HO $-CH_2-CH-COOH$ NH_2
Tryptophan	Trp, W	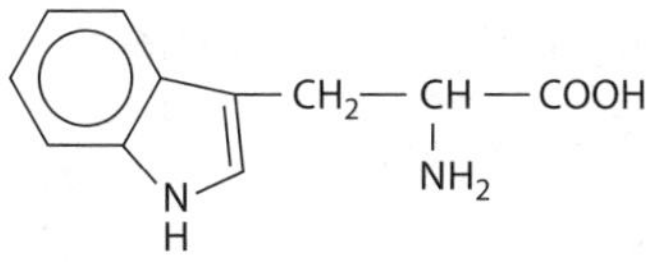 $CH_2-CH-COOH$ N H NH_2
Proline	Pro, P	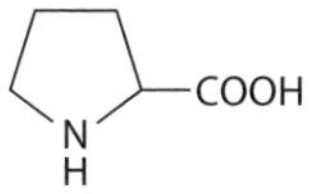 COOH N H
Hydroxyproline	Hyp	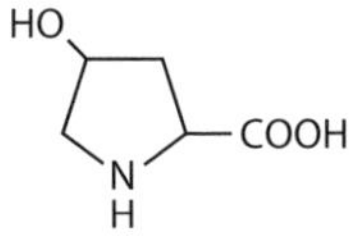 HO COOH N H

Note: The single-letter abbreviations are used as shorthand in delineating large protein sequences.

TABLE 8.2
Classification of Amino Acids Based on Polarity of the Functional Groups

Nonpolar R groups			
Alanine	Phenylalanine	Methionine	Leucine
Valine	Tryptophan	Proline	Isoleucine
Polar uncharged R groups			
Serine	Asparagine	Cysteine	Glycine
Threonine	Glutamine	Hydroxyproline	Tyrosine
Positively charged R groups			
Lysine	Hydroxylysine		
Arginine	Histidine		
Negatively charged R groups			
Aspartic acid			
Glutamic acid (GLA)			

TABLE 8.3
Amino Acids Classified according to Chemical Characteristics

Monoamino monocarboxylic	Glycine, alanine, valine, leucine, isoleucine
Diamino monocarboxylic (basic)	Arginine, lysine
Monoamino dicarboxylic (acidic)	GLA, aspartic acid
Sulfur containing	Cystine (and cysteine), methionine
Aromatic	Tyrosine, phenylalanine
Heterocyclic	Proline, hydroxyproline, histidine, tryptophan

because it relates to the functions of the amino acids in protein structures. Another classification that is frequently useful is based on the chemical character of the amino acids. This grouping is listed in Table 8.3. Nutritionists, while interested in the physical and chemical characteristics of the individual amino acids, classify the amino acids on the basis of whether the body can synthesize them in sufficient quantities to meet its need or whether the diet must provide them. For these purposes, then, amino acids are classified as essential or nonessential. The definition of essentiality rests with the species of animal in question and its physiological need. Felines, for example, require taurine, a metabolite of L-cysteine, as a component of their diets. In the adult human, arginine need not be in the diet.

However, during periods of high rates of protein synthesis, growth, for example, not enough arginine can be synthesized. Additional supplies must then be provided in the diet. Table 8.4 lists the essential and nonessential amino acids for adults.

Occasionally, through a mutation in one or more genes that encode enzymes needed for amino acid interconversion, certain of the nonessential amino acids cannot be synthesized. In these instances, the amino acid in question then becomes essential and must be provided in the diet. An example is the mutation in the gene for phenylalanine hydroxylase. There are four different mutations in this gene and all are clinically characterized by mental retardation. Phenylalanine hydroxylase catalyzes the conversion of phenylalanine to tyrosine. In the patient with phenylketonuria, tyrosine cannot be synthesized,

TABLE 8.4
Essential and Nonessential Amino Acids for Adult Mammals

Essential	Nonessential
Valine	Hydroxyproline
Leucine	Cysteine
Isoleucine	Glycine
Threonine	Alanine
Phenylalanine	Serine
Methionine	Proline
Tryptophan	GLA
Lysine	Aspartic acid
Histidine	Glutamine
Arginine[a]	Asparagine
	Hydroxylysine
	Tyrosine

[a] Not essential for maintenance of most adult mammals.

and thus it becomes an essential amino acid and must be provided in the diet. Phenylalanine metabolites other than tyrosine are made and accumulated, and it is this accumulation of metabolites that has neurotoxic effects on the central nervous system. These neurotoxic compounds destroy brain cells that, in turn, results in mental retardation. The condition can be managed if diagnosed early (within days of birth), and the diet is then restricted in its phenylalanine content. Care must be taken to provide the enough phenylalanine to support growth and development without providing excess amounts. Care too must be exercised to provide sufficient tyrosine to meet the needs of the growing child and then to provide the amino acid needs after growth has ceased.

Stereochemistry

Amino acids, like the simple sugars, exist as stereoisomers. Their absolute configuration, similarly, is related to the configuration of glyceraldehyde. The Fischer projection of D-glyceraldehyde shows the hydroxyl function on the α-carbon to the right. At a similar point in a D-amino acid, the amino function is to the right.

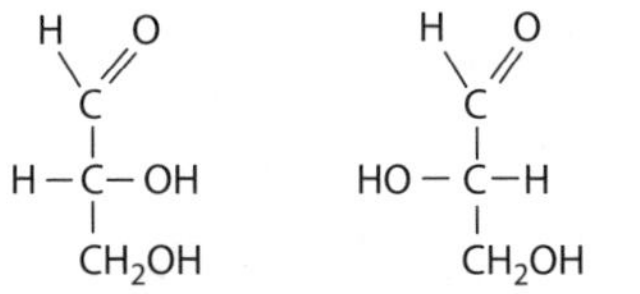

$$\begin{array}{c} \text{H}\quad\text{O} \\ \diagdown\;/\!/ \\ \text{C} \\ | \\ \text{H}-\text{C}-\text{OH} \\ | \\ \text{CH}_2\text{OH} \end{array} \qquad \begin{array}{c} \text{H}\quad\text{O} \\ \diagdown\;/\!/ \\ \text{C} \\ | \\ \text{HO}-\text{C}-\text{H} \\ | \\ \text{CH}_2\text{OH} \end{array}$$

D-glyceraldehyde L-glyceraldehyde

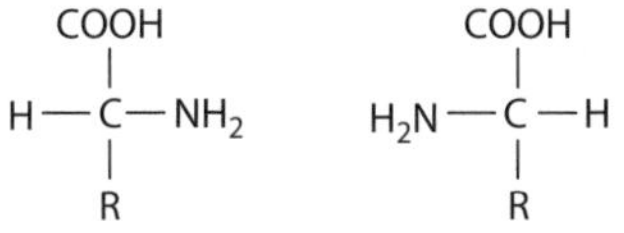

$$\begin{array}{c} \text{COOH} \\ | \\ \text{H}-\text{C}-\text{NH}_2 \\ | \\ \text{R} \end{array} \qquad \begin{array}{c} \text{COOH} \\ | \\ \text{H}_2\text{N}-\text{C}-\text{H} \\ | \\ \text{R} \end{array}$$

D-amino acid L-amino acid

All of the amino acids except glycine (which has no asymmetric carbon atom) possess optical activity. The amino acids of nutritional importance are all L-amino acids, whereas the nutritionally important sugars are of the D-series. Species differences exist in the utilization of L- versus D-amino acids. There are a number of D-amino acids that are of use to single cell organisms. Further, some D-amino acids combine to form potent antibiotics; gramicidin D and actinomycin D, for example, contain D-amino acids. Their utility as antibiotics rests with the fact that mammalian cells cannot absorb them as readily as microorganisms. These antibiotics are antimetabolites. That is, they are not degraded by the metabolic pathways. Because of this, they accumulate blocking metabolism and killing the cell.

Acid–Base Properties

Because amino acids possess acidic carboxyl and basic amino groups, they can function as either hydrogen acceptors or donors. At low pH, amino acids can exist in the fully protonated form:

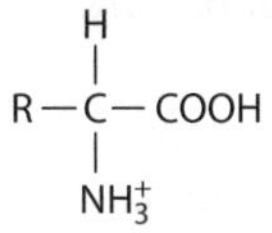

$$\begin{array}{c} \text{H} \\ | \\ \text{R}-\text{C}-\text{COOH} \\ | \\ \text{NH}_3^+ \end{array}$$

At higher pH levels, H^+ from the carboxyl function will be released and the amino acid exists as the dipolar ion,

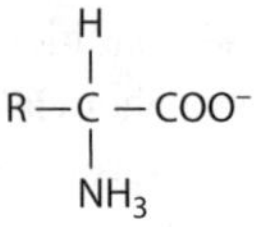

$$R-\overset{\displaystyle H}{\underset{\displaystyle NH_3}{\overset{|}{\underset{|}{C}}}}-COO^-$$

At even higher pH values, the amino function dissociates and the amino acid exists in the negatively charged form

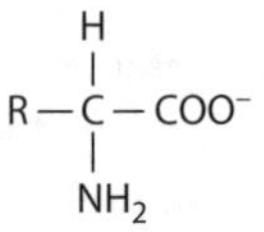

$$R-\overset{\displaystyle H}{\underset{\displaystyle NH_2}{\overset{|}{\underset{|}{C}}}}-COO^-$$

If the amino acid has more than one amino or carboxyl group, further dissociation can occur, and the range in pH over which this occurs is much broader. For example, aspartic acid exists at

$$\text{pH 1 as: } \begin{array}{l} COOH \\ | \\ CH_2 \\ | \\ CH\text{–}NH_3^+ \\ | \\ COOH \end{array}$$

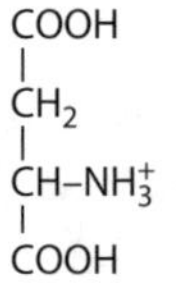

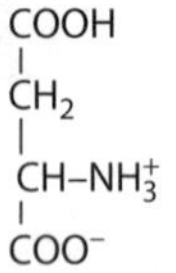

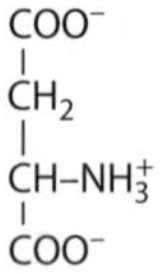

$$\text{at pH 3 as: } \begin{array}{l} COOH \\ | \\ CH_2 \\ | \\ CH\text{–}NH_3^+ \\ | \\ COO^- \end{array} \qquad \text{at pH 6-8 as: } \begin{array}{l} COO^- \\ | \\ CH_2 \\ | \\ CH\text{–}NH_3^+ \\ | \\ COO^- \end{array} \qquad \text{at pH 11 as: } \begin{array}{l} COO^- \\ | \\ CH_2 \\ | \\ CH\text{–}NH_2 \\ | \\ COO^- \end{array}$$

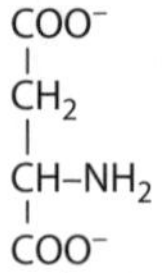

With each change in the form of the amino acid that occurs, from the lowest to the highest pH, a hydrogen ion is released. The capacity to accept or release hydrogen ions is characteristic of all amino acids; however, only a few (glutamate, aspartate, histidine, and, perhaps, arginine) serve as buffers with respect to the regulation of hydrogen ion concentration in the body. Glutamine is especially important because its metabolism yields bicarbonate, which serves in the regulation of pH. However, because free amino acids are in low concentrations relative to the other buffering systems in the body, their buffering power is much less important than that of the carbonate and phosphate buffering systems.

Reactions

Amino acids undergo characteristic chemical reactions at the carboxyl group, at the α-amino group, and at the functional groups of the side chains. Such characteristic reactions are particularly useful to the biochemist, for they assist in the quantitative determination of the amino acid composition and sequence in a given protein. These reactions are summarized in Table 8.5.

Among the reactions that the functional groups on the side chains of the amino acids undergo, those that involve the thiol or sulfhydryl group of cysteine are most important. This group is weakly acidic and quite reactive. It is very susceptible to oxidation by either oxygen in the presence of iron salts or by other oxidizing agents. When oxidized, cysteine is converted to cystine.

TABLE 8.5
Characteristic Chemical Reactions of Amino Acids

Reaction Name	Reagent	Use
Ninhydrin reaction	Ninhydrin	To estimate amino acids quantitatively in small amounts
Sanger reaction	1-Fluoro-2,4-dinitrobenzene	To identify the amino-terminal group of a peptide
Dansyl chloride reaction	1-Dimethylamino-napthalene (also called dansyl chloride)	To measure very small amounts of amino acids quantitatively
Edman degradation	Phenylisothiocyanate	To identify the terminal NH_2 group in a protein
Schiff base	Aldehydes	To measure labile intermediates in some enzymatic reactions involving α-amino acid substrates

In this conversion, two cysteine residues are joined together by a disulfide (–S–S–) bridge. Within the extracellular proteins, sulfhydryl groups react with one another to form disulfide bridges. These bridges stabilize the internal structure of the protein. Sulfhydryl groups also react with heavy metals to form mercaptides. This reaction is of great interest to the nutritionist. The protein–mineral interactions, or more truly mineral–sulfhydryl reactions, are important not only for an understanding of how minerals serve as cofactors in enzymatic reactions and for mineral transport into and out of cells but also for an understanding of the mechanisms involved in heavy metal intoxication. Figure 8.1 illustrates this reaction.

No discussion of the chemical reactions of the amino acids would be complete without discussing the formation of the peptide bond (Figure 8.2). Without question, this is the most important reaction of these compounds. The formation of peptide bonds involves the removal of one molecule

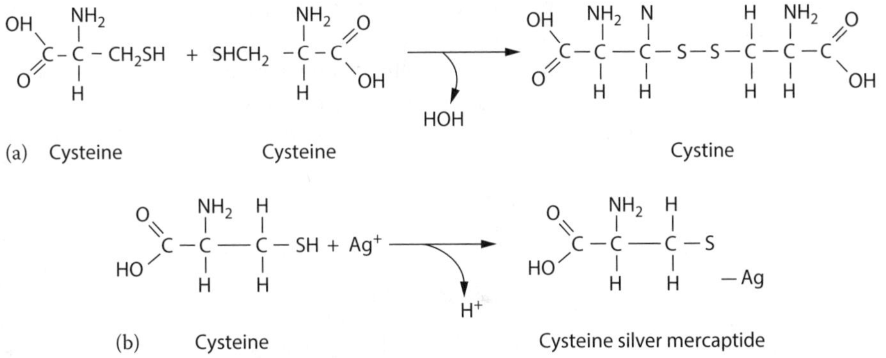

FIGURE 8.1 Examples of sulfhydryl group reactions. (a) Formation of disulfide bridge. (b) Formation of mercaptide.

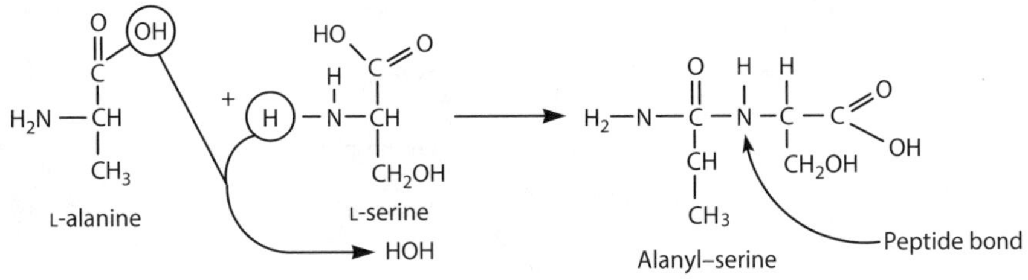

FIGURE 8.2 Formation of the peptide bond. Example: L-alanine + L-serine → alanyl–serine (a dipeptide).

of water with the resultant linkage between the carbon of one amino acid to the amino group of a second amino acid. Water is formed when the hydroxyl ion of the carboxyl group of one amino acid combines with a hydrogen atom from the amino group of a second amino group. Peptide bonding is the basis for the formation of peptides, polypeptides, and proteins and is the linkage used in the primary structure of any sequence of amino acids.

There are many possible combinations of the 20 amino acids commonly found in proteins. In a dipeptide that contains two different amino acids (A and B), two combinations are available: A–B and B–A. In a tripeptide with three different amino acids, six combinations are available if all three amino acids are used and each used only one time: A–B–C, B–A–C, A–C–B, B–C–A, C–A–B, and C–B–A. The number of possible combinations of the sequential arrangement of different amino acids is determined by the expression $n!$ (n factorial), when n is the number of different amino acids. If 20 amino acids are present in a protein, the number of possible combinations would be $20 \times 19 \times 18 \times 17 \times \ldots \times 1 = 2 \times 10^{18}$. The molecular weight of this molecule is about 2400 (average molecular weight of an amino acid × number of amino acids = 120 × 20), a relatively small protein. If the molecule were larger, and if the amino acids were used more than once, the number of possible combinations is increased even more. That nature can consistently reproduce the same protein, when there are so many choices of amino acids and sequences, is due to its dependence on the codes for each of these amino acids in the genetic material, DNA. These codes in turn dictate the sequence of amino acids in the protein being synthesized (see Chapter 7).

Amino Acid Derivatives

Creatine Phosphate

The energy needed to drive the energy-dependent reactions of the body is provided by the high-energy bonds of the adenine nucleotides, the guanine nucleotides, and the uridyl nucleotides. The concentrations of these nucleotides are carefully regulated, and their energy is metered out as needed. Short, quick bursts of energy from these nucleotides are not possible. However, Mother Nature has devised another compound, creatine phosphate, which can do just this. Creatine is formed from glycine, arginine, and *S*-adenyl methionine in a reaction sequence shown in Figure 8.3. It circulates in the blood and can be found in measurable quantities in the brain

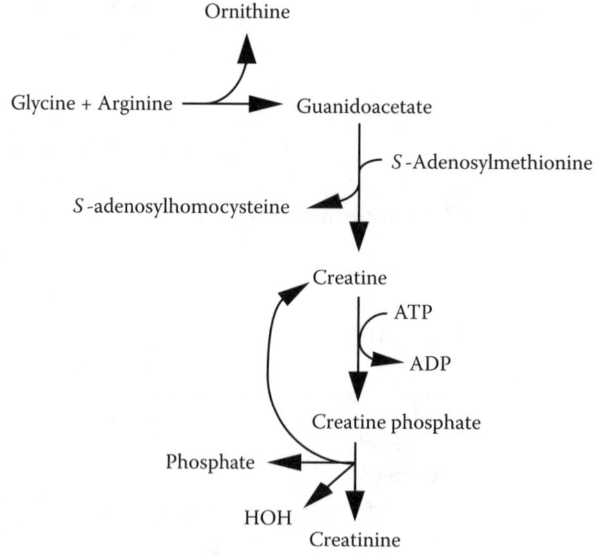

FIGURE 8.3 Formation of creatine phosphate.

and muscle. The creatine is phosphorylated to form creatine phosphate via the enzyme creatine phosphate. Creatine can be converted to creatinine by irreversible nonenzymatic dehydration. Upon hydrolysis, creatine phosphate will provide sufficient energy for muscle contraction. This hydrolysis yields creatine and inorganic phosphate. Some of the creatine can be rephosphorylated, while the remainder is converted to creatinine that then is excreted in the urine. Creatine phosphate has the same free energy of hydrolysis as ATP. Creatine phosphate is found primarily in muscle and provides the quick burst of energy needed each time a muscle contracts. Since the muscle activity produces the end product, creatinine, measuring creatinine allows for the estimation of the muscle mass.

Because creatinine excretion is reasonably constant from day to day, researchers use the amount of creatinine in the 24 h urine collection as an assurance of the completeness of the urine sample. Variations can occur if the usually sedentary subject has an unusually active day. A dramatic increase in muscle use will result in an increase in creatine phosphate breakdown and an increase in creatinine excretion.

Choline

Choline is a highly methylated compound synthesized from serine. Choline is an essential component of the neurotransmitter acetylcholine as well as an essential ingredient of the phospholipids phosphatidylcholine and sphingomyelin. These two phospholipids are integral parts of cell membranes. The phosphatidylcholine is on the outer aspect of the membrane, while other phospholipids (phosphatidylserine and phosphatidylethanolamine) are on the interior aspect of the cell membrane.

Polyamines

Certain amino acids can be decarboxylated to form the polyamines. Some polyamines are very short-lived compounds that are neurotransmitters. They are quickly broken down so as to limit their effects. The neurotransmitter catecholamines (epinephrine and norepinephrine) fall into this category of polyamines. Other polyamines, putrescine and spermine, bind nucleic acids and other polyanions. They have a role in cell division.

Peptides

Two amino acids joined together form a dipeptide, three form a tripeptide, and so on. Each amino acid in a chain is referred to as an amino acid residue. A chain of up to 100 amino acids joined together is called a polypeptide. If many amino acids are involved, then the compound is called a protein. Proteins have been identified that have as many as 300,000 amino acid residues and molecular weights in excess of 4×10^7.

The sequence of the amino acids in a given protein is represented by a sequential arrangement of abbreviations for each. For example, the polypeptide bradykinin is represented as Arg–Pro–Pro–Gly–Phe–Ser–Pro–Phe–Arg. The right-hand side of the chain represents the carboxyl terminal, while the left-hand side represents the amino-terminal. The systematic name for bradykinin is arginyldiprolylglyclyphenylalanyl–serylprolylphenylalanylarginine. This is very cumbersome so the systematic name is seldom used except when one wishes to give the amino acid sequence of a peptide. Otherwise, the common name is used. The amino acid sequence of a given peptide or protein can vary and its variation is controlled genetically. Many of the proteins of importance in nutrition have been sequenced and their DNA codes revealed.

PROTEIN STRUCTURE

Proteins are complex molecules having characteristic primary, secondary, tertiary, and quaternary structures. The primary structure is determined genetically as the particular sequence of amino acids in a given protein.

Under normal pH and temperature conditions, a protein is characterized not only by its amino acid sequence (its primary structure) but also by its 3D structure, that is, how the chain of amino acids twists and turns and what shape this long chain of amino acids assumes. This 3D shape, unique to each protein's particular amino acid sequence, is known as the *native conformation* of the protein. This assumption of shape may be spontaneous or may be catalyzed by enzymes and reflects the lowest energy state of the protein in its native environment. Protein conformation is usually divided into two categories: secondary and tertiary. The secondary and tertiary structures of a protein result from interactions between the reactive groups on the amino acids in the protein.

Secondary structure is the local conformation of the protein molecule. It is due to the formation of hydrogen bonds, disulfide bridges, and ionic bonds (in the case of the polar amino acids) between adjacent or nearby amino acids in an amino acid chain. As a result of these bonds, there is a regular recurring arrangement in space of the amino acids within the chain that can extend over the entire chain or only in small segments of it. Two kinds of periodic structures are found in proteins: the helix and the pleated sheet. In the helix, the amino acid chain can be viewed as wrapping itself around a long cylinder. The most common helical arrays are the α-helix and triple helix. The other periodic shape is the pleated sheet. It is essentially a linear array of the amino acid chain. All of these structures are stabilized by hydrogen bonding.

The tertiary structure is the regional conformation a protein molecule possesses; it develops after the secondary structure is established. It refers to how the amino acid chain bends or folds in three dimensions to form a compact, tightly packaged protein. It results from hydrogen bonding, disulfide cross-linkages, ionic bonds between polar amino acids, and interactions between hydrophobic R groups. This last feature tends to locate the hydrophobic R groups internally in the protein structure, away from the aqueous environment. A protein that clearly demonstrates a tertiary structure is hemoglobin. Some parts of the amino acid chains in this molecule form helices; others do not. This gives the molecule the fluidity to assume different 3D shapes along the chain: it will bend back upon itself to accomplish the maximum number of hydrogen bonds and disulfide bridges.

The quaternary structure refers to how groups of individual amino acid chains are arranged in relation to each other within a given protein. It is the structure that results when two or more polypeptide chains combine. The chains (subunits) may be different or identical, yet each subunit still possesses its own primary, secondary, and tertiary structure. The number of subunits in a protein may vary; some proteins have only two subunits, while others have more than 2000 subunits. The protein hemoglobin, for example, consists of four subunits and is one of the few proteins whose primary, secondary, tertiary, and quaternary structures are known. It contains four separate peptide chains: two chains that contain 141 amino acid residues and two chains that contain 146 amino acid residues. To each of these is bound a heme (iron) residue in a noncovalent linkage.

As a result of the various bonds that can form within a protein molecule, essentially two kinds of proteins exist: fibrous protein and globular protein. Fibrous proteins resemble long ribbons or hairs. They tend to be insoluble in most solvents and include such tough, resilient protein structures as collagen and elastin. Fibrous protein can have either the helical or pleated-sheet structure. Collagen is an example of the triple helix and silk an example of a pleated-sheet structure. Where the fibrous proteins appear to have a long *stringy* shape, globular proteins are roughly spherical or elliptical. Many enzymes and antibodies have a globular structure.

PROTEIN DENATURATION

One of the most striking characteristics of proteins is the response to heat, alcohol, and other treatments that affect their quaternary, tertiary, and secondary structures. This characteristic response is called *denaturation*. Denaturation results in the unfolding of a protein molecule, thus breaking its hydrogen bonds and the associations between functional groups; as a result, the 3D structure is lost. Denaturation affects many of the properties of the protein molecule. Its physical shape is changed, its solubility in water is altered, and its reactivity with other proteins may be lost. When denatured, the protein loses its biological activity. Heating will denature most proteins. As little as 15°C can denature some proteins. The majority of food proteins are denatured at heats in excess of 60°C. Some proteins are very heat stable (e.g., those found in thermophilic bacteria), while others are quite labile. A very good example of protein denaturation is the coagulation of egg white when heated. Heat denaturation, unless extreme, does not affect the amino acid composition of proteins and, indeed, may make these amino acids more available to the body. Heating provokes the unfolding or uncoiling of the protein and exposes more of the amino acid chain to the action of the proteolytic digestive enzymes. For this reason, many cooked proteins are of higher biological value (BV) than those same proteins consumed without heat treatment. If only mild denaturation occurs, it can be reversed. This process is called *renaturation.* If a protein is renatured, it will resume its original shape and biological activity.

CLASSIFICATION OF PROTEINS

Classification by Solubility and Prosthetic Groups

In addition to the conformational classification of proteins as described earlier, proteins have been classified on the basis of their solubility characteristics. As more and more information has been acquired about proteins, this classification system has become outmoded. However, because the vocabulary from this system has become so firmly entrenched in discussions of protein, it is necessary to be familiar with it. In this system, proteins are classed as simple or conjugated proteins. Simple proteins are those that contain only L-amino acids or their derivatives and no prosthetic group. Such proteins as albumin, histones, and protamines are examples of simple proteins.

Conjugated proteins contain some nonprotein substances linked by a bond other than an ionic bond. Since most proteins occur in cells in combination with prosthetic groups, conjugated proteins are the ones most nutritionists will recognize. Table 8.6 describes representative conjugated proteins.

Glycoproteins

A majority of the naturally occurring conjugated proteins are glycoproteins.[1] Sugar molecules are covalently bound to proteins, especially those proteins that are secreted from cells (mucin, for example) and those that compose the proteins found in the outer surface of the plasma membrane. Different types of covalent linkages have been found. The most common are the N-glycosidic linkages formed between asparagine amide and the sugar. Another common linkage is the O-glycosidic linkage between either the serine or threonine hydroxyl group and a sugar. Glycoproteins include the mucin in saliva as well as the conjugated proteins of plasma, collagen, ovalbumin (the major protein of egg white), and plant agglutinins. The glycoproteins range in size from a molecular weight

TABLE 8.6
Some Conjugated Proteins

Name	Prosthetic Group	Example
Lipoproteins	Neutral fats, phospholipids, cholesterol	Cell membranes; blood lipid–carrying proteins
Nucleoproteins	Nucleic acid	Chromosomes
Phosphoproteins	Phosphate joined in ester linkage	Milk casein
Hemoproteins	Iron	Catalase, hemoglobin, cytochromes
Flavoproteins	Flavin adenine nucleotide (FAD)	FAD-linked succinate dehydrogenase
Metalloproteins	Metals (not part of a nonprotein prosthetic group)	Ferritin
Glycoproteins	Carbohydrates	α-, β-, γ-globulins
Mucoproteins	Carbohydrates, hexosamines	Mucin

TABLE 8.7
Components of Glycoproteins

Sugars Found in Glycoproteins		Amino Acids That Bind to the Carbohydrates in Glycoproteins
Glucose	Acetylglucosamine	Asparagine
Galactose	Acetylgalactosamine	Serine
Mannose	Arabinose	Threonine
Fucose	Xylose	Hydroxylysine

of 15,000 to more than 1 million; the carbohydrate component of these proteins varies from 1% to 85%. Some of these proteins have uronic acids and are called proteoglycans.

Only 8 of the 100 or so carbohydrates that are known to occur in nature are found in glycoproteins (Table 8.7). These carbohydrates occur in chains containing no more than 15 saccharide units. Of the 20 amino acids in these proteins, only 4 (Table 8.7) actually bind to the carbohydrate moiety. The carbohydrates are linked to these amino acids by a nitrogen–oxygen glucosidic bond or through an oxygen bond. Some proteins contain small amounts of carbohydrate in loose association rather than as integral and characteristic parts of their structure. An example of this association is the glycosylated hemoglobin. In diabetes, blood glucose levels may fluctuate and exceed the normal range of 80–120 mg/dL. Some of this excess of glucose may be picked up by the hemoglobin and used to form glycosylated hemoglobin. Levels of glycosylated hemoglobin are used as indicators of the degree of control of glucose homeostasis. Normal levels of glycosylated hemoglobin range from 5.5% to 6.6%. Values above 7% indicate that blood glucose is not under tight control. Uncontrolled diabetes may be characterized by even higher levels of glycosylated hemoglobin.

Other peptidases are also glycoproteins. They are found in the plasma membranes of cells and serve in the release of neuropeptides and peptide hormones.[2] Many of them contain zinc. These peptidases have a homology (i.e., these proteins are similar to) with erythrocyte cell surface antigen and with the product of the PEX gene, which if mutated can result in X-linked hypophosphatemic rickets.

The function of the carbohydrate moiety of glycoproteins is not well defined. Some of the glycoproteins, those located on the exterior aspect of the plasma membrane, are part of the cell-recognition system. Others are essential to the immune mechanism as a component of globulin. The glycoprotein, C-reactive protein, is part of the system that responds to invading pathogens or to environmental stresses that in turn induce chronic low-grade inflammation. When C-reactive protein is elevated, there is insulin resistance.

Some dietary proteins such as those found in fish can reduce the levels of C-reactive protein.[3] The fish protein may be a good source of glutamine and arginine that in turn have immunomodulatory properties.[4] Patients with Crohn's disease (an autoimmune disease) have been studied. Biopsies of colonic tissue were cultured with arginine and glutamine. When incubated with these amino acids, there were reductions in the production of proinflammatory cytokines in association with reductions in nuclear factor-κB and p38 mitogen-activated protein kinase pathways.

In addition to their function within the immune system, glycoproteins are essential components of membrane active transport systems. Glycoproteins are important components of many receptors. These receptors are in the plasma membrane and in membranes of the organelles within the cells. The receptors that are part of the binding of cis and trans acting transcription factors on the DNA are also glycoproteins. Some hormones are glycoproteins; thyroid-stimulating hormone (TSH), follicle-stimulating hormone (FSH), and luteotropic hormone (LH) are examples.

Lipoproteins

Lipoproteins are multicomponent complexes of lipids and protein that form distinct molecular aggregates with approximate stoichiometry between each of the components.[5] In addition to proteins, they contain polar and neutral lipids, cholesterol, or cholesterol esters. The protein and lipid are held together by noncovalent forces. The protein component (apolipoprotein) is located on the outer surface of the micellar lipid structure, where it serves a hydrophilic function. Lipids, primarily hydrophobic molecules, are not easily transported through an aqueous environment such as blood. However, when they combine with proteins, the resulting combination becomes hydrophilic and can be transported in the blood to tissues that can use or store these lipids. The importance of these lipoproteins as carriers is discussed in Chapter 10.

Membrane lipoproteins, like the glycoproteins, are essential components of membrane transport systems and, as such, are important in the overall regulation of cellular activity.

Nucleoproteins

Nucleoproteins are combinations of nucleic acids and simple proteins. The protein usually consists of a large number of the basic amino acids. Nucleoproteins are ubiquitous molecules that tend to have very complex structures and numerous functional activities. All living cells contain nucleoproteins. Some cells, such as viruses, seem to be entirely composed of nucleoproteins.

Other Conjugated Proteins

The phosphoproteins and the metalloproteins are associations of proteins with phosphate groups or such ions as zinc, copper, and iron. The association of protein with phosphate may be fairly loose, as with the phosphate-carrying protein, or tight as with the phosphate in casein and the iron in ferritin.

Heme proteins sometimes are grouped with the metalloproteins because of the iron they contain. Flavoproteins are primarily enzymes and have as their prosthetic group a phosphate containing adenine nucleotide, which functions as an acceptor or donor of reducing equivalents.

Classification by Function

In addition to the system described above for the classification of proteins, the biochemist classifies these compounds on the basis of their function. Thus, proteins are classified as enzymes, storage proteins such as casein or ferritin, transport proteins such as hemoglobin, DNA-binding proteins such as the various transcription factors, contractile proteins such as myosin, immune proteins such as antibodies, toxin proteins such as the *Clostridium botulinum* toxin, hormones such as insulin, receptor proteins such as the insulin receptor, intracellular transporters such as the mobile glucose transporters, and structural proteins such as elastin and collagen. Nutritionists might not use this system for classifying food or body proteins, yet will want to understand these functions as part of their knowledge about the protein nutrient class.

Classification by Nutritive Value

In nutrition, we are interested in food proteins as sources of needed amino acids.[6,7] Those proteins that contain the essential amino acids in the proportions needed by the body are referred to as *complete proteins*. They are primarily of animal origin. Eggs, cheese, milk, meat, and fish are sources of complete protein. Proteins lacking in one or more essential amino acids or having a poor balance of amino acids relative to the body's need are *incomplete or imbalanced proteins*. These proteins are usually of plant origin, although some animal proteins are incomplete. The connective tissue protein called collagen, from which gelatin is prepared, lacks tryptophan; zein, the protein in corn, is low in lysine as well as tryptophan. Table 8.8 gives the protein content of some foods in the human diet.

Table 8.9 gives the amino acid content of several food proteins. The reader can find a more complete list of foods and their protein and amino acid content by using the USDA website for food composition (www.nal.usda.gov/foodcomposition). When food selection is limited and there

TABLE 8.8
Protein Content of Representative Foods in the Human Diet

Food (Serving Size)	Protein, Grams
Milk 244 g (8 oz)	8
Cheddar cheese, 84 g (3 oz)	21.3
Egg, 50 g (1 large)	6.1
Apple, 212 g (1–3¼″ diameter)	0.4
Banana, 74 g (1–8¾″ long)	0.2
Potato, cooked, 136 g (1 potato)	2.5
Bread, white, slice, 25 g	2.1
Fish, cod, poached, 100 g (3½ oz)	20.9
Oysters, 100 g (3½ oz)	13.5
Beef, pot roast, 85 g (3 oz)	22
Liver, pan fried, 85 g (3 oz)	23
Pork chop, bone in, 87 g (3.1 oz)	23.9
Ham, boiled, 2 pieces, 114 g	20
Peanut butter, 16 g (1 tablespoon)	4.6
Pecans, 28 g (1 oz)	2.2
Snap beans, 125 g (1 cup)	2.4
Carrots, sliced, 78 g (½ cup)	0.8

Source: www.nal.usda.gov/foodcomposition.

is a shortage of high-quality protein-rich foods, incomplete proteins can be combined so that all of the essential amino acids are provided. For example, corn or wheat and soy or peanut proteins can be combined in the same meal so that all of the essential amino acids are provided. When these proteins are combined and consumed in sufficient amounts, they will meet the amino acid needs of the consumer. This combination of incomplete proteins must be consumed within a relatively short time interval (less than 4 h) to obtain the appropriate and needed amounts of amino acids. Maximum benefit is obtained when the combination is consumed at the same time. Supplementation of incomplete proteins with missing amino acids has been suggested for populations consuming diets having a single dietary item as its main protein source. This supplementation is not very practical over a long period of time due to the cost of the pure amino acid supplement. Such populations are also likely to develop other nutritional disorders when their food supply is so limited.

Through selective plant breeding and the use of biotechnology, some of the plant foods listed in Table 8.9 have been improved to provide a better array of amino acids in their edible portions. A corn variety containing more lysine has been developed. This high-lysine corn shows promise for populations that have corn as a major food component. Other plant species have also been improved with respect to their amino acid content. However, some of these improved varieties may have special cultural requirements that economically challenged farmers cannot meet. Some of these cultivars may require added fertilizer, a very expensive item in such a farmer's budget. Agronomists, plant scientists, and agricultural economists continue to work to improve the nutritional value of the crops raised as well as improve crop yield. With judicious planning of food choices, nonetheless, it is possible to meet the protein and amino acid needs of populations subsisting on plant foods with little food from animal sources. Vegetarians, those who abstain from consuming nonplant foods, are particularly challenged in meeting their amino acid needs. Soy protein, peanut protein, dried beans, peas, lentils, and other protein-containing plant foods need to be combined to provide the appropriate amounts of the essential amino acids. For example, soy protein is low in methionine,

TABLE 8.9
Amino Acid Content of Several Food Proteins

Food	Tryptophan	Threonine	Isoleucine	Leucine	Lysine	Methionine	Cysline	Phenylalanine	Tyrosine	Valine	Arginine	Histidine	Alanine	Aspartic Acid	Glutamic Acid	Glycine	Proline	Serine
Milk	90	294	407	626	496	156	57	309	325	438	233	168	220	465	1491	126	709	376
Cheddar cheese	87	237	430	622	468	166	36	342	305	458	233	208	179	372	1745	98	731	384
Whole egg	103	311	415	550	400	196	146	361	269	464	410	150	0	438	773	221	265	525
Beef	73	276	327	512	546	155	79	257	212	347	403	217	361	583	946	387	308	262
Lamb	81	286	324	484	506	150	82	254	217	308	407	174	349	576	948	365	289	250
Bacon	65	210	274	500	403	97	73	298	161	298	427	169	0	589	702	589	331	242
Chicken	76	266	330	452	549	163	84	246	220	307	395	180	0	614	1004	418	0	0
Fish	62	271	317	472	548	182	84	232	169	333	352	0	0	551	796	345	381	193
Baked beans	61	295	314	524	381	64	19	359	179	336	270	20	0	0	0	0	0	0
Pecans	78	219	312	436	245	86	122	318	178	296	668	154	0	0	0	0	0	0
White bread	61	189	288	448	151	95	134	312	163	292	228	129	180	286	1980	202	675	0
Corn meal	38	249	289	810	180	116	81	284	382	319	220	129	622	776	1103	212	522	353
Rice	64	233	279	513	235	107	81	299	272	416	343	100	0	281	815	407	288	302
Banana	95	0	0	0	289	55	0	0	162	0	0	0	0	0	0	0	0	0
Oranges	39	0	0	0	221	33	0	0	0	0	0	0	0	0	0	0	0	0
Peas	52	229	287	390	295	50	68	240	152	256	555	102	183	596	442	202	0	0
Brussels sprouts	63	218	264	276	280	66	0	210	0	274	396	150	0	0	0	0	0	0
Potatoes	67	246	274	311	333	78	60	276	112	334	308	90	292	0	625	0	208	250

Source: From USDA, Handbook #8, *Amino Acid Composition of Foods*, U.S. Government Printing Office, Washington, D.C. 1963.

while corn is not. Corn is low in tryptophan and lysine. These two plant foods could be consumed in the same meal to provide all the needed amino acids.

In addition to the amino acid content, protein quality or rather the quality of the food containing the protein is classed according to its total protein content. Potatoes, for example, contain a very good distribution of essential and nonessential amino acids, yet, because the potato contains so little protein (1.7%), it is not considered a good protein source. One would have to consume a lot of potatoes (3.18 kg or ~7 lb) to meet one's daily amino acid and total nitrogen requirements.

PROTEIN ANALYSIS

The total protein content of food is estimated from the total nitrogen content of the food as determined by the classical Kjeldahl method. This method also determines nonprotein nitrogen as well; however, the amount of error in the method due to the inclusion of these compounds is very small. Most proteins contain about 16% nitrogen. To convert the nitrogen content to protein, one uses the following formula:

$$P_G = N_G \times 100/16 = N_G \times 6.25$$

where

P_G is the grams of protein in 100 g of food
N_G is the grams of nitrogen in 100 g of food

This conversion factor is an average factor. If more-exact figures are required, established conversion factors for each food category are available. For example, cereals generally have less protein nitrogen and more nonprotein nitrogen; thus, the conversion factor of 5.7 is used for cereal foods. On the other hand, milk has more protein nitrogen and the factor of 6.4 can be used. Generally speaking, because humans usually consume a mixed diet, the lower and higher factors tend to average out, and the value of 6.25 is acceptable when the total protein content of a day's food is determined in this way.

The amino acid determination of a protein has two phases: qualitative identification and quantitative estimation of the residues. The peptide bond that connects the amino acid residues is cleaved by acid, base, or enzyme-catalyzed hydrolysis to give a mixture of amino acids. The free amino acids are separated from one another and identified using chromatographic or electrophoretic techniques. Once separated and identified, each amino acid present can be determined quantitatively. Several of the reactions given in Table 8.5 can be used. These assays do not establish the sequence of the amino acids or the protein's primary structure, but merely tell how much of each amino acid is present. The sequence of amino acids can be determined by cleaving, one by one, the amino acids in the chain and following this cleavage with an analysis of the individual amino acids. Usually, high-performance liquid chromatography (HPLC) is used for this aspect of sequence analysis.

BIOLOGICAL VALUE OF DIETARY PROTEIN

Although the total protein (nitrogen) content can be readily determined, as can the amino acid content of the food, albeit with greater difficulty, the determination of the BV of a given protein within a food is far more difficult.[8] BV means how well the food is digested and absorbed and how well the component amino acids of the food meet the amino acid needs of the consumer. The BV of a food protein depends not only on its amino acid content but also on the needs of the consumer.[9] For example, the BV of a food for a rapidly growing child is quite different from that for a nongrowing adult. Growth carries with it a demand for particular amino acids as part of the total nitrogen requirement, whereas maintenance (as in the adult, nongrowing person) has a total nitrogen requirement with less stringent demands for specific amino acids.

There is also a species dependence to BV.[10] Chickens, because they grow feathers, need more sulfur-containing amino acids in their diets than humans. Thus, proteins having a higher proportion of sulfur-containing amino acids will have relatively higher BVs for chickens than for other species. Rats, the usual test animals in nutrition studies, grow fur, which contains a lot of arginine. This means that proteins rich in arginine will have a higher BV for rats than for humans.

A number of methods for assessing BV have been used. Each has its advantages and disadvantages. Using a holistic approach to assessing protein quality, H.H. Mitchell devised the nitrogen balance technique in 1924. This technique was based on Folin's definitions of endogenous and exogenous nitrogen excretion. By definition, the endogenous nitrogen comes from the nitrogen-containing excretory products synthesized in the body and not recycled. It is the unavoidable nitrogen loss. Exogenous nitrogen was defined as those nitrogen-containing products that are excreted in direct proportion to the amount of nitrogen consumed in the food. These are arbitrary definitions and there is some crossover between categories. They are, however, useful in the context of evaluating the biological usefulness of dietary protein. Endogenous nitrogen comes from the breakdown of body tissue and represents nitrogenous compounds produced as a result of one-way reactions. For example, when muscles contract, creatine phosphate breaks down to creatine and phosphate. While both the creatine and the phosphate can be recycled, some of the creatine is converted to creatinine and excreted in the urine. Its excretion is relatively constant, reflecting the muscle mass of an individual who is a normal healthy adult following a fairly regular daily routine. Other nitrogenous compounds considered to be in the endogenous category are uric acid, allantoin, 3-methyl histidine, and ammonia. Regardless of the dietary protein intake, excretion of these compounds by normal individuals with fairly uniform daily activity levels is relatively constant.

In contrast, exogenous nitrogen fluctuates in response to the dietary protein intake. The main compound providing this nitrogen is urea. Urea results when excess amino acids are deaminated. The body converts the $-NH_3$ to urea via the urea cycle and excretes the urea in the urine. Exogenous nitrogen is also found in the feces and represents undigested food protein. Fecal nitrogen represents not only the undigested–unabsorbed food but also the nitrogen of intestinal flora, desquamated intestinal cells, lubricants, and intestinal enzymes. There are species differences in these excretory patterns. While mammals excrete primarily urea, birds excrete uric acid as their major nitrogenous excretory product. Figure 8.4 illustrates the principle of nitrogen balance.

The nitrogen balance method assumes that a given protein, when fed at maintenance levels, will completely replace the protein being catabolized during the normal course of metabolic events in the body. It also assumes that all nitrogen gain and loss can be measured. Thus, for good-quality proteins, nitrogen balance (intake vs. excretion) should be zero for an adult individual, and for

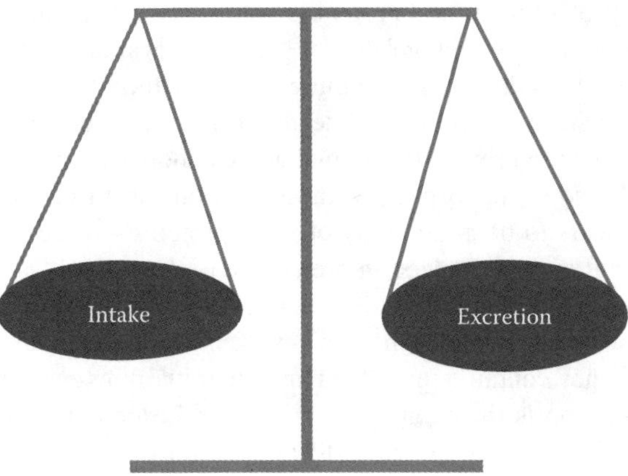

FIGURE 8.4 Nitrogen balance exists when the diet contains sufficient high-quality proteins to provide amino acids for the synthesis of proteins lost through degradation. It also exists when intake equals excretion.

poor-quality proteins, nitrogen balance will be negative. For growing individuals, good-quality proteins result in high nitrogen retentions, while poor-quality proteins result in low nitrogen retentions. The amount of protein retained can be determined by analyzing the total nitrogen content of the food, the feces, and the urine.

BV can thus be calculated as a ratio of the nitrogen retained to that absorbed multiplied by 100:

$$BV = 100 \times N \text{ retained/N absorbed} = 100 \times N_I - (N_{FT} - N_{FF}) - (N_{UT} - N_{UF})/N_I - (N_{FT} - N_{FF})$$

where

BV is the biological value
N_I is the nitrogen intake
N_{FT} is the fecal nitrogen during test period
N_{FF} is the fecal nitrogen during nitrogen-free period
N_{UT} is the urinary nitrogen during test period
N_{UF} is the urinary nitrogen during nitrogen-free period

In the original method, animals were fed a nitrogen-free diet for 7–10 days, and it was assumed that the nitrogen excreted during this period represented the endogenous nitrogen. The animals were then fed a diet containing the test protein at a level commensurate with their protein maintenance requirements for the same time interval. The nitrogen excreted during this period corrected for the nitrogen excreted during the nitrogen-free period was assumed to represent the exogenous nitrogen.

The method makes a lot of assumptions about overall protein metabolism, and these assumptions can account for some of the error associated with evaluating the quality of the test protein in this way. The method is noninvasive and very useful for work with humans. However, nitrogen can be lost via routes other than urine and feces. In hot climates or in physically active subjects, significant nitrogen losses can occur through sweat. On an adequate protein intake, it has been estimated that up to 10 g N/L can be lost. On an inadequate or low-protein diet, sweat losses can amount to 5 g N/L. Hair, nail, and menstrual losses can also contribute errors to the nitrogen balance technique. Usually sweat, hair, skin, and nail losses are ignored since they are minor in comparison with the urine and fecal losses, but, as mentioned, they do contribute to the error term for the method. Other errors in the method include the possibility of daily cumulative errors in the collection and analysis of the food, urine, and feces and the effects of prior poor nutritional status on the responses of the subject to this procedure. Good subject cooperation is essential to insure quantitative ingestion of the food and quantitative collection of the urine and feces.

The main disadvantage of this method is theoretical in character. The basic assumption of *replaceability* of body protein by a food protein is valid only when comparing good-quality proteins. When poor proteins such as zein, gelatin, or gluten are evaluated, unrealistically high values result. This overestimation results from the failure of the method to account for the mobilization of body protein to meet particular amino acid needs. If there is a deficiency of one or more of the essential amino acids in the test protein, the animal will catabolize body proteins in an effort to provide the missing amino acid to support the synthesis of vital short-lived proteins such as enzymes or hormones. There appears to be a hierarchy of body proteins—those that are most essential to the survival of the animal are synthesized in preference to those, such as muscle protein, that are not as essential. Similarly, those that are most essential to survival are *protected* from catabolism in favor of those proteins less essential to life. In any event, when the body proteins are mobilized, the needed amino acids they contain are utilized and the remaining ones are deaminated and used for energy. The amino group is then converted to urea and excreted, contributing to the urinary nitrogen level. The Mitchell nitrogen balance technique does not differentiate the source of the nitrogen in the excreta and, because of this, the technique is not as valid in evaluating incomplete proteins. Source differentiation could be accomplished through the use of isotopic markers that would allow the investigator to identify body proteins as distinct from food proteins. Heavy isotopes incorporated into the food protein as it is grown could identify the food nitrogen that was excreted. The use of heavy isotopes, however, is expensive as well as time consuming, so this variation in the Mitchell technique might not be frequently used. In efforts to circumvent the problem of overestimating the BVs of incomplete or imbalanced proteins, other methods, some of which are variations of the original nitrogen balance technique, have been proposed and used.

The nitrogen balance index (NBI) of Allison and coworkers relates the absorbed nitrogen to the nitrogen excretion of a separate but concurrent group of individuals fed a nitrogen-free diet. This technique requires less time than the Thomas–Mitchell method, but is subject to many of the same kinds of errors. Both methods suffer from the inaccuracies contributed by the methodological measure of the so-called endogenous nitrogen loss. Both methods assume that this loss is represented by the nitrogen excreted by the animal during the nitrogen-free period, when actually the feeding of such a diet accelerates protein loss rather than modeling the endogenous nitrogen excretion.

The dynamic state of the body proteins, that is, the constant need to synthesize proteins having a short half-life (see Chapter 6 for discussion of half-life), must be considered. This synthesis must be accommodated by the catabolism of tissue protein, a catabolic process unlikely to occur extensively if good-quality proteins are consumed. Because this overestimation of endogenous loss is more serious with proteins of poor quality, inconsistent BVs are obtained. This is particularly true when unrefined proteins or food mixtures are evaluated.

A more-accurate method for the evaluation of protein quality is one that actually measures the retention of nitrogen in the carcass from the ingested protein nitrogen. This is called the NPU-BV or NPU method. Using these methods that calculate BV from the change in carcass protein, groups of animals, usually rats, are fed diets containing graded amounts of the test protein or a nitrogen-free diet. After a period of 7–10 days, the animals are killed and the nitrogen content of the carcasses determined. Obviously, proteins of high quality will evoke a greater retention of nitrogen in the carcass than proteins of poor quality. Using this technique, BV can be calculated as follows:

$$\text{NPU} - \text{BV} = \text{B}_\text{F} - \text{B}_\text{K} + \text{I}_\text{K}/\text{I}_\text{F} \times 100$$

where

B_F is the carcass nitrogen of animals fed test protein diet
B_K is the carcass nitrogen of animals fed nitrogen-free diet
I_K is the absorbed nitrogen of animals fed nitrogen-free diet
I_F is the absorbed nitrogen of animals fed test protein diet

While this method has the obvious advantage of actually measuring nitrogen retention, its disadvantages are also obvious. Feeding a protein-free diet induces an exaggerated body protein loss. This method is inappropriate for large animals because of the technical difficulties associated with the determination of body composition and because of the excessive cost. Obviously, too, human studies would not be possible. However, conceptually, the method has merit, and several investigators have devised variations that are useful in a variety of species.

One variation that is useful in man is to measure the changes in body composition indirectly using heavy isotopes. The various methods for determining body composition changes can be used to evaluate proteins. For example, Steffee et al. used a stable isotope of nitrogen, ^{15}N, to study the rates of total body protein synthesis and breakdown as a response to variation in amounts of dietary protein. Constant infusions of ^{15}N-glycine allowed these investigators to assess the value of given proteins in the homeostatic situation where there is constant protein synthesis and breakdown. While a very useful technique, it is also very expensive and requires sophisticated techniques and equipment to make the appropriate measurements.

Another variation of the carcass retention method uses the naturally occurring radioactive isotope ^{40}K. The method measures the change in ^{40}K concentration in the adult body as a result of consuming a given protein for a period of 7–10 days. This method is based on the constancy of potassium as an intracellular ion. The concentration of potassium in the body can be directly related to the number of cells in the body and indirectly related to the protein in the body. Since a set percentage of this potassium exists as the naturally occurring radioactive isotope, measuring ^{40}K levels is a direct measure of body cell number and an indirect measure of body protein. If a poor-quality protein is consumed, ^{40}K levels will fall. If a good-quality protein is consumed, there will be no change. Again, while this method has the advantage of its applicability to humans, its disadvantage is the cost and availability of the whole-body counters needed to determine the presence of the isotope.

By far the easiest variation of the carcass retention method is the protein efficiency ratio (PER). In this method, carcass composition is not determined and it is assumed that the gain in body weight of a given animal is related to the quality of the protein fed. Thus, young growing animals are fed test protein–containing diets for a period of 28 days. The weight gain is computed and divided by the total protein intake.

The formula, PER = weight gain (g)/protein intake(g), is easy to use and the method requires no specialized expensive equipment. This is the method used for protein quality evaluation by most food companies and has been adopted by the regulatory agencies of the United States and Canada as their method of choice in evaluating the nutritional quality of foods. The ease and simplicity of the method, however, should not lull the reader into thinking that it is a *choice* method. PER can vary from species to species and, within a given species, from strain to strain. Examples of within-species variation in the PER of a given protein is shown in Table 8.10. Seven different strains of rats were fed the same diet for 4 weeks. PER was calculated at the end of each week. As can be seen in this table, the PER varied from week to week and between the seven strains. Variation can be introduced if levels of protein intake are higher or lower than 10% by weight. In addition, the methods make no allowance for the maintenance requirement of the animal. Values obtained from a variety of food proteins are nonlinear. That is, a protein having a PER of two may not have twice the nutritional value of a protein having a PER of one. Examples of the PER for a variety of food proteins is shown in Table 8.11.

A modification of the PER is the net protein ratio. This method attempts to account for the maintenance needs of the animal. In this method, two groups of animals are used. One is fed a nitrogen-free diet, the other the test diet. This modification is accompanied by all the pitfalls of using the nitrogen-free diets that were discussed earlier.

A variety of methods employing the assay of enzymes concerned with protein metabolism have been devised. The determination of the activity of transaminase, xanthine dehydrogenase, renal arginase, and others has been reported as indicators of protein quality. Unfortunately, these methods have not been rigorously tested and compared with the presently available whole-body methods.

TABLE 8.10
PER of a Test Protein as Calculated Using the Weight Gain of Rats from Seven Different Strains

	PER			
Rat Strain	**Week 1**	**Week 2**	**Week 3**	**Week 4**
Holtzman	4.14	3.94	3.61	3.50
Charles River	4.29	3.64	3.54	3.60
Sprague Dawley	4.31	3.76	3.32	3.36
Osborne-Mendel	4.20	3.52	3.24	3.39
Wistar	4.47	3.59	3.33	3.37
Wistar Lewis	3.69	3.64	3.37	3.28
SSB/PL (NIH)	3.80	3.37	2.96	2.47

TABLE 8.11
PER of Various Human Foods

Eggs	3.9–4.0
Fish	3.5
Milk	3.0–3.1
Beef	2.3
Soybeans	2.3
Beans	1.4–1.9
Nuts	1.8
Peanuts	1.7
Gluten	1.0
Rice	2.0
Corn	1.2

The holistic approach, while valuable and useful, is nonetheless time consuming and not particularly good for poor-quality proteins. It also is expensive. The aforementioned approaches have the advantage of digestibility and amino acid availability being given due consideration.

Attempts to circumvent the time and expense of whole-animal work have resulted in a number of techniques. One method, the amino acid score or chemical score is a nonbiological method and requires the amino acid analysis of the test protein. The amount of the most limiting amino acid (only the essential amino acids are considered) is related to the content of that same amino acid in a reference protein. In most cases, this reference is egg protein, however, a theoretical protein based on the amino acid requirements of the species in question could also be used.

While this method is quick and does not use animals, it makes no allowance for digestibility or availability of the constituent amino acids. This is a rather important aspect of protein nutrition. Some protein foods are poorly digestible; others contain compounds that interfere with absorption. For example, some amino acids form sugar–amino acid complexes that render the amino acids less available to the body. This occurs with the browning of baked goods such as bread; while bread is not considered a prime protein source, evaluation of its protein quality using the amino acid score would be in error due to the browning reaction.

A variation of this chemical method tries to account for digestibility.[12] In this method, test proteins are first digested in vitro using conditions resembling those in the gastrointestinal tract. The amino acid score is then determined on the products of this digestion. Another method is a variation of the amino acid–digestibility method. In this method the metabolic availability of essential amino acids is assessed. This amino acid oxidation indicator method has been used to evaluate the metabolic availability of sulfur amino acids in casein and soy protein.[4] Likely other essential amino acids can be evaluated this way, and the method might be useful in determining the BV of a variety of dietary proteins.

PROTEIN USE

Digestion

The daily protein intake plus that protein that appears in the gut as enzymes, sloughed epithelial gut cells, and mucins is almost completely digested and absorbed. This is a very efficient process that ensures a continuous supply of amino acids to the whole-body amino acid pool. Less than 10% of the total protein that passes through the gastrointestinal tract appears in the feces. If food contributes between 70 and 100 g of protein and the endogenous protein contributes another 100 g (range, 35–200 g), then about 1–2 g of nitrogen might be expected to be found in the feces. This is equivalent to 6–12 g protein. Of the dietary protein, the fecal protein might include the hard-to-chew or

TABLE 8.12
Digestive Enzymes and Their Target Linkages

Enzyme	Location	Target
Pepsin	Stomach	Peptide bonds involving the aromatic amino acids
Trypsin	Small intestine	Peptide bonds involving arginine and lysine
Chymotrypsin	Small intestine	Peptide bonds involving tyrosine, tryptophan, phenylalanine, methionine, and leucine
Elastase	Small intestine	Peptide bonds involving alanine, serine, and glycine
Carboxy-peptidase A	Small intestine	Peptide bonds involving valine, leucine, isoleucine, alanine
Carboxy-peptidase B	Small intestine	Peptide bonds involving lysine and arginine
Endopeptidase, aminopeptidase, dipeptidase	Cells of brush border	Di- and tripeptides that enter the brush border of the absorptive cells

hard-to-digest, tough, fibrous, connective tissue of meat or nitrogen-containing indigestible kernel coats of grains or particles of nuts that are not attacked by the digestive enzymes. For example, whole peanuts have a structure that is difficult to broach by the digestive enzymes. Unless chewed very finely, much of the nutritive value of this food may be lost. Peanut butter, on the other hand, is very well digested because its preparation ensures that its particle size is very small and is thus quite digestible.

The purpose of protein digestion is to liberate the amino acids from the consumed proteins.[11] Except for the period shortly after birth, the enterocyte cannot absorb intact proteins. Prior to gut closure, the neonate can absorb some proteins. Most of these proteins are immunoglobulins. The proteins found in the colostrum, or first milk, provide passive immunity to the newborn. After gut closure, only amino acids and small peptides can pass from the lumen of the gut into the bloodstream. Thus, the food proteins must be hydrolyzed into their component amino acids, dipeptides, and tripeptides. This is accomplished through a series of enzymes that have specific target linkages as their point of action. These enzymes are summarized in Table 8.12. The protein hydrolases, called peptidases, fall into two categories. Those that attack internal peptide bonds and liberate large peptide fragments for subsequent attack by other enzymes are called the endopeptidases. Those that attack the terminal peptide bonds and liberate single amino acids from the protein structure are called exopeptidases. The exopeptidases are further subdivided according to whether they attack at the carboxy end of the amino acid chain (carboxypeptidases) or the amino end of the chain (aminopeptidases). The initial attack on an intact protein is catalyzed by endopeptidases, and the final digestive action is catalyzed by the exopeptidases. The final products of digestion are free amino acids and some di- and tripeptides that are absorbed by the intestinal epithelial cells.

In contrast to carbohydrate and lipid digestion, which is initiated in the mouth with the salivary amylase and the lingual lipase, protein digestion does not begin until the protein reaches the stomach and the food is acidified with the gastric hydrochloric acid. The hydrochloric acid serves several functions. It acidifies the ingested food, killing potential pathogenic organisms. Unfortunately, not all pathogens are killed. Some are acid resistant or are so plentiful in the food that the amount of gastric acidification is insufficient to kill all of the pathogens. When this happens, the consumer is afflicted with a foodborne illness.

Hydrochloric acid (HCl) also serves to denature the food proteins, thus making them more vulnerable to attack by the pepsins, which are endopeptidases. The pepsins are a group of enzymes. The pepsins are released into the gastric cavity as pepsinogen. When the food entering the stomach stimulates HCl release and the pH of the gastric contents falls below two, the pepsinogen loses a 44-amino-acid sequence and forms pepsin A. Pepsin A attacks peptide bonds involving phenylalanine or tyrosine and several other enzymes that have specific attack points. The activation of the pepsins from pepsinogen occurs by one of two processes. The first, called autoactivation, occurs when the pH drops below five. At low pH, the bond between the 44th and 45th amino acid residue falls apart and the 44-amino-acid residue (from the amino terminus) is liberated. The liberated residue acts as an inhibitor of pepsin by binding to the catalytic site until pH 2 is achieved. The inhibition is relieved when this fragment is degraded. The second process is called autocatalysis and occurs when already active pepsin attacks the precursor pepsinogen. This is a self-repeating process that ensures ongoing catalysis of the resident protein. The cleavage of the 44-amino-acid residue, in addition to providing activated pepsin, has another purpose. That is, it serves as a signal peptide for cholecystokinin release in the duodenum. This then sets the stage for the subsequent pancreatic phase of protein digestion. Cholecystokinin stimulates both the exocrine pancreas and the intestinal mucosal epithelial cells. The intestinal cell releases an enzyme, enteropeptidase or enterokinase, which activates the protease trypsin released as trypsinogen by the exocrine pancreas. This trypsin not only acts on food proteins, it also acts on other preproteases released by the exocrine pancreas and activating them. Thus, trypsin acts as an endoprotease on chymotrypsinogen, releasing chymotrypsin; on proelastase, releasing elastase; and on procarboxypeptidase, releasing carboxypeptidase. Trypsin, chymotrypsin, and elastase are all endoproteases, each having specificity for particular peptide bonds as detailed in Table 8.13. Each of these three proteases has serine as part of their catalytic site, so any compound that ties up the serine will inhibit the activity of these proteases. Such inhibitors as diisopropylphosphofluoridate react with this serine and in so doing brings a halt to protein digestion.

Through the action of pepsin, trypsin, chymotrypsin, and elastase, numerous oligopeptides are produced that then are attacked by the amino and carboxypeptidases of the pancreatic juice and those on the brush border of the absorptive cells. One by one, the amino acids are liberated from the peptide chains, and one by one, they are absorbed and appear in the portal blood.

Absorption

Although single amino acids are liberated in the intestinal contents, there is insufficient power in the enzymes of the pancreatic juice to render all of the amino acids singly for absorption. The brush border of the absorptive cell therefore absorbs not only the single amino acid but also di- and tripeptides. In the process of absorbing these small peptides, it hydrolyzes them to their amino acid constituents. There is little evidence that peptides enter the bloodstream. There are specific transport systems for each group of functionally similar amino acids and di- and tripeptides. Most of the biologically important L-amino acids are transported by an active carrier system against a concentration gradient (see Figure 8.5).[12] This active transport involves the intracellular potassium ion and the extracellular sodium ion. As the amino acid is carried into the enterocyte, sodium also enters in exchange for potassium. This sodium must be returned (in exchange for potassium) to the extracellular medium. This return uses the sodium–potassium ATP pump. In several instances, the carrier is a shared carrier. That is, the carrier will transport more than one amino acid. Such is the case with the neutral amino acids and those with short or polar side chains (serine, threonine, and alanine). The mechanism whereby these carriers participate in amino acid absorption is similar to that described for glucose uptake (see the unit on carbohydrates). This mechanism is illustrated in Figure 8.5.

Metabolism

The amino acids leaving the absorptive cell enter a whole-body amino acid pool from which all cells withdraw amino acids for use in the synthesis of biologically important proteins, peptides, and amino acid derivatives. The peptides may be hormones or cytokines that are part of the various signaling systems found in the body.[13] Amino acids not used for peptide or protein synthesis can be deaminated and the carbon unit used for energy or for the synthesis of glucose or fatty acids. In humans consuming a fat-rich diet, very little fatty acid synthesis occurs. Amino acids can also be decarboxylated to form amines. Amines are quite potent compounds that act as intracellular effectors such as the neurotransmitters or as high-energy compounds such as creatine phosphate. The catabolism of the

TABLE 8.13
Some Protein and Peptide Compounds and their Function

Hormone	Source	Type	Function
Thyroid	Thyroid gland	Dipeptide	Regulates oxygen consumption by tissues
TSH	Pituitary	Polypeptide	Stimulates synthesis and release of thyroid hormone by the thyroid gland
Calcitonin	Thyroid gland	Polypeptide	Stimulates bone uptake of calcium
Parathyroid hormone	Parathyroid glands	Polypeptide	Raises serum calcium levels; lowers serum phosphorus levels; increases urinary phosphorus excretion; decreases urinary calcium excretion; activates vitamin D in renal tissue
Insulin	β-Cells of islets of Langerhans (pancreas)	Protein	Regulates glucose utilization; stimulates glucose uptake; influences lipid and protein synthesis
Glucagon	α-Cells of islets of Langerhans (pancreas)	Polypeptide	Rapid mobilization of hepatic glucose from glycogen; mobilizes fatty acids from adipose tissue stores; enhances hepatic glucose production from amino acids and glycerol
Somatostatin	D cells of islets of Langerhans (pancreas)	Polypeptide	Inhibits food passage along gastrointestinal system; decreases gall bladder release of bile; slows down uptake of nutrients from intestinal lumen; inhibit growth hormone release
Epinephrine	Adrenal medulla	Tyrosine derivative	Stimulates lipolysis; stimulates glycogen breakdown; increases vasodilation of arterioles of skeletal muscles and vasoconstriction of arterioles in skin and viscera
Norepinephrine	Adrenal medulla	Tyrosine derivative	Exerts an overall vasoconstriction effect on vascular system
ACTH	Pituitary	Polypeptide	Stimulates production and release of adrenal corticoid hormones
Antidiuretic hormone (ADH) (vasopressin)	Pituitary	Polypeptide	Promotes water conservation; controls water resorption by kidney; raises blood pressure
FSH	Anterior pituitary	Peptide	Controls testicular function; spermatogenesis; stimulates ovum production; enhances release of estrogen
LH (prolactin)	Anterior pituitary	Protein	Controls testicular function and spermatogenesis; stimulates ovum production; enhances release of estrogen
Growth hormone	Anterior pituitary	Protein	Stimulates growth of long bones and muscles; stimulates production of somatomedin
Gastrin	Gastric glands	Polypeptide	Stimulates acid and pepsin secretion; stimulates growth of gastric mucosa
Cholecystokinin	Intestine, pancreas	Polypeptide	Stimulates gall bladder contraction; stimulates pancreatic enzyme release
Secretin	Intestine, pancreas	Polypeptide	Stimulates pancreatic secretion; augments action of cholecystokinin
Leptin	Adipose tissue	Peptide (cytokine)	Signals the satiety center of the brain; suppresses appetite; stimulates UCPs and apoptosis

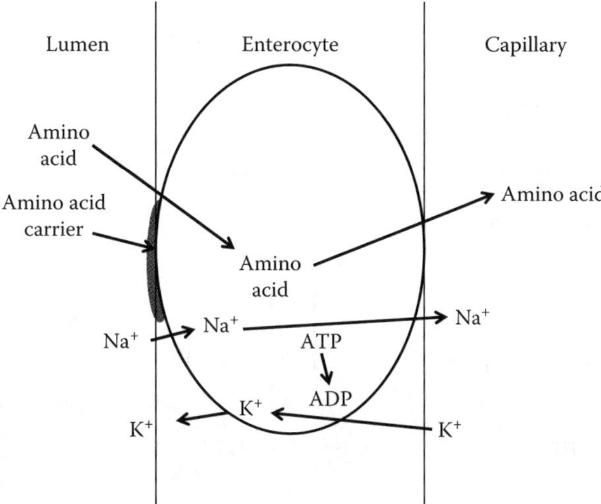

FIGURE 8.5 Carrier-mediated sodium-dependent amino acid transport. The amino acid enters the absorptive cell with sodium. The sodium is reticulated back to the lumen for reuse. The sodium is pumped out via the Na^+K^+ ATPase system. As the sodium leaves the cell, potassium flows back in and the electrolyte balance is maintained.

essential amino acids is shown in Figures 8.6 through 8.12. Amino acids that are deaminated send their $-NH_3$ group to the urea cycle shown in Figure 8.12. An important component of this cycle is arginine. It accepts acetyl Ca from the Krebs cycle and forms *N*-acetyl glutamate. The acetyl group is then released to form carbamoyl phosphate, which combines with ornithine to form citrulline. Citrulline passes into the mitochondria and when joined with aspartate reforms argininosuccinate. This is split to fumarate and arginine, which can form urea or ornithine or with the release of nitric oxide reforms into citrulline. The kinetics of the use of dietary arginine has been studied.[14] Using ^{15}N–^{15}N guanidol–arginine and isotope ratio mass spectroscopy, it was learned that ~60% of the ingested arginine was converted to urea with kinetics indicative of a first-pass splanchnic phenomenon. About 2% was used for nitric oxide production and the remainder was recycled into ornithine.

FUNCTIONS OF PROTEINS

A variety of proteins are found in the body. Each serves a specific function in the maintenance of life. Any loss in body protein, in effect, means a loss in cellular function. In contrast to lipids and carbohydrates, which have a body reserve to be used in times of need, the functioning body has no true protein reserve. Humans, when they are deprived of or insufficiently supplied with protein, will compensate for this dietary deficiency by catabolizing some, but not all, of their tissue proteins with a consequent loss in tissue functionality. If too much is lost, the body dies.

PROTEINS AS ENZYMES

From conception to death, living cells use oxygen and metabolize fuel. Cells synthesize new products, degrade others, and generally are in a state of metabolic flux. For these processes to occur, catalysts are needed to enhance each of the many thousands of reactions occurring in the cell. These catalysts, called enzymes, are proteins.[15] Enzymes make up the largest and most specialized class of proteins. Each enzyme is unique and catalyzes a specific kind of reaction. In the cell, enzymes are found in all the cellular compartments (cytoplasm, nucleus, mitochondria, etc.) as well as the membranes within and around the cell. The membrane-associated enzymes are part of the protein component of the cell wall. The location of an enzyme is one of its characteristics and dictates, in part, its role in metabolism.

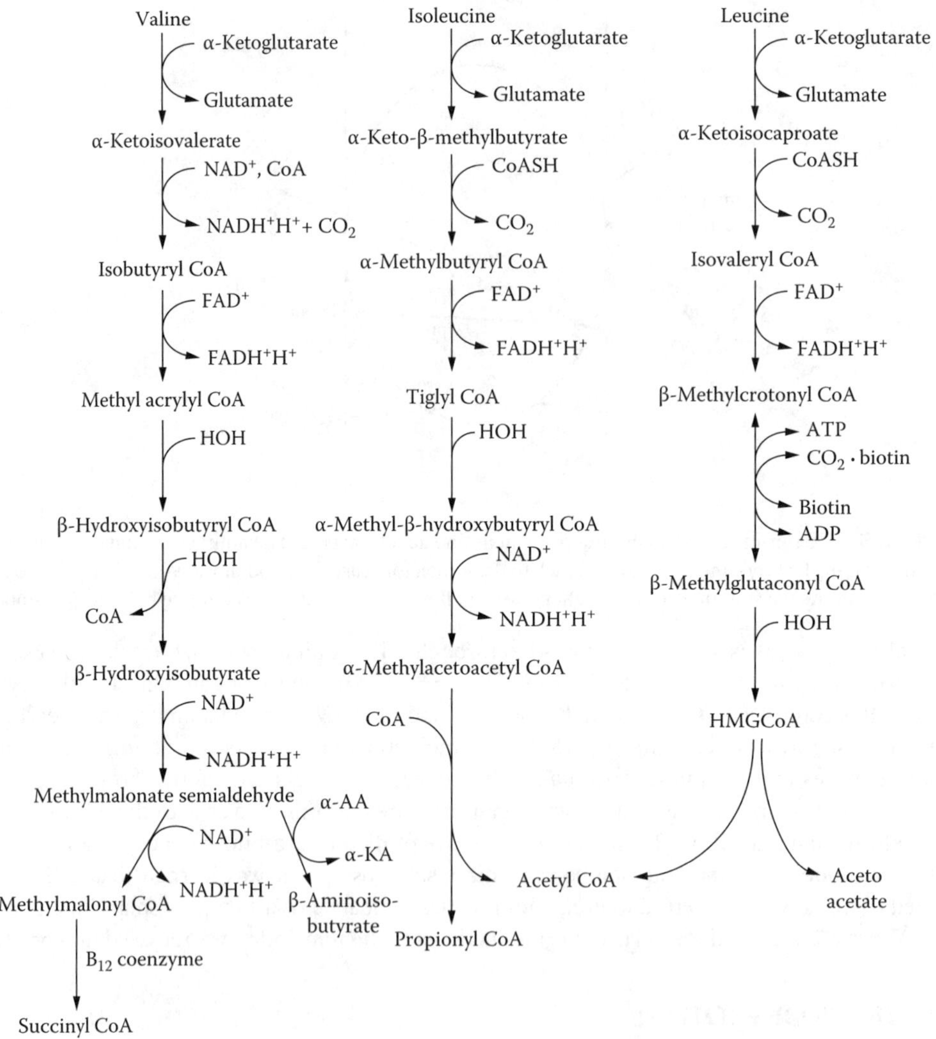

FIGURE 8.6 Catabolism of valine, isoleucine, and leucine.

Enzymes consist of specific sequences of amino acids. Should the sequence deviate, alterations in enzyme activity can be anticipated, unless, of course, the change in amino acid does not affect the active site of the enzyme or its molecular shape. The importance of the amino acid sequence is obvious and is related to the availability of R groups (on the amino acids) that will complement reactive groups on the substrate, the molecule on which the enzyme exerts its catalytic action. The catalytic function of the enzyme is intimately related to its amino acid sequence. Enzymes must possess a shape that will complement the molecular shape of the substrate in much the same way as a key fits into a lock. This shape, of course, is a function of the enzyme protein's primary, secondary, tertiary, and quaternary structure. Just as enzymes must have a specific shape, substrates must also have specific shapes to be catalyzed by their respective enzymes. This is the reason that only D-sugars or only L-amino acids can be metabolized by mammalian cells. These stereoisomers conform to the shape required by the enzyme that serves as its catalyst. While enzymes show absolute specificity, the specificity generally applies to only a portion of the substrate molecule. If the substrate is a small compound, this specificity applies to the entire molecule. If, however, the substrate is large and complex, the structural requirements are less stringent in that only that part of the substrate

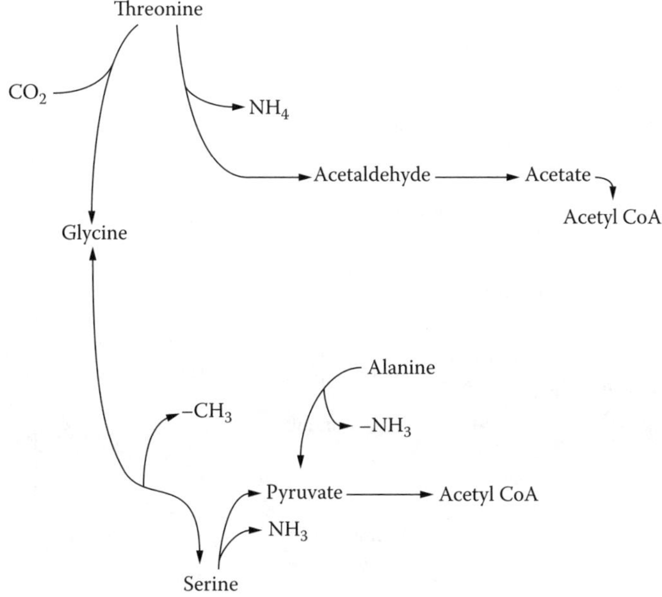

FIGURE 8.7 Catabolism of threonine showing its relationship to glycine, serine, and alanine.

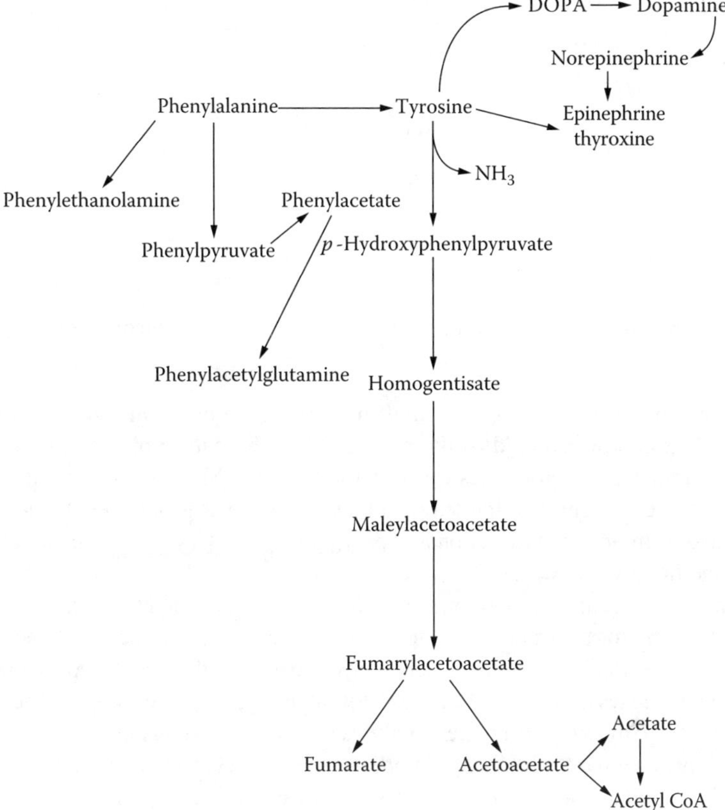

FIGURE 8.8 Catabolism of phenylalanine and its relationship to tyrosine as well as its use as a precursor of DOPA, thyroxine norepinephrine, and epinephrine.

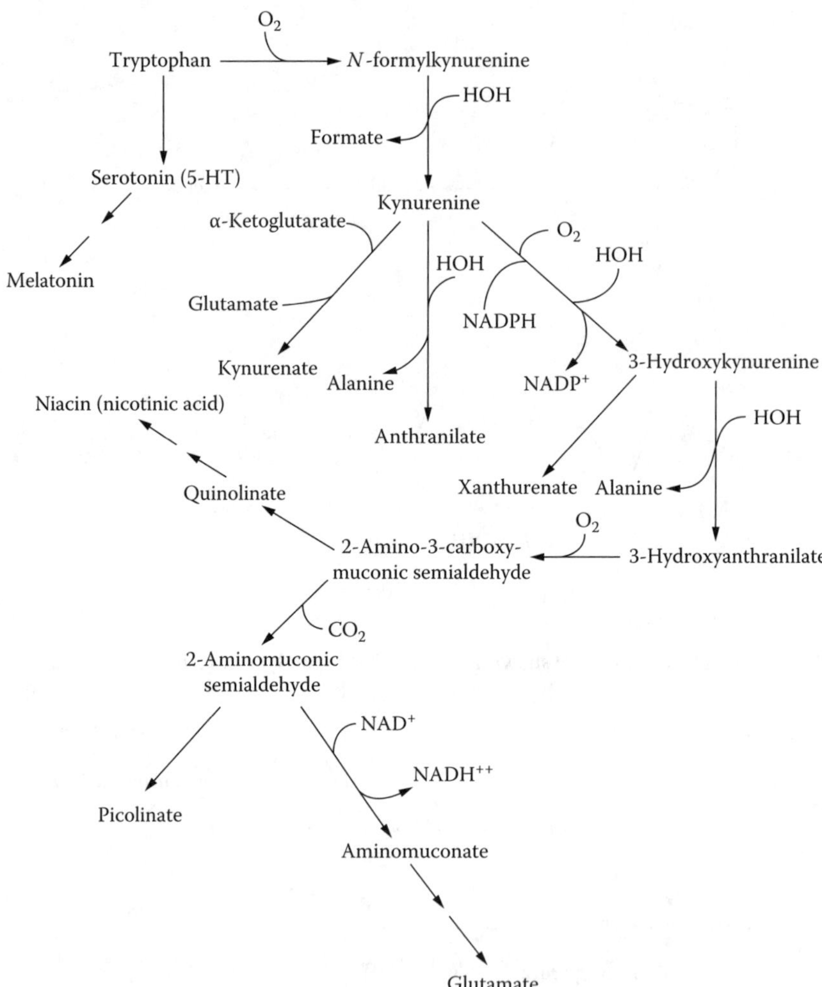

FIGURE 8.9 Tryptophan catabolism and its relationship to serotonin, melatonin, glutamate, alanine, and niacin.

involved in the enzyme–substrate complex must have the appropriate molecular arrangement. The portion of the substrate not involved in the reaction (i.e., the nature of the R group) need not be the appropriate conformation. How does this specificity work? Many substrate–enzyme complexes form with a three-point attachment that leaves a fourth atom or R group free. If the attachment site can be approached from only one direction and only complementary atoms can attach, the substrate molecule can bind in only one way.

Some enzymes are specific for only one substrate; others may catalyze several related reactions. While some are specific for a particular substrate, others are specific for certain bonds. This is called group specificity. For example, glycosidases act on glycosides (any glycoside), pepsin and trypsin act on peptide bonds, and esterases act on ester linkages. Within these groups, certain enzymes exhibit greater specificity than others. Chymotrypsin preferentially acts on peptide bonds in which the carboxyl group is a part of the aromatic amino acids (phenylalanine, tyrosine, or tryptophan). Enzymes such as carboxypeptidase or aminopeptidase catalyze the hydrolysis of the carboxy-terminal or amino-terminal amino acid of a polypeptide chain. This bond specificity rather than molecular specificity is useful to the animal in that it reduces the number of enzymes needed within the organism. Incidentally, these enzymes are very useful to protein chemists in their determination of the amino acid sequence of a given protein.

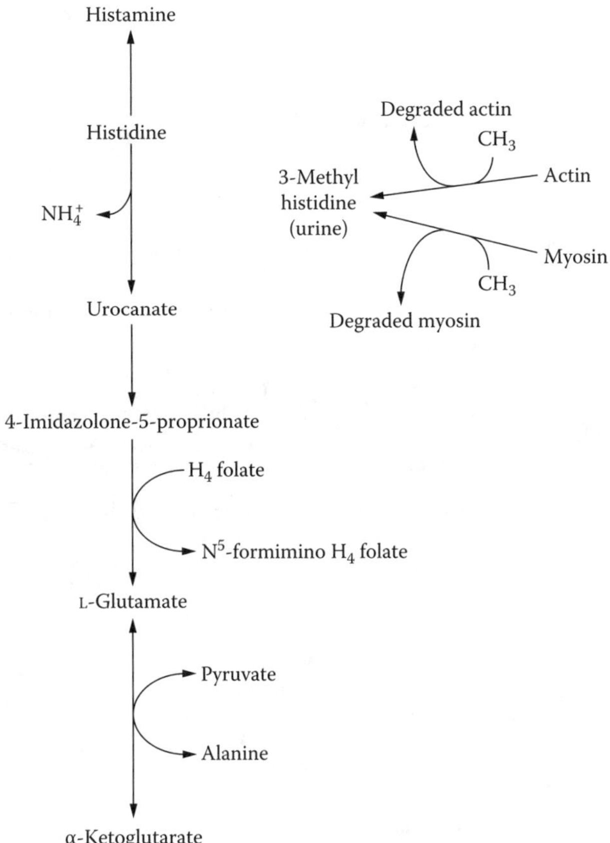

FIGURE 8.10 Histidine catabolism showing its relationship to histamine synthesis and also the unique catabolic pathway for histidine in the muscle protein.

Cells synthesize enzymes in much the same fashion as they synthesize other proteins, yet enzymes are relatively short lived. Cells must continually synthesize their enzymes if they are to survive. A variety of signals serve as stimulants or inhibitors of this synthesis. One of these signals is the substrate. An excess of substrate will not only activate any preexisting enzyme in the cell but will also serve to stimulate enzyme synthesis. The substrate may act at the level of mRNA transcription or at the level of translation or protein assembly. Hormones such as insulin, thyroid hormone, and glucocorticoid may also serve in this way to stimulate enzyme synthesis and/or activation. Hormonal inhibition of enzyme synthesis also occurs and serves as an internal regulator of the synthetic process.

Proteins as Carriers and Receptors

A wide variety of compounds is carried in the blood between tissues and organs of the body. Some of the compounds require a specific protein for their transport. Not only is this protein necessary for the transport of compounds insoluble in blood, but it is also necessary to protect these compounds from further reactions during the transport process. Some of the membrane proteins are carriers, some are both carriers and enzymes, and still others are receptors. Both intracellular and extracellular carriers and receptors have been identified. Receptors were discussed in Chapter 6.

The plasma proteins that can have a carrier function are the albumin and the α- and β-globulins. Perhaps the best studied of the plasma proteins are those associated with the transport of lipid, since these lipoproteins (carriers plus lipids), when elevated, appear to be related to the development

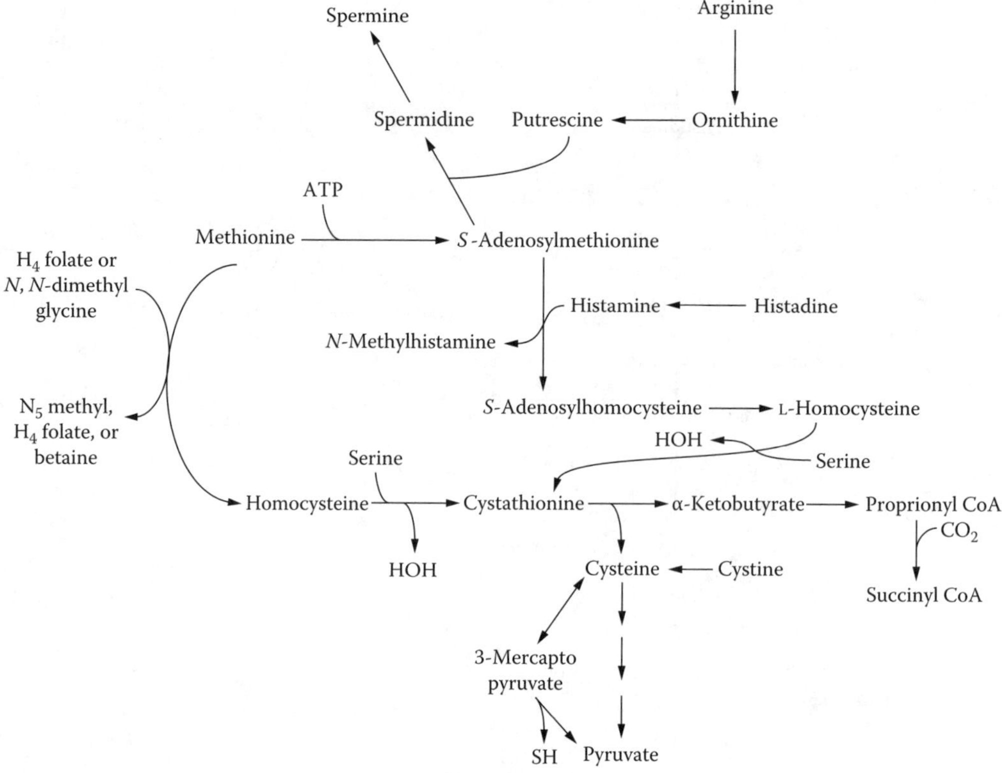

FIGURE 8.11 Methionine metabolism and its relationship to a number of important metabolic intermediates. Note the conversion of methionine to homocysteine that requires folacin. Also note the cystine to cysteine conversion and the histidine to histamine conversion that are parts of the pathway for methionine catabolism.

of cardiovascular disease (see Chapter 10). These lipoproteins make up about 3% of the plasma proteins. They are loose associations of such lipids as phospholipids, triacylglycerols, and cholesterols and represent an example of how proteins function as carriers.

In addition to serving as carriers of lipids, some of the globulins in the plasma can combine stoichiometrically with iron and copper as well as with other divalent cations. These combinations are called metalloproteins. The globulins serve to transport these cations from the gut to the tissues where they are used. The monovalent cations, sodium and potassium, do not need carriers, but many minerals do.

Many hormones and vitamins require transport or carrier proteins to take them from their point of origin to their active site. In addition, there are intracellular transport proteins, such as those in the mitochondrial membrane, that are responsible for the transfer of metabolites between the mitochondrial and cytosolic compartments. Finally, there are transport proteins that carry single molecules. The classic example is, of course, hemoglobin, the red cell protein responsible for the transport of oxygen from the lungs to every oxygen-using cell in the body.

Proteins as Regulators of Water Balance

As substrates and solutes are transferred or exchanged across membranes, water has a tendency to follow in order to maintain equal osmotic pressure on each side of the membrane. If osmotic pressure is not maintained, the individual cells either shrink from lack of internal water or burst from too much. The balance of water between the intracellular and extracellular compartments is closely regulated.

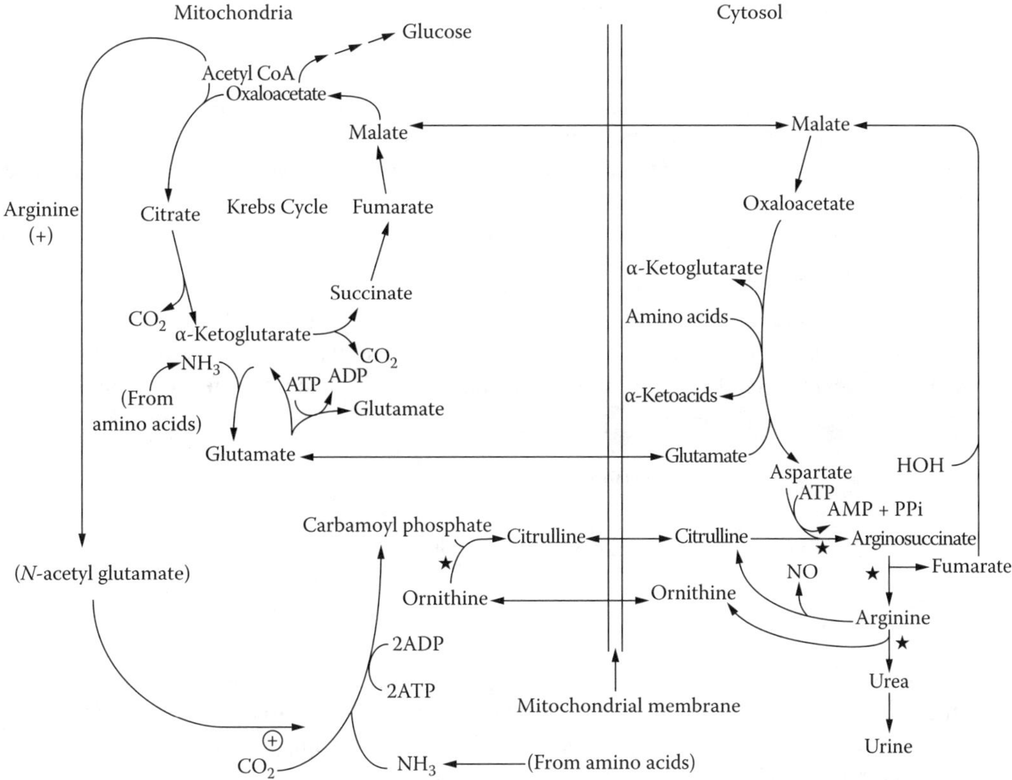

FIGURE 8.12 The urea cycle. Note the use of two ATPs for every NH_3 initially used in the synthesis of carbamoyl phosphate in the mitochondrion. More ATPs are used in the cytosolic portion of the cycle that in turn produces urea that can then be excreted in the urine.

One of the most carefully controlled points of water balance is across the capillary membrane, where a close balance is maintained between the osmotic pressure of the blood plasma, the interstitial fluids, and the cells and the hydrostatic pressure exerted by the pumping action of the heart. The total osmotic pressure of the plasma and of the intra- and extracellular fluids is the result of its content of inorganic electrolytes, its organic solutes, and its proteins. The concentrations of the electrolytes and organic solutes in plasma, interstitial fluid, and cells are substantially the same, so that the contribution to the osmotic pressure by these substances is practically equal. However, since there are more proteins in plasma than in the cells, plasma exerts an osmotic pressure on the tissue fluids. The result of this inequity of solutes is the drawing of fluids from the tissue spaces and from the cells into the blood. Opposing this force is the hydrostatic pressure exerted by the pumping action of the heart, which moves fluids from the blood into the tissue spaces and into the cells. The hydrostatic pressure is greater on the arterial side of the capillary loop than on the venous side. There is an interplay among these four kinds of pressure—blood osmotic pressure, tissue osmotic pressure, blood hydrostatic pressure, and tissue hydrostatic pressure. This interplay results in a filtration of solutes and metabolites and the transfer of oxygen from the arterial blood into the tissues and cells it supplies and on the venous side, a resorption from the tissue space of CO_2, metabolites, and solutes back into the blood supply.

Albumin plays a more significant role in maintaining the osmotic pressure than the other blood proteins because of its size and abundance. In the blood, there are more albumin molecules than other serum proteins and thus, albumin has a considerable influence on osmotic pressure. Malnourished individuals are characterized by a reduction in serum proteins. With fewer proteins in the serum, water leaks out into the interstitial space and accumulates. The condition known as edema results. The edema of protein deficiency may also be the result of the body's inability to synthesize the protein hormones, particularly ADH, which plays a role in controlling water balance. Edema not involving protein deficiency can also result from other factors such as increased blood pressure or renal disease, but the edema that results in these situations is a result of factors other than the plasma proteins. The effect of protein is on the distribution of water among the various body compartments, rather than on the total body water.

Proteins as Biological Buffers

Proteins have the ability to accept or donate hydrogen ions and by so doing they serve as biological buffers. In blood, there are three important buffering systems: plasma proteins, hemoglobin, and carbonic acid–bicarbonate. The equilibrium reactions for each of these buffering systems are as follows:

$$\text{HProtein} \leftrightarrow \text{H}^+ + \text{Protein}$$

$$\text{H}_2\text{CO}_3 \leftrightarrow \text{H}^+ + \text{HCO}_3^-$$

$$\text{HHb} \leftrightarrow \text{H}^+ + \text{Hb}^-$$

The first of these buffering systems, the plasma proteins, can function as a weak acid/salt buffer when the free carboxyl groups on the protein dissociate or as a weak base/salt buffer when the free amino groups dissociate. Although the buffering ability of the plasma protein is extremely important in maintaining blood pH, it is not as important as the other two systems.

The second buffering system, carbonic acid–bicarbonate, is extremely effective because there are reactions that follow this equilibrium that will regulate either acids or bases. The H_2CO_3 level in plasma never goes too high because it is in equilibrium with CO_2 ($H_2CO_3 \leftrightarrow CO_2 + H_2O$), which is expelled by the lungs. In blood, this equilibrium proceeds very quickly because of the presence of carbonic anhydrase, an enzyme found in red blood cells. If the carbonic acid–bicarbonate reaction goes in the opposite direction, the concentration of the HCO_3^- so formed will be regulated by the kidneys.

The third important buffering system in blood results from hemoglobin. Hemoglobin has six times the buffering power of the plasma proteins. It functions well as a buffer for three reasons. First, it is present in large amounts. Second, it contains 38 histidine residues, which are good buffers because they can dissociate to H^+ and the imidazole group. Third, hemoglobin exists in the blood in two forms, reduced hemoglobin and oxyhemoglobin. The imidazole groups of reduced hemoglobin dissociate less than those of oxyhemoglobin; thus, it is a weaker acid and a better buffer.

Hemoglobin's role in maintaining blood pH is extremely important and is best appreciated by understanding the transport of oxygen and carbon dioxide during respiration through the blood. Oxyhemoglobin is formed when each of the four ferrous ions in hemoglobin reversibly combines with one O_2 molecule. The reaction between oxygen and hemoglobin is written as $Hb + O_2 \rightarrow HbO_2$. The combination is not an oxygenation reaction because iron stays in the positive two-oxidation state. Instead, there is a loose association that exists between the oxygen and hemoglobin molecules.

At an oxygen tension of at least 100 mmHg, hemoglobin is almost completely saturated with oxygen. This curve has a sigmoid shape rather than linear, because after the first oxygen molecule is added to the hemoglobin, the affinity for the second is increased, the second increases the affinity for the third, etc. This increase in affinity results because, as the O_2 is taken up, the two β-chains move closer together. As O_2 is given up, they move farther apart. When fully saturated, as it is at normal physiologic conditions, each gram of hemoglobin contains 1.34 mL of oxygen. In a normal 100 mL of blood, there are about 15 g of hemoglobin and, hence, 20 mL of oxygen.

In addition to the oxygen carried in the blood in association with hemoglobin, there is additional oxygen present that is dissolved in the blood. Henry's law states that this concentration is a linear function of the pressure of the oxygen. Only 0.4 mL of oxygen is in the blood by being dissolved there and, thus, the major source of oxygen in the blood is hemoglobin.

As the cells consume the oxygen carried to them by hemoglobin, the oxygen tension falls, the oxyhemoglobin more readily dissociates, and the saturation of the hemoglobin falls. At about 50 mmHg, hemoglobin rapidly *unloads* its oxygen. In the tissues, oxygen tension is about 40 mmHg. This tension is below that necessary for unloading to occur and a gradient of high to low oxygen tension exists that facilitates the passage of oxygen to the tissues. This gradual change in oxygen content of the blood can be followed visually. Leaving the lungs, the blood is bright red. As it moves through the vascular system toward the periphery, the blood gradually darkens, and by the time it returns to the lungs, it has a bluish hue, a color characteristic of deoxygenated hemoglobin and the reason that persons lacking good respiratory exchange have a bluish tinge to their skin.

The CO_2 that is expired by the cells is transported in three forms. That which diffuses into the red blood cells is rapidly hydrated to H_2CO_3 by the presence of the carbonic anhydrase. The H_2CO_3 then dissociates into H^+ and HCO_3. The H^+ is neutralized primarily by hemoglobin and the bicarbonate diffuses into the plasma. This is the form in which most expired CO_2 is carried. The hemoglobin is present primarily in the blood in the reduced form by the time significant quantities of carbon dioxide are present so it can better function as a buffer. Some CO_2 that diffuses into red blood cells is not converted into bicarbonate ion but instead reacts with the amino groups of proteins, principally hemoglobin, to form carbamino compounds:

$$CO_2 + R-N{<}^{H}_{H} \rightleftharpoons R-N{<}^{H}_{COOH}$$

Reduced hemoglobin forms the carbamino compounds more readily than does oxyhemoglobin. The third form of CO_2 is that which is dissolved; it will exist as carbonic acid. It makes up only a small fraction of the total amount of CO_2 present. CO_2 present as carbonic acid will lower the blood pH. The CO_2 that diffuses into the plasma also exists in these three forms. The carbamino compounds will form with the plasma proteins. Much less CO_2 is hydrated to form carbonic acid in plasma than in red blood cells because the carbonic anhydrase enzyme is located only in red blood cells. And, finally, a small amount of dissolved CO_2 is present in blood.

There is a much greater rise in the HCO_3^- concentration in red blood cells than in plasma. As a result, HCO_3^- will diffuse into the plasma. This presents the problem of maintaining electrochemical neutrality. It is accompanied by a diffusion of chloride ions from the plasma to the red blood cells. This phenomenon is known as the chloride shift. Since CO_2 transport will occur primarily in venous blood, the chloride content of venous blood is higher than that of arterial blood. At the lungs, when venous blood becomes arterial, all these reactions are reversed. Occasionally, these reactions are perturbed and the acid–base balance is not maintained. Under normal conditions, the carbonic acid/bicarbonate ratio is maintained at 1:20. When the CO_2 levels rise, carbonic acid levels rise and respiratory acidosis occurs. Conversely, when CO_2 levels fall, respiratory alkalosis occurs. By adjusting inspiration and expiration, respectively, small rises and falls in CO_2 levels can be adjusted, and the ratio of carbonic acid to bicarbonate remains constant. The kidney, through increasing its resorption of bicarbonate, can also assist in the regulation of this buffer system.

Large shifts in the acid–base balance that originate not in the respiratory system but rather as a result of metabolic alterations also occur. The prime example is the metabolic acidosis that occurs in the severe, uncontrolled diabetic. As a result of the lack of insulin, the metabolic fuel, glucose, cannot be used. The body then uses an alternate fuel, fatty acids. Fatty acid oxidation in the diabetic results in an accumulation of ketone bodies—acetone, acetoacetate, and β-hydroxybutyrate. Normally, these substances are further oxidized to produce CO_2 and water. However, because so much fatty acid is being oxidized, its completion to CO_2 and water does not occur and the ketone bodies accumulate. These are acidic and must be neutralized. All of the buffering systems are mobilized, but eventually they will not be able to compensate for this gradual increase in ketone bodies. The pH will fall, the enzymes that work at pH 7.4 will be appreciably less active, and the hemoglobin will become less able to carry oxygen. Unless treated with insulin, the patient will become comatose (lack of oxygen to the brain) and die.

Metabolic alkalosis is not nearly as common as metabolic acidosis. However, it can occur in persons having prolonged bouts of both diarrhea and vomiting. This is a result of the loss of the stomach acid, hydrochloric acid (the chloride ion), and the loss of potassium ions. Alkalosis can also occur in individuals who consume large quantities of alkali, as might occur in persons with peptic ulcers who self-medicate with antacids. In any event, the elevated blood pH may result in slow and shallow breathing, lowered serum calcium and potassium levels, and muscle tetany (prolonged contractions). Buffering activity is not limited to the blood. The carbonic acid–bicarbonate buffering system is active in interstitial fluids. Intracellular buffers include the proteins and organic phosphates.

While the blood pH is maintained within a fairly narrow range through the systems just described, the urine pH can vary considerably depending on the metabolic state of the individual. The kidney and the urinary tract can tolerate a greater fluctuation in pH than can other tissues. Nonetheless, a number of buffer systems are also active in this tissue. In the kidney, although little buffering is done by the proteins, the bicarbonate buffer system is particularly active in the extracellular fluid. Once urine is produced, little effort is made to buffer its pH; it can vary from 4.7 to 8.0. The bladder and urinary tract are constructed so that this broad pH range is tolerated with little effect on the metabolism that occurs in these tissues.

Proteins as Structural Elements

The lipid component of the membrane is discussed in Chapter 10. Analysis of the liver cell membrane has shown that this membrane contains 50%–60% protein, 35% lipid, and 5% carbohydrate. The carbohydrate present is found primarily in the membrane glycoproteins. These glycoproteins serve as receptors as well as cell-recognition proteins. The protein portion of the membrane is so oriented that its hydrophilic aspects are also in proximity to the intracellular and extracellular fluids. The protein molecules are interspersed within the lipids and lend both structural stability and fluidity to the membrane.

Membrane function depends on how the proteins are placed in the membrane and on the fluidity that results from the combination of proteins in a lipid mixture. As indicated earlier, the lipid portion of the membrane needs to be fairly unsaturated. If saturated, a more rigid crystalline structure will form. By being fluid and less rigid, these lipids can allow the proteins to change their shape in response to ionic changes. Thus, these proteins can function as enzymes, carriers, or receptors, for the large variety of materials binding, entering, or leaving the cell.

How can these proteins serve in this fashion? Recall the protein conformation. The R groups of the amino acids project both in and out from the conformation and interact to form hydrogen bonds and disulfide bridges, however briefly, with compounds in proximity to them. Proteins that react with materials external to the cell may change their conformation and, in so doing, change their position within the membrane structure so that the reactive site changes from facing outward to the extracellular environment to facing inward toward the intracellular environment. Once facing inward, the material temporarily attracted to the membrane protein might be more attracted to another protein within the cell and *let go* of the membrane protein. Of course, this explanation is very simplistic. Transport into and out of cells probably involves many other reactions, a source of energy, and cations and/or anions for exchange. Yet this simplified explanation may be sufficient to explain the passage of a number of materials through the cell membrane. The reactive groups of the amino acid side chains, the R groups of the *structural* membrane proteins, may also serve as identifiers or facilitators of reactive sites. Proteins serve as receptors for materials, such as insulin, that do not usually enter the cell. Insulin, also a protein, has reactive side chains protruding from it just as reactive side chains protrude from the proteins in the membrane. These two reactive groups interact and the binding of the insulin to the receptor occurs. Again, this is a very simplistic explanation of receptor action. In the instance of insulin, the receptor is probably a glycoprotein.

In addition to the function of proteins in the cell membrane as a structural element and as functional units, proteins are important intracellular structural units. Muscle is 20% protein, 75% water, and 5% inorganic material, glycogen, and other organic compounds. The major proteins in muscles are myosin, a large globular protein, and actin, a smaller globular protein. These two proteins plus the filamentous tropomyosin and troponin are the structural proteins of the muscles. The muscle proteins are characterized by their elasticity, which in turn contributes to the contractile power of this tissue.

Perhaps one of the most important structural functions of protein is that related to skin and connective tissue. The skin is composed of epithelial tissue that not only covers the exterior of the body but lines the gastrointestinal tract, the respiratory tract, and the urinary tract. One of the proteins found in the skin is melanin. Melanin is a tyrosine derivative and provides the pigmentation or color to the skin. Persons unable to form this pigment are albinos and their disease is called albinism. Three separate genetic errors have been identified as causes for albinism.

Another of the proteins found in skin is keratin, which is the protein that forms hair, nails, hooves, feathers, or horns. Each of these structures is slightly different from the others, but all contain keratin. This protein is insoluble in water and is resistant to most digestive enzymes. It has a high percentage of cystine.

Connective tissue holds all of the various cells and tissues together. It contains two distinct types of proteins: collagen and elastin. Collagen is the principal solid substance in white connective tissue.[16] It contains a high percentage of proline, hydroxyproline, and glycine. It is difficult to degrade this protein and, like hair, it is relatively inert metabolically. Even in protein-deficient states, the body will synthesize collagen and elastin, and these proteins will not be catabolized for needed amino acids. Incidentally, although the body does not readily catabolize collagen, this protein can be degraded to a limited degree by boiling in acid. It is then converted to gelatin. The collagen of bone, skin, cartilage, and ligaments differs in chemical composition from that of the white fibrous tissue that holds individual cells together within muscle, liver, and other organs. Elastin and chondroalbumoid are two other proteins in the connective tissue. They are present in small amounts and serve as part of the structural protein. Finally, bones and teeth belong to the structural protein class because they start out with a matrix protein (*ground substance*) into which various amounts of minerals are deposited.

Proteins as Lubricants

The mucus of the respiratory tract, the oral cavity, the vaginal tract, and the rectal cavity reduces the irritation that might be caused by materials moving through these passages. This mucus is a mucoprotein, a conjugated protein that contains hexosamine. Proteins as lubricants also surround the joints and facilitate their movement. Should these lubricants be absent, or present but with substantial decreases in their fluidity through the deposition of minerals, skeletal movement may be difficult and painful.

Proteins in the Immune System

Proteins such as γ-globulin serve to protect the body against foreign cells. The immunoglobulins produced by lymphocytes are large polypeptides having more than one basic monomeric unit. These proteins differ in their amino acid structure, which affects their secondary, tertiary, and quaternary structures. Just as the amino acid sequence of an enzyme determines substrate specificity, the amino acid sequence of the immunoprotein assures antigen–antibody specificity. The synthesis of particular immunoglobulins has been much studied. It is now well accepted that initiation of synthesis by the lymphocyte requires the binding of an antigen (a foreign protein) to the cell surface at particular locations called antigen receptors. As with other receptors on other cells, there must be a good conformational *fit* between the site and the antigen. Once the immunoglobulin is synthesized, it will bind with the foreign protein, immobilizing it, and the complex antigen–antibody will be formed.

Proteins in the Endocrine System: Hormones

Hormones serve as internal messengers regulating the ebb and flow of a variety of cellular functions. As internal signals, hormones regulate such processes as heartbeat, vascular contraction, salt conservation, glucose uptake and utilization, glucose production, and oxygen consumption as well as other processes. Hormones can be viewed as system regulators.

Hormones are substances that are released into the bloodstream by a tissue or organ and have an action distal to that tissue. Not all hormones are proteins. Some are peptides, some are steroids, some are small polypeptides, and some are amino acid derivatives. All, however, serve as coordinators of activity in specific tissues. Some of the protein hormones are listed in Table 8.13.

The actions of many of these hormones are mediated by specific interactions with specific proteins in the membrane or cytosol or certain of the organelles within the cell. These proteins are called receptors (see Chapter 6). In turn, the hormones themselves are released via a cascade of sequential reactions that usually begin in the central nervous system, followed by signals generated in the hypothalamus, then the pituitary, and finally by the endocrine cell itself.[16–19] This cascaded signaling system is a means to amplify the response to a specific stimulus. For example, an individual is suddenly exposed to a dangerous situation—perhaps an explosion or an oncoming car or a charging bull. The person perceives the danger and responds to it. The response involves the central nervous system as well as other systems that are involved in the fight-or-flight response to danger. Figure 8.13 illustrates this signal cascade system.

Other stimuli may originate from the environment and likewise elicit a systemic response. Specific foods or nutrients can also evoke such cascades as discussed in Chapter 4 with respect to food intake regulation. This regulation involves a variety of signals from both the CNS and the gut. In summary, stimuli from the environment elicit specific electrical or chemical signals. These are generated by the hypothalamus that either directly or indirectly (via releasing hormones) stimulates the anterior pituitary, which directly or indirectly signals the target endocrine cell to synthesize or release its hormone, which has the needed effect on metabolism. Not all hormone-releasing mechanisms use all steps in this cascade. Sometimes, short loops are used that bypass some of the

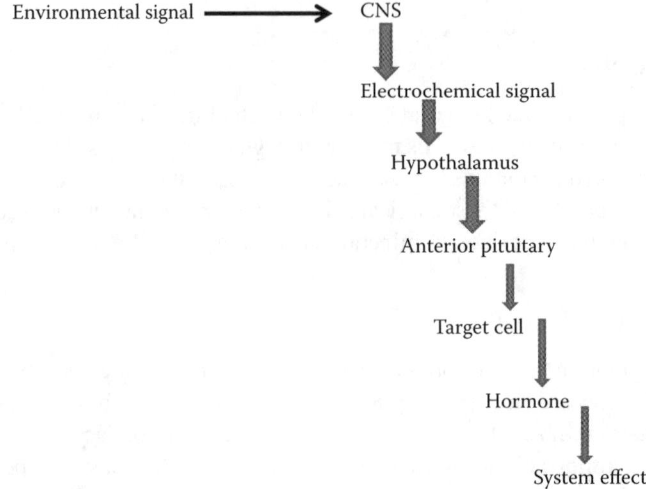

FIGURE 8.13 Signaling cascade that begins with an initial signal originating in the environment and ends with a whole-body systemic response.

initial steps in the cascade. In addition, there is some negative feedback involved that tells the target endocrine cell that enough hormones have been released.

Some of the peptide and protein hormones in the body are listed in Table 8.13. Others, notably the cytokines, are discussed in Chapters 4 and 6. The local hormones (the eicosanoids) are discussed in Chapter 10. In general, hormones function through one of several mechanisms:

1. They induce enzyme synthesis by stimulating mRNA transcription. Protein hormones bind to specific DNA sites and promote the transcription of mRNA. An increase in mRNA synthesis leads to an increase in enzyme protein synthesis. Hormones acting in this way are thought to be functioning as modifiers of gene expression.
2. Hormones stimulate enzyme synthesis through enhancing the translation of messenger RNA. Growth hormone, a small protein, appears to act in this fashion.[20]
3. Hormones directly activate enzymes by either changing the phosphorylation state of the cell or one of its compartments or changing the flux of ions as cofactors in the reactions.
4. Hormones activate membrane transport systems, which have G proteins as part of their structures.

In the cascade system illustrated in Figure 8.6, hormones or signals must emanate from one level of the cascade to the next for the system to work. The precision of the signaling system depends largely on the specificity of the signal for its target. Some hormones are more specific than others. In general, the protein and peptide hormones are more specific than the steroid hormones. The polypeptide hormones bind to their cognate receptors lodged in the plasma membrane. These receptors generally penetrate the membrane and have a tyrosine-rich tail protruding into the cytosol (see Chapter 6). Part of the hormone–receptor binding and subsequent cellular events involves G proteins. Not all of these hormone–receptor cascades use G proteins. The G proteins serve as the signal transducer for the hormone, stimulating a subsequent series of metabolic events that may involve the enzymes adenyl cyclase or phospholipase C and the calcium ion. The calcium ion plays a role in exocytosis, may be active in the exchange of metabolites across intracellular membranes, or may itself be a signal molecule.

While the details of the synthesis of all of these peptide and protein hormones have yet to be elucidated, some pathways are well known. The synthesis of thyroxine from tyrosine by the thyroid gland (Figure 8.8) and of dopamine, epinephrine, and norepinephrine, also from tyrosine, by the adrenal medulla is established (Figure 8.14). A cascade of signals is needed for the release of these hormones. The synthesis of the pancreatic hormones and of the more complicated protein hormones is not clear. The enzymes needed for some of these synthetic pathways have been described as having some of the control points in the synthetic pathways. This is a very active area for research in endocrinology, as is the study of the signal transduction systems that explain the actions of each of these hormones. One of the more interesting observations is that several of the peptide hormones are encoded together in a single gene and that many copies of the same message can exist. As shown in Figure 8.15, one gene has been found to encode adrenocorticotropic hormone (ACTH), β-lipotropin, α-lipotropin, alpha-melanocyte-stimulating hormone (α-MSH), β-MSH, corticotropin-like peptide (CLIP), β-endorphin, and some of the enkephalins and proopiomelanocortin. Not all are generated by the same tissue or cell type but occur separately, generated by specific signals in specific cells. In the earlier example, one of the gene products, ACTH, is produced and released by the anterior pituitary under the control of the corticotropin-releasing hormone (CRH). Enzymes are present in the corticotrophic cells that cleave the amino acid sequence of proopiomelanocortin at specific sites releasing ACTH and β-lipotropin into the circulation. These products can be cleaved further by cells of the pars intermedia to produce and release α-MSH, CLIP, α-lipotropin, and β-endorphin. α-Lipotropin and β-endorphin can be split further to produce β-MSH and Met-enkephalin (Figure 8.15). The reason that all these gene products arise from the same initial compound has to do with the unique location in the different cell types of specific proteases that act on specific

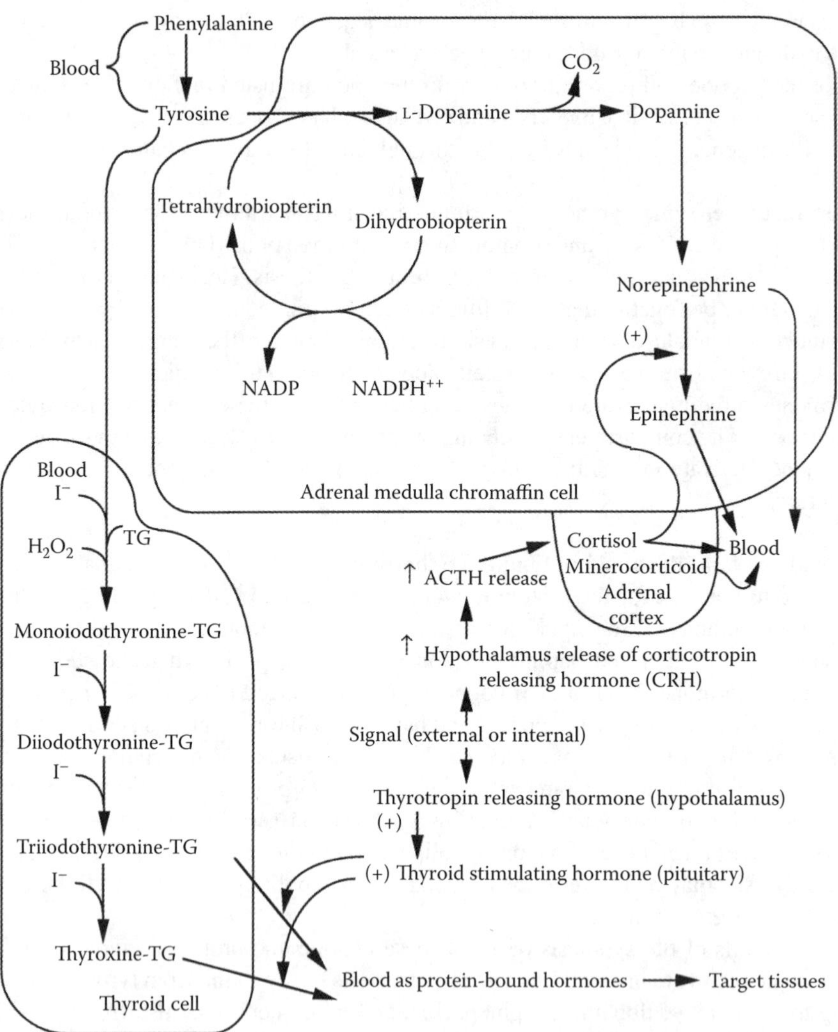

FIGURE 8.14 Tyrosine in the circulation enters specific cells of either the thyroid or adrenal glands. This tyrosine is used to make thyroid hormone and the catecholamines. These hormones are released into the circulation and are carried to their target cells, where they have their effects. Thyroxine synthesis occurs as a sequential iodination of tyrosine residues contained by the protein thyroglobulin (TG). At the target tissue, thyroxine is deiodinated to its active form, triiodothyronine.

linkages and thus release these smaller peptides into the circulation. Only a few cell types possess these specific proteases.

Other hormones are also encoded together. Just as ACTH and β-lipotropin are components of the proopiomelanocortin, so too are other hormones split off from prohormone molecules. Vasopressin and neurophysin II arise from the same molecule. Oxytocin and neurophysin I also have the same parent peptide. Although the earlier examples are all peptide hormones, no doubt we will find that nonhormone peptides can arise in a similar fashion. Amino acids in the circulation enter a vast array of cell types, each of which has many uses for these amino acids.

Proteins as Signaling Molecules

Already described are the hormones that are released as signals to other tissues. However, proteins and peptides also serve as part of a variety of signaling systems. The G proteins, for example, are

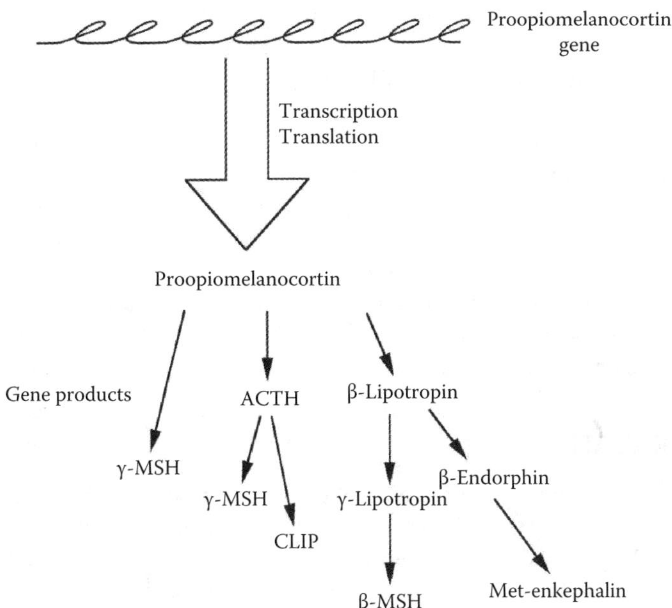

FIGURE 8.15 One gene encodes several signal peptides depending on the cell type and the signals generated to synthesize one or more of these products; ACTH and β-lipotropin gene products are under the control of CRH, whereas α-MSH, CLIP, γ-lipotropin, and β-endorphin gene products in the pituitary are under the control of dopamine. MSH, melanocyte-stimulating hormone; CLIP, corticotropin-like intermediary peptide.

intimately involved in signals perceived extracellularly and transmitted intracellularly. G proteins are involved in the signal transmission process. They are intracellular proteins that bind either GDP or GTP as part of their function.[21] Peptides (cytokines) serve as signals sent from one tissue to another. Amino acid amines can also serve as signals. Histamine, for example, is involved in allergic reactions, headache, hypotension, cardiac arrhythmia, and the group of intense allergic reactions by sensitive people to certain allergens.[22,23] Glutamine, while not truly a signaling compound as it is the most abundant α-amino acid in the body,[24] seems to signal cell protein synthesis.[25,26] Glutamine is essential for the optimal growth of cells and seems to be an important component for the normal recovery from illness and injury. Lastly, glutathione, a tripeptide, serves an important role in the response to oxidative stress, detoxification reactions, cell proliferation, and in some instances in the response to hormones. In these functions, it may indeed be a signaling peptide.[27] *DNA-directed protein synthesis* is described and discussed in Chapter 7.

PROTEIN TURNOVER

Protein turnover consists of two processes: synthesis and degradation. Synthesis is described in Chapter 7. The proteins synthesized by the body have a finite existence. They are subject to a variety of insults and modifications. Some of these modifications, touched upon as metabolic control processes, have been discussed—a prohormone is converted to an active hormone, an enzyme is activated or inactivated with the addition or removal of a substituent, and so forth. Thus, a dynamic state within the body exists with respect to its full complement of peptides and proteins. Some proteins have very short lifetimes and very rapid turnover times; other proteins are quite stable and long lived.[18] Their turnover time is quite long. The estimate of the life of a protein, that is, how long it will exist in the body, is its half-life (see Chapter 6). A half-life is that time interval that occurs when half of the amount of a compound synthesized at time X will have been degraded. Given the dynamic state of metabolism, some of these time estimates will be very short. Half-lives of biologically active compounds are very difficult to estimate, yet the concept is handy when one is trying to understand and quantitate the turnover of body protein. Hormones are examples of short-lived proteins. They may be released, serve their function, and be degraded within a very short period (seconds to minutes to hours) of time. The protein of the lens is an example of the latter; once synthesized, the lens protein is not degraded or recycled. Adult humans have a daily turnover of about 1%–2% of their total body protein. Most of this is muscle protein because the largest group of body proteins is found in muscle. Accretion of muscle mass means that protein synthesis is greater than protein degradation.[28] Age as well as exercise can affect this balance as can the quality of the ingested protein.[29] The control of this balance of synthesis versus degradation (positive nitrogen balance) rests at the level of gene transcription.[28,29] Apparently, the signals for growth and muscle protein accretion turn on the transcription of genes encoding the various muscle proteins.[20,29–31]

PROTEIN DEGRADATION

Protein degradation ultimately results in amino acids that are usually recycled. There are some exceptions to this general rule; histidine in the muscle protein is methylated and excreted as 3-methyl histidine. This 3-methyl histidine cannot be reused and thus is an indication of muscle breakdown. It is often used as an indicator of excess protein catabolism as happens in malnutrition or in such clinical states as thyrotoxicosis[32] or trauma.[28,33] Most of the products of protein degradation (the liberated amino acids) join the body's amino acid pool, from which the synthetic processes withdraw their needed supply. It is estimated that 75%–80% of the liberated amino acids are reused.

Different proteins are degraded at different rates. The rates of degradation are determined not only by the physiological status of the individual but also by the amino acid composition of the protein in question. High rates of degradation of the structural proteins mean that considerable structural rearrangement is occurring. For example, during starvation, structural proteins are degraded at higher rates than during nonstarvation. Prolonged trauma also elicits accelerated structural protein degradation.[28,33] Short-lived proteins such as those mentioned earlier as proteins, enzymes, or receptors have in common regions rich in proline, glutamate, serine, and threonine. These amino acids, when clustered, provide a target for rapid degradation.

The process of degradation first reduces the protein to peptides and then reduces these peptides to their constituent amino acids. Two major pathways are used for this process. Extracellular, membrane, and long-lived intracellular proteins are degraded in the lysosomes by an ATP-independent pathway. Short-lived proteins as well as abnormal proteins are degraded in the cytosol using ATP and ubiquitin. This pathway is illustrated in Figure 8.16.

Protein degradation in the cytosol requires energy from ATP and the highly conserved 76 amino acid protein called ubiquitin.[17,32–37] Proteins that are to be degraded via the ubiquitin-dependent pathway are derivatized by several molecules of ubiquitin. The ubiquitin is attached by nonpeptide bonds between the carboxy terminus of ubiquitin and the D-amino groups of lysyl residues in the protein. This requires ATP.

Although the proteases of digestion are important to the degradation of dietary protein, they have no role in the intracellular protein degradation. Intracellular proteases hydrolyze internal peptide bonds. This is followed by the action of carboxy- and aminopeptidases, which remove single amino acids from the carboxy end or the amino end of the peptides.

Proteins in the extracellular environment are brought into the cell by endocytosis.[38–41] This is a process similar to pinocytosis, where the cell membrane engulfs and encapsulates the extracellular material. Endocytosis occurs at indentations in the plasma membrane that are internally coated with a protein called clathrin. As in pinocytosis, the extracellular protein is surrounded by the plasma membrane to form an intracellular vesicle that, in turn, fuses with a lysosome. Degradation then occurs via calcium-dependent proteases called calpains or cathepsin. Both the Golgi and the

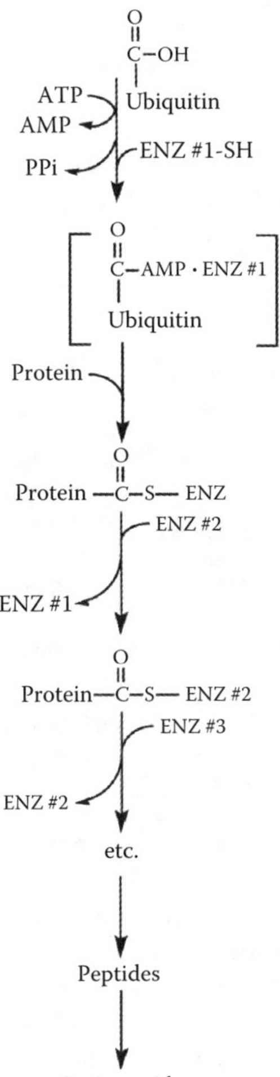

FIGURE 8.16 General pathway for intracellular protein degradation.

endoplasmic reticulum are involved in providing proteases that degrade peptide fragments that arise during the maturation of proteins in the secretory pathway.[39,40]

The rate of degradation varies from protein to protein and this rate is determined by the amino acid at the amino end of the protein amino acid chain. Proteins with short half-lives are degraded quickly and have terminal regions rich in proline, glutamate, serine, and threonine. Proteins with long half-lives are degraded slowly and therefore have slower turnover times.

Those amino acids in the body's amino acid pool that are neither used for peptide or protein synthesis nor used to synthesize metabolically important intermediates are deaminated, and the carbon skeletons are either oxidized or used for the synthesis of glucose or fatty acids. Very little fatty acid synthesis occurs in humans consuming 20%–30% of their energy as fat. There are three general reactions for the removal of NH_3 from the amino acids:

1. They can be transaminated with the amino group transferred to another carbon chain via amino transaminases.
2. They can be oxidatively deaminated to yield NH_3.
3. They can be deaminated through the activity of an amino acid oxidase.

Figure 8.17 illustrates these general reactions.

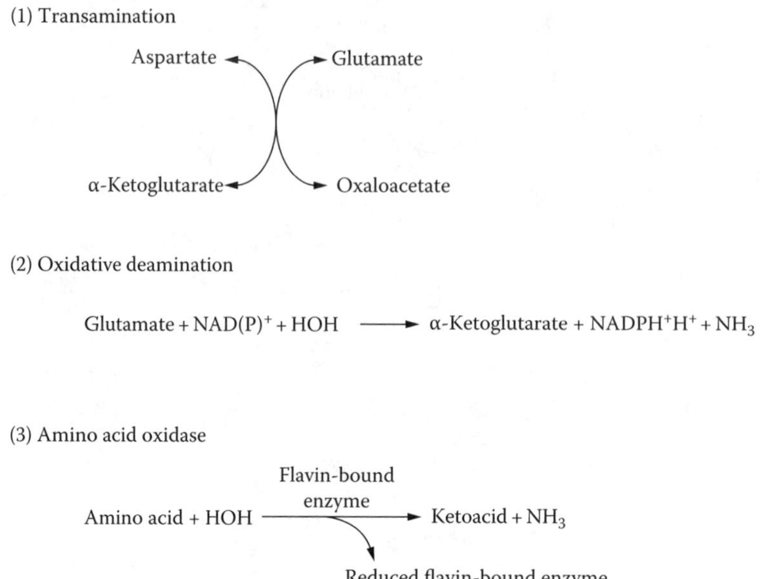

FIGURE 8.17 Amino acid reactions that result in the removal or transfer of the amino group.

PROTEIN INTAKE RECOMMENDATIONS

Human protein and amino acid requirements have been studied for well over 100 years using a variety of techniques. Nutrition scientists have collected data on the quantity of protein foods consumed versus health, growth, and weight gain of various populations. The assumption was made that whatever *healthy* people ate was probably what kept them healthy and should, therefore, be used as a standard of comparison for other diets. These standards, with respect to protein, were invariably high for populations having an abundance of meat, milk, poultry, and fish in their diets. Voit and Atwater, around the turn of the twentieth century, found intakes of 118 and 125 g of protein per day, respectively, for adult men and termed these intakes as desirable.

As nutrition developed as a science, more-accurate methods for assessing nutrient needs were developed. Among these methods were those for assessing the intake and excretion of nitrogen compounds. These methods made possible the development of the concepts that today's scientists use to determine the nutrient requirements of humans as well as other species. Hence, the term requirement means the amount of a nutrient that must be consumed to provide for the needs for that nutrient. In terms of protein, the requirement for dietary protein is that amount that can completely replace the body protein that is destroyed by the body in the course of living. It is influenced by age, genetics, environmental temperature, energy intake, gender, micronutrient intake, infection, activity, previous diet, trauma, pregnancy, and lactation. The latest recommendations for protein intake can be found in the NIH website for dietary reference intakes (DRIs). For many years, the recommended dietary allowance (RDA) for protein was set at 1 g/kg body weight for the average adult male. He was assumed to weigh 70 kg (about 155 lb) so the RDA was 70 g/day. With an ever-increasing database that the Nutrition Board of the National Research Council can use for its recommendations, the RDA for protein was adjusted downward about every 5 years. At present, protein intake recommendations are given as a DRI rather than RDA. This is a set of recommendations for the protein intake by various age and life stage groups. The intake is given as grams protein per kilogram body weight per day. This is an expression that makes allowances for differences in body size. It presumes that the dietary protein is coming from a mixed diet containing a reasonable amount of good-quality proteins. For persons subsisting on mixtures of poor-quality proteins, this recommendation may not be adequate. Table 8.14 gives the current DRI for protein for different age groups.

TABLE 8.14
DRIs for Protein

Life-Stage Group	Intake Recommendation (g/kg/day)
Infants, 7–12 months	1.0
Children, 1–3 years	0.87
Children, 4–8 years	0.76
Males, 9–13 years	0.76
14–18 years	0.73
19–30 years	0.66
31–50 years	0.66
51–70 years	0.66
>70 years	0.66
Females, 9–13 years	0.76
14–18 years	0.71
19–30 years	0.66
31–50 years	0.66
51–70 years	0.66
>70 years	0.66
Pregnancy, 14–18 years	0.88
19–30 years	0.88
31–50 years	0.88
Lactation, 14–18 years	1.05
19–30 years	1.05
31–50 years	1.05

Source: www.nap.edu.

AGE

A protein intake in excess of maintenance needs is required when new tissue is being formed. Certain age periods, that is, rapid growth, require more dietary protein than other periods.[42–44] Age differences in protein turnover (protein flux) as well as protein synthesis explain some of the effects of age on protein need. Table 8.15 gives figures for humans at different ages. Premature infants (those infants born before their 10-lunar-month gestation time) grow at a very rapid rate and require between 2.5 and 5 g/protein/kg/day if they are to survive. Pregnancy also is a period of rapid growth. During the last trimester, the protein needs of the pregnant female increase to support the growth of the fetus. After the baby is born, the mother must also increase her protein intake to support lactation and the baby's nutrient needs.

TABLE 8.15
Age Effects on Nitrogen Flux That Reflects Protein Flux and Protein Synthesis Rate per Day

Age	Protein (N) Flux mg (N/kg/h)	Total Body Protein Synthesis (g/kg/day)
Newborn	124 ± 46	17.4 ± 9.9
Infant	65 ± 7	6.9 ± 1.1
Young adult	26 ± 2	3.0 ± 0.2
Elderly	19 ± 2	1.9 ± 0.15

Studies of full-term infants have indicated that a protein intake of 2–2.5 g/kg/day resulted in a satisfactory weight gain and that further increases in protein intake did not measurably improve growth. Older infants and children whose growth rate is not as rapid as the premature or newborn infant require considerably less protein (~1.25 g/kg/day). As growth rate increases during adolescence, the need for protein increases. Again, this can be related to the demands for dietary amino acids to support the growth process. As humans complete their growth, the need for protein decreases until it arrives at a level that is called the maintenance level. It is at this level that the concept of body protein replacement by dietary protein applies. During the growth period, it is very difficult to separate the requirements for maintenance from those of growth. The impulse for growth is so strong that it will occur in many instances at the expense of the maintenance of body tissues. For example, protein-malnourished children will continue to grow taller even though their muscles, as well as other tissues, show evidence of wastage due to dietary protein deficiency. Growth carries with it not only a total nitrogen requirement but also a particular amino acid requirement. Maintenance, on the other hand, appears to have only a total protein requirement. Adults can make a number of short-term adjustments in their protein metabolism that can compensate for possible inequities or imbalances in amino acid intake as long as the total protein requirement is met. The young growing animal and the pregnant and lactating adult are not that flexible. The essential amino acid requirements are age dependent. Histidine, although it can be synthesized in sufficient quantities by the adult to meet maintenance needs, is not synthesized in great enough amounts to support growth. Thus, histidine is an essential amino acid for the infant and growing child. This is due to the nature of the growth process. Methionine, another essential amino acid, is particularly important to the infant and the pregnant female.[43,44] Inadequate intakes by these groups will result in metabolic imbalances of homocysteine.[44] Hyperhomocysteinemia during pregnancy has been linked to the development of neural tube defects in the infants, preeclampsia, miscarriage, and premature delivery.[44] Low protein intakes of pregnant women can have epigenetic effects on the progeny.[45] At the other end of the life span, there are effects on protein need and metabolism. In the senescent individual, there is a loss of skeletal muscle mass (sarcopenia), cachexia (wasting disease), and inactivity.[46] There are also losses in other body proteins. In part, this is due to the gradual accumulation of errors in the genetic code of the aging individual. Studies of humans from newborn to 80 years of age have shown that there is a graduate increase in the number of base deletions in the mitochondrial genome. This may be due to the wide variety of genomic insults that occur over a life span. Exposure to ultraviolet light, noxious chemicals, drugs, or changes in the food supply can all affect the fidelity of the genome. These insults inflict their damage randomly so no one instance is responsible for the age effect, yet altogether there can be subtle and cumulative effects on gene expression and these, in turn, can affect the efficiency and fidelity of the gene products. Thus, metabolic processing of food materials loses its efficiency. The elderly person, although synthesizing less protein than the young growing person, may not synthesize this protein accurately. This, in turn, means a decline in function. Does this mean that the elderly may have an increase in protein need? We don't know. Until recently, this portion of the population had not been well studied vis-à-vis protein need.

Environmental Temperature

As environmental temperatures rise or fall above or below the range of thermic neutrality, animals begin to increase their energy expenditure to maintain their body temperature. In environments that are too warm, vasodilation occurs along with sweating and increased respiration. All of these mechanisms are designed to cool the body and all require an increase in the basal energy requirement as expressed per unit of body surface area. In cool environments, vasoconstriction and shivering occur in an effort to warm the body and prevent undue heat loss. Again, an increase in basal energy requirement is observed. Smuts, in 1934, found that nitrogen requirements were related to basal energy requirements. Through the study of a large number of species, he concluded that 2 mg nitrogen was required for every basal kilocalorie required when the energy requirement was expressed on a surface area basis. Thus, any increase in basal energy needs due to changes in environmental temperature will, because of the relationship between protein and energy, be accompanied by an increase in the protein requirement for maintenance. In addition, profuse sweating, as it occurs in very warm environments, carries with it a nitrogen loss that must be accounted for in the determination of minimal protein needs.

Previous Diet

The effects of previous diet on the determination of protein requirements may be rather profound. If, for example, the subjects selected for studies on protein needs have been poorly nourished prior to the initiation of the study, their retention of the protein during the study will be greater than would be observed in subjects who have been well nourished prior to the initiation of the study. In other words, malnourished subjects have a higher protein requirement than well-nourished subjects. This, of course, raises the issue of whether there are body protein reserves. Many investigators have observed that animals fed a protein-free diet exhibit a *lag* before their nitrogen excretion level is minimized; during this phase, the animal is metabolizing its protein reserve. Other investigators maintain that there is no such thing as a protein reserve or store. These investigators maintain that every protein in the body has a function, and if some of these proteins are lost, there is a loss in body function. Support for this concept is seen in the reduced ability of protein-depleted animals to fight infection or respond to the metabolic effects of trauma. Whether one believes that there is such an entity as a protein reserve may depend upon whether one perceives a difference between an optimal protein intake and a minimum protein intake. This difference may relate more to a personal opinion on how nutrient requirements should be defined. Some nutritionists believe in stating the absolute minimum requirement to sustain life and then adding on increments for each body function above mere survival; this is known as the particulate approach. Other nutritionists believe that one cannot separate and quantitate the individual requirements of each function beyond survival. They advocate a protein intake sufficient for optimal function of the animal; this is known as the integrative approach. The particulate and integrative approaches have their merits when argued intellectually. However, since man does not merely exist, many human nutritionists tend to take the integrative approach to human nutrition requirements in their determination of protein needs.

Physical Activity

Research on protein needs for muscular work had its beginning in 1863 when Von Leiberg postulated that muscle as protein was destroyed with each contraction of the muscle. On this basis, he recommended that heavy muscular work required a heavy protein diet. This theory has been amply disproved, yet even today, many believe that a protein-rich diet will contribute to athletic prowess. Today, we know that muscle contraction does not result in destruction of the muscle. It does, however, require energy in the form of ATP, glucose, and fatty acids and does result in the breakdown of creatine phosphate to creatine, some of which is then converted to creatinine, a nitrogenous waste product excreted in the urine.

As the energy requirement is increased to support the increase in muscular activity, so too is the protein requirement in much the same manner as described earlier for the effects of temperature. In a number of studies, the athletic performance of subjects could not be directly related to the quantity of protein consumed above that determined to be the requirement for those subjects. When subjects were fed less than their respective protein requirements, their muscular efficiencies were reduced unless a vigorous training program was included as part of the experiment's protocol. Since most of the studies were of short duration and since muscle protein has a relatively long half-life, the lack of any demonstrable effect of protein intake on muscle performance (aside from the energy/protein relationship) is not surprising. Other factors such as sex, pregnancy, lactation, and trauma affecting the protein requirement have been studied.[47] As can be anticipated, males, due to their greater physical activity and larger body size, have a larger protein requirement than females; pregnancy, lactation, and trauma all increase the protein requirement.

Protein Deficiency

One of the most common nutritional disorders in the world today is the deficiency of protein. Both adults and children are affected as the populations in the less-developed nations of the world exceed their food supply. Instances of deficiency in the United States have also been observed. Due to the ubiquitous nature of protein and its role in bodily function, protein deficiency is characterized by a number of symptoms. In many situations, not only is protein lacking in the diet but the energy intake is also insufficient. For this reason, it is difficult to segregate symptoms due solely to protein deficiency from those due solely to energy deficit. Acute energy deprivation affects skeletal muscle protein synthesis and associated intracellular signaling proteins in adults and likely in children. In children, one can observe the different symptoms and visualize them all as parts of a continuum called protein–energy or protein–calorie malnutrition (PEM or PCM) rather than distinctly different nutritional disorders. Kwashiorkor, a disease initially observed in Africa, was first regarded as a dietary state where only protein was deficient, not energy. Marasmus, on the other hand, was regarded as a dietary state where both protein and energy were deficient. Today, as mild and moderate cases of these two diseases are treated, it has become apparent that the symptoms of one may intermingle with the other so that a clear-cut diagnosis is impossible. For every severe case of either kwashiorkor or marasmus that is identified, treated, and cured, there are probably another 99 people who are not diagnosed and treated and who will, if they survive, experience lifelong effects from their early nutritional deprivation.

Kwashiorkor

Kwashiorkor usually affects young children after they weaned from their mother's breast. The children are usually between 1 and 3 years old; they are weaned because their mothers have given birth to another child or is pregnant and cannot support both children. If the children have no teeth, they are given a thin gruel. This may be a fruit, vegetable, or cereal product mixed with water; it is not usually a good protein source. Cultural food practices or taboos may further limit the kinds and amounts of protein given to the child. Concurrent infections, parasites, seasonal food shortages, and poor distribution of food among the family members may also contribute to the development of kwashiorkor. The deficiency develops not only because of inadequate intake but also because, at this age, the growth demands for protein and energy are high.

Growth failure is the single most outstanding feature of protein malnutrition. The child's height and weight for his age will be less than that of his well-nourished peer. Tissue wastage is present but may not be apparent if edema is also present. The edema begins with the feet and legs and gradually presents itself in the hands, face, and body. If edema is advanced, the child may not appear underweight but many appear *plump*. This plumpness can be ascertained as edema by feel. If a thumb were to be pressed on the surface of the foot or ankle and then removed, the depression would remain for a short time. This is edema. It is thought to result from insufficient ADH production and insufficient serum and tissue proteins needed to maintain water balance.

Protein-deficient children are usually apathetic, have little interest in their surroundings, and are listless and dull. These children are usually *fussy* and irritable when moved. Mental retardation may or may not result. Hair changes are frequently observed. Texture, color, and strength are affected. Black, curly hair may become silkier, lusterless, and brown or reddish-brown in color. Lesions of the skin are not always present, but if present, they give the appearance of old flaky paint. Depigmentation or darkly pigmented areas may develop, with a tendency for these areas to appear in places of body friction such as the backs of legs, groins, and elbows. Diarrhea is almost always present. The diarrhea may be a result of the inability of the body to synthesize the needed digestive enzymes so that the food that is consumed can be utilized, or it may be the result of concurrent infections and parasites. In rats fed protein-free diets, significantly less intestinal enzyme activity has been measured. Anemia due to an inability to synthesize hemoglobin as well as red blood cells is invariably present. Hepatomegaly (enlarged liver) is usually observed.

In children consuming energy-sufficient–protein-insufficient diets, the enlarged liver is usually fatty because the child is unable to synthesize the proteins needed to make the transport proteins that, in turn, are needed to transport the lipids out of the liver. Studies with rats and chickens have shown that protein deficiency also results in decreases in a variety of hepatic enzymes, a decrease in hepatic RNA and DNA content, a reduction in spleen size, a decrease in antibody formation, a decrease in urea cycle activity and urea production, and a decrease in the levels of plasma amino acids. All of these symptoms can be related to the various functions of proteins as discussed in the earlier section.

Marasmus

Although children of all ages and adults can suffer from a deficiency of both energy and protein, the marasmic child is usually less than one year old. In developing countries, a common cause for marasmus is a cessation of breastfeeding. Milk production by the mother may have stopped because of the mother's poor health, or the mother may have died, or there may be a desire on the part of the mother to bottle-feed her infant rather than breastfeed. This decision to bottle-feed may be made for a variety of reasons. The mother may view bottle-feeding as a status symbol, or she may be forced to work to earn a living and may be unable to have her baby with her, or she may not be able to lactate. While under optimal conditions of economics and sanitation, the bottle-fed child may be well fed; in emerging nations, this is not always true. The mother may not be able to buy the milk formula in sufficient quantities to adequately nourish the child, she may overdilute the milk, or she may use unsafe water and unsanitary conditions to prepare the formula for the child. This, plus the insufficient nutrient content, often precipitously leads to the development of marasmus, a form of starvation characterized by growth failure with prominent ribs, a characteristic monkey-like face, and matchstick limbs with little muscle or adipose tissue development; tissue wastage but not edema is present. Whereas the kwashiorkor child has a poor appetite, the marasmus child is eager to eat. The child is mentally alert but not irritable. Anemia and diarrhea are present for the same reasons as in kwashiorkor. The skin and hair appear to be of normal color.

The treatment of both kwashiorkor and marasmic children must be approached with due care and caution. Because their enzymes for digestion and their protein absorption and transport systems are less active, feeding these children with large quantities of good-quality protein would be harmful. Their diets must be gradually enriched with these proteins to allow their bodies sufficient time to develop the appropriate metabolic pathways to handle a better diet. Giving these children solutions of either predigested proteins or solutions of amino acids may be of benefit initially, but these solutions, too, must be used with care. If the amino acids in excess of immediate use are deaminated, and if the pathway for synthesizing urea is not fully functional, ammonia can accumulate in the child and become lethal. Schimke has shown that, in the rat, up to 3 days are needed to increase the activities of the urea cycle enzymes. The rat has a much faster metabolic rate than the human, so one would anticipate that a much longer period of time would be necessary for a similar induction in humans.

One must be concerned about the enzymes of not only the malnourished child but also protein-depleted children who are unable to synthesize adequate amounts of the protein hormones that regulate and coordinate their use of dietary nutrients. In addition, protein deprivation affects the structures of the cell and hormone receptors, further dampening the effectiveness of those hormones produced. Children with marasmus or kwashiorkor have been shown to have decreased blood sugar levels, decreased serum insulin and growth hormone levels, and, in marasmus, decreased thyroid hormone levels. Additional hormonal changes have been observed, but their relevance to treatment has not been ascertained. Most likely, these changes in the levels of the protein-, peptide-, or amino acid–derived hormones are reflective of the reduced synthesis of them as a result of a shortage of incoming amino acids. Changes in the steroid hormones probably reflect the response of the child to the stress of deprivation.

PROTEIN AND AMINO ACID INTERACTIONS WITH OTHER NUTRIENTS

Recently, it has come to the attention of nutrition scientists that there can exist nutrient interactions that can have either negative or positive effects on the nutrients concerned.[49] For example, the availability of iron from food depends on its source. Soybean protein contains an inhibitor of iron uptake. Diets such as those in Asia contain numerous soybean products, and iron absorption is adversely affected by this soybean inhibitor. Tannins, phytates, certain fibers (not cellulose), carbonates, phosphates, and low protein diets also adversely affect the apparent absorption of iron. In contrast, ascorbic acid, fructose, citric acid, high-protein foods, lysine, histidine, cysteine, methionine, and natural chelates, that is, heme, all enhance the apparent absorption of iron.

Two types of iron are present in the food, namely, heme iron, which is found principally in animal products and nonheme iron, which is inorganic iron bound to various proteins in plants. Most of the iron in the diet, usually greater than 85%, is present in the nonheme form. The absorption of nonheme iron is strongly influenced by its solubility in the upper part of the intestine. Absorption of nonheme iron depends on the composition of the meal and is subject to enhancers of absorption such as animal protein and reducing agents such as vitamin C. On the other hand, heme iron is absorbed more efficiently. It is not subject to these enhancers. Although heme iron accounts for a smaller proportion of iron in the diet, it provides quantitatively more iron to the body than dietary nonheme iron.

Zinc will form complexes with phosphate groups (PO_4^-), chloride (Cl^-), and carbonate groups (HCO_3^-) as well as with cysteine and histidine. Zinc can sometimes be displaced on the zinc fingers of DNA-binding proteins (receptors) by other divalent metals.[49] Iron, for example, has been used to displace zinc on the DNA-binding protein that also binds estrogen. This protein binds to the estrogen response element of the DNA promoter region encoding estrogen-responsive gene products. When this occurs in the presence of H_2O_2 and ascorbic acid, damage to the proximate DNA, the estrogen response element, occurs. It has been suggested that in this circumstance of an iron-substituted zinc finger, free radicals are more readily generated with the consequence of genomic damage. This suggestion has been offered as an explanation of how excess iron (iron toxicity) could instigate the cellular changes that occur in carcinogenesis.

As ions, minerals react with charged amino acid residues of intact proteins and peptides. Table 8.16 provides a list of minerals and the amino acids with which they react. Depending on their valence state, these electrovalent bonds can be very strong or very weak associations or anything in between. The marginally charged ion (either an electron acceptor or an electron donor) will be less strongly attracted to its opposite number than will an ion with a strong charge.

The formation of mineral–organic compound bonds is also seen when one examines the roles of minerals in gene expression. Almost every mineral is involved in one or more ways. Zinc cysteine or histidine linkages form the zinc fingers that bond with certain base sequences of DNA, thereby affecting transcription. Mineral–protein complexes serve as cis or trans acting elements that enhance or inhibit promoter activity and/or RNA polymerase II activity. Minerals can bond either by themselves or in complexes with proteins to inhibit or enhance translation.

TABLE 8.16
Mineral–Amino Acid Interactions

Minerals	Amino Acid
Calcium	Serine, carboxylated GLA
Magnesium	Tyrosine, sulfur-containing amino acids
Copper	Histidine
Selenium	Methionine, cysteine
Zinc	Cysteine, histidine

There are also interactions and competitions between dietary amino acids in the small intestine. The amino acid carriers (carriers that transport amino acids from the lumen into the absorptive cell) will transport more than one amino acid.[12] Neutral amino acids share a common carrier as do those with short or polar side chains (serine, threonine, and alanine). There is also a carrier for phenylalanine and methionine and one specific for proline and hydroxyproline. Similarly, there are carriers that transport amino acids across the blood–brain barrier, and there is some competition among amino acids for these carriers. For example, tryptophan competes with tyrosine for entry through the blood–brain barrier. Both tryptophan and the aromatic amino acids (phenylalanine and tyrosine) serve as precursors of neurotransmitters, and a competition between them for transport may have a role in the regulation of the balance of these transmitters in the body. Sulfur-containing amino acids are spared by each other, that is, methionine is spared by cysteine.

In intermediary metabolism, there appears to be an interaction between leucine, isoleucine, and valine. All are branched chain amino acids and share the same enzymes for their metabolism. All are needed to support protein synthesis. Should one be in a short supply, the rate of protein synthesis will fall.

VEGETARIAN DIETS

Vegetarianism is rapidly growing in popularity. Technically defined, vegetarians are individuals who do not eat any meat, poultry, or seafood.[50] Estimates on the number of vegetarians in the United States vary greatly according to the definition of vegetarianism provided in the survey. True vegetarians make up about 2.8% of the population, representing approximately 5.7 million adults. A higher percentage of teenagers than adults follow a vegetarian diet.

Many people consider themselves to be vegetarian when they eat meals consisting of nonflesh foods several days a week. Others will claim to be vegetarians when they consume fish or poultry but not red meat such as beef, pork, or lamb. Table 8.17 lists the types of vegetarian diets and

TABLE 8.17
Types of Vegetarian Diets

Vegan	Consumes nuts, fruits, grains, legumes, and vegetables. Does not consume animal-based food products, including eggs, dairy products, red meats, poultry, or seafood. Some vegetarians may avoid foods with animal processing (honey, sugar, vinegar, wine, beer).
Lacto-vegetarian	Consumes milk and other dairy products, nuts, fruits, grains, legumes, and vegetables. Does not consume eggs, red meats, poultry, or seafood.
Ovo-vegetarian	Consumes eggs, nuts, fruits, grains, legumes, and vegetables. Does not consume milk or dairy, red meats, poultry, or seafood.
Lacto-ovo vegetarian	Consumes milk and other dairy products, eggs, nuts, fruits, grains, legumes, and vegetables. Does not consume red meats, poultry, or seafood.
Pollo-vegetarian[a]	Not technically considered a vegetarian type of diet, although often referred to as *vegetarian* in popular culture. Consumes milk and other dairy products, eggs, nuts, fruits, grains, legumes, vegetables, and poultry.
Peche-vegetarian also called pesco- and pecto-vegetarian[a]	Not technically considered a vegetarian type of diet, although often referred to as *vegetarian* in popular culture. Consumes milk and other dairy products, eggs, nuts, fruits, grains, legumes, vegetables, and seafood.
Omnivore	Consumes from a wide variety of foods, including meats, grains, fruits, vegetables, legumes, and dairy products. Individuals who consume red meats (beef, pork, lamb, etc.), poultry, seafood, or any still or once living nonplant-based matter are not vegetarians.

Source: Plaisted Fernandez, C. et al., Vegetarian diets in health promotion and disease prevention, in: *Handbook of Nutrition and Food*, Berdanier, C.D., Dwyer, J., Heber, D., eds., 3rd edn., CRC Press, Boca Raton, FL, 2013, pp. 403–436.

[a] This is not technically a vegetarian diet, although it is often referred as such.

describes what foods are excluded. Some are more restrictive than others. The more restrictive the diet, the more likely it will be deficient in essential nutrients.

Most of the nutrition–health risks associated with vegetarianism are really those associated with the strict vegetarian diet (veganism). The more liberal forms of this diet choice (lacto-vegetarians, ovo-vegetarians, or lacto-ovo vegetarians) usually are less risky. The health risks are not unique to vegetarians, however, as they can be found in people following an imbalanced omnivorous diet. Typical vegetarian diets are rich in many beneficial nonnutritive factors such as dietary fiber and phytochemicals.

A common misconception about a vegetarian diet concerns protein. Individuals following a lacto-ovo vegetarian diet rarely have to worry about protein. Even adult vegans eating a reasonably balanced diet with adequate calories can meet their protein needs if the protein sources are mixed to provide an optimal amino acid supply. It is much more likely that a dietary deficiency of a micronutrient would occur, rather than a protein deficiency. Deficiencies in vitamin B_{12} have been reported as well as deficient intakes of calcium and other micronutrients.[50] Children are particularly vulnerable with respect to malnutrition when required by parents or caregivers to follow a vegan diet. The more liberal diets do not pose as much risk with respect to children; nonetheless, care must be taken to assure adequate intakes of the essential nutrients by all who follow these food intake patterns.

Long-term vegetarians have been studied with respect to their antioxidant status and disease risks. Compared to nonvegetarians, vegetarians had less oxidative biomarkers and lower coronary heart disease risk profiles.[51,52] They also had lower risks for cataract formation[53] and lower rates of hospitalization for ischemic heart disease.[54] Comparing casein protein to soy protein in feeding studies with humans showed similar results. Those consuming soy protein had lower blood lipids, lower low-density lipoprotein, lower levels of biomarkers for inflammation, and lower levels of homocysteine.[55–58]

RENAL DISEASE

The kidneys play a vital role in the maintenance of normal blood volume and pressure, water balance, and acid–base balance. Approximately one-fourth of the cardiac output is filtered through the kidneys each minute. The kidneys play important roles in red cell synthesis as well as bone mineralization. They are a major excretory organ in that they are important to the urinary excretion of the waste products of absorption and metabolism. Waste products include ammonia, urea, creatinine, phosphorus, water, sodium, and potassium. Their role in bone mineralization has to do with the activation of vitamin D that, in turn, regulates calcium and phosphorus deposition in the bone. The kidneys produce the hormone erythropoietin. Deficiency of this hormone results in profound anemia. Should the kidneys fail, a plethora of problems develop that, if untreated, will result in death.

The role of the kidneys as an excretory organ is important to protein nutrition. Urea as well as other nitrogenous end products is excreted by the kidneys in the urine. If this excretion does not take place, these end products of protein metabolism accumulate and become toxic. Renal disease is most often a gradual process and may be secondary to other diseases such as cardiovascular disease and diabetes mellitus.[59–63] There are two major types of renal disease. The acute, inflammatory disease, nephritis, may be sudden and secondary to pathogen invasion. In this instance, renal failure is abrupt. Immediate attention is needed. Frequently, the patient is placed on dialysis until the pathogenic condition can be corrected. Once corrected, the kidneys may begin to function once again. However, sometimes this does not occur.

The chronic condition, nephropathy, may develop gradually sometimes secondary to diabetes mellitus and/or cardiovascular disease. Again, this can be either acute or chronic. Nephrotic syndrome is a dysfunction of the glomerular capillaries. Symptoms include urine losses of plasma proteins, low serum albumin, edema, and elevated blood lipids. In acute renal failure, the nephrons lose function and the glomerular filtration rate (GFR) drops. Symptoms include increased blood urea nitrogen, catabolism, negative nitrogen balance, elevated electrolytes, acidosis, increased blood pressure, and fluid overload. Nephrotic syndrome and acute renal failure are usually reversible conditions. In chronic renal disease, the GFR declines gradually. In early stages, compensation occurs by enlarging the remaining nephrons. Following a low-protein diet that reduces the workload of the kidneys assists the patient. Symptoms similar to those in acute renal failure appear when the kidney is at 75% of its normal function. When the GFR is 10% or less of the normal rate, the patient is considered to be in end-stage renal disease. Dialysis is started to replace diminished kidney function. Electrolytes, fluids, anemia, and diet are monitored monthly. Some patients in end-stage renal failure receive a kidney transplant. This restores kidney function and the patient is able to return to a more liberal diet. The terms for the different renal disease conditions are listed and defined in Table 8.18.

Patients with acute or chronic renal disease may become malnourished. Protein–energy imbalances worsen this prognosis regardless of disease stage. There may be a significant depletion in visceral protein stores and weight loss. Common manifestations include edema, uremia, hypertension, anemia, and metabolic acidosis. The medical nutrition therapy for kidney failure becomes increasingly complex as the renal disease advances. The diet prescription is matched to the stage of renal failure in order to keep the diet at liberal as possible. The stages of chronic renal disease are listed in Table 8.19.

Chronic renal insufficiency is the ninth leading cause of death in the United States.[60] The most common cause of this problem is diabetes mellitus. Both type 1 and type 2 diabetes patients are affected making diabetes the leading cause of end-stage renal disease. Both genetic and environmental factors contribute to this development. Hypertension likewise contributes to the pathophysiology of renal disease and is often associated with obesity as well as diabetes. When all three

TABLE 8.18
Definition of Terms Used in Renal Disease

Term	Explanation
Acute renal failure	Sudden onset secondary to shock, trauma, hypertension, and exposure to nephrotoxic substances of bacteria. Reversible in many cases.
Azotemia	Elevated concentrations of nitrogenous wastes in blood serum.
Chronic renal failure (CRF) or insufficiency (CRI)	Gradual progression terminating with end-stage renal disease requiring dialysis or transplant. Causes include obstructive disease of the urinary tract like congenital birth defects, systemic diseases such as diabetes mellitus or systemic lupus erythematosis, glomerular disease, and overdosing on analgesic medications. Patients follow an increasingly restricted diet as renal failure progresses.
Hemodialysis	Removal from blood of the waste products of metabolism; uses a semipermeable membrane and a dialysis machine. This process takes 3–6 h three times per week in an outpatient clinic or hospital. Some patients, with appropriate training and assistance, can dialyze at home. Hemodialysis patients follow a diet restricted in sodium, potassium, phosphorous, and fluids.
Nephrotic syndrome	Failure of the glomerular basement membrane to filter waste products appropriately. Large amounts of protein are found in the urine. Patients frequently have edema secondary to hypoalbuminemia.
Peritoneal dialysis	Removal of the waste products of metabolism by perfusion of a sterile dialysate solution throughout the peritoneal cavity. This method of dialysis can be done at home. Dialysate exchanges are performed several times per day or continuously at night with the aid of a peritoneal dialysis machine. Peritoneal dialysis patients follow a liberalized diet as dialysis happens daily. The diet is normally a low-sodium diet.
Uremia	A toxic systemic syndrome caused by retention of high levels of urea.

Source: Thomas, L. and Poole, R., Renal nutrition, in: *Handbook of Nutrition and Food*, Berdanier, C.D., Feldman, E.B., Dwyer, J., eds., 2nd edn., CRC Press, Boca Raton, FL, 2007, pp. 815–832.

TABLE 8.19
Chronic Renal Disease Stages

Stage	Description	GFR (mL/min/1.73 m^2)
1	Kidney damage with normal or increased GFR	≥90
2	Kidney damage with mildly decreased GFR	60–90
3	Moderately decreased GFR	30–59
4	Severely decreased GFR	15–29
5	Kidney failure	≤15 or on dialysis

Source: Collins, A.J., *Am. J. Kidney Dis.*, 59, evii, 2012.

TABLE 8.20
Blood Pressure Classifications in Adults

Category	Systolic Pressure	Diastolic Pressure (mmHg)
Normal	<120	<80
Prehypertension	120–139	80–89
Stage 1 hypertension	140–159	90–99
Stage 2 hypertension	≥160	≥100

Source: National Heart Lung and Blood Institute, *Hypertension*, 42, 1206, 2003.

conditions develop, the patient also develops cardiovascular disease. The sequence of events leading up to the development of renal disease is complicated. The triad of hypertension, obesity, and cardiovascular disease often is complicated by the gradual onset of renal insufficiency.

Polycystic renal disease is one of the most common genetic disorders in renal disease. It is characterized by the formation of cysts in the kidneys and when enlarged may interfere with renal function. The formation of stones in the kidneys also interferes with normal renal function especially if the stones become lodged in the collecting ducts and vessels leading to the bladder. This is a very painful situation. Sometimes, surgical removal is mandated, but if the stones are very small, they can be dissolved and can be passed out of the body in the urine. Sometimes, stones too large to be passed out in the urine can be broken down to a smaller size suitable for passing. Ultrasound waves have been used for this option.

Hypertension, as mentioned earlier, is one of the leading causes of renal disease due to the damage to the renal vasculature caused by the high blood pressure. When the blood pressure is elevated, there is also high intraglomerular pressure and this impedes glomerular filtration. Protein is excreted in the urine (called microalbuminuria or proteinuria). It is the first sign of renal dysfunction. Careful control of blood pressure (systolic/diastolic < 120/80) through medication as well as through lifestyle changes (attaining appropriate body weight, exercise, increased consumption of vegetables and fruits and reduced consumption of meat, and reducing stress) can mitigate the risk for hypertension-mediated renal disease. Table 8.20 provides the classification and staging of hypertension in adults over the age of 18. Sodium intake can also affect the development of hypertension. A low salt intake can be of benefit to some individuals (see Chapter 13).

INTEGRATION OF THE METABOLIC FEATURES OF PROTEIN NUTRITION

In the preceding section, protein malnutrition and PEM or starvation and protein nutrition problems associated with renal disease have been characterized. Throughout this chapter, the chemical and biochemical nature of proteins has been discussed in detail. But how does the body *know* when to synthesize a new protein or degrade a resident one? What messages are sent and received that integrate these anabolic and catabolic processes? How does the body cope with its ever-changing environment—of which nutrition is but a part?

Recall that some of the amino acids that are contained by the dietary protein can be decarboxylated and converted to amines. These amines are potent neurotransmitters. That is, they are capable of eliciting system responses via activation of certain neurons or neuronal pathways. Some of these systemic responses include the release of hormones that have positive effects on protein synthesis. An example might be the signals to the pituitary to release growth hormone that, when bound to its cognate membrane receptor, elicits a cascade of intracellular signals that, in turn, migrate to the nucleus and serve as instigators of protein synthesis. Providing that sufficient ATP and amino acids are available, protein synthesis will be stimulated. Another example might be the chronic ingestion of a high-sugar diet that stimulates insulin release. The insulin plus the glucose plus several other factors instigates the synthesis of enzyme proteins needed to metabolize this sugar load. Initiation and cessation of feeding are an example of a system response to changing levels of the neurotransmitter serotonin. Likely, other neurotransmitters are involved as well (see Chapter 5). Through the action of neurotransmitters, other systems can be activated or suppressed, and these systems might include sleep or voluntary activity or other such whole-body actions. These responses will have effects on the need for energy and, because the energy need is tightly linked to the protein need, effects on the latter should be expected.

The dietary protein, once consumed, stimulates the release of a variety of gut hormones. These hormones likewise elicit systemic responses as outlined in the section on digestion and absorption. Further, once amino acids are liberated through the action of the digestive enzymes, these amino acids, as substrates for enterocyte carriers (see section on absorption), not only stimulate the carrier activity (substrate activation) but also are involved in the synthesis of the carrier itself by the enterocyte. This is not an uncommon phenomenon. A number of high-turnover proteins, that is, enzymes, carriers, and hormones, have their synthesis dictated by rising levels of the substrates upon which they act. Hence, rising levels of cytosolic citrate in the cell might be expected to instigate the transcription of the messenger RNA for ATP citrate lyase, the enzyme that catalyzes the formation of acetyl CoA and oxaloacetate from citrate and CoA with a concomitant hydrolysis of ATP to ADP and phosphate. So, too, might one expect to find in the enterocyte an increase in the mRNAs for those proteins that are responsible for the transport of the amino acids into the enterocyte via carrier-mediated mechanisms. Thus, we see multiple roles for the amino acids found in the dietary proteins. These roles are not restricted to just the enterocyte. Other cells, tissues, and organs also are affected. The enzymes that are responsible for amino acid metabolism are likewise synthesized or degraded in response to the levels of those amino acids on which they work. The expression of the genes that encode these enzymes may be unique to a given cell type, tissue, or organ or may be universal. Uniqueness of gene expression means that factors other than the substrate are operative in the regulation of that expression. For example, muscle cells cannot complete the oxidation of histidine, which is liberated as muscle protein is degraded during muscle contraction and relaxation. Even though the muscle cell contains the same DNA as every other cell type, the expression of those genes responsible for the complete deamination and oxidation of histidine (see Figure 8.10) does not occur despite the rising levels of histidine. Instead, this histidine is methylated and excreted in the urine. In few other cell types does this methylation occur; histidine is usually metabolized. However, the expression of the gene for the enzyme responsible for histidine methylation is *turned on* by its substrate, histidine, and its affinity for this substrate as well as its activity as a catalyst exceeds that of any other enzyme in the muscle cell that might use histidine. As the muscles are increased in activity and size, the amount of methylated histidine found in the urine also increases. Here, then, is a complete loop. The histidine in the food is transported to the muscle that uses it to synthesize myosin and actin, and when that muscle is actively working, myosin and actin are degraded, with 3-methyl histidine appearing in the urine. Histidine has acted as a signal for the expression of genes coded for its transport, for its incorporation into muscle protein, and for its methylation and excretion. It has also served as a substrate for all of these processes.

Each of the amino acids, as well as every other nutrient consumed as part of the diet, likewise has multiple roles. In and of themselves, amino acids serve as signals of metabolic processes, or they can serve as substrates for the synthesis of proteins that act as carriers, receptors, enzymes, hormones, or structural materials.

The complexity of these interacting roles of amino acids as neurotransmitters, as enzyme activators, as inducers of gene expression, and as substrates for a multitude of synthetic and degradative reactions is enormous. Yet the brain and other vital organs signal each other such that integration of function occurs and a comprehensive metabolic pattern emerges. When the body is without sufficient nutrient intake to sustain normal body function, it has a hierarchy in place that controls amino acid use so that more-important functions are maintained at the expense of less-important ones. Hence, in the protein-malnourished child, the symptoms of weight loss, skin lesions, and hair changes are observed, while the activity of metabolic enzymes and hormones is conserved.

Protein synthesis is energetically very expensive as well as being dependent on amino acid availability. Thus, protein synthesis is also suppressed in a hierarchical manner.[11] Skin cells and hair cells are not replaced, due to this decreased protein synthesis, as rapidly as in the well-nourished individual, hence the skin lesions and hair changes that typify protein malnutrition. Energy conservation and protein conservation similarly are preserved. The synthesis and release of hormones that accelerate protein breakdown and use are suppressed via effects of diet deprivation on the brain, peptides that signal food-seeking behavior are maintained, gut motility is suppressed so as to retard the passage of food from mouth to anus and extract as much nourishment as possible from that food, body activity is diminished to reduce energy expenditure (the symptom of lethargy), and sleep time is increased for the same reason. All of these defenses against death due to starvation are directed by the central nervous system and executed by the secretions of the endocrine organs. In turn, these defenses are activated when the body senses, via the gut cells, that insufficient food has been consumed.

Some of these defenses can be compromised by additional problems in the environment. If the drinking water is contaminated, the reduction in gut passage time as a defense is negated by pathogen-induced diarrhea. This results in a loss of gut contents and abrasion of the cells lining the intestinal tract. In this instance, the person is less able to cope with an inadequate food supply. The coordination of the defense against death due to starvation is disrupted by the stress response (also coordinated by hormones) to the invading pathogens. Such stress elicits a signal from the pituitary that stimulates an outpouring of the catecholamines and steroidal hormones by the adrenals. These hormones mobilize muscle protein, body fat stores, and glycogen stores needed for the synthesis of antibodies to the pathogens as well as for the synthesis of replacement enterocytes and the conservation of electrolytes and water. Because such syntheses require energy, amino acids, and a number of micronutrients—all of which may be in short supply—it is easy to understand why malnourished individuals are more vulnerable to environmental contaminants and why the resultant disease is far more severe.

The interaction of disease and nutritional state can have lasting effects on body function. Hence, it is not uncommon to observe short stature in populations whose food supply is inadequate. Growth, a reflection of protein synthesis that in turn is dependent on an adequate energy, protein, and micronutrient intake, is suppressed because growth is lower on the hierarchical scale of body functions that are preserved in times of need. When the food supply changes and becomes reliably abundant with a variety of foods, including sources of good-quality protein, then the genetic potential for body size is fully realized. The average height of the population increases from one generation to the next and the body fat stores are maintained at capacity. The latter feature may not be deemed to be desirable (see Chapter 3). Thus, the protein in the food that in turn supplies the needed amino acids to support the synthesis of all of the functional proteins in the body is a critical consideration for all living creatures. Without dietary protein, life cannot exist.

SUMMARY

1. Protein is a required macronutrient. It consists of the nitrogenous compounds called amino acids. There are many different kinds of protein.
2. The number and kinds of the amino acids in protein determine its BV as a nutrient.
3. Some of the amino acids can be synthesized in the body; others cannot. Those that cannot be synthesized in sufficient quantities to meet need are called essential amino acids. The others are called nonessential amino acids.
4. Dietary proteins must be digested by specific gastrointestinal enzymes into their constituent amino acids. These amino acids join the body amino acid pool and are then used to synthesize needed body proteins.
5. The genetic heritage of the individual determines the sequence of amino acids in the body proteins.
6. Proteins serve many functions in the body. They are structural elements, hormones, signals, enzymes, components of the immune system, receptors, transporters, and other bodily components.

LEARNING OPPORTUNITIES

CASE STUDY 8.1 Steven Has a Belly Ache

Steven is a 45-year-old store manager who is complaining of a burning, gnawing pain, moderately severe, almost always in the epigastric region. The pain is absent when he wakes up in the morning but appears about midmorning. It is relieved by food but recurs 2–3 h after a meal. This pain often wakes him up during the night. Endoscopic examination of his GI tract showed normal stomach anatomy but craters and inflammation were observed in the duodenum. Gastric analysis demonstrated that the gastric juice pH fell to 1.9 with pentagastrin stimulation (6 μg/kg s.c.). Fasting serum gastrin levels were normal.

Analyze this situation: What is the problem? How did it develop? What management recommendations would you suggest?

CASE STUDY 8.2 Julia Is Thin

Julia is 28 years old. She is 5′6″ tall and weighs 103 lb. She has had intermittent bouts of diarrhea, painful abdominal cramping, bloating, and lots of flatus. She is tired all the time and her boss has reprimanded her for not completing her assigned work in a timely manner. Julia has a hard time keeping warm. She wears a sweater all the time even in the middle of the summer. Julia is quite discouraged and her mom suggests that she go to the doctor for a complete physical checkup. Her blood workup reveals hemoglobin level at 8.2 g/dL, red cell count 3.8 million/mm^3, hematocrit 30%, ferritin 18 μg/mL, red cell folate 200 nmol/L, and B_{12} 100 pg/L. The doctor orders a bone scan using DEXA and this reveals a measure of osteoporosis. The doctor then suggests that Julia fill out a food intake form. A dietitian evaluates the results and cannot find any indication that Julia is inadequately nourished. The doctor scratches his head for an appropriate diagnosis when suddenly, as Julia is in his office, she has to make a rush visit to the lady's room. For some reason, Julia had failed to mention her gastrointestinal problems. Now, it becomes obvious that an endoscopy and biopsy of the intestine are needed. The endoscopy examination revealed that the villi of the small intestine are shortened and in some areas were flattened and inflamed. Now the doctor needs to know why this occurred so he orders a scraping of the lining of the intestine as well as an immune system workup. The results of these tests show an increase in MHC class II molecules, and these molecules do not have a normal shape. Further tests show that these molecules react to the proteins in wheat, rye, and barley but not to corn or rice. What do you think is the problem here? If you were involved in this case, what would you suggest as the reason for these physical signs and symptoms?

MULTIPLE-CHOICE QUESTIONS

1. Essential amino acids
   a. Cannot be synthesized in the body
   b. Include methionine, phenylalanine, and tryptophan
   c. Include threonine, valine, and leucine
   d. All of the above
2. The absence of active phenylalanine hydroxylase means
   a. Tyrosine becomes an essential amino acid
   b. Phenylalanine intake must be limited
   c. The individual may become mentally retarded
   d. All of the above
3. Gastrointestinal enzymes include
   a. Lactase
   b. Glucokinase
   c. Pepsin
   d. None of the above
4. The BV of good-quality proteins
   a. Is easily determined
   b. Is greater than a tryptophan-deficient protein
   c. Is tedious to determine
   d. Is largely inaccurate
5. Signal molecules are
   a. Hormones, minerals, and cytokines
   b. Found in specific cells
   c. Required as a source of energy
   d. All of the above

REFERENCES

1. Hartree, A.S., Renwick, A.G. (1992) Molecular structures of glycoprotein hormones and functions of their carbohydrate components. *Biochem. J.* 287: 665–679.
2. Turner, A.J., Tanzawa, K. (1997) Mammalian membrane metallopeptidases: NEP, ECE, KELL, and PEX. *FASEB J.* 11: 355–364.
3. Ouellet, V., Weisnagel, S.J., Marois, J., Bergeron, J., Julien, P., Gougeon, R., Tchernof, A., Holub, B., Jacques, H. (2008) Dietary cod protein reduces plasma C-reactive protein in insulin resistant men and women. *J. Nutr.* 138: 2386–2392.
4. Lecleire, S., Hassan, A., Marion-Letellier, R., Antonietti, M., Savoye, G., Bole-Feysot, C., Lerebours, E., Ducrotte, P., Dechelotte, P., Coeffier, M. (2008) Combined glutamine and arginine decrease proinflammatory cytokine production by biopsies from Crohn's patients in association with changes in nuclear factor-kB and p38 mitogen-activated protein kinase pathways. *J. Nutr.* 138: 2481–2485.
5. Olson, E.N. (1988) Modification of proteins with covalent lipids. *Prog. Lipid. Res.* 27: 177–197.
6. Harper, A.E., Yoshimura, N.N. (1993) Protein quality, amino acid balance, utilization and evaluation of diets containing amino acids as therapeutic agents. *Nutrition* 9: 460–469.
7. Humayun, M.A., Elango, R., Moehn, S., Ball, R.O., Pencharz, P.B. (2007) Application of the indicator amino acid oxidation technique for the determination of metabolic availability of sulfur amino acids from casein versus soy protein isolate in adult men. *J. Nutr.* 137: 1874–1879.

8. Young, V.R., Marchini, J.S. (1990) Mechanisms and nutritional significance of metabolic responses to altered intakes of protein and amino acids with reference to nutritional adaptation in humans. *Am. J. Clin. Nutr.* 51: 270–289.
9. Lobley, G.E. (1993). Species comparisons of tissue protein metabolism: Effects of age and hormonal action. *J. Nutr.* 123: 337–343.
10. Mitchell, H.H. (1962) *Comparative Nutrition of Man and Domestic Animals*, vol. 2. Academic Press, New York, pp. 129–191.
11. Darragh, A.J., Hodgkinson, S.M. (2000) Quantifying the digestibility of dietary protein. *J. Nutr.* 130: 1850S–1856S.
12. Kilberg, M.S., Stevens, B.R., Novak, D.A. (1993) Recent advances in mammalian amino acid transport. *Annu. Rev. Nutr.* 13: 137–166.
13. Wu, G. (2009) Amino acids: Metabolism, functions and nutrition. *Amino Acids* 37: 1–17.
14. Mariotti, F., Petzke, K.J., Bonnet, D., Szezepanski, I., Bos, C., Huneau, J.-F., Fouillet, H. (2013) Kinetics of the utilization of dietary arginine for nitric oxide and urea synthesis: Insight into the arginine-nitric oxide metabolic system in humans. *Am. J. Clin. Nutr.* 97: 972–979.
15. Aragon, J., Sols, A. (1991) Regulation of enzyme activity in the cell: Effect of enzyme concentration. *FASEB J.* 5: 2945–2950.
16. Van der Rest, M., Garrone, R. (1991) Collagen family of proteins. *FASEB J.* 5: 2814–2823.
17. Bounpheng, M.A., DSimas, J.J., Dodds, S.G., Christy, B.A. (1999) Degradation of Id proteins by the ubiquitin-proteasome pathway. *FASEB J.* 13: 2257–2264.
18. Glenney, J.R. (1992) Tyrosine-phosphorylated proteins: Mediators of signal transduction from tyrosine kinases. *Biochem. Biophys. Acta* 1134: 113–127.
19. Putney, J.W., Bird, G. (1993) The inositol phosphate-calcium signaling system in non excitable cells. *Endocr. Rev.* 14: 610–631.
20. Baumann, G. (1993) Growth hormone binding proteins. *Proc. Soc. Exp. Biol. Med.* 202: 392–400.
21. Neubig, R.R. (1994) Membrane organization in G-protein mechanisms. *FASEB J.* 8: 939–946.
22. Maintz, L., Novak, N. (2007) Histamine and histamine intolerance. *Am. J. Clin. Nutr.* 85: 1185–1196.
23. Sicherer, S.H. (2007) Food allergy. In: *Handbook of Nutrition and Food* (C.D. Berdanier, E.B. Feldman, J. Dwyer, J., eds.), 2nd edn. CRC Press, Boca Raton, FL, pp. 1111–1124.
24. Watford, M. (1993) Hepatic glutaminase expression: Relationship to kidney-type glutaminase and to the urea cycle. *FASEB J.* 7: 1468–1474.
25. Low, S.Y., Rennie, M.J., Taylor, P.M. (1997) Signaling elements involved in amino acid transport responses to altered muscle cell volume. *FASEB J.* 11: 1111–1117.
26. Neu, J., Shenoy, V., Chakrabarti, R. (1996) Glutamine nutrition and metabolism: Where do we go from here? *FASEB J.* 10: 829–837.
27. Lu, S.C. (1999) Regulation of hepatic glutathione synthesis: Current concepts and controversies. *FASEB J.* 13: 1169–1183.
28. Dice, J.F. (1987) Molecular determinants of protein half-lives in eukaryotic cells. *FASEB J.* 1: 349–357.
29. Vary, T.C., Lynch, C.J. (2007) Nutrient signaling components controlling protein synthesis in striated muscle. *J. Nutr.* 137: 1835–1843.
30. Tang, J.E., Phillips, S.M. (2009) Maximizing muscle protein anabolism: The role of protein quality. *Curr. Opin. Clin. Nutr. Metab.* 12: 66–71.
31. Vary, T.C., Deiter, G., Lynch, C.J. (2007) Rapamycin limits formation of active eukaryotic initiation factor 4F complex following meal feeding in rat hearts. *J. Nutr.* 137: 1857–1862.
32. Yates, R.O., Connor, H., Woods, H.F. (1981) Muscle protein breakdown in thyrotoxicosis assessed by urinary 3-methylhistidine excretion. *Ann. Nutr. Metab.* 25: 262–267.
33. Wolfe, R.R., Jahoor, F., Hartl, W.H. (1989) Protein and amino acid metabolism after injury. *Diabetes Metab. Rev.* 5: 149–164.
34. Ciechanover, A., Schwartz, A.L. (1994) The ubiquitin-mediated proteolytic pathway: Mechanisms of recognition of the proteolytic substrate and involvement in the degradation of native cellular proteins. *FASEB J.* 8: 182–191.
35. Obin, M., Shang, F., Gong, X., Handelman, G., Blumberg, J., Taylor, A. (1998) Redox regulation of ubiquitin-conjugating enzymes: Mechanistic insights using the thiol-specific oxidant diamide. *FASEB J.* 12: 561–569.
36. Haas, A.L., Siepmann, T.J. (1997) Pathways of ubiquitin conjugation. *FASEB J.* 11: 1257–1268.
37. Hicke, L. (1997) Ubiquitin-dependent internalization and down regulation of plasma membrane proteins. *FASEB J.* 11: 1215–1226.

38. Wilkinson, K.D. (1997) Regulation of ubiquitin-dependent processes by deubiquitinating enzymes. *FASEB J.* 11: 1245–1256.
39. Sommer, T., Wolf, D.H. (1997) Endoplasmic reticulum degradation: Reverse protein flow of no return. *FASEB J.* 11: 1227–1233.
40. Grune, T., Reinheckel, T., Davies, K.J. (1997) Degradation of oxidized proteins in mammalian cells. *FASEB J.* 11: 526–534.
41. Rapoport, T.A. (1991) Protein transport across the endoplasmic reticulum membrane: Facts, models, mysteries. *FASEB J.* 5: 2792–2798.
42. Elango, R., Humayun, M.A., Ball, R., Pencharz, P.B. (2012) Protein requirement of healthy school-age children determined by the indicator amino acid oxidation method. *Am. J. Clin. Nutr.* 94: 1545–1552.
43. Huang, L., Hogewind-Schoonenboom, J.E., van Dongen, M.J.A., de Groof, F., Voortman, G.J., Schierbeek, H., Twisk, J.W.R. et al. (2012) Methionine requirement of the enterally fed term infant in the first month of life in the presence of cysteine. *Am. J. Clin. Nutr.* 95: 1048–1054.
44. Dasarathy, J., Gruca, L.L., Bennett, C., Parimi, P., Duenas, C., Marczewski, S., Fierro, J.L., Kalhan, S.C. (2010) Methionine metabolism in human pregnancy. *Am. J. Clin. Nutr.* 91: 357–365.
45. Jia, Y., Cong, R., Li, R., Yang, X., Sun, Q., Parvizi, N., Zhao, R. (2012) Maternal low-protein diet induces gender-dependent changes in epigenetic regulation of glucose-6-phosphatase gene in newborn piglet liver. *J. Nutr.* 142: 1659–1665.
46. Evans, W.J. (2010) Skeletal muscle loss: Cachexia, sarcopenia, and inactivity. *Am. J. Clin. Nutr.* 91: 1123S–1127S.
47. Hoffer, L.J., Bistrian, B.R. (2012) Appropriate protein provision in critical illness: A systematic and narrative review. *Am. J. Clin. Nutr.* 96: 591–600.
48. Pasiakos, S.M., Vislocky, L.M., Carbone, J.W., Altieri, N., Konopelski, K.M., Freake, H.C., Anderson, J.M., Ferrando, A.A., Wolfe, R.R., Rodriguez, N.R. (2010) Acute energy deprivation affects skeletal muscle protein synthesis and associated intracellular signaling proteins in physically active adults. *J. Nutr.* 140: 745–751.
49. Berdanier, C.D. (2013) Nutrient-nutrient interactions. In: *Handbook of Nutrition and Food* (C.D. Berdanier, J. Dwyer, D. Heber, eds.), 3rd edn. CRC Press, Boca Raton, FL, pp. 243–248.
50. Plaisted Fernandez, C., Adams, K.M., Kohlmeier, M. (2013) Vegetarian diets in health promotion and disease prevention. In: *Handbook of Nutrition and Food* (C.D. Berdanier, J. Dwyer, D. Heber, eds.), 3rd edn. CRC Press, Boca Raton, FL, pp. 403–436.
51. Szeto, Y.T., Kwok, T.C., Benzie, I.F. (2004) Effects of a long term vegetarian diet on biomarkers of antioxidant status and cardiovascular disease risk. *Nutrition* 20: 863–866.
52. Boor, S.K., Valachovicova, M., Blazicek, P., Parrak, V., Babinska, K., Heidland, A., Krajcovicova-Kudlackova, M. (2006) Association of metabolic syndrome risk factors with selected markers of oxidative status and microinflammation in healthy omnivores and vegetarians. *Mol. Nutr. Food Res.* 50: 858–868.
53. Appleby, P.N., Allen, N.E., Key, T.J. (2011) Diet, vegetarianism and cataract risk. *Am. J. Clin. Nutr.* 93: 1128–1134.
54. Crowe, F.L., Appleby, P.N., Travis, R.C., Key, T.J. (2013) Risk of hospitalization or death from ischemic heart disease among British vegetarians and nonvegetarians: Results from the EPIC-Oxford cohort study. *Am. J. Clin. Nutr.* 97: 597–603.
55. Crouse, J.R., Morgan, T., Terry, J.G., Ellis, J., Vitolins, M., Burke, G.L. (1999) A randomized trial comparing the effect of casein with that of soy protein containing varying amounts of isoflavones on plasma concentrations of lipids and lipoproteins. *Arch. Intern. Med.* 159: 2070–2076.
56. Campbell, C.G., Brown, B.D., Dufner, D., Thorland, W.G. (2006) Effects of soy or milk protein during a high fat feeding challenge on oxidative stress, inflammation, and lipids in healthy men. *Lipids* 41: 257–265.
57. Tonstad, S., Smerud, K., Hoie, L. (2002) A comparison of the effects of 2 doses of soy protein or casein on serum lipids, serum lipoproteins and plasma total homocysteine in hypercholesterolemic subjects. *Am. J. Clin. Nutr.* 76: 78–84.
58. Nelausen, K., Meinertz, M. (1999) Lipoprotein(a) and dietary proteins: Casein lowers lipoprotein(a) concentration as compared to soy protein. *Am. J. Clin. Nutr.* 69: 419–425.
59. Martins, D., Norris, K., Heber, D. (2013) Nutrition in renal disease and hypertension. In: *Handbook of Nutrition and Food* (C.D. Berdanier, J. Dwyer, D. Heber, eds.), 3rd edn. CRC Press, Boca Raton, FL, pp. 901–909.
60. Thomas, L., Poole, R. (2007) Renal nutrition. In: *Handbook of Nutrition and Food* (C.D. Berdanier, E.B. Feldman, J. Dwyer, eds.), 2nd edn. CRC Press, Boca Raton, FL, pp. 815–832.

61. Centers for Disease Control (2012) Summary health statistics for U.S. adults: National Health Interview Survey, 2010. Vital and Health Statistics, Series 10, Number 252. National Center for Health Statistics, Hyattsville, MD.
62. Collins, A.J., Foley, R.N., Chavers, B. et al. (2012) U.S. renal data system 2011 annual data report. *Am. J. Kidney Dis.* 59: evii.
63. National Heart Lung and Blood Institute. (2003) The 7th report of the Joint National Committee on Prevention, Detection, Evaluation and Treatment of High Blood Pressure (JNC 7). *Hypertension* 42: 1206–1212.
64. USDA. Handbook #8, Amino acid composition of foods, U.S. Government Printing Office, Washington, D.C.

9 Carbohydrates

Carbohydrates provide as much as 60% of the daily energy intake. The percentage of the diet that is carbohydrate varies inversely with economic conditions and with the percentage of the diet that is fat and protein. As a general rule, carbohydrate-rich foods are less expensive than fat- and protein-rich foods. Hence, as people have more disposable income, they tend to buy and consume fewer cereals, breads, fruits, and vegetables and buy more meat, butter (or margarine), milk, and eggs. This is not always true, however. Over the last decade, education about the possible health risks of high intakes of fatty foods and the health benefits of high-fiber intakes, as well as the benefits of consuming fruits and vegetables, has altered the eating habits of many consumers. This, in turn, has had an impact on the percentage of intake provided by this macronutrient class.

The term carbohydrate originated in the late 1800s with the idea that there existed naturally occurring compounds composed of carbon, hydrogen, and oxygen, which could be represented as hydrates of carbon. For instance, glucose ($C_6H_{12}O_6$), sucrose ($C_{12}H_{22}O_{11}$), and starch $(C_6H_{10}O_5)n$ could all be represented by the general formula $Cx(H_2O)y$. This definition was too rigid, however, because it excluded such common compounds that could be classed as carbohydrates such as deoxyribose, a component of DNA, ($C_5H_{10}O_4$) and ascorbic acid, a vitamin, ($C_6H_8O_6$). This definition included the compound acetic acid ($C_2H_4O_2$), which, strictly interpreted, is not a carbohydrate. To overcome these exclusions, a better definition was developed, that is, carbohydrates are polyhydroxy aldehydes or ketones and their derivatives.

CLASSIFICATION

Carbohydrates are divided into three major classes: monosaccharides, oligosaccharides, and polysaccharides. A monosaccharide consists of a single polyhydroxy aldehyde or ketone unit. An oligosaccharide contains two to ten monosaccharide units. The upper limit on the number of monosaccharides in an oligosaccharide is not rigorously defined. Disaccharides, composed of two monosaccharides, are the most common dietary oligosaccharides. A polysaccharide contains many monosaccharides.

STRUCTURE AND NOMENCLATURE

Monosaccharides

Monosaccharides, called simple sugars, have the empirical formula $(CH_2O)n$, where n is 3 or more. Although monosaccharides may have as few as three or as many as nine carbon atoms, those of interest to the nutritionist have five or six. The carbon skeleton is unbranched, and each carbon atom, except one, has a hydroxyl group and a hydrogen atom. At the remaining carbon atom, there is a carbonyl group. If the carbonyl function is on the last carbon atom, the compound is an aldehyde and is called an aldose; if it occurs at any other carbon, the compound is a ketone and is called a ketose. These structures are illustrated in Figure 9.1.

The simplest monosaccharide is the three-carbon aldehyde or ketone triose. Glyceraldehyde is an aldotriose; dihydroxyacetone is a ketotriose. Successive chain elongation of trioses yields tetroses, pentoses, hexoses, heptoses, and octoses. In the aldoseries, these are called aldotriose, aldotetrose, aldopentose, aldohexose, etc.; in the ketoseries, they are ketotriose, ketotetrose, ketopentose, ketohexose, etc. Figure 9.2 shows the D-aldose monosaccharides that have three to six carbons.

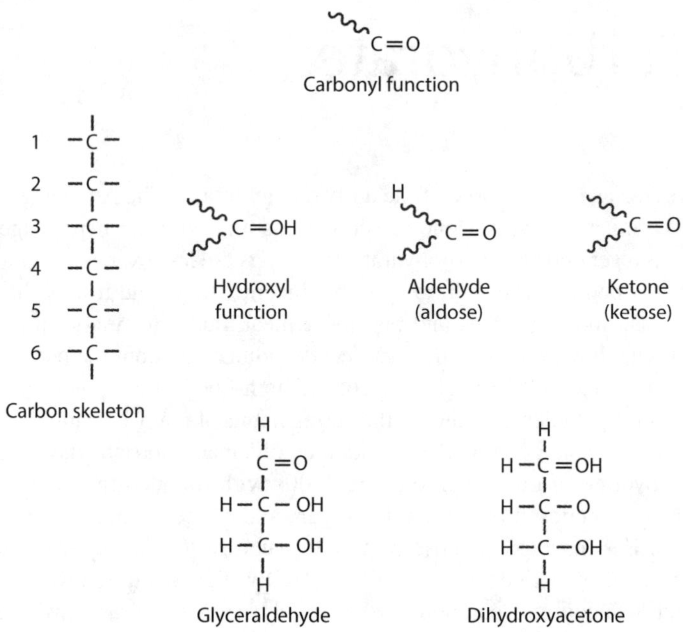

C=O
Carbonyl function
1
2
3
4
5
6
Carbon skeleton
C=OH
Hydroxyl function
H
C=O
Aldehyde (aldose)
C=O
Ketone (ketose)
H
C=O
H−C−OH
H−C−OH
H
Glyceraldehyde
H
H−C=OH
H−C−O
H−C−OH
H
Dihydroxyacetone

FIGURE 9.1 Structures of monosaccharides.

Aldotriose
D-glyceraldehyde
Aldotetrose
D-erythrose
D-threose
Aldopentose
D-ribose
D-arabinose
d-xylose
D-lyxose
Aldohexose
D-allose
D-altrose
D-glucose
D-mannose
D-gulose
D-idose
D-galactose
D-talose

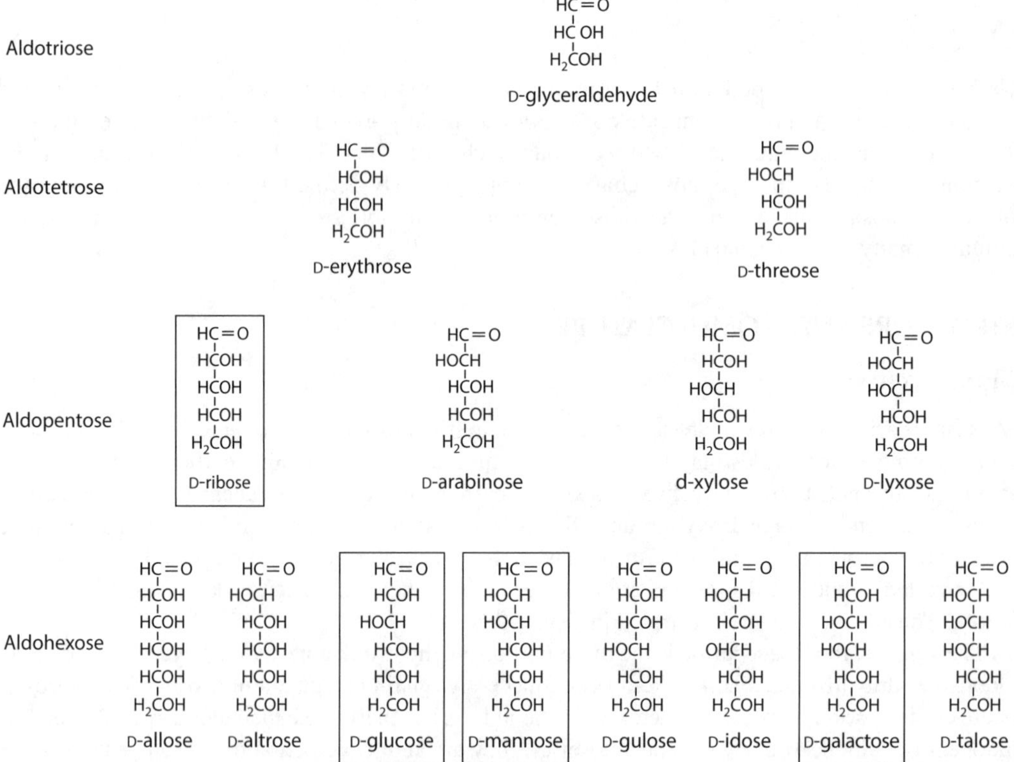

FIGURE 9.2 D-Aldoses having three to six carbon atoms. Those of the greatest biological significance are enclosed in boxes.

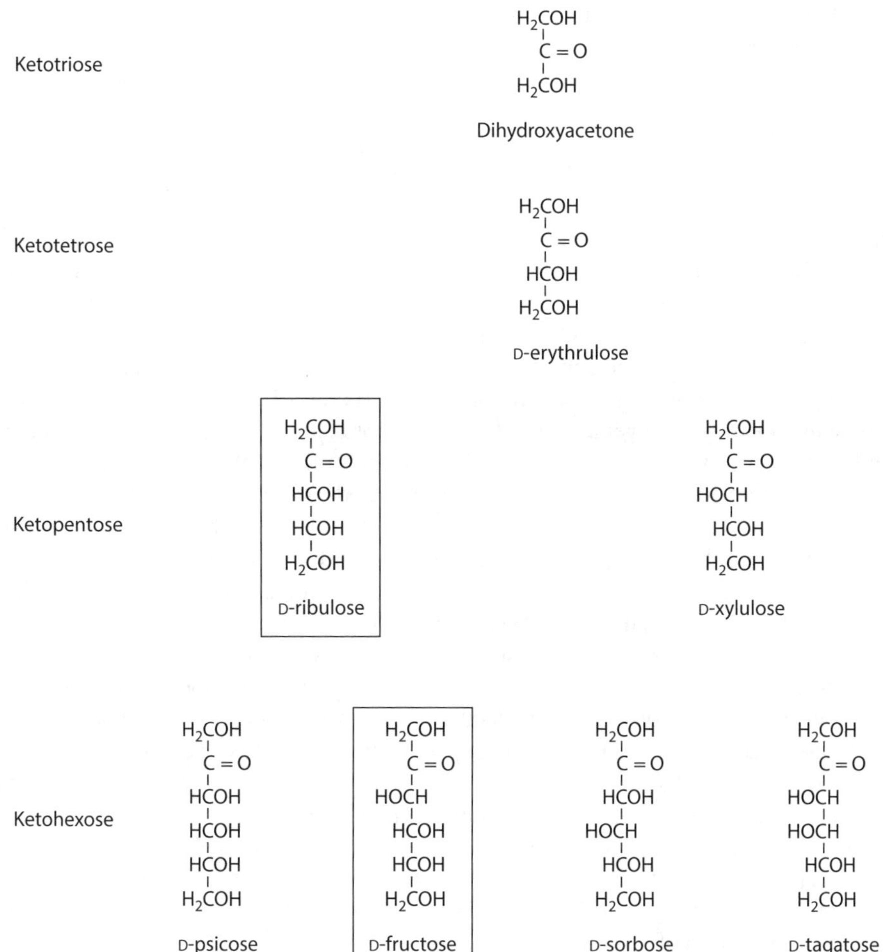

FIGURE 9.3 D-Ketoses having three to six carbon atoms. Those of the greatest biological significance are enclosed in boxes. Ketoses are sometimes named by inserting *-ul* into the name of the corresponding aldose. D-Ribulose, for example, is the ketopentose corresponding to the aldopentose D-ribose.

Figure 9.3 illustrates the corresponding D-ketoses. Within a given series of the same number of carbon atoms, these molecules differ only in the arrangement of the hydrogen atom and the hydroxyl group about the carbon atoms. Compare, for example, glucose and mannose—the configuration of the hydrogen and hydroxyl group about each of the carbons is the same except for carbon 2. In glucose, the hydroxyl function is to the right; in mannose, it is to the left. Two sugars that differ only in the configuration about one carbon atom are referred to as epimers. D-glucose and D-mannose are epimers with respect to the number 2 carbon atom; D-mannose and D-talose are epimers with respect to the number 4 carbon atom.

Configuration and conformation are two frequently used terms that are easily confused. *Configuration* is the arrangement in space of atoms or groups of atoms of a molecule that can be changed only by breaking and making bonds. *Conformation* is the arrangement in space of atoms or groups of atoms of a molecule that can arise by rotation about a single bond and that are capable of a finite existence.

The common monosaccharides are white crystalline compounds, freely soluble in water but insoluble in such nonpolar solvents as benzene and hexane. Most of them have a sweet taste and are by far the most abundant of the simple sugars. Of these, glucose, fructose, and galactose are most often found in foods, frequently as members of disaccharides or polysaccharides. Mannose is occasionally found, but only in complexes that are poorly digested. Aldopentoses are important components of DNA and RNA; derivatives of triose and heptose are intermediates in carbohydrate metabolism.

Stereoisomeric Forms

All of the monosaccharides, except dihydroxyacetone, contain at least one asymmetric carbon atom, which, in the simplest sense, is one to which four different constituents are attached. Molecules that possess an asymmetric center can exist in stereoisomeric forms.

Stereoisomers have the same structural framework but differ in the spatial arrangement of the various substituent groups. Stereoisomers include *cis* and *trans* forms (chair and boat forms) and epimers. They are different from structural isomers. Structural isomers have different structural frameworks; the bonding arrangements for the component atoms are different. C_4H_8 is the molecular formula for the two structural isomers (D-erythrose and D-threose) shown in Figure 9.3.

For example, glyceraldehyde may occur in either the D or the L stereoisomer. D and L stereoisomers bear the same relationship to each other as one's right and left hands; if both hands are laid flat on a table and the right hand slid on top of the left hand, the right hand does not cover the left (note that thumbs stick out in opposite directions). When the chemical structure for each of these molecules is written as projection formulas, their differences are obvious—the hydroxyl group and the hydrogen atom on the asymmetric carbon reverse positions; these two compounds are mirror images of each other. Mirror-image forms of the same compound are called enantiomers. Pairs of enantiomers (the D and L stereoisomers of a molecule) possess the same chemical and physical properties except for rotating plane-polarized light in opposite but equal directions; that is, the values of their specific rotation have opposite signs. A note of caution, however, a D or an L used in the name of a sugar molecule does not refer to the sign of its optical rotation; these letters specify the absolute configuration of the molecule. If one desires to include the sign of optical rotation in the molecular name, a (+) for dextrorotary, rotation to the right, or (–) for levorotary, rotation to the left, is used. For example, the specific rotation of the D-glyceraldehyde is 14°; hence, its name is D-(+)-glyceraldehyde; D-lactic acid has a specific rotation of –3.8 and is called D-(–)-lactic acid.

By convention, a carbohydrate belongs to the D-series if, when it is written in the projection formula with the aldehyde or hydroxyketone group at the top, the hydroxyl group on the next to the last carbon is to the right; conversely, if the molecule is written exactly as just described except for the fact that the hydroxyl group on the next to the last carbon is written to the left, it belongs to the L-series. A molecule that possesses n asymmetric carbons has $2n$ as the upper limit of the number of stereoisomers. The aldohexose series has four asymmetric carbon atoms; thus, it has 16 stereoisomers or eight pairs of enantiomers. One of these pairs is α-D-glucose and α-L-glucose.

In nature, D-monosaccharides are much more abundant than l. Most mammalian cells require D-sugar because they are unable to metabolize the L form. However, a few L monosaccharides can be found; among the most important are L-rhamnose and L-sorbose. Glucose is often called dextrose because the stereoisomer almost always rotates plane-polarized light to the right; it is dextrorotary. Similarly, fructose is often called levulose because its most common natural form is levorotary.

Anomeric Forms

In the section on stereoisomeric forms, glucose was referred to as α-D-glucose instead of D-glucose. The presence of the Greek letter alpha (α) adds another dimension to the structure of carbohydrates. This feature can be more readily understood if one realizes that aldehydes and ketones can add hydroxyl groups at the carbonyl function. If water is added, the unstable hydrate of the aldehyde is formed. If alcohol is added, a hemiacetal is first formed followed by the formation of a full acetal (or simple acetal) and the elimination of water. Ketones undergo

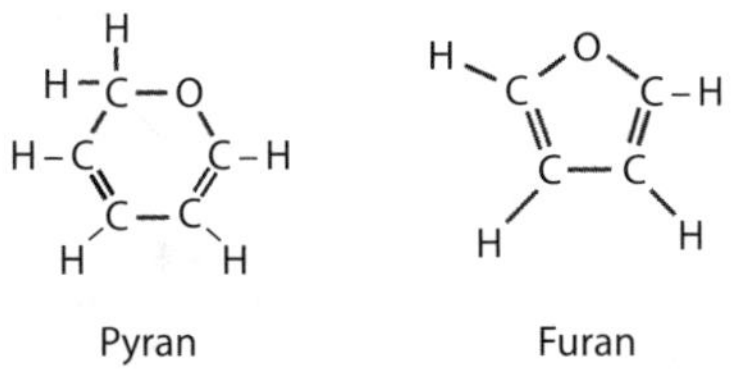

Pyran Furan

FIGURE 9.4 Structural representations of pyran and furan rings.

similar reactions but form hemiketals or ketals. The hemiketal, having four different constituents, is an asymmetric carbon atom; it exists in one of two stereoisomeric forms.

In the case of carbohydrates, the same hemiacetal formation can occur, but it will be an intramolecular reaction and a ring is produced. A six-membered ring, containing five carbon atoms and one oxygen atom is called pyranose (after pyran). A five-membered ring, containing four carbons and one oxygen, is called a furanose (after furan). Figure 9.4 illustrates these two structures. As with aldehydes, this addition reaction in a carbohydrate produces an asymmetric carbon atom; it is referred to as the anomeric carbon. We now have two monosaccharides that differ only in their configuration about the anomeric carbon; they are called anomers and are referred to as α- and β-forms. In the α-form, the hydroxyl group is below the plane of the ring to which it is attached. In the β-form, it is above. This ring closure is illustrated for D-glucose and D-fructose in Figure 9.5.

The monosaccharides in the body undergo a number of reactions. These reactions produce five general groups of products as shown in Table 9.1.

Oligosaccharides

Oligosaccharides consist of 2–10 monosaccharides joined with a glycosidic bond. The bond is formed between the anomeric carbon of one sugar and any hydroxyl function of another. If two monosaccharides are bonded in this manner, the resulting molecule is a disaccharide; if three, a trisaccharide; if four, a tetrasaccharide, etc.

Disaccharides

Of the oligosaccharides, by far the most prevalent in nature are the disaccharides. Of dietary significance are lactose, maltose, and sucrose. Lactose, the sugar found in the milk of most mammals (it is lacking in the milk of the whale and the hippopotamus), consists of a D-galactose and D-glucose joined with a glycosidic linkage at carbon 1 of galactose and carbon 4 of glucose. Lactose is a reducing sugar. The glycosidic linkage between galactose and glucose is symbolized by α (1 → 4). An important characteristic of lactose is its ability to promote the growth of certain beneficial lactic acid–producing bacteria in the intestinal tract. These bacteria have a possible role in the displacement of undesirable putrefactive forms of bacteria. Lactose also enhances the absorption of calcium.

Maltose, also known as malt sugar, contains two glucose residues. The glycosidic linkage is α (1 → 4). Cellobiose, the repeating disaccharide unit of cellulose, and gentiobiose are two other disaccharides that have as their repeating units D-glucose. In cellobiose, the glycosidic linkage is β (1 → 4); in gentiobiose, it is β (1 → 6). Since all have free anomeric carbons, they are reducing sugars. The β-linkage cannot be broken by the intestinal enzymes but are approachable by the intestinal flora.

Sucrose, also known as table sugar, cane sugar, beet sugar, or grape sugar, is a disaccharide with glucose and fructose linked through the anomeric carbon of each monosaccharide. Because neither anomeric carbon is free, sucrose is a nonreducing sugar. It is not a hemiacetal and does not undergo mutarotation. In dilute acid or in the presence of the enzyme invertase, sucrose hydrolyzes into its constituent monosaccharides. The hydrolysis of sucrose to D-glucose and D-fructose is called

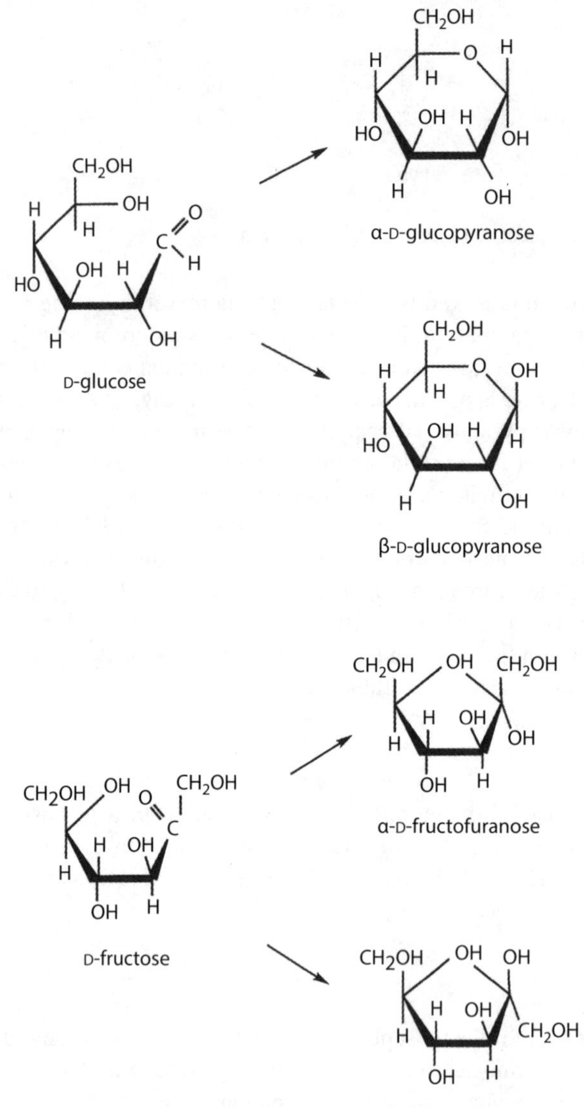

FIGURE 9.5 Ring closure of D-glucose and D-fructose to make the pyranose and furanose forms.

TABLE 9.1
Reaction Products of Monosaccharides

Product	Example
Phosphoric acid esters	Glucose-6-phosphate
Polyhydroxy alcohols	Sorbitol
Deoxy sugars	Deoxyribose
Sugar acids	Gluconic acid
Amino sugars	Glucosamine

inversion because it is accomplished by a change in the sign of specific rotation from dextro (+) to levo (–) as the equimolar mixture of glucose and fructose is formed; this mixture is called invert sugar. The development of an enzyme that will isomerize D-glucose to D-fructose has proven to be commercially valuable. It provides a method of obtaining a product known as high-fructose corn syrup, similar to invert sugar and containing no sucrose.

Invert sugar syrups are available commercially at varied levels of inversion. They are sweeter than sucrose at comparable concentrations. This greater sweetness reflects the D-fructose component of the syrup and is an important and critical feature. When sucrose is used in the preparation of acidic foods, some inversion invariably takes place. For instance, if it is used to sweeten fruit drinks, it is completely inverted within a few hours. In soft drinks, there is also a considerable amount of inversion. Honey is a largely invert sugar. While bees collect sucrose from flowers, they have an enzyme that inverts the sucrose. Honey, however, is not pure glucose and fructose; it also contains sucrose, water, and small quantities of flavor extract peculiar to the flower from which the sucrose is obtained.

In general, the disaccharides, while of importance as dietary sources of carbohydrates, have few metabolic functions. They are hydrolyzed into their component monosaccharides by enzymes located in the brush border of the enterocyte of the small intestine. These monosaccharides are then converted to glucose, the body's primary metabolic fuel. Some of the hydrolysis takes place in the lumen of the small intestine, while most takes place within the absorptive cell.

Two oligosaccharides are of nutritional interest. These are stachyose and raffinose. Stachyose, a tetrasaccharide, is composed of two molecules of D-galactose, one of D-glucose, and one of D-fructose. It is found in certain foods, particularly those of legume origin. It is usually found with raffinose (fructose, glucose, and galactose) and sucrose. The human digestive tract does not possess an enzyme that can hydrolyze either stachyose or raffinose. Evidently, however, these sugars are fermented in the lower intestinal tract by the intestinal flora to some short-chain fatty acids and some other metabolites. The fermentation of these oligosaccharides is thought to be responsible for the unwanted flatus (gas produced and released by the intestinal tract) that frequently follows the ingestion of foods containing these compounds. Dried legumes (peas and beans) are good sources of raffinose and stachyose.

Polysaccharides

Polysaccharides (also known as glycans) are compounds consisting of large numbers of monosaccharides linked by glycosidic bonds; they are analogous in structure to oligosaccharides. Some have as few as 30 monosaccharides. However, most of the polysaccharides found in nature have a high molecular weight; they may contain several hundreds or even thousands of monosaccharide units. Polysaccharides differ from one another in the nature of their repeating monosaccharide units, in the number of such units in their chain, and in the degree of branching. The polysaccharides that contain only a single kind of monosaccharide or monosaccharide derivative are called homopolysaccharides; those with two or more different monomeric units are called heteropolysaccharides. Often, homopolysaccharides are given names that indicate the nature of the building blocks: for example, those that contain mannose units are mannans; those that contain fructose units are called fructans. The important biological polysaccharides are the storage polysaccharides, the structural polysaccharides, and the mucopolysaccharides.

Storage Polysaccharides

Among plants, the most abundant storage polysaccharide is starch. It is deposited abundantly in grains, fruits, and tubers in the form of large granules in the cytoplasm of cells; each plant deposits a starch characteristic of its species. Starch exists in two forms: α-amylose and amylopectin. α-Amylose makes up 20%–30% of most starches and consists of 250–300 unbranched glucose residues bonded by α (1 → 4) linkages. The chains vary in molecular weight from a few thousand to 500,000. The molecule is twisted into a helical coil. Amylopectin, which the remainder of the starch in a plant comprises, is highly branched. Its backbone consists of glucose residues with α (1 → 4) glycosidic linkages; its branch points are α (1 → 6) glycosidic bonds. Although the structure of amylopectin is shown in Figure 9.6 as being linear, it too exists as a helical coil.

When amylose is broken down in successive stages either by the enzyme amylase or by the action of dry heat, as in toasting, the resulting polysaccharides of intermediate chain length are called *dextrins*. Amylopectin, when broken down by the same methods, does not cleave at its branch points. Its end product is a large, highly branched product called *limit dextrin*.

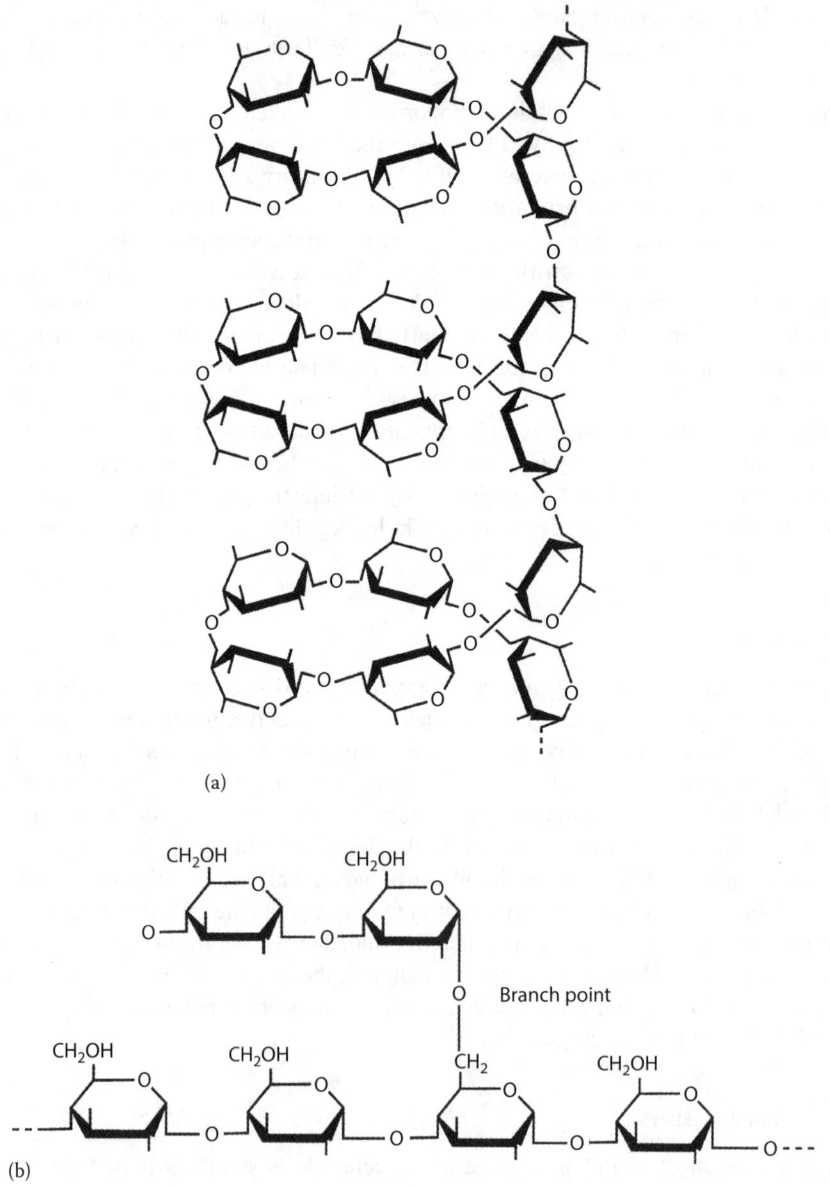

(a)

CH_2OH CH_2OH O Branch point CH_2OH CH_2OH CH_2 CH_2OH

(b)

FIGURE 9.6 Structures of storage polysaccharides: (a) the helical coil of amylose and (b) An α(1 → 6) branch point in amylopectin.

Other homopolysaccharides are found in plants, bacteria, yeast, and mold as storage polysaccharides. Dextrans, found in yeast and bacteria, are branched polysaccharides of D-glucose with their major backbone linkage α (1 → 6). Inulin, found in artichokes, consists of D-fructose monomers with β (2 → 1) glycosidic linkages. Mannans are composed of mannose residues and are found in bacteria, yeasts, mold, and higher plants.

Among animals, the storage polysaccharide is glycogen. Glycogen is stored primarily in the liver and muscles. Like amylopectin, glycogen is a branched polysaccharide of D-glucose with a backbone glycosidic linkage of α (1 → 4) and branch points of α (1 → 6). However, its branches occur every 8–10 residues, as compared with every 12 for amylopectin. Glycogen is of no importance as a dietary source of carbohydrate. The small amount of glycogen in an animal's body when it is slaughtered is quickly degraded during the postmortem period.

Structural Polysaccharides

Cellulose is the most abundant structural polysaccharide in the plant world. Fifty percent of the carbon in vegetables is cellulose; wood also is about 50% cellulose and cotton is nearly pure cellulose. It is a straight chain polymer of D-glucose with β (1 → 4) glycosidic linkages between the monosaccharides. Cellobiose, a disaccharide, is obtained on partial hydrolysis of cellulose. The molecular weight of cellulose has been estimated to range from 50,000 to 500,000 (equivalent to 300 to 3,000 glucose residues). Cellulose molecules are organized in bundles of parallel chains, called fibrils. These fibrils are cross-linked by hydrogen bonding; the chains of glucose units are relatively rigid and are cemented together with hemicelluloses, pectin, and lignin.

Hemicellulose bears no relation structurally to cellulose. It is composed of polymers of D-xylose having β (1 → 4) glycosidic linkages with side chains of arabinose and other sugars. Pectin is a polymer of methyl D-galacturonate. Pectin is found in fruit and is the substance needed to make jelly out of cooked fruit. The juice plus sucrose plus the pectin form a gel that is stable for many months at room temperature. Pectin is a nonabsorbable carbohydrate that has pharmacological use as well. It is a key component, together with kaolin (clay), of an antidiarrheal remedy.

There are other structural polysaccharides found in nature. Chitin is a polysaccharide that forms the hard skeleton of insects and crustaceans and is a homopolymer of *N*-acetyl-D-glucosamine. Agar, derived from sea algae, contains D- and L-galactose residues, some esterified with sulfuric acid, primarily with 1 → 3 bonds; alginic acid, derived from algae and kelp, contains monomers of D-mannuronic acid; and vegetable gum (gum guar) contains D-galactose, D-glucuronic acid, rhamnose, and arabinose. These are used as food stabilizers by the food-processing industry. Algin derivatives, for example, are used to stabilize the emulsions of salad dressings; gum guar is frequently used to stabilize processed cheese products. It acts to retard the separation of the solids from the fluid component in such products.

Mucopolysaccharides

The mucopolysaccharides are heteropolysaccharides that are components of the structural polysaccharides found at various places in the body. Mucopolysaccharides consist of disaccharide units in which glucuronic acid is bound to acetylated or sulfurated amino sugars with glycosidic β (1 → 3) linkages. Each disaccharide unit is bound to the next by a β (1 → 4) glycosidic linkage. Thus, they are linear polymers with alternating β (1 → 3) and β (1 → 4) linkages. Hyaluronic acid is the most abundant mucopolysaccharide. It is the principal component of the ground substance of connective tissue and is also abundant in the synovial fluid in joints and the vitreous humor of the eye. The repeating unit of hyaluronic acid is a disaccharide composed of D-glucuronic acid and *N*-acetyl-D-glucosamine; it has alternating β (1 → 3) and β (1 → 4) glycosidic linkages. The molecular weight is several million.

Another mucopolysaccharide that forms part of the structure of connective tissue is chondroitin. It differs from hyaluronic acid only in that it contains *N*-acetyl-D-galactosamine residues rather than *N*-acetyl-D-glucosamine ones. The sulfate ester derivatives of chondroitin, chondroitin sulfate A and chondroitin sulfate C, are major structural components of cartilage, bone, cornea, and other connective tissue. Types A and C have the same structure as chondroitin, except for a sulfate ester at carbon atom 4 of the *N*-acetyl-D-galactosamine residue on type A and one at carbon atom 6 of type C.

Heparin is a mucopolysaccharide that is similar in structure to hyaluronic acid, in that it contains residues of D-glucuronic acid. However, in heparin, these residues contain varying portions of both sulfate and acetyl groups. Its structure is not entirely known. It is a blood anticoagulant.

Sources of Carbohydrate

Carbohydrates are constituents of all living cells. As such, one could anticipate finding one or more carbohydrates in almost any food of importance to humans. Practically speaking, however, foods from animal sources contain few carbohydrates. Milk, with its high lactose content, is the only significant animal source of carbohydrate. Cow's milk contains 4.8% lactose; human milk, 7%. Eggs, scallops, and oysters contain small amounts of carbohydrate. Foods from plant sources, on the other hand, contain large amounts of carbohydrates. Oranges, bananas, and apples are good sources of fructose. Potatoes and cereal grains are good sources of starch. The percentage of carbohydrate in several common foods can be seen in Table 9.2. A more complete list of foods and the carbohydrates they contain can be found in the *Tables of Food Composition* maintained by the USDA and can be accessed using the USDA website (www. nal.usda.gov/foodcomposition).

The sugar content of several fresh fruits and vegetables is given in Table 9.3. The starch content is not shown. Canned and frozen fruits often contain sugar in addition to that which occurs naturally. This sugar is used in processing the fruit to preserve the structure, color, and flavor of the fruit. Thus, canned and frozen fruits may have more sugar in them than when eaten fresh and unprocessed. The high-fructose corn syrup solutions are also used in soft drinks to add body without affecting or masking flavors. Canners and preservers choose these syrups because they penetrate the fruit easily and preserve its natural form, flavor, and color.

TABLE 9.2
Carbohydrates in Common Foods

Item	%
Fruits and vegetables	5–20
Milk (depending on species)	5
Shellfish	<1
Fish	<1
Lean pork	<1
Ice cream, cake, pie	40–50
Lunch meat	<5
Cheese, roast beef	<1
Peanut butter, bacon	<10
Nuts	<10
Butter, margarine	0
Salad oil	0
Sugar	100

Source: http://www.nal.usda.gov/fnic/foodcomp/data.

TABLE 9.3
Free Sugar Content (g/100 g Fresh Weight) in Fruits and Vegetables

Item	Glucose	Fructose	Sucrose	Maltose	Raffinose	Stachyose
Apple	1.17	6.04	3.78	Trace		
Beans, lima	0.04	0.08	2.59		0.20	0.59
Beans, snap	0.48	1.30	0.28		0.26	
Broccoli	0.73	0.67	4.24			
Peach	0.91	1.18	6.92	0.12		
Strawberry	2.09	2.40	1.03	0.07		

Source: http://www.nal.usda.gov/fnic/foodcomp/data.

TABLE 9.4
Fiber Content in Common Foods

Item	Fiber (g/100 g)
Almonds	2.6
Apples	0.9
Beans, lima	1.8
Beans, string	1.0
Broccoli	1.5
Carrots	1.0
Flour, whole wheat	2.3
Flour, white wheat	0.3
Noodles, dry	0.4
Oat flakes	1.4
Pears	1.5
Pecans	2.3
Popcorn	2.2
Strawberries	1.3
Walnuts	2.1
Wheat germ	2.5

Source: K. Diem and C. Letner, eds., *Tables of Food Composition, Scientific Tables*, 7th edn., CIBA-Geigy, Ardsley, New York, 1974.

In addition to the sugars and starches, plants contain cellulose, hemicellulose, pectin, and lignin (a noncarbohydrate). These carbohydrates provide fiber, or indigestible residues. Table 9.4 gives the amounts of crude fiber in many common foods. By definition, crude fiber is the residue of plant food left after extraction by dilute acid and alkali. The exact amount of fiber that a food can provide is the subject of some dispute.[3–6] In the past, chemical analyses of foods have provided values for the amount of crude fiber in specific foods. However, the term *crude fiber* is not the same as the indigested carbohydrate that appears in the feces. While cellulose, plant fibers, and other so-called nondigestible carbohydrates are not digestible by the enzymes located in the upper portion of the intestine, the intestine contains flora that can partially degrade some of these food components. This degradation provides fatty acids and other useful compounds that are then absorbed by the lower small intestine and colon. Several methods of analysis for dietary fiber are available, but none truly assess and quantitate the amount of fiber that is truly not used. As mentioned, several of the nondigestible carbohydrates provide useful substrates to the colon flora and thus should not be considered as nondigestible carbohydrate.

DIGESTION AND ABSORPTION

Once a carbohydrate-rich food is consumed, digestion begins. In the mouth, the food is chewed and mixed with saliva, which contains α-amylase. This amylase begins the digestion of starch by attacking the internal α-1,4-glycosidic bonds. It will not attack the branch points having α-1,6-glycosidic bonds; hence, the salivary α-amylase will produce molecules of glucose, maltose, α-limit dextrin, and maltotriose. The α-amylase in saliva has an isozyme with the same function in the pancreatic juice. The salivary α-amylase is denatured in the stomach as the food is mixed and acidified with the gastric hydrochloric acid. As the stomach contents move into the duodenum, it is called chyme. The movement of chyme into the duodenum stimulates pancreozymin release. This gut hormone acts on the exocrine pancreas stimulating it to release pancreatic juice into the duodenum. Pancreozymin has another name: cholecystokinin. The two names were given before it was realized that the two different functions, the stimulation of the release of pancreatic juice from the exocrine pancreas and bile from the gall bladder, were performed by the same hormone. This hormone is secreted by the epithelial endocrine cells of the small intestine, particularly the duodenum. Its release is stimulated by amino acids in the lumen and by the acid pH of the stomach contents as it passes into the duodenum. The low pH of the chyme also stimulates the release of secretin, which, in turn, stimulates the exocrine pancreas to release bicarbonate and water so as to neutralize the acidity of the stomach contents as they are moved into the small intestine. This neutralization then optimizes the environment for the activity of the digestive enzymes located on the surface of the luminal cell. Both cholecystokinin and secretin have roles in the regulation of food intake (see Chapter 4).

The disaccharides in the diet are hydrolyzed to their component monosaccharides. Lactose is hydrolyzed to glucose and galactose by lactase; sucrose is hydrolyzed to fructose and glucose, and maltose is hydrolyzed to two molecules of glucose. Table 9.5 lists these enzymes together with their substrates and products. One of these enzymes, lactase, declines in activity after weaning. In rodents, this decline is regulated at the level of transcription by factors in addition to the cessation of milk consumption.[7–9] This may also occur in humans; however, the identity of these regulatory substances has not been fully elucidated. Many adult humans in the world are lactose intolerant. African-Americans and Asian-Americans are disproportionately affected compared to people from the northern parts of Europe.[10,11] Some of this intolerance is due to a culture that dictates the lack of consumption of fluid milk after weaning. According to a report from the National Institutes of Health,[12] the prevalence of this intolerance is not as great as thought. Many people self-report this problem that in fact do not have lactose intolerance. Because milk contains so many essential nutrients in addition to lactose, it would be useful to understand the development of the disorder. The regulation and decline of lactase activity is not well understood, and many people who do not like milk maintain that they are lactose intolerant when in fact they are not.

However, there are indeed people who cannot tolerate the lactose in milk and milk products. Food processors have developed lactose-free milk, and this should be a benefit to such individuals.

TABLE 9.5
Enzymes of Importance to Carbohydrate Digestion

Enzyme	Substrate	Products
α-Amylase	Starch, amylopectin, glycogen	Glucose, maltose, maltotriose, limit dextrins
α-Glucosidase	Limit dextrin	Glucose
Lactase	Lactose	Galactose, glucose
Maltase	Maltose	Glucose
Sucrase	Sucrose	Glucose, fructose

Some people can tolerate small amounts of milk without digestive upset, so therapy for these individuals consists simply of restricting their milk intakes. Fermented products such as yogurt and cheese are lactose-free since the fermentation process uses the lactose as a carbohydrate fuel. Lactose-intolerant people can consume these nutritious foods while varying amounts of fresh milk induce the typical symptoms of diarrhea and flatulence.

Lactulose, the alcohol form of lactose, is sometimes prescribed to relieve constipation. It is also used to relieve the symptoms of hepatic cancer. In both instances, the lactulose is in a liquid form. If the individual is lactose intolerant, using lactulose to relieve the constipation might not be a good choice.

As mentioned, starch digestion begins in the mouth with salivary amylase. It pauses in the stomach as the stomach contents are acidified but resumes when the chyme enters the duodenum and the pH is raised. The amylase of the pancreatic juice is the same as that of the saliva. It attacks the same bonds in the same locations and produces the same products: maltose, maltotriose, and the small polysaccharides (average of eight glucose molecules) the limit dextrins. The limit dextrins are further hydrolyzed by α-glucosidases on the surface of the luminal cells. The mucosal maltase-glucoamylase plays a crucial role in starch digestion and in the subsequent flux of glucose through glycolysis.[13] The carbohydrates, whose bonds are not attacked by α-amylase or α-glucosidase, are then passed to the lower part of intestine where they are attacked by the enzymes of the intestinal flora. Most of the products of this digestion are used by the flora themselves; however, the microbial metabolic products may be of use. The flora can produce useful amounts of short-chain fatty acids and lactate as well as methane gas, carbon dioxide, water, and hydrogen gas. The carbohydrates of legumes typify the substrates these flora use. Raffinose, which is an α-galactose 1 → 6 glucose 1 → 2 β-fructose and trehalose, and α-glucose 1 → 1 α-glucose are the typical substrates from legumes for these flora. The flora will also attack portions of the fibers and celluloses that are the structural elements of fruits and vegetables. Again, some useful metabolic products may be produced, but the bulk of these complex polysaccharides have indigestible β-linkages and are largely untouched by both intestinal and bacterial enzymes. These indigested, unavailable carbohydrates serve very useful functions:

1. They provide bulk to the diet, which in turn helps to regulate the rate of food passage from mouth to anus.
2. They act as adsorbents of noxious or potentially noxious materials in the food.
3. They assist in the excretion of cholesterol and several minerals, thereby protecting the body from overload.

Populations consuming high-fiber diets have a lower incidence of colon cancer, fewer problems with constipation, and, as a general rule, lower serum cholesterol levels.

Once the monosaccharides are released through the action of the aforementioned enzymes, they are absorbed by one of several mechanisms. Glucose and galactose are absorbed by an energy-dependent, sodium-dependent, carrier-mediated mechanism.[14,15] This mechanism is termed *active transport* because glucose is transported against a concentration gradient. Because the transport is against a concentration gradient, energy is required to *push* the movement of glucose into the enterocyte. This transport is diagrammed in Figure 9.7. Glucose and galactose appear to compete for the same active transport system. They also compete for a secondary transporter, a sodium-independent transporter (the glucose transporter GLUT 2) found in the basolateral surface of the enterocyte membrane. The two transporters differ in molecular weight. The sodium-dependent transporter has a molecular weight of 75 kDa, while the sodium-independent transporter weighs 57 kDa. This sodium-independent transporter is a member of a group of transporters called GLUT 1, 2, 3, or 4.[14–20] Each of these transporters is specific to certain tissues (Table 9.6). They are sometimes called mobile GLUTs because, when not in use, they reside in the endoplasmic reticulum. Under the appropriate conditions, they move from the endoplasmic

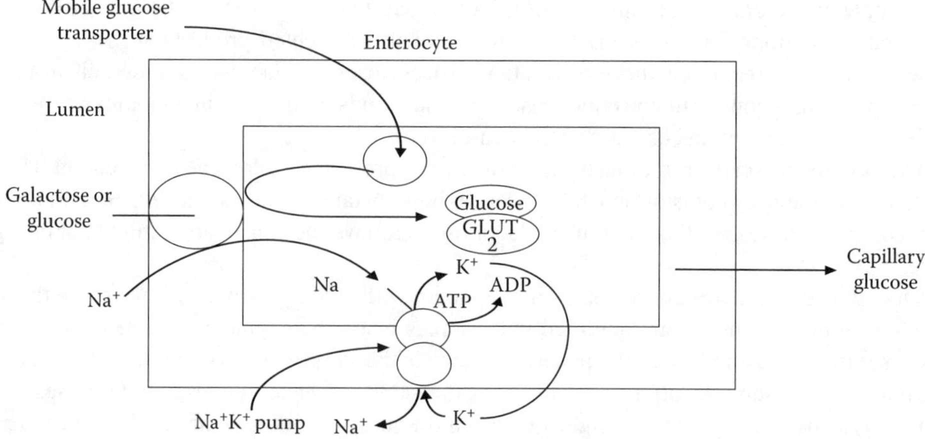

FIGURE 9.7 Two systems are used for glucose uptake by the enterocyte. One is the active transport of glucose from the lumen into the enterocyte that uses the energy-dependent Na^+K^+ exchange to facilitate the movement of glucose across the cell membrane. The other uses a mobile GLUT 2 to move the glucose through the cell to the capillary side of the enterocyte.

TABLE 9.6
Location of the Glucose Transporters

Transporter	Location
GLUT 1	Ubiquitous but found mainly in brain, erythrocytes, placenta, kidneys, and cultured cells. Is not particularly responsive to insulin regulation
GLUT 2	Liver, β-cells of pancreas, kidney, intestine
GLUT 3	Ubiquitous in human tissue, central nervous system, placenta
GLUT 4	Adipose tissue, heart, skeletal muscle
GLUT 5	Jejunum, spleen
GLUT 6	Brain, spleen, leukocytes
GLUT 7	Endoplasmic reticulum

reticulum to the plasma membrane, where they fuse with the plasma membrane and bind glucose. Upon binding, the transporter and its associated glucose are released from the membrane and then disassociate. The transporter returns to its storage site and the glucose is phosphorylated for entry into glycolysis. In addition to the preceding listed transporters, there are three others. GLUT 5 functions as a fructose transporter in the jejunum and spleen. GLUT 6 functions in the brain, spleen, and leukocytes, and GLUT 7 serves as a transporter of glucose-6-phosphate in the endoplasmic reticulum.

Fructose is not absorbed via an energy-dependent, active transport system, but by GLUT 5 via facilitated diffusion.[20,21] This process is independent of the sodium ion and is specific for fructose. In the enterocyte, much of the absorbed fructose is metabolized so that little fructose can be found in the portal blood even if the animal is given an intraluminal infusion of this sugar. On the other hand, an intraluminal infusion of sucrose will result in measurable blood levels of fructose. The reason that this occurs may be due to the location of sucrase on the enterocyte. Rather than extending out into the lumen as do the other disaccharidases that are anchored to the enterocyte by a glycoprotein, sucrase is more intimately anchored. The sucrose molecule then is closely embraced by the enzyme, which, in turn, facilitates both the hydrolysis of sucrose and the subsequent transport of its constituent monosaccharides. Thus, both monosaccharides enter the enterocyte simultaneously. If the diet is particularly rich in sucrose, the rise in both glucose and fructose in the portal blood will be measurable. This has some interesting consequences, as will be discussed later in the section on metabolism.

Of the other monosaccharides present in the lumen, passive diffusion is the means for their entry into the enterocyte. Pentoses, such as those found in plums or cherries and other minor carbohydrates, will find their way into the system only to be passed out of the body via the urine if the carbohydrate cannot be used.

METABOLISM

Once absorbed by the intestinal cell, glucose passes into the portal blood and circulates first to the liver and then throughout the body.[22–26] Glucose is the universal and, in many cases, the preferred fuel for almost all cells. It enters the pathways of intermediary metabolism as glucose-6-phosphate. (See review at the front of this book for the details of these pathways.) Even though a human being consumes almost as much energy from carbohydrate as from fat, the body prefers to oxidize the carbohydrate and store the fat. However, there are times when the intake energy is insufficient to maintain the body. At these times, the body uses its energy store. Some of this store (less than a day's need) can be provided by glycogen, a polymer of glucose. Hence, glucose in excess of immediate oxidative need is used to synthesize glycogen in the muscle and liver. Once the glycogen stores are filled, surplus glucose from the diet can be converted to fatty acids and stored as triacylglycerols in the adipose fat depots. In times of need, this fat can be oxidized, as can the stored glycogen. For those cells having an absolute requirement for glucose (certain brain cells), this important fuel can be provided through glycogenolysis or synthesized via gluconeogenesis in the liver and kidney. All of these processes (see Figure 9.8), including food intake regulation (see Chapter 4), glucose oxidation, lipid oxidation, fatty acid synthesis, glycogenesis, glycogenolysis, and gluconeogenesis, are under genetic, dietary, and hormonal control. This control is carefully integrated so that normal blood glucose levels are maintained at 100 ± 20 mg/dL (4–6 mmol/L). Excursions below (as during starvation) or above (as immediately after a meal or sugary treat) this range may occur. If the excursion is of short duration, there is no cause for alarm. However, if these excursions are more prolonged, then, depending on the reason for these excursions, medical assistance may be required.

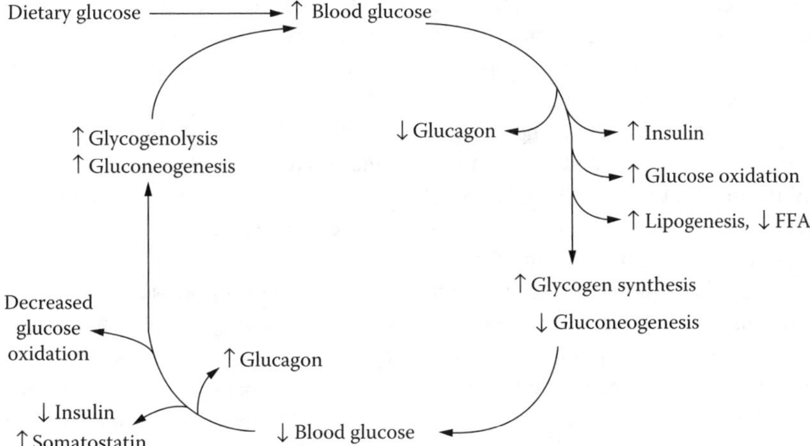

FIGURE 9.8 Overview of glucose metabolism. As blood glucose levels rise due to the influx of dietary glucose, blood insulin levels rise and glucagon levels fall. Glucose oxidation increases, as does glycogenesis and lipogenesis. Gluconeogenesis falls. As the blood glucose levels fall, these processes reverse. Glucagon levels rise, insulin falls; glycogenolysis and gluconeogenesis rise, peripheral glucose oxidation decreases.

Glucose Homeostasis

Soon after food is consumed, digested, and absorbed, blood glucose levels rise. Glucose is a hydrophilic compound and can circulate freely in the bloodstream without the need for a special carrier. However, as a hydrophilic compound, it cannot penetrate the plasma membrane surrounding the cells of the body without help. The mechanism for glucose entry is dependent on the hormone insulin and on proteins called GLUTs. As was discussed in the absorption of glucose by the enterocyte, there are seven of these proteins.[14–20] GLUT 1 has a Km that ranges from 16.9 to 26.2 mM. Under the same conditions, GLUT 2 has a low affinity for glucose and a Km between 3.9 and 5.6 mM. GLUT 3 has a Km of 10.6 and GLUT 4 has a Km of 1.8–4.8 mM. The GLUT 2 transporter transports fructose. Its activity is regulated by glucose concentration and by triiodothyronine. Some cell types have only one of these proteins, while others have more than one.

The transporters differ slightly in their structure yet have large areas of homology. As mentioned, they also differ in their affinity for glucose. GLUTs 3 and 4 have a higher affinity for glucose than does GLUT 1. These higher affinities assure that glucose transport will be maximal in tissues containing these isoforms even when the substrate levels are relatively low. This is particularly important to the CNS since glucose is its main energy source. GLUT 2 has the lowest affinity for glucose, and the rate of transport of glucose via this carrier is directly proportional to the change in blood glucose concentration. This has importance in the absorption of glucose by the enterocyte, as described in the section on digestion and absorption. It means that the intestinal cell has a fail-safe glucose uptake system—one that is energy dependent and another that is not. In addition, when the body is in the postprandial state (after a meal has been consumed) and blood glucose levels are high, there is a net flux of glucose into the hepatocytes and islet cells of the pancreas because of the presence of the GLUT 2 transporter. It is not particularly active unless blood glucose levels are elevated. In contrast, when the body is starving, intracellular glucose levels rise as a result of increased glucose production via gluconeogenesis and glycogenolysis. When the intracellular glucose levels rise, GLUT 2 can work in the opposite direction transporting glucose out of the liver cell for transport to cells lacking significant glucose production capacity. Table 9.6 lists the transporters and their locations. As mentioned in the section on absorption, the GLUT is referred to as a mobile transporter because, when it is not in use, it is sequestered in an intracellular pool. When needed, it leaves its storage site, moves to the interior aspect of the plasma membrane, forms a loose bond with the membrane, picks up the glucose molecule, and moves it through the membrane into the cytosol, whereupon the glucose can be phosphorylated and metabolized. Figure 9.9 is a cartoon of how these transporters work when the recruitment of the transporter is responsive to insulin signaling.

The action of insulin is initiated when it binds to its plasma membrane insulin receptor. The insulin receptor extends through the plasma membrane and has an intrinsic protein kinase as part of its structure. When insulin binds to the receptor, almost instantly, autophosphorylation of the receptor occurs with phosphate groups from ATP attached to the exposed tyrosine residues. Phosphorylation of the tyrosine residues requires the movement of the calcium ion from its storage site on the endoplasmic reticulum. This mobilization of calcium occurs when phosphatidyl inositol triphosphate (PIP_3) and diacylglycerol (DAG) are produced from the membrane phospholipid phosphatidylinositol (PI). In turn, the DAG stimulates the temporary binding of Ca^{++} to the kinase to facilitate the phosphorylation of the tyrosine residues. All of these reactions result in a change in the phosphorylation state of the transporter in its storage site facilitating its release and migration to the interior aspect of the plasma membrane. This, then, accomplishes the goal of moving the glucose from the bloodstream into the cell for its appropriate use.

Not all cells mobilize their GLUTs under the influence of insulin. Some use a different mechanism. Brain cells are an example, as are the β-cells in the islets of Langerhans in the pancreas. These cell types have stringent requirements for glucose as their principal metabolic fuel, yet their use and transport of glucose is independent of insulin bound to a plasma membrane receptor.

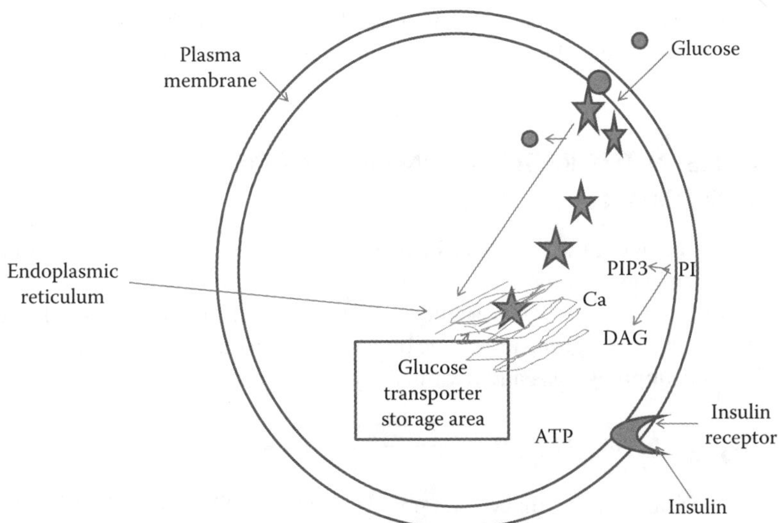

FIGURE 9.9 As blood glucose levels rise, the β-cell of the pancreas releases insulin that binds to its receptor on the surface of the target cell and signals the release of the mobile GLUT from its storage site. The transporter (star) migrates to the plasma membrane, picks up the glucose (circles), transports it to the cytosol, and releases it. Both the PIP cycle and the Ca^{++} are involved.

The presence of GLUTs in a wide variety of tissues has been ascertained by a number of scientists, yet the details of their recruitment and the signals necessary for this recruitment are not fully known. As mentioned, insulin bound to its receptor on the plasma membrane is essential to the entry of glucose into insulin-dependent cells. When a person (or animal) consumes a glucose-rich food, the blood glucose rises.[27,28] This glucose stimulates the pancreatic β-cells in the islets of Langerhans to release insulin. How the GLUT is recruited is not known, but when glucose enters the cytosol of the β-cell via GLUT 2, it is phosphorylated to glucose-6-phosphate by the enzyme glucokinase (GK). It is thought that this phosphorylation step provides the signal to the β-cell to release insulin from its insulin store. Aberrations in pancreatic GK result in impaired insulin release and subsequent impairment in the use of glucose. Again, exactly how this signal is generated is not known. The phosphatidyl inositol phosphate (PIP) cycle is involved, as is the tyrosine kinase and the calcium ion, but information is lacking on the specifics of the mechanism. The transport of glucose into the pancreatic β-cell and the subsequent release of insulin via the Golgi complex also involve the calcium, sodium, and potassium ions and ATP.

As the blood glucose levels fall because of the insulin-stimulated use of glucose, less glucose is transported into the β-cell and thus less insulin is released. In turn, all of the various cells that use glucose will have less glucose to use as well as less insulin bound to its receptors. In the fully fed state, insulin is the key to normal glucose oxidation or conversion to glycogen or fatty acids.[22] However, in the absence of continuous feeding, the body must adjust its metabolism to ensure a continuous fuel supply.[29] Other hormones such as the gut hormones, epinephrine, glucagon, somatostatin, and glucocorticoids now play key roles as the blood glucose falls. These hormones switch metabolism from glucose disposal to blood glucose maintenance. First, they exert an anti-insulin action at insulin target cells by interfering with insulin-stimulated glucose uptake. In so doing, they promote insulin resistance. That is, the cells are resisting the positive effects of insulin on glucose uptake and oxidation via glycolysis. Second, these hormones provide signals that enhance glycogenolysis and gluconeogenesis to provide glucose to those cells that need it. The enhancement of glycogenolysis in the liver precedes that of gluconeogenesis, since glycogen is more readily available than are the substrates for gluconeogenesis. In addition, glycogenolysis is energetically less expensive than is gluconeogenesis. Third, lipolysis and fatty acid oxidation are enhanced to provide energy and glycerol for glucose synthesis. All of these inhibitions and enhancements are coordinated so that the blood glucose level remains within the normal range of 80–110 mg/dL (4–6 mmol/L).

ABNORMALITIES IN THE REGULATION OF GLUCOSE HOMEOSTASIS: DIABETES MELLITUS

Just as we have learned about the details of intermediary metabolism through the study of genetic anomalies in these pathways, so too have we learned about the regulation of glucose homeostasis through the study of a large number of genetic errors that result in the disease diabetes mellitus. Diabetes mellitus is the largest group of genetic disorders that afflict humans. The prevalence of this disorder is rising as better diagnosis and treatment modalities are developed.

Prevalence of Diabetes

The number of Americans having diabetes is growing (Figures 9.10 and 9.11).[30–35] It has increased by 42% in the last decade. In part, this is due to better care and management of the disease, thus prolonging the lives of those with the disease. It is also due to earlier diagnosis of the disease and to the fact that as the population with diabetes grows and reproduces, the genetic traits carried by

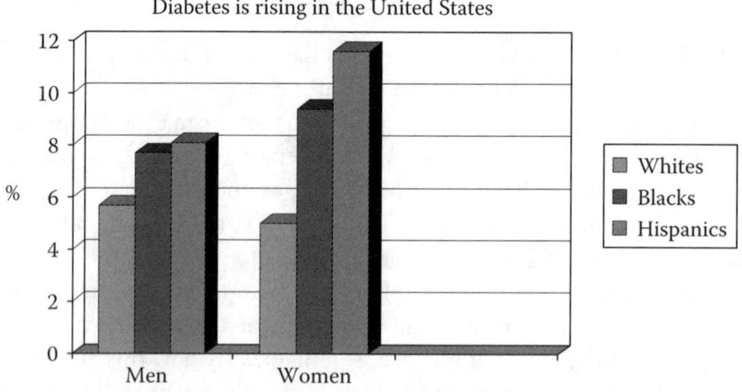

FIGURE 9.10 Estimated age-adjusted prevalence of physician-diagnosed diabetes in adults 20+ years of age segregated by gender and race.[34] The ADA estimates that another 40% of people with diabetes are undiagnosed. Altogether, 13.4% of the population have or are likely to have the disease.

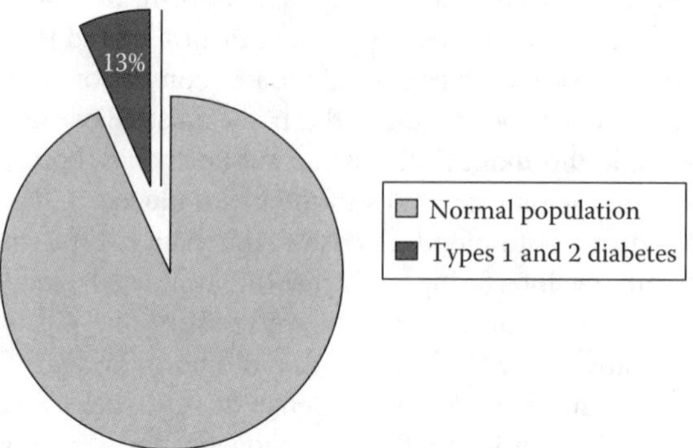

FIGURE 9.11 Distribution of people with diabetes in the United States.

these people are passed on to their progeny. Often, people with diabetes are also obese. Obesity is a growing problem in the United States. In some instances, obesity precedes diabetes, and in some, the two conditions develop simultaneously.

Approximately 10,240,000 Americans have physician-diagnosed diabetes. The American Diabetes Association (ADA) estimates that perhaps many more people have the disease but are undiagnosed.[32] Approximately 798,000 new cases are diagnosed each year. Death due to diabetes ranks seventh in the top ten causes of death in the United States. Diabetes as a contributory cause of death is rising. Diabetes death rates were 24.2/100,000 population for white males, 47.0/100,000 for black males, 19.5/100,000 for white females, and 48.8/100,000 for black females. Two-thirds of people with diabetes die of some form of vascular disease. This includes heart disease and stroke. More than 60% of people with end-stage renal disease are people with diabetes. Within the total population in the United States, there are groups that have an even higher prevalence rate of diabetes than those shown earlier for black and Caucasian populations. The Pima Indians in Arizona have a prevalence of 60% of the adult population. Hispanic Americans aged 50 years or older have a prevalence of 25%–30%. Diabetes is two to three times more common in Mexican American and Puerto Rican adults than in non-Hispanic Caucasian adults.[32]

The prevalence of diabetes depends on the diagnostic criteria used for identification. The newest criteria are those of the ADA.[36] These are modifications of those previously recommended by the NDDG[34] and WHO.[35] These criteria are shown in Table 9.7. The ADA expert committee recognized that there may be deviants in people who fail to meet these criteria yet may not be considered normal. This group is defined as having fasting blood glucose levels ≥110 mg/dL (6.1 mmol/L) but ≤126 mg/dL (7.0 mmol/L) or 2 h values in the oral glucose tolerance test of ≥140 mg/dL (7.8 mmol/L) but ≤200 mg/dL (11.1 mmol/L). People who fall into this category have impaired glucose tolerance but are not yet considered to have diabetes. They may progress to diabetes or may remain impaired and never progress to diabetes.

Figures 9.10 and 9.11 show population figures with all causes and types of diabetes lumped together. Figure 9.12 shows the distribution of the different types of diabetes within the population with this disease. Not included are people with gestational diabetes and people for whom the diabetes is secondary to another disorder. Of the total population with diabetes mellitus, about 10% have the disease as a result of pancreatic insulin-production failure either due to autoimmune disease or secondary to a viral infection. Approximately 80% develop the disease as a response to

TABLE 9.7
Criteria for the Diagnosis of Diabetes Mellitus

(1) A1C ≥ 6.5%. The test should be performed in a laboratory using a method that is NGSP certified and standardized to the DCCT assay.[a]

OR

(2) Fasting blood glucose ≥126 mg/dL (7.0 mmol/L). Fasting is defined as no food intake for at least 8 h.[a]

OR

(3) Two-hour plasma glucose ≥200 mg/dL (11.1 mmol/L) during an oral glucose tolerance test.[a] The test should be performed as described by WHO[6] using a glucose load containing the equivalent of 75 g anhydrous glucose dissolved in water.

OR

(4) In a patient with classic symptoms of hyperglycemia or hyperglycemic crisis, a random plasma glucose ≥200 mg/dL (11.1 mmol/L).

Source: American Diabetes Association, American diabetes association: Clinical practice recommendations, *Diabetes Care*, 36, S1–S103, 2013.

[a] These measures should be repeated on a different day to confirm diagnosis.

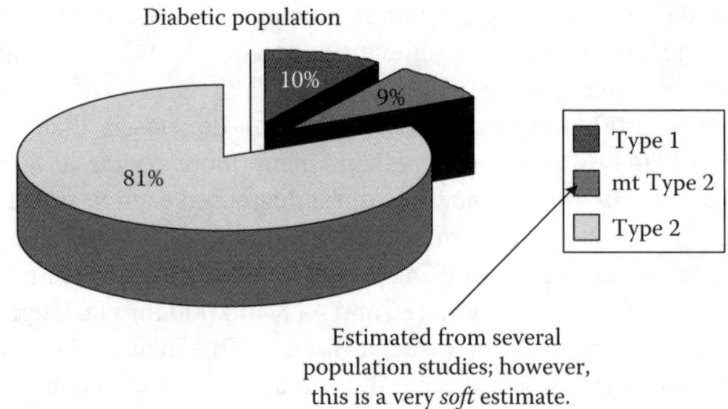

FIGURE 9.12 Distribution of people with different forms of diabetes. (From Prevalence of diabetes, impaired fasting glucose, and impaired glucose tolerance in US adults. NHANES III, 1988–1994, *Diabetes Care*, 21, S1–S144, 1998; National Center for Chronic Disease Prevention and Health Promotion, http://www.cdc.gov/diabetes/statistics/surv199/chap2/table0.1htm.)

one or more failures in the target tissues: liver, muscle, and/or adipose tissue. An additional 0.1% to 9% develop the disease as a consequence of mitochondrial failure. This estimate of the number of people with mitochondrial diabetes is a very *soft* figure because very few population studies have been conducted to document its prevalence.

While the number of people with type 1 diabetes has remained fairly constant since insulin replacement therapy was made possible, the number of people with type 2 diabetes is rapidly rising. In part, this is due to the rising prevalence of obesity and in part due to more active population screening and better treatment of the disease.

Clinicians divide the population with diabetes based on the therapy needed upon diagnosis; however, there is some blurring of this separation. Patients requiring hormone replacement upon disease recognition are type 1 patients, while those whose disease can be initially managed with diet, exercise, and/or oral medications are type 2 patients. In children, type 1 diabetes is of rapid onset and hormone replacement plus careful management of diet and activity is essential to the survival of the child. In adults, the division between type 1 and type 2 patients is sometimes unclear because type 2 patients might not be diagnosed early in their disease development. These patients may have progressed to islet cell exhaustion prior to diagnosis and thus require insulin replacement for survival.

Glucose Tolerance Test[36]

Although diabetes is a collection of diseases arising for a variety of reasons, its diagnosis is based on the results of a glucose tolerance test. Glucose tolerance is tested by giving the person a bolus (usually 1 g/kg body weight) of glucose in solution and monitoring the blood glucose level before and at 30 min intervals after the glucose bolus. Variations in the procedure have been developed for screening purposes. A single fasting blood sample may be examined for its glucose content, or a fasting plus a 2 h post meal blood sample may be examined, or the test may be 5 h in duration rather than the usual 2 h. The type of test is usually determined by the patient's symptoms and the family history. In normal nondiabetic fasted individuals, administration of a bolus of glucose elicits a typical rise then fall in blood glucose levels. In contrast, diabetic individuals may have an elevated fasting blood glucose level and/or may have a failure to appropriately reduce the glucose level after the test dose.

Abnormal glucose tolerance is defined in several ways: there may be a departure from the normal fasting blood glucose level (80–110 mg/dL, 4–6 mmol/L), and/or postchallenge values may be excessively high (exceeding 250 mg/dL) and/or fail to return to the prechallenge blood glucose level by 120 min after the challenge. Blood insulin values may exceed normal in some individuals, and this is interpreted as a sign of target tissue insulin resistance. These individuals are referred to as hyperinsulinemic. They may be hyperinsulinemic yet have normal blood glucose levels and normal glucose tolerance.

Genetics and Diabetes Mellitus

Currently, the number of genetic mutations thought to be responsible for the development of this disease is in excess of 300, depending on the definitions used for the disease. Type 2 diabetes, while more prevalent, has a more diverse genetic origin than does type 1 diabetes (Table 9.8). The number of genetic mutations thought to be responsible depends on the definitions used for the disease. A computer search of the Online Mendelian Inheritance in Man (http://www.OMIM.org, accessed February 14, 2013) revealed 338 entries of mutations associated with diabetes. Some of these mutations phenotype as other diseases that have diabetes as a secondary feature. A number of these are relatively rare diseases. Some of the reports relate to mutations associated with type 1 diabetes, while others associate with type 2 diabetes or with mitochondrial diabetes. Quite a bit of information suggests that the phenotypic expression of those mutations that associate with type 2 diabetes can be modified by environmental factors. Environmental influences may explain the discrepancy between the frequencies of the genotypes and phenotypes. That is, far more people have these mutations in their genome than the number of people who actually develop the disease diabetes mellitus.

TABLE 9.8
Mutations That Associate with Type 1 and Type 2 Diabetes Mellitus

Gene	Comments
Nuclear DNA	
Hepatic nuclear transcription factor 4α (MODY 1)	Subjects have impaired insulin secretion. 44 different mutations in this gene have been reported.[37,39]
GK (MODY 2)	Subjects are generally nonobese.[40–48]
Hepatic transcription factor 1α (MODY 3)	Hypertension and type 2 are found in this genotype, which is polymorphic.[41–43]
Glycogen synthase	Activation of the enzyme is impaired.[49]
Glucagon receptor	Susceptibility to type 2 is variable among different population groups.[50,51]
Insulin and the insulin receptor	Several mutations reported.[52–58]
	Associated with peripheral insulin resistance in some type 2 subjects.
IRS-1	Results in a signal transmission defect associated with insulin resistance.[59,60]
Mitochondrial α-glycerol 3 phosphate dehydrogenase	Associated with type 2 and with impaired mitochondrial function.[61]
GLUTs 1–4	Associated with both obesity and type 2 diabetes.[14–20]
Mitochondrial DNA[a 62–65]	
$tRNA^{leu}$	7 Mutations have been found that associate with diabetes.
ND 1	11 Mutations have been reported.
ND 2, ND 3, ND 4	1 Mutation in each of these genes has been reported.
$tRNA^{Cys, Ser, Lys}$	1 Mutation in each of these genes has been reported.
$tRNA^{thr}$	4 Mutations have been found.
D-Loop[b]	3 Mutations have been reported.
COX II	2 Mutations have been reported.
ATPases 6,8	4 Mutations have been reported.

[a] Mutations in the mitochondrial genome that associate with diabetes are heteroplasmic, that is, there is mixture of normal and abnormal DNAs in each cell. The percentage of the abnormal determines the degree to which the function of that cell is impaired.

[b] Promoter regions for the 13 structural genes found in the mitochondrial genome are found here.

In some of these mutations, there is an association with both obesity and diabetes. This means that if the food supply is abundant and people with these genotypes consume excess food that in turn results in excess body fat stores, they will become diabetic. If food is scarce, people with these genotypes do not become obese, nor do they become diabetic. Thus, if the people with these genotypes are physically active, they may not become obese and diabetic. Here is an example of the interaction of diet and exercise with one or more of the diabetes-associated gene mutations. In addition, there may be certain dietary constituents that may be particularly active with respect to enhancing or suppressing the phenotypic expression of the diabetes genotype. Studies in rodents have suggested that this may occur and these results may be applicable to humans.

There are additional groupings (not shown in Figure 9.12) that refer to specific circumstances. One is the diabetes that develops during pregnancy (gestational diabetes) that either disappears after pregnancy or goes on as type 2 diabetes. The other is impaired glucose tolerance (described above) that may or may not proceed into type 2 diabetes. In each of these instances, the patients are managed as though they were diabetic. Careful attention is paid to the diet as well as to physical activity. In the pregnant woman, as gestation proceeds, there may be a requirement for insulin supplementation. The physician will monitor this very carefully. Most obstetricians will observe the growth and development of the fetus and terminate the pregnancy as soon as it is apparent that the fetus can be delivered (by caesarian usually) and will do well. By paying careful attention to this problem, it is hoped that the unusually large baby typical of gestational diabetes can be avoided as well as the problem of neonatal hypoglycemia. Neonatal hypoglycemia is a response to the mother's inability to fully use glucose; the fetal islet cells respond to this by producing insulin in amounts larger than needed by the fetus. When the child is born, this insulin production must be downregulated to avoid the potentially dangerous hypoglycemia that could develop.

Type 1 Diabetes

Insulin deficiency is the result of β-cell loss. It is characterized by high blood glucose levels (hyperglycemia) that in turn result in the excessive thirst (polydipsia), excessive urine production (polyuria), and rapid weight loss. The body fat stores are raided, but fatty acid oxidation is incomplete. As a result, acetone, β-hydroxybutyrate, and acetoacetate, products of incomplete fatty acid oxidation, accumulate. These are the ketone bodies. Elevated blood levels of these ketones (ketonemia) are observed, as is an elevated urinary excretion (ketonuria). Rising levels of ketones increase the need for buffering power, since they tend to lower pH. Acidosis is a characteristic feature of diabetes. Not only are the fat stores raided, but so too is the body protein. Proteolysis (body protein breakdown) is enhanced and the amino acids thus liberated are used for energy or as substrates for intracellular glucose synthesis. The ammonia released as a product of the deamination of these amino acids assists in the buffering of the accumulating ketones. However, this ammonia is in itself cytotoxic, so the body must increase its capacity to convert it to urea. Humans with uncontrolled diabetes thus are characterized by a loss in body protein, an increase in blood and urine levels of ammonia, an increase in urea synthesis, a negative nitrogen balance, a loss in fat store, elevated blood and urine levels of glucose, and elevated levels of fatty acid oxidation products. Some of these metabolic products are also excreted via the lungs in the expired air. The breath of an uncontrolled diabetic has the aroma of the ketones—somewhat like the aroma of fingernail-polish remover.

Two causes of pancreatic insulin-production failure have been identified: destructions of the islet cells due to autoimmune disease and/or to viruses. In each of these instances, the genetic heritage of the individual plays a role. In both, the immune system is involved.

Autoimmune Disease

Autoimmune diabetes can be accompanied by a number of other diseases; multiple endocrine failures are not uncommon. This means that autoimmune diabetes can be found in a person who also develops psoriasis, rheumatoid arthritis, or thyroiditis (inflammation of the thyroid gland).

In autoimmune diabetes, there may be an immune tolerance that is particularly difficult to break. This is because the body may lack antibody specificity. Antibodies can be raised that will react to a group of closely related compounds in an instance of *mistaken identity*. Usually, an antibody reacts to a single antigen rather than to a group of closely related antigens. In autoimmune disease, the body tolerates a range of exposures to these antigens before it reacts. Thus, the term immune tolerance means that the individual will tolerate a wide range of exposures to an antigen or group of antigens before a systemic immunologic reaction is elicited. This is not the same thing as food allergies or skin allergies or localized reactions to allergens. Neither should this term immune tolerance be confused with diseases of the immune system per se.

Autoimmunity is characterized by an increase in the number of T cells. The T cell originates in the thymus and is a type of cell that is an essential component of the immune system. The B cell originates in the bone marrow and produces antibodies in response to an antigen. T cells interact with B cells in order to initiate antibody production. In some instances, the recognition is nonspecific. That is, antibodies are produced that react to a group of related antigens. In autoimmune disease, this is what happens. There is a loss in antigen recognition specificity and the immune system reacts to a group of related compounds. Some of these are self-proteins, while others are from the environment. In each situation, the self-proteins are destroyed and the cells that produce them are destroyed as well. In the instance of the β-cells, the immune system is responding to proteins in these cells and thus is destroying them. Immunosuppression drugs can interfere with this destruction, but the use of such drugs has its own set of problems, such as kidney disease or increased susceptibility to infectious disease. The immunologic response is initiated when the T-cell receptor recognizes an antigen on the correct histocompatibility complex on the surface of the antigen-presenting cell. Transmission of this signal to the nucleus of the cell involves the calcium ion, a complex of related proteins, and the PI cycle, which is responsible for the movement of the calcium ion from the intracellular store to where it is needed. Antigens are then produced. Figure 9.13 illustrates the immune system.

Autoimmune disease can result when mutations in the genes that encode the various components of the immune system occur and the body's own protein is recognized as foreign. The body then develops antibodies that effectively destroy that protein.

Several cell surface proteins (Table 9.9) have been found to elicit antibody production.

The autoimmune destruction of the β-cell is associated with one or more mutations in the genes that encode the major histocompatibility complex (MHC). These genes have been mapped to the short arm of chromosome 6 and comprise approximately 2×10^6 nucleotides. Mutations in these genes have been divided into two classes (I and II) and are further identified by letter designations. There are so many genes that it would be impossible to list them all in this text. Suffice it to say that

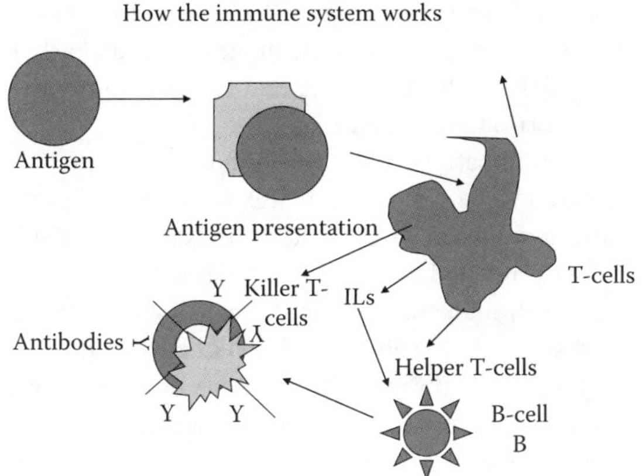

FIGURE 9.13 Schematic for the immune system.

TABLE 9.9
Autoantigens That Elicit Islet Cell–Reactive Antibodies in Humans with Autoimmune Type 1 Diabetes Mellitus

Autoantigen	Comments
GAD	Antibodies present before clinical state develops
Insulin (58,000 kDa, 51 amino acids)	Antibodies found after diagnosis
Insulin receptor	Antibodies found after diagnosis
38,000 Mr	Antibodies develop in patients with insulinoma
RIN polar	Antibodies that are related to those formed in response to certain gangliosides
52,000 Mr	Antibodies present before clinical state develops; likely the same as GAD
Carboxypeptidase H	Cell surface autoantigen and a major protein in insulin secretory granules
ICA 12/ICA 512	Putative islet cell antigens
PM-1 60,000 Mr	A 24-amino acid peptide that may be a polyclonal activator of autoreactive T cells
IAAb (antialgAb)	Anti-immunoglobulin antibodies that appear prior to IDDM[a]
C-peptide	Antibodies found after IDDM diagnosis

[a] IDDM, type 1 insulin-dependent diabetes mellitus.

class II HLA genes are more closely linked to autoimmune diabetes than are class I HLA genes. In rodents (db/db mice and BB rats), several mutations in the MHC region have been identified that express themselves as autoimmune diabetes mellitus. These rodents have been studied extensively and have helped scientists understand the process of the disease.

The development of autoimmune diabetes is associated with an inflammation of the pancreatic islet cells (insulitis). In insulitis, CD4 and CD8 T cells, B cells, macrophages, and killer T cells have all been found. The presence of these marker cells indicates that an immunologic reaction is taking place. In humans with autoimmune diabetes, islet cell antibodies to cytoplasmic self-proteins were reported in 1974. Following this initial report, many different antibodies reacting to a variety of self-proteins and non-self-proteins have been reported. Glutamic acid decarboxylase (GAD), an enzyme found in β-cells that catalyzes the synthesis of the neurotransmitter gamma amino butyric acid (GABA), has been shown to be an antigen. Islet β-cells, like neuronal cells, possess a mechanism for hormone release that depends on a specific trophic stimulus. GABA and GAD are components of this secretion signaling system, as is GLUT2, and the enzyme, GK, and the mitochondrial oxidative phosphorylation (OXPHOS) system that produces ATP. ATP and the calcium ion are major players in the insulin-release mechanism.

Autoantibodies to GAD have been observed prior to the development of the clinical type 1 diabetes, and the presence of these antibodies has been suggested as an early indication of the disease. The gene for GAD has been cloned, characterized, and mapped to chromosome 10. Two isoforms (a 65 kDa form and a 67 kDa form) have been isolated, and a single gene encodes each. While antibodies to GAD have been found in patients with autoimmune diabetes, the GAD itself is not abnormal nor has its gene been found to be abnormal. It was then concluded that these antibodies were reacting to a similar protein but not to the GAD protein. This is where the loss of antigen specificity is shown. Antibodies are being generated to a protein similar to but not identical to the GAD protein.

Although GAD antibodies can indicate incipient type 1 diabetes, these antibodies are also elevated in other autoimmune diseases in the absence of diabetic symptoms; yet, in each disease, there are distinct differences in epitope recognition. This suggests that the autoantigen is being presented to the T cells and the B cells by different mechanisms. However, so many have been reported that it is difficult to assign causality to any of them. For example, islet cell antibodies to plasma insulin C-peptide have been reported in adults having diabetes for at least 10 years. Antibodies to insulin have been found in newly diagnosed children but not in their high-risk relatives. This suggests that these antibodies are a result, not a cause, of the disease. As mentioned, GAD antibodies have been reported to occur prior to the development of diabetic symptoms, so it is possible that they may serve as an early marker of autoimmune disease.

Diabetes Secondary to Viral Infections

Epidemiologists have noted that following epidemics of diseases such as flu (influenza), there are upsurges in the numbers of people with newly diagnosed type 1 diabetes.[66–70] Not all people who develop flu develop diabetes, nor have all people who develop type 1 diabetes had their disease preceded by flu. Other infections (mumps, rubella) can also precede diabetes. Infections due to cytomegalovirus, the Epstein–Barr virus, the picornaviruses (which include several strains of encephalomyocarditis virus—the foot-and-mouth disease virus), and a number of the coxsackie B viruses can precede diabetes in susceptible individuals. These persistent infections can cause damage in addition to the typical lytic effect that occurs during the acute phase. Damage can take the form of producing (or inducing) small changes in cell proteins that change the function of the protein or change the recognition of this protein as a normal cell constituent. These slightly modified self-proteins then are recognized as foreign, and an antibody is produced to destroy it. One such protein is the islet cell surface (ICS) protein. Antibodies to ICS have been found in virally infected humans. Viruses also induce the production of cytokines such as interferon, the interleukins, and tumor necrosis factor. These substances alter the immune response by regulating the expression of β-cell antigens and thus contribute to the development of insulitis. The mechanisms whereby viruses induce diabetes have been the subject of considerable speculation.

There appears to be a genetic determination of susceptibility to these infections that probably involves genes that encode the various components of the immune system. This explains why some humans may develop diabetes secondary to a viral infection, while others do not. Notkins and coworkers have demonstrated that susceptibility is compatible with a single gene acting in an autosomal recessive manner.[69] The mode of action of such a gene would be to control specific virus receptors on the β-cell membrane or perhaps to control the membrane permeability to such viruses, thus facilitating the incorporation of the viral DNA into the β-cell DNA and altering its function. Fluorescein labeling of viral antibody has confirmed the entry of the coxsackie B virus into β-cells, as well as changes in β-cell mRNA. Here is another example of an interaction between the environment and genetics. If the genetic material is such that the immune system is somewhat incompetent in its response to a particular virus, then the viruses will inflict serious damage on the β-cell. In persons with a fully competent immune system, such damage does not occur. Evidence of virus-induced diabetes in humans has been gathered through postmortem studies of pancreatic tissue excised from children with fatal viral infections.[70] Of the 250 children studied, seven had a coxsackie B infection, and of these, four had significant β-cell destruction and evidence of acute or chronic inflammation in the islet tissue. Whether immunization against these viruses is possible and will prevent this disorder is a significant research problem.

MUTATIONS ASSOCIATED WITH TYPE 2 DIABETES

Insulin Release

Although rare, persons with mutations in the gene for the pancreatic glucose–sensing enzyme GK have provided insights into how insulin is released by the pancreatic β-cell.[37–48] The β-cell GK plays a pivotal role in the cascade of events leading to the release of the insulin molecule by the β-cell (see subsequent discussion of maturity-onset diabetes of the young [MODY]). There are several important players: the GLUT 2, the GK enzyme, and the mitochondrial system (OXPHOS) that produces the energy (ATP) needed for both insulin synthesis and release, for the movement of the sodium

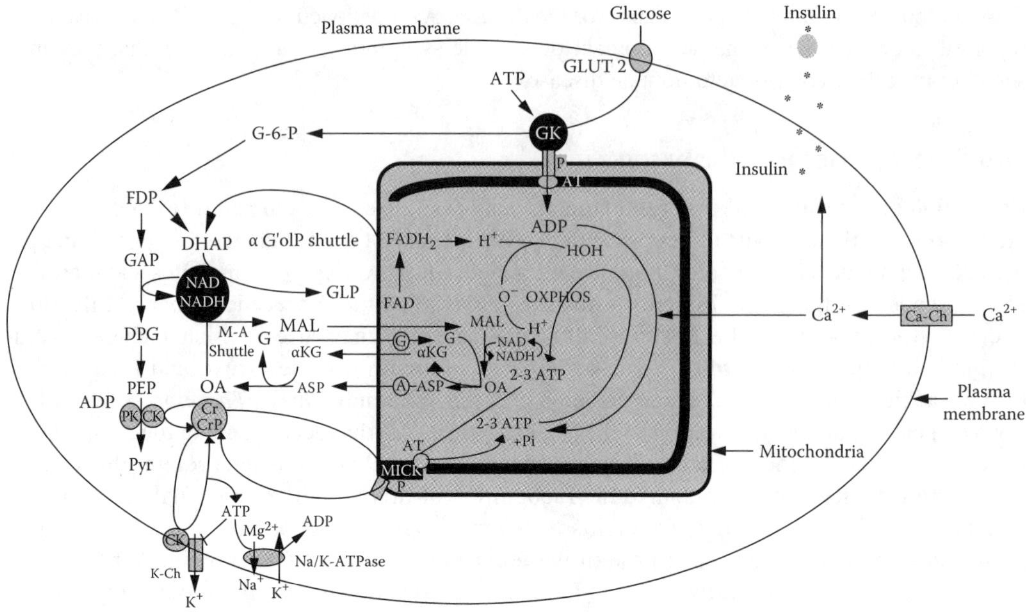

FIGURE 9.14 Proposed mechanism for the release of insulin by the pancreatic β-cell. Abbreviations used are those for glucose metabolism: GLUT 2, mobile GLUT 2; ATP, adenine triphosphate; G6P, glucose-6-phosphate; FDP, fructose diphosphate; GAP, glyceraldehyde phosphate; PEP, phosphoenolpyruvate; DHAP-α G'olP shuttle, glycerol phosphate shuttle; MAL, malate; OXPHOS, oxidative phosphorylation. The inner compartment shown here is the mitochondrial compartment.

(Na^+), potassium (K^+), and calcium (Ca^{++}) ions and for the Na^+K^+ATPase.[27] Shown in Figure 9.14 is a proposed mechanism whereby the islet cell is stimulated to release insulin.

Rising levels of glucose in the blood promotes the uptake of this glucose by the β-cell. The GLUT 2 facilitates its entry and the ATP-dependent GK facilitates the phosphorylation of this glucose. If either the GLUT or the GK is abnormal due to a mutation in the genes that encode either of these proteins, then the glucose-sensing system that is part of the insulin-release process will not work appropriately, and the β-cell will not respond appropriately to the glucose signal. Actually, numerous mutations have been reported for the GK gene, yet altogether these many mutations are thought to account for less than 0.1% of the population with diabetes mellitus. Indeed, there is some argument as to whether these people should be included in type 1 category rather than type 2. Usually, they are thought to have type 2 diabetes because although abnormal, the islets do respond to some secretagogues such as amino acids (leucine, glutamine, arginine) and fatty acids (palmitate) as well as some metabolites (inosine and membrane-permeant analogs of pyruvate and succinate) and do produce and release insulin.[27,28] Again, lifestyle choice determines whether hormone supplements are required for the successful management of the disease.

Maturity-Onset Diabetes of the Young

Within the category of type 2 diabetes (Table 9.8) is a subgroup called MODY. People with this form of diabetes have a problem with the responsiveness of the pancreas to changes in blood glucose level. The islet cells do not adequately sense blood glucose change and therefore do not release appropriate amounts of insulin in response. There are three major groups of mutations that phenotype as MODY. One group (MODY 1) has mutations in the gene for hepatic nuclear factor 4α.[37,38] A second group has mutations in the gene for pancreatic GK (MODY 2),[39–45] and a third group (MODY 3) has mutations in the gene for hepatic nuclear factor 1α.[46,48] The hepatic nuclear factors are thought to serve as DNA transcription enhancers in the islet cell and other cells as well and are abbreviated HNF 1 or 4α. As can be seen in Table 9.8, MODY is associated with a large number of mutations. Theoretically, people with the MODY gene mutations could, through appropriate food choice, avoid diabetic symptoms. With problems in glucose sensing, these people would benefit from diets that do not challenge the islet cells with excessive loads of glucose. Using low-glucose (as well as other simple sugars that can be converted to glucose) diets, these patients could reduce the metabolic problems associated with the sensing of blood glucose by the islet cell. A diet with glucose coming from complex carbohydrates would be a benefit to these people because it would provide a leveling of glucose influx from the diet. Also, a diet where the major energy sources are proteins and fats might be useful since these foods also do not stress the islet cell. There are some amino acids, some metabolites, and some fatty acid analogs that stimulate insulin release, but these substances do this using sensing systems that do not involve the GK reaction.

The MODY mutations are inherited as autosomal dominant traits. While all MODY patients have an islet cell secretory defect, MODY 1 and MODY 3 patients also manifest a defective responsiveness to the glucose-lowering effect of insulin. Thus, they are classed as insulin resistant. If given a dose of insulin, this insulin is less effective in lowering blood glucose than a person without these genetic defects. This is because the hepatic transcription factors 1α and 4α affect the transcription of several of the genes that encode the enzymes of intermediary metabolism. These enzymes are critical to the appropriate oxidation of glucose, and if less than optimally active, glucose will not be as easily oxidized, hence the apparent reduction in glucose uptake and use by the target tissues. Indeed, some of the common hepatic nuclear factor 4α variants are associated with high serum lipids and metabolic syndrome.[37]

Genetic Errors in Insulin Structure

In addition to failure of the islet cell to release insulin in response to a glucose signal, the possibility exists that the islet cell may not be producing insulin in the appropriate amino acid sequence to have full biological activity. Insulin gene mutations have been documented in both humans and mice. These mutations result in a variety of amino acid substitutions and have a variety of effects on insulin action. These mutations are very rare. Steiner et al.,[58] for example, studied a number of families with aberrant insulin genes. Ten families were studied that had single-point mutations that resulted in amino acid substitutions in the proinsulin molecule. Six of these substitutions resulted in the secretion of defective insulin molecules due to changes within the A or B chains. These changes resulted in molecules that were immunoreactive but did not bind adequately to the plasma membrane insulin receptor on the adipocyte. Four additional families were found to have insulin gene mutations that prevented the recognition of the C-peptide–A chain dibasic cleavage site and its removal. When insulin is ready for release, a fraction of this large molecule is split off. This fraction is called the C-chain or C-peptide. If not removed, proinsulin circulates in the blood. It is 1/40 to 1/60 times as active as insulin. The aberrant proinsulin molecule may have the appropriate β-cell–processing protease but not the appropriate C-peptide recognition site. Families with this genetic error have high levels of proinsulin in the blood.

The variability of the insulin gene in a group of phenotypically normal individuals has been studied. Although several variants have been found, none were considered mutants. That is, the base pair substitutions that coded for specific amino acids in the insulin molecules were in places that did not affect the conformation of the molecule or the active site of the insulin molecule nor affect the cleavage of proinsulin to active insulin. The variety of base pair substitutions and subsequent amino acid substitutions in the insulin molecule appears to be large, yet the impact of these aberrations (if they can be called aberrations) is very small or nonexistent. However, should substitutions occur that affect proinsulin cleavage or reactive sites in the insulin molecule as described earlier, then diabetes would develop. Whether the diabetes is type 1 or type 2, would, as mentioned, depend on the nature of the defect.

Mitochondrial Diabetes

There is a third form of the disease that does not follow Mendelian genetics; it is the diabetes that occurs due to a mutation in the mitochondrial genome (see Table 9.8).[62–65] Mutation in this genome results in an impaired production of ATP. ATP is essential to the synthesis of insulin in the islet cell and also is essential to the activity of the glucose-sensing enzyme GK and to the release of insulin in response to the glucose signal (Figure 9.14). ATP is also essential to intermediary metabolism. In patients with these mutations, diabetes may be secondary to more serious neuromuscular disease or to neuronal disease that occurs due to a shortfall in ATP for the neuronal pathways. These pathways are exquisitely dependent on adequate ATP supplies. The central nervous system is the largest consumer of ATP followed by pancreatic islet cells and renal cells. Diabetes occurs in patients whose mutation burden is not high enough to manifest the severe neuronal or neuromuscular diseases. Recognition of diabetes as a phenotype for mitochondrial DNA mutation has been fairly recent so the numbers of people with diabetes due to this cause are poor estimates at best. Furthermore, diabetes itself can cause mitochondrial DNA mutations,[64] and it is difficult to assign causality to the mutation without familial studies that show that the appearance of the mutation appears before the appearance of the signs and symptoms of diabetes. Current estimates of the number of people with diabetes due to a mitochondrial mutation vary from 0.1% to 10% of the population with diabetes (Figure 9.12).

Peripheral Insulin Resistance

Insulin resistance due to mutations in the genes for the insulin receptors in fat cells, muscle cells, and liver cells has been reported. Insulin receptors have been isolated and their structures analyzed and sequenced. It is generally agreed that the receptor is synthesized as a single polypeptide precursor of 1382 amino acids that contains a signal peptide of 27 amino acids, the α-subunit of 735 amino acids (including four basic amino acids of the processing site), and the β-subunit of 620 amino acids. After glycosylation, processing, and disulfide bonding, it is expressed as a heterotetramer composed of two α-subunits with a molecular weight of 95,000. The α-subunit is entirely located on the exterior aspect of the plasma membrane, while the β-subunit extends through the plasma membrane into the cytoplasm. The human insulin receptor gene is located on chromosome 19. It consists of 22 exons. The α-subunit is encoded by the first 120 kb and includes a signal peptide, an insulin-binding region, and a cysteine-rich region. The β-subunit is encoded by the last 30 kb. As mentioned, this subunit is the portion of the receptor molecule that crosses the plasma membrane. It has a proreceptor-processing site and the final portion of the unit of the receptor molecule consists of tyrosine kinase. When insulin binds to the α-subunit, autophosphorylation occurs, resulting in activation of tyrosine kinase. If the DNA coding for the receptor protein has mutated such that lysine, an important amino acid for ATP binding and receptor activity, is replaced by arginine, alanine, or methionine, the receptor is no longer able to mediate insulin action. Thus, lysine is a critical component of the ATP-binding site. Clusters of tyrosine residues are also critical to the autophosphorylation process. If tyrosine is replaced by phenylalanine, again, receptor activity is compromised. Other mutations in the code for the receptor protein that affect its amino acid sequence have been reported.[51–56] These mutations (depending on their location) likewise can affect the activity of the receptor and, in turn, can explain insulin resistance.

A person with insulin resistance may *not* develop abnormal glucose tolerance if (1) the individual is physically active and/or (2) the pancreas is able to sustain an abnormally high insulin output and (3) the person maintains a low body fat. In this circumstance, the individual may be insulin resistant and hyperinsulinemic, but not hyperglycemic or having abnormal glucose tolerance. Eventually, the islet β-cells may not be able to sustain this high insulin output, and the insulin resistance will then progress to abnormal glucose tolerance and subsequently to the diabetic hyperglycemic state. Physical activity stimulates the noninsulin-dependent entry of glucose into the exercising muscle.

This reduces the level of circulating glucose and thus assists in maintaining normal glucose homeostasis. In addition, the very active individual will be less likely to accumulate excess fat stores, and this too contributes to the maintenance of glucose homeostasis. The ADA recommends that people with diabetes exercise 2.5 h/week with an exercise that raises the heart rate to 50%–70% of capacity. Many activities can do this, not just the traditional jogging or cycling activity.[71]

One feature of type 2 diabetes is excess fat stores. With enlarged fat cells, there is resistance of the cell to the effects of insulin.[72] When the fat cell becomes enlarged, it loses its responsiveness to the action of insulin in facilitating the entry of glucose into that fat cell. For decades, it has been known that overly fat people who are insulin resistant can reverse their condition by restricting their energy intake, thereby reducing their excess fat store. When the adipocyte returns to its normal size, it becomes normally responsive to the action of insulin. For many years, it was thought that the enlarged fat cell receptor defect was simply due to a distortion of the plasma membrane insulin receptor brought about by the increased fat store. In some instances, this may be true. However, it is now thought that the resistance of the enlarged fat cell favors its smaller neighbors that bind insulin normally.

In addition to mutations in the genes for the insulin receptor, mutations in the downstream signaling (the INS-1 system) have been found.[60] These mutations result in impaired signal transduction from the receptor to the downstream reactions that metabolize glucose in the cell. Mutations in the genes for this system result in impaired glucose use. Signals generated when insulin binds to its receptor on the plasma membrane are needed for the recruitment of the GLUTs from their storage sites on the endoplasmic reticulum to the plasma membrane and thus transport glucose into the cell and present it to the various enzymes for metabolism. As the aforementioned, aberrations in the genes for the GLUTs likewise can associate with diabetes particularly that associated with obesity. Finally, mutations in the mitochondrial genome can affect the amount of ATP available for glucose metabolism. Again, glucose metabolism will be aberrant and this aberration fits the description of diabetes.

While the information provided in Table 9.8 is useful in understanding the genetic basis of diabetes, it is altogether possible that the mutations listed here are merely characteristic of the disorder not causal. Some of these mutations have been identified as being associated with the diabetic state, and some of the mutations cause other metabolic problems that in turn elicit abnormalities in glucose metabolism. In other words, not all of the mutations listed here are truly causal. The ADA[34,36] reminds diabetologists that there are numerous reasons why diabetes develops and only some of these reasons are genetic in nature. Endocrine diseases such as Cushing's disease (adrenal steroid hypersecretion) have diabetes as its secondary characteristic. When the primary disease is managed, diabetes disappears. There are other instances as well of diabetes appearing as a secondary consequence of a primary disease. In fact, most of the mutations in the mitochondrial genome could be classified in this way.[62–65,73] Mutations in this genome when mutation load is high elicit some very serious diseases involving the central nervous system, the neuromuscular system, and the sensory system as well as intermediary metabolism. When the mutation load is high, these primary diseases receive the clinician's attention. That diabetes also develops is a secondary concern. Lastly, those mutations that phenotype primarily as obesity may also have diabetes as a secondary condition. If obesity could be managed (fat stores are reduced), then diabetes might be mitigated. However, most of the cases of genetic obesity are extremely difficult to manage if the mutations have occurred in the genes that encode components of the food intake regulation system. The Prader–Willi syndrome is a prime example of this type of genetic disorder. Persons with this disorder have insatiable appetites and become exceedingly obese. Diabetes is a secondary consequence of this massive obesity that shortens the life span of the affected individual.

However, there are mutations that elicit both obesity or excessive fat stores and diabetes. Examples here are the mutations in the genes that encode the intracellular GLUTs 1–4. Mutations in one or more of these genes can phenotype as both excessive fatness and diabetes. It is a condition that could be viewed not as the primary/secondary related condition but as a coequal syndrome. Both diabetes and excess fat stores develop at similar times. If there is insulin resistance, there will be a reduction in the insulin effect on the mobilization of the GLUTs.[20,74] Similarly, if the transporter gene(s) is aberrant, although there is sufficient insulin bound to the receptor site, glucose is inadequately transported into the cell due to the GLUT gene mutation and hence is inadequately metabolized. Furthermore, if there is a defect in GLUT, there is an increase in intramyocellular lipid metabolism as well as a reduction in muscle glycogen synthesis.[74] The fatty metabolites lead to a defect in insulin receptor substrate (IRS-1) signaling through serine/threonine phosphorylation. This results in muscle insulin resistance and the appearance of diabetes. A similar mechanism is proposed for liver where an aberration of the hepatic GLUT gene could lead to a fatty liver and reduced mitochondrial function mostly attributed to a reduction in mitochondrial density.

Animal Models for Humans with Type 2 Diabetes

Much of what we have learned about diabetes has come from studies of animals that develop the disease.[75,76] Type 1 diabetes can be mimicked through chemical ablation of the islet cells using either surgical ablation of the pancreas or the administration of either alloxan or streptozotocin. Alloxan is a powerful oxidizing chemical. It works by attacking the β-cells of the pancreas. There is one mouse model that is resistant to alloxan.[75] Alloxan-resistant mice have an equally powerful antioxidant system that suppresses the oxidant action of alloxan. This suggests that there may be humans that are diabetes resistant for the same reason. They may possess sufficient antioxidant power to suppress the oxidant actions on the pancreas of a variety of insults from intermittent anoxia, viral attack, or certain chemicals in the environment. There are also animals that become diabetic through a spontaneous mutation in their genome. These animal models are listed in Table 9.10.

Animals that are genetically obese usually overeat, and studies of the neuroendocrine influence on food intake have suggested that, in part, the genetic error in these animals may reside in the satiety signaling system in the brain.[77] In the obese ob/ob mouse, the mutation involves the production of the satiety signaling cytokine leptin. In the db/db mouse and the fa/fa rat, the mutation is that of the gene for the leptin receptor. In all of the animal models for obesity described to date that have hyperphagia as a part of its character, the satiety signal leptin is either missing or ineffective due to an aberrant leptin receptor.

There could be other aberrant signals and receptors as well. Adiponectin is a candidate for its role in satiety signaling. If in low amount, fatty acid oxidation is faulty. Adiponectin seems to play a role in stimulating metabolism and metabolic turnover. Low levels of adiponectin are associated with obesity and insulin resistance as well as with a condition known as polycystic ovary syndrome (PCOS).[78–82] Variants in the adiponectin gene and in the adiponectin receptor gene are associated with overall adiposity especially in the abdomen.[83]

Lastly, animal models of type 2 diabetes have been produced through genetic engineering.[84,85] In these animals, an aberrant gene is inserted into a fertilized egg. Transgenic mice have been produced harboring aberrant genes for the insulin receptor, the IRS-1, hexokinase, GLUT 1 or 4, PEPCK (the rate-limiting enzyme in gluconeogenesis, phosphoenolpyruvate carboxykinase), and one of the G proteins (the protein that inhibits adenylyl cyclase). No doubt other transgenic mice have been constructed as well allowing researchers to learn how single mutations can phenotype as diabetes and whether environmental manipulations such as dietary variation can affect phenotypic expression. Knockout mice have also been produced allowing researchers to learn the function of some of the more obscure proteins involved in pancreatic function and glucose homeostasis. In these models, a specific gene is removed from the fertilized egg that encodes a specific protein. Knockout models for the GLUTs as well as some of the signaling molecules such as IRS-1 have been produced. Recently, a knockout mouse in which the gene for resistin was reported.[86] Resistin is an adipocyte-secreted protein that circulates at increased levels in obesity. Acute administration of resistin to normal mice results in an impaired glucose tolerance. This was found to be due to an effect of resistin on glucose production via an increased expression of the gene for PEPCK.

TABLE 9.10
Animal Models for Type 2 Diabetes Mellitus and Characteristics

1. Low-dose chemical (streptozotocin and alloxan) treatment that reduces the capacity of the insulin-producing cells of the pancreas.
2. C57BL/KS db/db mouse; initially hyperinsulinemic and hyperphagic; obese; hyperglycemic; insulin resistant. When β-cells collapse and necrotize, mice are hypoinsulinemic, hyperglycemic, and ketotic and have a shortened life span.
3. BL/6J ob/ob mouse; defective leptin gene; obese, insulin resistant, hyperinsulinemic; when the ob gene is placed on the BL/Ks background, the features are not as severe.
4. Agouti or yellow obese mouse; obese trait is a dominant trait and only heterozygotes exist. Homozygosity is lethal. Hyperglycemia, hyperphagia, enlarged adrenals.
5. KK mouse; hyperphagia, moderate obesity, hyperglycemia.
6. PBB/Ld mouse; latent obesity and hyperglycemia, insulin resistance, hyperlipidemia.
7. NZO mouse; obese; mild hyperglycemia and hyperinsulinemia.
8. Zucker fa/fa rat; hyperphagic, hyperglycemic, insulin resistant.
9. BBZ/Wor rat; cross between Zucker and autoimmune diabetic BB rat; divergent progeny segregate into lean and obese phenotypes.
10. SHR/N-cp rat; hypertensive, hyperglycemic, obese.
11. BHE/Cdb rats; hyperglycemic at maturity; early hyperinsulinemia that subsides to hypoinsulinemia; models the human with diabetes due to mitochondrial mutation.
12. Spiny mice (*Acomys cahirinus*); obese, β-cell hypertrophy; with age, β-cells collapse with onset of hypoinsulinemia, ketosis, hyperinsulinemia, and early death.
13. Psammomys obesus (sand rat); obese, insulin resistant, hyperinsulinemia, at midlife islets are depleted and symptoms of diabetes appear followed by early death.
14. Chinese hamster (*Cricetulus griseus*); four gene mutations seem to be involved; hyperphagic, obese, hyperglycemic, insulin resistant.
15. Djungarian hamster (*Phodopus sungorus*) and South African hamster (*Mystromys albicaudatus*) are spontaneously diabetic but have not been genetically characterized.

Population Surveys Relating Diet to Diabetes

West and Kalbfleisch[87] were among the first to suggest that diet played a role in the development of diabetes. Sixteen countries were surveyed examining adults over the age of 30. They found a positive association between the prevalence of diabetes and the intake of both fats and sugars. There was a negative association of diabetes with total carbohydrate intake and correlations between diabetes and serum cholesterol and with body fat. This was one of the first papers to point out the relationship between nutritional status and diabetes.

Following the NHANES observations of rises in both obesity and type 2 diabetes, a number of surveys of different population groups were conducted. Wirfalt et al.[88] examined the relationship between food patterns and five components of the metabolic syndrome in Sweden. They reported that consumption of high sugar, bread, cheese, cake, and alcoholic beverages was associated with increased development of metabolic syndrome. Metabolic syndrome is a combination of indicators for diabetes, obesity, and cardiovascular disease. In women, increased dairy food consumption provided a protective effect with respect to type 2 diabetes. They concluded that there may be gender differences in how different foods affect metabolic consequences with respect to diabetes. The studies of van Dam et al.[89] asked a somewhat similar question. They found that following a prudent diet reduced the risk for developing type 2 diabetes and that following a *nonprudent* diet together with inactivity had the reverse effect especially in men. Mennen et al.[90] reported that increased bread and/or dairy product consumption might be related to an increased risk of developing metabolic syndrome. In contrast, Alvarez-Leon et al.[8] reported on an inverse relationship between dairy food intake and hypertension, stroke, and colorectal cancer. Mensink[91] followed this with a summary of the epidemiological evidence supporting a negative association of dairy food consumption and the development of type 2 diabetes. Those populations consuming dairy products were at less risk to develop type 2 diabetes as well as metabolic syndrome than populations consuming a low dairy food diet. Meyer et al.[92] reported that there was an inverse relationship between the incidence of type 2 diabetes and the intake of vegetable fat as well as with the substitution of polyunsaturated fat for saturated fat in the daily diet of older women in Iowa. Lopez-Ridaura et al.[93] reported that after adjusting for age, body mass index, physical activity, family history, and hypercholesterolemia at baseline, the relative risk of developing type 2 diabetes in women was 0.66, while for men, it was 0.67 comparing the highest to the lowest of magnesium intakes. These findings suggested that there was a negative association between magnesium intake and diabetes risk. That is, at higher magnesium intake, the risk of developing diabetes falls. Song et al.[94,95] and Ma et al.[96] reached a similar conclusion through estimating magnesium intakes and measuring insulin levels or examining the data from the Insulin Resistance Atherosclerosis Study (IRAS). In another population study using 12,700 participants without evidence of diabetes, serum magnesium levels were inversely correlated with fasting serum insulin, plasma glucose, plasma high-density lipoproteins, and diastolic and systolic blood pressure. These findings were similar to those reported by Humphries et al.[97] and Rosolova[98] suggesting that since dairy foods provide so much magnesium (~16% of the daily magnesium intake), these foods would be beneficial with respect to insulin action and glucose homeostasis. It should be noted that one of the secondary effects of diabetes is a weakening or demineralization of the bones.[99–104] Some of this bone demineralization can be reversed with good insulin treatment and good glucose control as well as a regular exercise program. Exercise on its own can assist in glucoregulation.[104,105]

In the CARDIA study, young (18–30 years of age) adults were examined over 10 years to determine associations between the consumption of dairy products, obesity, and the development of insulin resistance.[106] They found that the consumption of dairy products was inversely related to the development of insulin resistance. In a continuing survey of the nutrient contributions of dairy products, Weinberg et al.[107] reported that the consumption of these foods was associated with higher intakes of micronutrients without any adverse effects on either the fat intake of these people or their cholesterol intake.

Berkey et al.[108] studied adolescents with respect to dairy intake, dietary calcium intake, and body weight gain. Those subjects consuming the most dairy food gained the least weight. Multivariant analysis of milk, dairy fat, calcium, and total energy intake suggested that energy intake was the most important predictor of weight gain by these adolescents. Liu et al.[109] examined the food intakes of calcium and vitamin D of 10,066 middle-aged and older women and the prevalence of metabolic syndrome. Dietary vitamin D was inversely associated with metabolic syndrome, but this effect was not independent of the calcium intake. A similar relationship was reported for the consumption of dairy foods and metabolic syndrome. The report was seconded by Azadbakht et al.[110] in Iranian adults. Those consuming more dairy food were less likely to develop metabolic syndrome. Rajpathak et al.[111] reported on the long-term (12 years) weight gain in men. When the data were adjusted for potential confounders, there was no association between a change in calcium intake or dairy food intake and weight gain. These data did not support the hypothesis that an increase in calcium intake or dairy consumption could result in a lower long-term weight gain in men.

Prospective Studies Linking Food Intake to a Reduction in Type 2 Diabetes

Salmeron et al.[112] prospectively followed 84,204 women aged 34–59 with no history of diabetes, cardiovascular disease, or cancer. They were particularly interested in the role of fat (both type and amount) in the development of diabetes. They found no association between total fat, monounsaturated fatty acids, and saturated fatty acids and type 2 diabetes. They did note that trans fatty acids increase and polyunsaturated fatty acids reduce the risk for diabetes. Song et al.[95] asked a similar question with respect to red meat intake and type 2 diabetes. An increase in red meat consumption was related to an increase in risk for type 2 diabetes. Liu et al.[113] and also Choi et al.[114] conducted a prospective study of dairy intake and the risk of type 2 diabetes. They found an inverse relationship between the two.

Dietary Intervention in Diabetes

As pointed out earlier, diabetes is often associated with obesity. Thus, it should come as no surprise that intervention strategies that target obesity will have an effect on the time course of diabetes development. Marshall et al.[115] studied 134 subjects with impaired glucose tolerance. Those subjects consuming 40.6% of their intake energy as fat were less likely to proceed onto type 2 diabetes than those subjects consuming 43.4% of their daily energy intake as fat. These authors concluded that the level of fat consumption significantly affected diabetes risk even after correcting for obesity and markers for abnormal glucose metabolism. The implication is that the fat intake can significantly affect the time course for diabetes development.

King and Dowd[116] as well as Stern,[117] Melander,[118] and Kumar et al.[119] have reviewed the literature on the prevention of type 2 diabetes. Table 9.11 provides a summary of some of these studies.

From the diet perspective, reduction in the conversion of impaired glucose tolerance to type 2 diabetes was reduced from 29% to 13% in Swedish subjects through the limitation of energy intake from carbohydrates and fats. [120] Similar results were obtained in another study also conducted in Sweden.[121] In this second study, subjects were instructed in diet choices as well as in an exercise protocol. Annual assessments of the subjects showed that over the 6 years of the study, the rate of conversion from glucose intolerance to type 2 diabetes was reduced to 50%. A number of studies all directed toward increasing physical activity and reducing body fatness have shown that it is possible to intervene with the process of diabetes development where it is associated with excess fat stores or obesity.

The research to date suggests that clinicians should not only focus on the reduction in body fat stores but also pay attention to the various risk factors for cardiovascular disease. As noted in the introduction on the prevalence of diabetes, people with diabetes have five times the risk of developing cardiovascular disease as people without diabetes. Hence, intervention strategies should also include those tactics that will reduce the likelihood of a cardiovascular event. In view of the

TABLE 9.11
Intervention Studies

Investigators	Subjects/Origin	Study Length	Intervention/Outcome
O'Dea [123]	Aus. aborigines	7 weeks	Reversion to trad. lifestyle resulted in an improvement in GTT
Sartor et al. [120]	Swedish adults	10 years	Reduced energy intake/reduced conversion to diabetes
Ericsson et al. [121]	Swedish adults	6 years	Reduced energy intake, increased exercise/ reduced conversion to diabetes
Viswanathan et al. [125]	Offspring of diabetic parents	4 years	Weight control and exercise diabetes onset delayed
Ericsson et al. [121]	Overweight adults	1 year	Weight control, lifestyle advice/weight loss, no effect on diabetes
Pan et al. [125]	Chinese adults	6 years	Diet advise and/or exercise/weight loss and diabetes delay
Knowler et al. [126]	3234 adults	2.8 years	Placebo or metformin or weight loss and exercise; delay in diabetes

observation that more obesity is being observed in children and adolescents, it would appear that these age groups should be studied to determine if the interventions found successful in adults would be successful in children as well.

Several intervention trials have been conducted that addressed cardiovascular risk factors in children. The CATCH Multicenter Trial was a school-based research study that had as its objective the effectiveness of changes in school lunches, physical education, smoking policy curricula, and family activities.[117] The percentage saturated fat and total fat were reduced in the diets of those subjects in the intervention group. Physical activity was also increased. This trial lasted 3 years and involved 5016 third grade students. While the objectives of reducing fat intake and increasing physical activity were achieved, there were no significant differences between the control and intervention groups in blood pressure, body size, or blood cholesterol. In another study, the Heart Start Study, children in the third grade were again used, and again the goal was to reduce diet fat intake and increase physical activity.[113] This was achieved and again few differences in cardiovascular risk factors were noted in these children. As with the CATCH Trial, diabetes was not assessed but the hoped for outcome was that in modifying diet and physical activity in a child, one could have an effect on that child as he or she matures. Habits adopted as a child might have a long-term effect on subsequent adult health behavior such that a delay in the development of heart disease and also diabetes might occur. Intervention studies per se in children with respect to type 2 diabetes have not been conducted primarily because this has not been a child health problem until recently. Now with the early onset of obesity, these studies are needed.

Are there other strategies that could modify the phenotypic expression of a diabetes genotype? In BHE/Cdb rats having a diabetes genotype in the mitochondrial genome, feeding these rats an egg-based diet resulted in a delay in the onset of impaired glucose tolerance.[122,127–129] Rats of this strain fed a 10% fat diet where the fat was beef tallow lived longer and had a delay in the development of diabetic renal disease than those animals fed a 10% corn oil or a 9% fish oil and 1% corn oil diet. Those fed the fish oil diet had the shortest life spans and early onset of renal lesions.[123] Even though extra vitamin E was provided to these animals, free radical production was increased in the fish oil and corn oil fed rats. Oxidative capacity clearly had a role in the lesions that developed in these rats that in turn shortened their life spans. Longevity studies in humans with this kind of strict dietary regimens have not been conducted, yet it is known that oxidative capacity, as well as lipotoxicity, does occur. Some have suggested that free radical damage to the mitochondrial DNA could explain some of the secondary symptoms occurring in people with diabetes.[124] Lee[64] has proposed that diabetes itself damages DNA through an increase in free radical production and that this damage could be part of the downward spiral of tissue damage that occurs in people with diabetes.

In humans with defects in insulin receptors, the strategy logically would be that of reducing the glucose-stimulated need for insulin bound to the fat cell, liver cell, or muscle cell. Diets low in simple sugars and diets that maintain (or attain) ideal body weight should be used. This strategy would also be useful in those with mutations in the gene for glycogen synthesis. The objective would be to decrease the need to synthesize glycogen by keeping the carbohydrate intake relatively unrefined and low in amount. In persons having mutation(s) in the GLUTs and mutations in the mitochondrial genome, the strategy would be to increase the fluidity of the plasma and intracellular membranes. Such a strategy would maximize the activity of the insulin receptors through inducing a more fluid membrane. The receptors are membrane bound, and their activity is dependent on the fluidity of the lipid in which they are embedded. Several studies have been conducted showing that dietary fat type will have this effect. In diabetes-prone BHE/Cdb rats fed fish oil, insulin sensitivity was increased via an effect on glucose uptake by the fat cell.[130,131] The type of fat in the diet fed to these rats affected glucose homeostasis, insulin receptor number, and binding activity and glucose uptake and oxidation.[132,133] Ryan et al.[134] showed that humans provided a Mediterranean diet had an improvement in their insulin sensitivity, which these investigators attributed to a diet-induced change in membrane composition that in turn influenced membrane fluidity and function. The Mediterranean diet is an oleic acid–rich diet. Oleic acid is a monounsaturated fatty acid (18:1). This fatty acid is one of the most common fatty acids found in dairy fat. Thus, if a Mediterranean diet could have this effect, there is no doubt that ingestion of dairy fat would have the same effect. The mol% of oleic acid in dairy fat is about ~26.5%. The only fatty acid in greater concentration in dairy fat is palmitic acid (16:0) at ~29 mol%.[135]

Where there are mutations in the gluconeogenic pathway, the strategy would be to avoid prolonged periods without food necessitating the upregulation of gluconeogenesis that in turn contributes glucose to the circulation in excess. In this scenario, the problem is not in the gluconeogenic pathway itself but in the factors that control it. Upregulation is a common feature in diabetes, and part of the problem in glucose homeostasis management is the downregulation of this pathway. Several of the oral hypoglycemic drugs recently developed have this as their pharmaceutic objective.

For those patients with diabetes due to mutations in the MODY genes, the diet prescriptions might be different (see discussion on MODY). These people might need to increase their fat and protein intake to gain better control of their glucose metabolism. This may also be true for those who develop diabetes due to an error in the mitochondrial genome.

Increasing physical activity in most of the people with genotypes that phenotype as diabetes would potentiate the diet strategies because it would not only increase energy expenditure but also would increase the noninsulin-dependent use of glucose by the muscles. This is not a good strategy with respect to those afflicted with mutations in the mitochondrial genome. These persons usually are unable to sustain significant muscle activity because the mutations result in malfunctioning mitochondria that are so needed for muscular activity.

Overall Management of Both Type 1 and Type 2 Diabetes

The most effective diet plan to manage diabetes is the one that has been individualized to meet the needs of the patient taking into account that patient's personal likes and dislikes as well as the eating plan that best maintains that particular person's blood glucose within normal limits.[36] The strategy includes balancing food intake against exercise and the maintenance of blood glucose within normal limits. As the patient is adjusting their food plan and activity schedule, they are asked to monitor their blood glucose levels. They soon come to realize what foods they can tolerate well with little effect on overall glucose control. They also learn what foods are not well tolerated. Patients should keep a diary to help them remember what works and what does not work. Because it is not possible to detect the genetic reason for their diabetes, this kind of trial and error food plan development will be the next best plan for their disease management.

The general dietary recommendations are that of the USDA Food Plate. With this as the backbone, the ADA recommends the spacing of meals throughout the day avoiding binge eating or eating one or two large meals. A three-meal pattern plus a small snack is preferred to the two-meal pattern followed in many households (no breakfast, small lunch, large dinner). The distribution of energy from fats, carbohydrates, and proteins is important. Ten to twenty percent of the energy intake should be from protein with the remainder coming from fats and carbohydrates. Contrary to the historical position of the ADA on the food management of the person with diabetes, there is no prohibition of certain foods. Rather, there is the recommendation that the diet be designed to satisfy the patient yet keep the energy intake at a level commensurate with ideal body weight. In some instances, this means energy intake restriction needed to reduce the body fat stores of the patient. The ADA recommends that the person with diabetes should try to keep their saturated fat intake to 10% of total calories. For those patients with diabetes due to mutations in the MODY genes, the diet prescriptions might be different. These people might need to increase their fat intake to gain better control of the glucose metabolism. This may also be true for those who develop diabetes due to an error in the mitochondrial genome. Again, individualization of the food management plan will allow for such adjustments. At this time, there are no studies that show that certain foods are more efficacious in the management of diabetes in humans than other foods.

OTHER HEALTH CONCERNS IN CARBOHYDRATE NUTRITION

There are a number of genetic errors in glycolysis, shunt activity, gluconeogenesis, and glycogen synthesis and use that phenotype as disorders in carbohydrate metabolism (see Chapter 7). Most of these are very rare.

Fiber

A number of years ago, several scientists noticed that populations whose traditional diets were rich in fibrous food had low incidences of colon cancer as well as heart disease and diabetes mellitus. They compared these diets to those typically consumed by people in the United States and Europe and suggested that the health status of these populations was related to their high-fiber diets. With the consumption of high-fiber diets, the feces were bulkier, moister, and more frequent than when low-fiber diets were consumed. These reports attracted a lot of attention and a plethora of high-fiber foods appeared in the marketplace. People began to consume these products in the hope of having similar benefits conferred. It is not clear that such benefits have been acquired.

Dietary fiber refers to those carbohydrates that are indigestible and unabsorbed. The component glucose moieties are joined by β-linkages rather than α-linkages. They may also contain additional substituents, but their chief characteristic is that of nondigestibility by the α-amylases of the mammalian gastrointestinal system. These nondigestible carbohydrates are plant products and fall into five major categories: celluloses, hemicelluloses, lignins, pectins, and gums. The first three provide bulk to the gastrointestinal contents due to their property of absorbing water. The increased bulkiness of the gut contents stimulates peristalsis and results in shorter passage time and more frequent defecation. In addition to the water-holding property, fibers of the lignin type adsorb cholesterol, aiding in its excretion in the feces. Pectins and gums also influence gastric emptying but in the opposite direction. These fiber types form gels that slow gastric emptying and interfere with the absorption of sugars, starches, and also fats. The fibers, collectively, help to lower the level of serum cholesterol while increasing its excretion. It is for these reasons that nutritionists encourage the consumption of fiber-rich plant foods. Fruits are good sources of pectin, while cereal grains and the woody parts of vegetables are good sources of the celluloses, hemicelluloses, and lignins. Dried beans and oats are good sources of gums. The inclusion of foods containing all of these fiber types will no doubt be of benefit with respect to intestinal transit time and may also result in a small decrease in cholesterol absorption. This may have some impact on cholesterol balance. If fiber increases cholesterol excretion and reduces cholesterol recirculation, a small decrease in serum cholesterol level may occur. However, since cholesterol synthesis may rise to compensate for decreased absorption and reabsorption, the net effect with respect to cardiovascular disease development may be minor indeed.

The increased transit speed of high-fiber diets may be of benefit to those people susceptible to colon cancer. The fiber not only adsorbs cholesterol and hastens its excretion but also adsorbs potentially noxious components of the ingesta, hastening their excretion as well. Thus, carcinogenic compounds have less time for exposure to colon cells and thus less opportunity to convert a normal cell to a cancer cell.

Finally, as with all comparisons of population groups, one must be careful in the interpretation of the data. Yes, a certain primitive group has less degenerative disease than we do in the United States, and yes, the diet contains more fiber. Is this a cause-and-effect scenario? No, it is not. The picture is incomplete without observations on the incidence of other diseases, the average life span, the availability of clean water, immunizations, medical care, and observations on other aspects of lifestyle that can affect disease development.

Ethanol

Alcoholic beverages have been consumed by humans since the dawn of history. They have been used to ease anxiety, to promote social interaction, and as a vehicle to dominate others. Ethanol, the alcohol in beverages, is the quantitative end product of yeast glycolysis. Small amounts can be synthesized in mammalian cells. Thus, ethanol is a drug, a food, and a metabolite. It has been estimated that upward of 90 million Americans consume alcoholic beverages every day and that about 10% of these people are addicted to its consumption. This affliction is called alcoholism.

There are genetic components of alcoholism and it may well be that alcoholism is truly a disease that is a result of a diet–gene interaction.[136–138] The dietary ingredient in this instance is alcohol; the gene is as yet unidentified. However, there is ample evidence in the literature that supports the concept that the tendency toward alcoholism is inherited. Studies of twins reared by adoptive parents as well as multigeneration studies of families give support to this idea. An alcoholic is more likely than a nonalcoholic to have an alcoholic relative. At least 33% of alcoholics have an alcoholic parent. This has been observed in adopted individuals where the biological parent was unknown to the alcoholic and so the parent's proclivities were not taught. Studies of monozygotic (identical) and dizygotic (fraternal) twins indicated a high degree of concordance for alcoholism. If one twin became an alcoholic, the other twin also became one if that twin chose to consume alcohol. The concordance was greater in the identical twins than in the fraternal twins. While scientists agree on the heritable nature of alcoholism, no one gene or group of genes has been identified and found culpable for the disorder.

Ethanol, once consumed, is rapidly absorbed by simple diffusion. The diffusion is affected by the amount of alcohol consumed, the regional blood flow, the body surface area, and the presence of other foods. The different segments of the gastrointestinal tract absorb ethanol at different rates. Absorption is fastest in the duodenum and jejunum; slower in the stomach, ileum, and colon; and slowest in the mouth and esophagus. The rate of absorption by the duodenum depends on gastric-emptying time, which, in turn, depends on the kinds and amounts of foods consumed with the ethanol. Certain drugs may also influence gastric-emptying time and thus influence absorption. Complete absorption may vary from 2 to 6 h. The type of beverage can influence ethanol absorption. Ethanol from beer is absorbed slower than that found in whisky, which is slower than gin and red wine. Of course, pure ethanol is absorbed the fastest of all.

Once absorbed, ethanol is rapidly distributed between the intracellular and extracellular compartments. This is because ethanol is completely miscible in water and thus freely travels any place water travels. The uptake of ethanol by the fat depots is minimal. Ethanol crosses the plasma membranes but, in so doing, changes them. When ethanol is in contact with a protein, it denatures it. Thus, large and frequent ethanol exposures result in damage to proteins both within and around the cells. The most damaged tissue is the liver, since ethanol is carried directly to this tissue via the portal blood. While gut cells are also damaged, these cells have such a rapid turnover time (less than 7 days) that such damage due to intermittent ethanol consumption is not as long lasting as the damage that happens in the liver. Liver cells, in contrast, have a longer half-life and, once damaged, do not repair as readily. Alcoholic liver disease is a major cause of death among those who drink heavily.

Ethanol diffuses from the blood to the alveolar air so the ethanol content of expired air bears a constant relationship to pulmonary arterial blood ethanol levels. The partition coefficient is 2100:1. This means that 2100 mL of expired air contains the same amount of ethanol as 1 mL of blood. If the blood contains 100 mg of ethanol, the expired air will contain 232 ppm. This is the basis for the *breathalyzer* tests for intoxication. Intoxication occurs at 150 mg/100 mL of blood but most states prosecute drivers having blood levels exceeding 100 mg/dL.

Of the ethanol consumed, 90%–98% is oxidized to carbon dioxide and water. The rest is excreted as ethanol in the breath or in the urine. The metabolism of ethanol is shown in Figure 9.15. The rate of oxidation is fairly constant at about 10–20 mg/mL. This indicates that the first rate-limiting

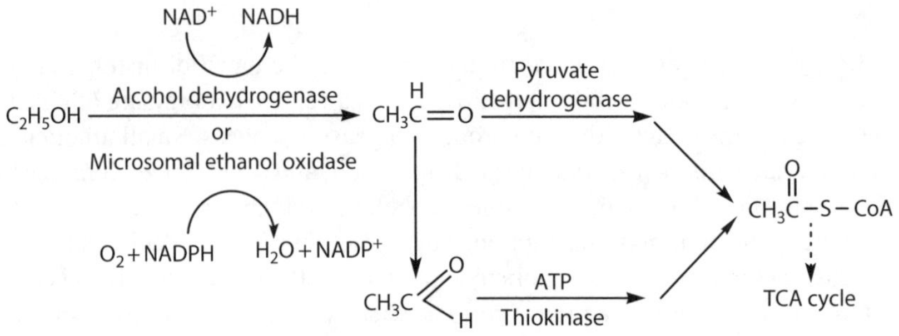

NAD+ NADH
Alcohol dehydrogenase or Microsomal ethanol oxidase
C_2H_5OH → $CH_3C(H)=O$
O_2 + NADPH → H_2O + $NADP^+$
Pyruvate dehydrogenase
CH_3CHO — ATP, Thiokinase →
$CH_3C(=O)-S-CoA$
TCA cycle

FIGURE 9.15 Metabolism of ethanol by the hepatocyte.

reaction catalyzed by alcohol dehydrogenase is saturated at this level. This is a zero-order reaction. The average rate at which alcohol can be metabolized is about 10 mL/h (or 7 g/h). The ethanol in 4 oz of whisky requires 5–6 h to metabolize completely to CO_2 and water. One mole of ethanol requires 16 moles of ATP for its conversion to CO_2 and HOH.

While ethanol is distributed throughout the body, the liver is the chief site for its oxidation.[139–143] As mentioned, the first rate-limiting reaction is catalyzed by alcohol dehydrogenase and converts ethanol to acetaldehyde. Acetaldehyde is quite damaging to cellular proteins and part of the hepatic injury found in alcoholics is due to this metabolite. It binds covalently to protein, impairs the microtubular assembly and the mitochondrial respiratory chain, depletes pyridoxine supplies, stimulates inappropriate collagen synthesis, inhibits DNA repair, and downregulates the transcription of the gene for microsomal triglyceride transfer. Ethanol interferes with the cell's signaling systems associated with the phospholipases C and D. Acetaldehyde is also produced when ethanol is metabolized by the microsomal ethanol oxidizing system (MEOS). This system uses peroxide (H_2O_2) and produces a molecule of water as well as the acetaldehyde. The acetaldehyde is converted to acetate, which can be either joined with a CoA or released to the circulation. If too much acetate is released, acidosis develops.

Acetyl CoA can either be used for fatty acid synthesis or be shuttled into the mitochondria via carnitine to be oxidized as through the citric acid cycle. A fatty liver typifies the alcoholic. The fatty liver may progress to alcoholic hepatitis, cirrhosis, liver failure, and death. The fatty liver is due to accelerated hepatic fatty acid synthesis as well as due to an ethanol-induced impairment in hepatic lipid output. If the hepatocyte accumulates too much lipid, the cell will burst and die. Areas of dead tissue within the liver are known as *cirrhosis*. When too much tissue dies, the liver may cease to function and the alcoholic dies.

In addition to the direct effects of ethanol on cell function, there are a number of auxiliary health concerns related to ethanol consumption. People who consume large quantities of ethanol find that their needs for thiamin, niacin, pyridoxine, and pantothenic acid increase dramatically. The alcoholic frequently manifests symptoms of beriberi, pellagra, and other deficiency diseases. In part, this is due to the increased need for these vitamins when ethanol is metabolized and in part because alcoholics may choose to consume alcoholic beverages in preference to nourishing food. Those alcoholics who continue to eat nourishing food in addition to consuming ethanol do not develop overt deficiency diseases as frequently. Nonetheless, the nutritionist should be aware of ethanol-induced increases in the needs for the B vitamins.

Finally, there is another concern with respect to ethanol consumption. That is the development of fetal malformations in women who drink ethanol during pregnancy. In 1973, eight cases of unrelated children were described having similar congenital defects. Particularly noticeable were the facial malformations involving eye placement and nose and mouth development. All of these children had mothers who were alcoholic. In a subsequent report, it was noted that alcoholism in mothers was associated with an increased incidence of spontaneous abortions, premature delivery of fetuses that were poorly developed for their gestational age, and infants born with respiratory distress syndrome. Many of these children failed to grow and develop normally with full intellectual capacity. Various learning disabilities (partial hearing or visual loss) also characterized these children. How the ethanol affects fetal development, particularly the development of the central nervous system, is not known. Yet awareness of the potential damage of ethanol to the developing embryo and fetus should dictate abstinence prior to and during the gestational period.

CARBOHYDRATE NEEDS

Carbohydrates are not considered essential nutrients aside from their use as providers of energy. Through gluconeogenesis, the body can usually synthesize sufficient glucose to sustain its absolute need for this fuel. Those cells that require other monosaccharides likewise can synthesize them. The mammary gland, for example, can convert glucose to galactose and use it (joined to glucose) to make the milk sugar lactose. The seminal vesicles likewise can isomerize glucose to fructose to meet the need for this particular monosaccharide for sperm production. Thus, the traditional definition of nutrient essentiality is not met. Neither a normal human nor members of other animal species need to consume glucose in any set amount if synthesis is sufficiently active to meet the need and if the diet provides sufficient gluconeogenic precursors. It has been estimated that an average human uses about 125 g of glucose per day to sustain neural activity. If this glucose is supplied by gluconeogenesis, 40% will come from lipid precursors and 60% will come from protein components. As mentioned earlier, this synthesis is very expensive with respect to the energy needed and, more importantly, with respect to the amount of dietary protein that must be consumed in order to support glucose synthesis. If no dietary carbohydrate is consumed, more than 155 g of protein (2–3 times the usual protein need) must be consumed to provide the 75 g of the 125 g glucose per day that is needed.

Are there circumstances where this is not true? Are there times when glucose serves a vital function that is in addition to its role as an energy provider? The answer to these questions is yes. Just as the growing child needs dietary arginine, while the adult does not, the traumatized or septic patient needs glucose, when otherwise this need could be met by gluconeogenesis.

In trauma or sepsis, the energy requirement is greatly increased because these conditions elicit a stress response (see Chapter 1). This response means an increase in levels of the catabolic hormones, which are anti-insulin hormones as well as anti-inflammatory hormones. The stress hormones mobilize body protein and fat stores to provide the means for repair of injured tissues. When this catabolic response is prolonged (days to weeks), it must be reversed or patients could die if their protein and energy stores are insufficient to sustain the prolonged mobilization. If sufficient glucose is provided in a hypertonic solution via a central vein such as the subclavian, it can reverse this catabolic response. This treatment is called parenteral nutrition. This will minimize the loss in body muscle mass. The effect of this hypertonic solution of glucose is to overcome (through mass action) the anti-insulin effects of the catabolic hormones and thereby stimulate glycolysis and glycogenesis and inhibit proteolysis and lipolysis.

The questions are as follows: how much carbohydrate (glucose) is needed to have the aforementioned effect, and how long should glucose be provided at this high level? The estimates vary. If the liver is functioning normally, 50%–80% of the energy intake should have the desired anticatabolic effect. This would mean a 5%–30% increase over the usual carbohydrate intake of 45%–55% of the total energy intake, presuming that the patient can and will eat. This is not always possible. The patient may be in a coma or may have a broken jaw, or the injury or sepsis may involve the gastrointestinal tract. In such instances, all needed nutrients, including glucose, must be supplied by the parenteral route. This creates other kinds of problems with respect to our knowledge about micronutrient needs in the absence of the protective role of the gastrointestinal system. Micromineral needs are especially difficult to manage under these circumstances. Humans need small amounts of most of these nutrients. If supplied in excess, a toxic state can develop.

With respect to the absolute amount of glucose that must be provided to the traumatized or septic patient, the estimates vary from 4 g/kg body weight (280 g/day/70 kg man) to 7 g/kg body weight (490 g/day/70 kg man). This would provide between 1120 and 1960 kcal (4686–8200 kJ) from glucose per day. The period of administration of this high level of glucose to achieve anticatabolism has been estimated to be from 4 days to 2 weeks. After this period, a more normal distribution of macronutrients may be more appropriate. While this glucose is being provided, the patient should also be monitored with respect to their insulin status. Some patients may require insulin supplementation to avoid hyperglycemic and diabetes-like symptoms.

SUMMARY

1. Carbohydrates provide a significant percentage of the total energy needed by the body.
2. There are many different carbohydrates segregated into monosaccharides, disaccharides, polysaccharides, and other compounds. Carbohydrates are found in every living cell but are more common in foods of plant origin than in foods of animal origin.
3. Most food carbohydrates consist of monosaccharides either by themselves or joined to other monosaccharides joined together by α-bonds. Those containing β-bonds are not digestible but serve as roughage. These carbohydrates serve as digestive aids improving the movement of the ingesta along the gastrointestinal tract. They also adsorb noxious materials assisting in their excretion in the feces.
4. After digestion, the component monosaccharides are absorbed. Glucose is absorbed via an energy- and sodium-dependent transport system.
5. Glucose is either catabolized to CO_2 and HOH after absorption or converted to glycogen or metabolized to substrates for fatty acid synthesis.
6. Glucose use is mediated by the hormone insulin.
7. The lack of insulin or the response to insulin results in diabetes mellitus.
8. Diabetes mellitus is the largest group of genetic diseases to afflict humans. More than 300 mutations have been reported that associate with this disease.
9. The uncontrolled consumption of alcohol results in alcoholism. This disease affects overall metabolism as well as the function of the central nervous system.

LEARNING OPPORTUNITIES

CASE STUDY 9.1 Herbert Is on a Food Supplement Kick

Herbert has type 1 diabetes mellitus. He is 40 years old and has had the disease for about 30 years. He has managed his glucose homeostasis very well but lately has developed an interest in the natural food movement. He has immersed himself in their literature and has learned that vitamins and minerals are important to good health. As a diabetic, he has always known that he must carefully manage what he eats so as to balance his food intake against the insulin he injects on a regular basis. But having achieved middle age, he has become very health conscious. He has begun taking a multivitamin supplement as well as several mineral supplements to boost his magnesium, calcium, iron, copper, and chromium intake. After a few days of beginning to consume all these supplements, he notices that he has diarrhea every midmorning. This is a real change in his usual pattern and the diarrhea has affected his glucose control. What is the problem here? Explain.

CASE STUDY 9.2 Sylvia, Raymond, and Reginald Have a Fat Mother with Type 2 Diabetes

Sylvia, Raymond, and Reginald are siblings. In their early thirties, they live in close proximity to each other frequently joining their mother for Sunday dinner and other family events. Their mother is an excellent cook who always encouraged her children to clean their plates of very generous portions. Sylvia was the first to notice that their mom was getting heavier than she had been. In fact, Sylvia tried to get her mother to join her in an exercise club. Mom did not want to do this because she was tired enough as it was and did not think she had what it took to go to an exercise session three to four times a week. Sylvia was dedicated to her exercise program. She even signed up for additional activities and decided to begin to train for marathon running. It was hard at first but eventually she became fit enough to run her first race. Mom was on the sidelines cheering her on until she collapsed into a chair. Sylvia became alarmed. She got her mom to an urgent care center as soon as she could. Mom was transported to the local hospital. Her blood work revealed a glucose level of over 500 mg/dL. She had indeed gained a lot of weight and her entry weight was 375 lb. She was not very tall so this meant that she was very fat indeed. Over the years, Sylvia had become used to seeing her mother always with a glass of iced tea or some beverage close at hand. She had also noticed how frequently her mom had to use the bathroom. Unfortunately, Sylvia did not connect the dots. She did not realize, until mom collapsed, that her mom had become diabetic. The hospital stay put it all together. Mom had type 2 diabetes. The doctor first started mom on metformin to see if oral medication would get the glucose level down. This did not work so he then prescribed insulin injections and mom was instructed on how to inject herself and how to check her blood glucose. A diabetes educator worked with her to help her develop a food plan that she liked. The clinicians also began a mild exercise program with mom's consent. Sylvia agreed to help mom adjust to this new lifestyle, and mom got her glucose under control. Sylvia began to look at her brothers. Although Raymond was 35 and Reginald was 39, she noticed that they were both becoming increasingly fatter and sedentary. Where they used to play touch football on Sunday afternoons at family gatherings, now, they were content to watch a game on TV. Sylvia worried that they were going to follow in mom's footsteps. What do you think? What should Sylvia do? What strategies might work?

MULTIPLE-CHOICE QUESTIONS

1. Monosaccharides include
   a. Sucrose, maltose, and cellulose
   b. Fructose, glucose, and galactose
   c. Lactose, mannose, and sucrose
   d. All of the above
2. The chief metabolic fuel for the brain is
   a. Fructose
   b. Glucose
   c. Ethanol
   d. Fatty acids
3. The glucose transporter is
   a. Found in the liver
   b. Found in the enterocytes
   c. Found in the muscle
   d. All of the above

4. Diabetes mellitus is
   a. A genetic disorder
   b. Caused by obesity
   c. Due to a lack of exercise
   d. Due to poor eating habits
5. Alcoholism
   a. Is a genetic disorder
   b. Can be avoided with alcohol abstinence
   c. Increases micronutrient needs
   d. All of the above

REFERENCES

1. http://www.nal.usda.gov/fnic/foodcomp/data.
2. Diem, K., Latmer, C. (1974) *Tables of Food Composition*, 7th edn. CIBA-Geigy, Ardsley, NY, pp. 241–266.
3. Goering, H.K., van Soest, J.P. (1970) Forage fiber analysis. In: *Agriculture Handbook No. 379*, Agriculture Research Service, U.S. Department of Agriculture, U.S. Government Printing Office, Washington, DC.
4. McCrane, R.A., Widdowson, E.M., and Shackelton, L.B. (1936) The nutritive value of fruits, vegetables, and nuts. Medical Research Council Special Report Series No. 213, London, U.K.
5. Southgate, D.A.T. (1969) Determination of carbohydrates in food. II. Unavailable carbohydrates. *J. Sci. Food Agric*. 20: 331–335.
6. van Soest, P.J., McQueen, R.W. (1973) The chemistry and estimation of fibre. *Proc. Nutr. Soc*. 32(1936): 123.
7. Montgomery, R.K., Buller, H.A., Rings, E.H.H., Grand, R.J. (1991) Lactose intolerance and the genetic regulation of intestinal lactase-phlorizin hydrolase. *FASEB J*. 5: 2824–2832.
8. Alvarez-Leon, E.E., Roman-Vinas, B., Serra-Majem, L. (2006) Dairy products and health: A review of the epidemiological evidence. *Br. J. Nutr*. 96(Suppl 1): S94–S99.
9. Petry, K.G., Reichardt, J.K.V. (1998) The fundamental importance of human galactose metabolism: Lessons from genetics and metabolism. *Trends Genet*. 14: 98–102.
10. (2009) Lactose intolerance and African Americans: Implications for the consumption of appropriate intake levels of key nutrients. *J. Nat. Med. Assoc*. 101: 3S–22S.
11. Nicklas, T.A., Qu, H., Hughes, S.O., Wagner, S.E., Foushee, H.R., Shewchuk, R.M. (2009) Prevalence of self reported lactose intolerance in multiethnic sample of adults. *Nutr. Today* 44: 222–227.
12. (2008) Lactulose. AHFS consumer medication information. http://www.ncbi.nlm.nih.gov/books. Accessed October 30, 2013.
13. Nichols, B.L., Quezada-Calvillo, R., Robayo-Torres, C.C., Ao, Z., Hamaker, B.R., Butte, N.F., Marini, J., Jahoor, F., Sterchi, E.E. (2009) Mucosal maltase-glucoamylase plays a crucial role in starch digestion and prandial glucose homeostasis of mice. *J. Nutr*. 139: 684–690.
14. Gould, G.W., Bell, G.I. (1990) Facilitative glucose transporters: An expanding family. *TIBS* 15: 18–23.
15. Olson, A.L., Pessin, J.E. (1996) Structure, function and regulation of the mammalian facilitative glucose transporter gene family. *Ann. Rev. Nutr*. 16: 235–256.
16. Baily, D.L., Horuk, R. (1988) The biology and biochemistry of the glucose transporter. *Biochem. Biophys. Acta* 947: 541–590.
17. Barnard, R.J., Youngren, J.F. (1992) Regulation of glucose transport in skeletal muscle. *FASEB J*. 6: 3238–3244.
18. Joost, H.G., Weber, T.M. (1989) The regulation of glucose transport in insulin sensitive cells. *Diabetologia* 32: 831–838.
19. Kahn, B.B., Pedersen, O. (1992) Tissue specific regulation of glucose transporters in different forms of obesity. *Proc. Soc. Exp. Biol. Med*. 200: 214–217.
20. Thong, F.S., Dugani, C.B., Klip, A. (2005) Turning signals on and off: GLUT 4 traffic in the insulin signaling pathway. *Physiology* 20: 271–284.
21. Bowman, B.A., Forbes, A.L., White, J.S., Glinsman, W.H., eds. (1993) Health effects of dietary fructose. *Am. J. Clin. Nutr*. 58: 721S–823S (Special issue).
22. Cherrington, A.D. (1999) Control of glucose uptake and release by the liver in vivo. *Diabetes* 48: 1198–1214.

23. Beale, E.G., Clouthier, D.E., Hammer, R.E. (1992) Cell-specific expression of cytosolic phosphoenolpyruvate carboxykinase in transgenic mice. *FASEB J.* 6: 3330–3337.
24. Nandan, S.D., Beale, E.G. (1992) Regulation of phosphoenolpyruvate carboxykinase mRNA in mouse liver, kidney, and fat tissues by fasting, diabetes and insulin. *Lab. Sci.* 42: 473–477.
25. Nordlie, R.C., Bode, A.M., Foster, J.D. (1993) Recent advances in hepatic glucose-6 phosphatase regulation and function. *Proc. Soc. Exp. Biol. Med.* 203: 274–285.
26. Short, M.K., Clouthier, D.E., Schaefer, I.M., Hammer, R.E., Magnuson, M.A., Beale, E.G. (1992) Tissue specific, developmental, hormonal and dietary regulation of rat phosphoenolpyruvate carboxykinase-human growth hormone fusion genes in transgenic mice. *Mol. Cell. Biol.* 12: 1007–1020.
27. Henquin, J.-C., Dufane, D., Nenquin, M. (2006) Nutrient control of insulin secretion in isolated normal islet cells. *Diabetes* 55: 3470–3477.
28. Las, G., Mayorek, N., Dickstein, K., Bar-Tana, J. (2006) Modulation of insulin secretion by fatty acyl analogs. *Diabetes* 55: 3478–3485.
29. Elwyn, D.H., Bureztein, S. (1993) Carbohydrate metabolism and requirements for nutritional support. *Nutrition* 9: 50–66; 164–175; 255–267.
30. (2013) 2011 national diabetes fact sheet. Centers for Disease Control. http://www.cdc.gov/diabetes/pubs/estimates. Accessed October 31, 2013.
31. (1998) Prevalence of diabetes, impaired fasting glucose, and impaired glucose tolerance in US adults. NHANES III, 1988–1994. *Diabetes Care* 21: S1–144.
32. National Center for Chronic Disease Prevention and Health Promotion. http://www.cdc.gov/diabetes/statistics/surv199/chap2/table0.1htm.
33. Diabetes in Hispanic Americans. NIDDK http://www.niddk.nih.gov/health/diabetes/pubs/hispan/hispan.htm.
34. Leong, A., Dasgupta, K., Chaisson, J.-L., Rahme, E. (2013) Estimating the population prevalence of diagnosed and undiagnosed diabetes. *Diabetes Care* 36: 3002–3009.
35. (1985) World Health Organization: Diabetes mellitus: Report of a WHO Study Group. World Health Organization (Technical Report Serial No. 727), Geneva, Switzerland.
36. American Diabetes Association. (2013) American diabetes association clinical practice recommendations. *Diabetes Care* 36: S1–S103.
37. Velho, G., Froguel, P. (1998) Genetic, metabolic, and clinical characteristics of maturity onset diabetes of the young. *Endocrinology* 138: 233–239.
38. Chiu, K.C., Tanizawa, Y., Permutt, M.A. (1993) Glucokinase gene variants in the common form of NIDDM. *Diabetes* 42: 579–582.
39. Weissglas-Volkov, D., Huertas-Vazquez, A., Suviolahti, E., Lee, J., Plaisier, C., Canizales-Quinteros, S., Tusie-Luna, T., Aguilar-Salinas, C., Taskinen, M.-R., Pajukanta, P. (2006) Common hepatic nuclear factor 4α variants are associated with high serum lipid levels and the metabolic syndrome. *Diabetes* 55: 1970–1977.
40. Velho, G., Blanche, H., Vaxillaire, M., Bellanne-Chantelot, C., Pardini, V.C., Timsit, J., Passa, P. et al. (1997) Identification of 14 new glucokinase mutations and description of the clinical profile of 42 MODY-2 families. *Diabetologia* 40: 217–224.
41. Vaxillaire, M., Rouard, M., Yamagata, K., Oda, N., Kaisaki, P.J., Boriraj, V.V., Chevre, J.C. et al. (1997) Identification of nine novel mutations in the hepatocyte nuclear factor 1 alpha gene associated with maturity-onset diabetes of the young (MODY3). *Hum. Mol. Genet.* 6: 583–586.
42. Hattersley, A.T., Turner, R.C., Permutt, M.A. (1993) Linkage of type 2 diabetes to the glucokinase gene. *Lancet* 339: 1307–1310.
43. Vionnet, N., Stoffel, M., Takeda, J., Yasuda, K., Bell G.I., Zouali, H., Leasge, S. et al. (1992) Nonsense mutation in the glucokinase gene causes early-onset non-insulin-dependent diabetes mellitus. *Nature* 356: 721–722.
44. Stoffel, M., Froguel, P.H., Takeda, J., Zouali, H., Vionnet, N., Nishi, S., Weber, I.T.. et al. (1992) Human glucokinase gene: Isolation, characterization, and identification of two missense mutations linked to early onset-non insulin-dependent (type 2) diabetes mellitus. *Proc. Natl. Acad. Sci. USA* 89: 7689–7702.
45. Shimada, F., Makino, H., Hashimoto, H. (1993) Type 2 (non-insulin -dependent) diabetes mellitus associated with a mutation of the glucokinase gene in a Japanese family. *Diabetologia* 36: 433–437.
46. Chevre, J.C., Hani, E.H., Boutin, P., Vaxillaire, M., Blanche, H., Vinnet, N., Pardini, V.C. et al. (1998) Mutation screening in 18 Caucasian families suggest the existence of other MODY genes. *Diabetologia* 41: 1017–1023.
47. Hansen, T., Eiberg, H., Rouard, M., Vaxillaire, M., Muller, A.M., Rasmussen, S.K., Fridberg, M. et al. (1997) Novel MODY3 mutations in the hepatocyte nuclear factor-1 alpha gene: Evidence for a hyperexcitability of pancreatic beta-cells to intravenous secretagogues in a glucose-tolerant carrier of a P447L mutation. *Diabetes* 46: 726–730.

48. Frayling, T.M., Bulamn, M.P., Ellard, S., Appleton, M., Dronsfield, M.J., Mackie, A.D., Baird, J.D. et al. (1997) Mutations in the hepatocyte nuclear factor-1 alpha gene are a common cause of maturity-onset diabetes of the young in the U.K. *Diabetes* 46: 720–725.
49. St-Onge, J., Joanisse, D.R., Simoneau, J.-A. (2001) The stimulation-induced increase in skeletal muscle glycogen synthetase content is impaired in carriers of the glycogen synthetase XbaI gene polymorphism. *Diabetes* 50: 195–198.
50. Zhang, Y., Wat, N., Stratton, I.M., Warren-Perry, M.G., Orho, M., Groop, L., Turner, R.C. (1996) UKPDS 19: Heterogeneity in NIDDM: Separate contributions of IRS-1 and beta 3-adrenergic-receptor mutations to insulin resistance and obesity respectively with no evidence for glycogen synthase gene mutations. *Diabetologia* 39: 1505–1511.
51. Kadowaki, T., Kadowaki, H., Rechler, M.M. (1990) Five mutant alleles of the insulin receptor gene in patients with genetic forms of insulin resistance. *J. Clin. Invest*. 86: 254–264.
52. Odawara, M., Kadowaki, T., Yamamoto, R. (1989) Human diabetes associated with a mutation in the tyrosine kinase domain of the insulin receptor. *Science* 245: 66–68.
53. Taylor, S.I., Cama, A., Accili, D., Barbetti, F., Quon, M.J., De La Luz Sierra, M., Suzuki, Y. et al. (1992) Mutations in the insulin receptor gene. *Endocr. Rev*. 13: 566–595.
54. Taylor, S.I., Kadowaki, H., Accili, D., Cama, A., McKeon, C. (1990) Mutations in the insulin receptor gene in insulin resistant patients. *Diabetes Care* 13: 257–279.
55. Makino, H., Taire, M., Shimada, F., Hasimoto, N., Suzuki, Y., Nozaki, O., Hatanaka, Y., Yoshida, S. (1992) Insulin receptor gene mutation: A molecular and functional analysis. *Cell. Signal*. 4: 351–363.
56. Cama, A., Sierra, M.L., Ottini, L. (1991) A mutation in the tyrosine kinase domain of the insulin receptor associated with insulin resistance in an obese woman. *J. Clin. Endocrinol. Metab*. 73: 894–901.
57. Olansky, L., Janssen, R., Welling, C., Permutt, M.A. (1992) Variability of the insulin gene in American Blacks with NIDDM. *Diabetes* 41: 742–749.
58. Steiner, D.F., Tager, H.S., Chan, S.J., Nanjo, K., Sanke, T., Rubenstein, A.H. (1990) Lessons learned from molecular biology of insulin gene mutations. *Diabetes Care* 13: 600–609.
59. Utsunomiya, N., Ohagi, S. Sanke, T., Tatsuta, H., Hanabusa, T., Nanjo, K. (1998) Organization of the human carboxypeptidase E gene and molecular scanning for mutations in Japanese subjects with NIDDM or obesity. *Diabetologia* 41: 701–705.
60. Rondinone, C.M., Wang, L.-M., Lonnroth, P., Wesslau, C., Pierce, J.H., Smith, U. (1997) Insulin receptor substrate (IRS) 1 is reduced and IRS 2 is the main docking protein for phosphatidyl inositol 3-kinase in adipocytes from subjects with NIDDM. *Proc. Natl. Acad. Sci. USA* 94: 4171–4175.
61. MacDonald, M.J., Brown, L.J., Hasan, N.M., Stoffel, M., Dills, D.G. (1997) Single stranded conformational polymorphism analysis of mitochondrial glycerol phosphate dehydrogenase gene in NIDDM. *Diabetes* 46: 1660–1661.
62. van den Ouweland, J.M.W., Lemkes, H.H.P.J., Ruitenbeek, W., Sandkuijl, L.A., de Vildjer, M.F., Struyvenberg, P.A.A., van de Kamp, J.J.P., Maassen, J.A. (1992) Mutation in mitochondrial $tRNA^{Leu(UUR)}$ gene in a large pedigree with maternally transmitted type II diabetes mellitus and deafness. *Nat. Genet*. 1: 368–371.
63. Mathews, C.E., Berdanier, C.D. (1998) Noninsulin dependent diabetes mellitus as a mitochondrial genomic disease. *Proc. Soc. Exp. Biol. Med*. 219: 97–108.
64. Lee, H.K. (2005) Mitochondria in diabetes mellitus. In: *Mitochondria in Health and Disease* (C. Berdanier, ed.) Taylor & Francis, Boca Raton, FL, pp. 377–454.
65. Gerbitz, K.-D., Gempel, K., Brdiczka, D. (1996) Mitochondria and diabetes. *Diabetes* 45: 113–126.
66. Yoon, J.-W., Austin, M., Onodera, T., Notkins, A.L. (1979) Virus induced diabetes mellitus. Isolation of a virus from the pancreas of a child with diabetic ketoacidosis. *N. Eng. J. Med*. 300: 1173–1179.
67. Yoon, J.-W. (1995) A new look at viruses in Type 1 diabetes. *Diabetes Metab. Rev*. 11: 83–107.
68. Leiter, E.H., Wilson, G.L. (1988) Viral interactions in pancreatic β cells. In: *Pathology of the Endocrine Pancreas* (D. Ripeleers, P. Lefebore, eds.). Springer-Verlag, Berlin, Germany, pp. 8–105.
69. Notkins, A.L., Yoon, J.W., Onodera, T., Toniolo, A., Jenson, A.B. (1981) Virus-induced diabetes mellitus. In: *Perspectives in Virology XI* (M. Pollard, ed.). Alan R. Liss, Inc., New York, pp. 141–162.
70. Jensen, B.A., Rosenberg, H.S., Notkins, A.L. (1980) Postmortem tissue changes in children with fatal viral infections. *Lancet* 2: 354–358.
71. Roberts, S.S. (2007) Aerobic exercise. *Diabetes Forecast* Spring: 15–17.
72. Belfiore, F., Iannello, S. (1998) Insulin resistance in obesity: Metabolic mechanisms and measurement methods. *Mol. Genet. Metab*. 65: 121–128.

73. Asman, Y.W., Stump, C.S., Short, K.R., Coenen-Schimke, J.M., Guo, ZK., Bigelow, M.L., Nair, K.S. (2006) Skeletal muscle mitochondrial functions, mitochondrial DNA copy numbers, and gene transcript profiles in type 2 diabetic and non diabetic subjects at equal levels of low or high insulin and euglycemia. *Diabetes* 55: 3309–3319.
74. Morino, K., Petersen, K.F., Shulmaan, G.I. (2006) Molecular mechanisms of insulin resistance in humans and their potential links with mitochondrial dysfunction. *Diabetes* 55(Suppl. 2): S9–S15.
75. Mathews, C.E., Leiter, E.H., Spirina, O., Bykhovskaya, Y, Gusdon, A.M., Ringquist, S., Fischel-Ghodsian, N. (2005) mt-Nd2 Allele of the ALR/Lt mouse confers resistance against both chemically induced and autoimmune diabetes. *Diabetologia* 48: 261–267.
76. Shafrir, E. (1992) Animal models of non-insulin dependent diabetes. *Diabetes Metab. Rev*. 8: 179–208.
77. Fisler, J.S., Warden, C.H. The current and future search for obesity genes. *Am. J. Clin. Nutr*. 85: 1–2.
78. Ducluzeau, P.H., Cousin, P. Malvoisin, E., Bornet, H., Vidal, H., Laville, M., Pugeat, M. (2003) Glucose to insulin ratio rather than sex hormone binding globulin and adiponectin levels is the best predictor of insulin resistance in nonobese women with polycystic ovary syndrome. *J. Clin. Endocrinol. Metab*. 88: 3626–3631.
79. Ardori, M.S., Rouzi, A.A. (2005) Plasma adiponectin and insulin resistance in women with polycystic ovary syndrome. *Fertil. Steril*. 83: 1708–1716.
80. Sieminska, L., Marek, B., Kos-Kudla, B., Niedziolka, D., Kajdaniuk, D., Nowak, M., Glogowska-Szelag, J. (2004) Serum adiponectin in women with polycystic ovarian syndrome and its relation to clinical, metabolic, and endocrine parameters. *J. Endocrinol. Invest*. 27: 528–534.
81. Spranger, J., Mohlig, M., Wegewitz, U., Ristow, M., Pfeiffer, A.F., Schill, T., Schlosser, H.W., Brabant, G., Schofl, C. (2004) Adiponectin is independently associated with insulin sensitivity in women with polycystic ovary syndrome. *Clin. Endocrinol*. 61: 738–746.
82. Sepilian, V., Nagamani, M. (2005) Adiponectin levels in women with polycystic ovary syndrome and severe insulin resistance. *J. Soc. Gynocol. Invest*. 12: 129–134.
83. Loos, R.J.F., Ruchat, S., Rankinen, T., Tremblay, A., Perusse, L., Bouchard, C. (2007) Adiponectin and adiponectin receptor gene variants in relation to resting metabolic rate, respiratory quotient and adiposity related phenotypes in the Quebec Family Study. *Am. J. Clin. Nutr*. 85: 26–34.
84. Joshi, R.L., Lamonthe, B., Bucchini, D, Jami, J. (1997) Genetically engineered mice as animal models for NIDDM. *FEBS Lett*. 401: 99–103.
85. Plum, L., Wunderlich, F.T., Baudler, S., Krone, W., Bruning, J.C., (2004) Transgenic and knockout mice in diabetes research: Novel insights into pathophysiology, limitations, and perspectives. *Physiology* 20: 152–161.
86. Rangwala, S.M., Rich, A.S., Rhoades, B., Shapiro, J.S., Obici, S., Rosetti, L., Lazar, M.A. (2004) Abnormal glucose production due to chronic hyperresistinemia *Diabetes* 53: 1937–1941.
87. West, K.M., Kalbfleisch, J.M. (1971) Influence of nutritional factors on the prevalence of diabetes. *Diabetes* 20: 99–108.
88. Wirfalt, E., Hedblad, B., Gulberg, B., Mattisson, I., Andrein, C., Rosander, U., Janzon, L., Bergland, G. (2001) Food patterns and components of the metabolic syndrome in men and women: A cross-sectional study within the Malmo diet and Cancer cohort. *Am. J. Epidemiol*. 154: 1150–1159.
89. van Dam, R.M., Hu, F.B., Rosenberg, L., Krishnan, S., Palmer, J.R. (2006) Dairy calcium and magnesium, major food sources and the risk of type 2 diabetes in US black women. *Diabetes Care* 29: 2238–2243.
90. Mennen, L.I., Lafay, L., Feskins, E.J.M., Novak, M., Lepinay, P., Balkau, B. (2000) Possible protective effect of bread and dairy products on the risk of metabolic syndrome. *Nutr. Res*. 20: 335–347.
91. Mensink, R.P. (2006) Dairy products and the risk to develop type 2 diabetes or cardiovascular disease. *Int. Dairy J*. 16: 1001–1004.
92. Meyer, K.A., Kushi, L.H., Jacobs, D.R., Folsom, A.R. (2001) Dietary fat and incidence of type 2 diabetes in older Iowa women. *Diabetes Care* 24: 1528–1535.
93. Lopez-Ridaura, R., Willett, W.C., Rimm, E.B., Liu, S., Stampfer, M.J., Hu, F.B. (2004) Magnesium intake and risk of type 2 diabetes in men and women. *Diabetes Care* 27: 134–140.
94. Song, Y., Manson, J.E., Buring, J.S., Liu, S. (2004) Dietary magnesium intake in relation to plasma insulin levels and risk of type 2 diabetes. *Diabetes Care* 27: 59–65.
95. Song, Y., Manson, J.E., Buring, J.E., Liu, S. (2004) A prospective study of red meat consumption and type 2 diabetes in middle aged and elderly women: The Women's health study. *Diabetes Care* 27: 2108–2115.

96. Ma, B., Lawson, A.B., Liese, A.D., Bell, R.A., Mayer-Davis, J. (2006) Dairy, magnesium, and calcium intake in relation to insulin sensitivity: Approaches to modeling a dose dependent association. *Am. J. Epidemiol.* 164: 449–458.
97. Humphries, S., Kushner, H., Falkner, B. (1999) Low dietary magnesium is associated with insulin resistance in a sample of young nondiabetic Black Americans. *Am. J. Hypertens.* 12: 747–756.
98. Rosolova, H., Mayer, O., Jr, Reaven, G.M. (2000) Insulin-mediated glucose disposal is decreased in normal subjects with relatively low plasma magnesium concentrations. *Metabolism* 49: 418–420.
99. Dixit, P.K., Ekstrom, R.A. (1980) Decreased breaking strength of diabetic rat bone and its improvement by insulin treatment. *Calcif. Tissue Int.* 32: 195–199.
100. Rosholt, M.N., Hegarity, P.V.J. (1981) Mineralization of different bones in streptozotocin-diabetic rats: Study on the concentration of eight minerals. *Am. J. Clin. Nutr.* 34: 1680–1685.
101. Lau, A.L., Failla, M. (1984) Urinary excretion of zinc, copper and iron in the streptozotocin-diabetic rat. *J. Nutr.* 114: 224–233.
102. Failla, M. (1983) Trace element metabolism in the chemically diabetic rat. *Biol. Trace Elem Res.* 5: 275–284.
103. Devlin J.T., Horton, E.S. (1986) Potentiation of the thermic effect of insulin by exercise: Differences between lean, obese, and non insulin dependent diabetic men. *Am. J. Clin. Nutr.* 43: 884–890.
104. Zinman, B., Murray, F.T., Vranic, M., Albisser, A.M., Leibel, B.S., McClean, P. Marlis, E.B. (1977) Glucoregulation during moderate exercise in insulin treated diabetics. *J. Clin. Endocrinol. Metab.* 45: 641–652.
105. Giacca, A., Groenewoud, Y., Tsui, E., McClean, P., Zinman, B. (1998) Glucose production, utilization, and cycling in response to moderate exercise in obese subjects with type 2 diabetes and mild hyperglycemia. *Diabetes* 47: 1763–1770.
106. Pereira, M.A., Jacobs, D.R., Van Horn, L., Slattery, M.L., Kartashov, A.I., Ludwig, D.S. (2002) Dairy consumption, obesity and the insulin resistance syndrome in young adults: The CARDIA study. *JAMA* 24: 2018–2089.
107. Weinberg, L.G., Berner, L.A., Groves, J.E. (2004) Nutrient contributions of dairy foods in the United States, Continuing Survey of Food Intakes by individuals, 1994–1996. *J. Am. Diet. Assoc.* 104: 895–902.
108. Berkey, C.S., Rockett, H.R., Willett, W.C., Colditz, G.A. (2005) Milk, dairy fat, dietary calcium, and weight gain: A longitudinal study of adolescents. *Arch. Pediatr. Adolesc. Med.* 159: 543–550.
109. Liu, S., Song, Y., Ford, E.S., Manson, J.E., Buring, J.E., Ridker, P.M. (2005) Dietary calcium, vitamin D and the prevalence of metabolic syndrome in middle aged and older U.S. women. *Diabetes Care* 28: 2926–2932.
110. Azadbakht, L., Mirmiran, P., Esmaillzadeh, A., Azizi, F. (2005) Dairy consumption is inversely associated with the prevalence of metabolic syndrome in Tehranian adults. *Am. J. Clin. Nutr.* 82: 523–530.
111. Rajpathak, S.N., Rimm, E.B., Rosner, B., Wilett, W.C., Hu, F.B. (2006) Calcium and dairy intakes in relation to long-term weight gain in US men. *Am. J. Clin. Nutr.* 82: 559–566.
112. Salmeron, J., Hu, F.B., Manson, J.E., Stampfer, M.J., Colditz, G.A., Rimm, E.B., Willett, W.C. (2001) Dietary fat intake and risk of type 2 diabetes. *Am. J. Clin. Nutr.* 73: 1019–1029.
113. Liu, S., Choi, H.K., Fod, E., Song, Y., Klevak, A., Buring, J.E., Manson, J.E. (2006) A prospective study of dairy intake and the risk of Type 2 diabetes. *Diabetes Care* 29: 1579–1584.
114. Choi, H.K., Willett, W.C., Stampfer, M.J., Rimm, E., Hu, F.B. (2005) Dairy consumption and risk of type 2 diabetes mellitus in men: A prospective study. *Arch. Intern. Med.* 165: 997–1003.
115. Marshall, J.A., Shetterly, S., Hoag, S., Hamman, R.F. (1994) Dietary fat predicts conversion from impaired glucose tolerance to NIDDM. *Diabetes Care* 17: 50–56.
116. King, H., Dowd, J.E. (1990) Primary prevention of type 2 diabetes mellitus. *Diabetologia* 33: 3–8.
117. Stern, M.P. (1991) Primary prevention of type 2 diabetes mellitus. *Diabetes Care* 14: 399–410.
118. Melander, A. (1996) Review of previous impaired glucose tolerance intervention studies. *Diabetes Metab.* 13: S20–S22.
119. Kumar, V.V.R., Adamson, U., Ostenson, C.-G. (2000) Primary prevention of type 2 diabetes: A review of the current state. *Int. J. Diab. Metab.* 8: 41–49.
120. Sartor, G., Schersten, B., Carstrom, S., Melander, A., Norden, A., Persson, G. (1980) Ten year follow-up of subjects with impaired glucose tolerance. Prevention of diabetes by tolbutamide and diet regulation. *Diabetes* 29: 41–49.
121. Eriksson, J., Lindstrom, J., Valle, T., Aunola, S., Hamalainen, H., Hanne-Parikka, P. (1999) Prevention of type 2 diabetes in subjects with impaired glucose tolerance The Diabetes Prevention Study (DPS) in Finland. Study design and I year interim report on the feasibility of the lifestyle programme. *Diabetologia* 42: 793–801.

122. Stone, E.J., Osganian, S.K., McKinlay, S.M., Wu, M.C., Webber, L.S., Luepker, R.V., Perry, C.L., Parcel, G.S., Elder, J.P. (1996) Operational design and quality control on the CATCH multicenter trial. *Prev. Med.* 25: 384–399.
123. O'Dea, K. (1984) Marked improvement in carbohydrate and lipid metabolism in diabetic Australian Aborigines after temporary reversion to traditional life style. *Diabetes* 33: 596–603.
124. Ericsson, K.-F., Lindgarde, F. (1991) Prevention of type 2 diabetes by diet and physical exercise. *Diabetologia* 34: 891–898.
125. Viswanathan, M., Snehalatha, C., Viswanathan, V., Vidyavathi, P., Indu, J., Ramachandran, A. (1997) Reduction in body weight helps to delay the onset of diabetes even in non-obese with strong family history of the disease. *Diabetes Res. Clin. Prac.* 35: 107–112.
126. Pan, X.R., Li, G.W., Hu, Y.H., Wang, J.X., Yang, W.Y., An, Z.X. (1997) Effects of diet and exercise in preventing NIDDM in people with impaired glucose tolerance. The Da Qing IGT and diabetes study. *Diabetes Care* 20: 537–544.
127. Berdanier, C.D., Kras, K., Wickwire, K., Hall, D.G. (1998) Whole egg diet delays the age related impaired glucose tolerance of BHE/Cdb rats. *Proc. Soc. Exp. Biol. Med.* 219: 28–36.
128. Berdanier, C.D., Johnson, B., Hartle, D.K., Crowell, W. (1992) Lifespan is shortened in BHE/Cdb rats fed a diet containing 9% menhaden oil and 1% corn oil. *J. Nutr.* 122: 1309–1317.
129. Schrauwen, P., Hesselink, M.K.C. (2004) Oxidative capacity, lipotoxicity, and mitochondrial damage in type 2 diabetes. *Diabetes* 53: 1412–1417.
130. Pan, J.-S., Berdanier, C.D. (1991) Effect of dietary fat on hepatocyte insulin binding and glucose metabolism in BHE rats. *J. Nutr.* 121: 1820–1826.
131. Pan, J.-S., Berdanier, C.D. (1991) Effect of dietary fat on adipocyte insulin binding and glucose metabolism in BHE rats. *J. Nutr.* 121: 1811–1819.
132. Kim, M.-J.C., Pan, J.-S., Berdanier, C.D. (1993) Glucose homeostasis in thyroxine treated rats fed corn oil or hydrogenated coconut oil. *J. Nutr. Biochem.* 4: 20–26.
133. Kim, M.-J.C., Berdanier, C.D. (1998) Nutrient-gene interactions determine mitochondrial function: Effect of dietary fat. *FASEB J.* 12: 243–248.
134. Ryan, M., McInerney, D., Owens, D., Collins, P., Johnson, A., Tomkin, G.H. (2000) Diabetes and the Mediterranean diet: A beneficial effect of oleic acid on insulin sensitivity, adipocyte glucose transport and endothelium-dependent vasoreactivity. *QJM* 93: 85–91.
135. Jensen, R.J. (2000) Fatty acids in milk and dairy products In: *Fatty Acids in Foods and Their Health Implications* (C.K. Chow, ed.). Marcel Dekker, New York, pp. 109–123.
136. Devor, E.J., Cloninger, C.R. (1989) Genetics of alcoholism. *Ann. Rev. Genet.* 23: 19–39.
137. Thacker, S.B., Veech, R.L., Vernon, A.A., Rutstein, D.D. (1984) Genetic and biochemical factors relevant to alcoholism. *Alcohol. Clin. Exp. Res.* 8: 375–383.
138. Harris, R.A., Allan, A.M. (1988) Alcohol intoxication: Ion channels and genetics. *FASEB J.* 3: 1689–1695.
139. Lieber, C.S. (1993) Herman Award Lecture, 1993: A personal perspective on alcohol, nutrition and the liver. *Am. J. Clin. Nutr.* 58: 430–442.
140. Hoek, J.B., Thomas, A.P., Rooney, T.A., Higashi, K., and Rubin, E. (1992) Ethanol and signal transduction. *FASEB J.* 6: 2386–2396.
141. Dicker, E., Cederbaum, A.I. (1988) Increased oxygen radical-dependent inactivation of metabolic enzymes by liver microsomes after chronic ethanol consumption. *FASEB J.* 2: 2901–2906.
142. Lin, M.C., Li, J.-J., Wang, E.-J., Princler, G.L., Kauffman, F.C., Kung, H.-F. (1997) Ethanol down-regulates the transcription of microsomal triglyceride transfer protein gene. *FASEB J.* 11: 1145–1152.
143. Smith, G.N., Patrick, J., Sinervo, K.R. (1991) Effects of ethanol exposure on the embryo-fetus: Experimental considerations, mechanisms, and the role of prostaglandins. *Can. J. Physiol. Pharmacol.* 69: 550–569.

10 Lipids

The third macronutrient group consists of lipids. They are energetically more dense than carbohydrates having more than twice the energy value of carbohydrate per gram. Americans consume approximately 32%–42% of their total energy intake as lipid. Lipids make up a group of compounds that are, in general, insoluble in water and soluble in nonaqueous solvents. They are present in varying amounts in all living cells. Nerve cells and adipose cells are rich in lipid; muscle cells and epithelial cells have less.

In addition to being a very important source of energy, lipids serve a variety of other needs. They perform a basic role in the structure and function of biological membranes. In the body, they are the precursors of a variety of hormones and also act as some important cell signals.

CLASSIFICATION

Lipids are relatively soluble in such solvents as ether, chloroform, benzene, and some alcohols. Additionally, some lipids are saponifiable; others are not. Saponifiable lipids, when treated with alkali, undergo hydrolysis at the ester linkage, resulting in the formation of an alcohol and a soap (fatty acids combined with hydroxide). Triacylglycerol (TG) (triglyceride), for example, when treated with sodium hydroxide, is hydrolyzed yielding a mixture of soaps and free glycerol. Traditionally, saponifiable lipids have been classified into three groups (A, B, C), each with subgroups.

A. Simple lipids: esters of fatty acids with various alcohols
   1. Fats: esters of fatty acids with glycerol (acylglycerols)
   2. Waxes: esters of fatty acids with long chain alcohols
   3. Cholesterol esters

B. Compound lipids: esters of fatty acids that contain substituent groups in addition to fatty acids and alcohol
   1. Phospholipids: esters of fatty acids, alcohol, a phosphoric acid residue, and usually an amino alcohol, sugar, or other substituent
   2. Glycolipids: esters of fatty acids that contain carbohydrates and nitrogen (but not phosphoric acid). In addition to fatty acids and alcohol
   3. Lipoproteins: loose combinations of lipids and proteins

C. Derived lipids: substances derived by saponification from these groups

Two other terms are frequently used in the classification of lipids but are not a division of the system just described. These are the neutral and polar lipids. Neutral lipids are uncharged lipids and include TGs, cholesterol, and cholesterol esters. Polar lipids have positive and negative charges on certain atoms of the molecule. Examples of these are the phospholipids that are the lipids in the cell membrane. Phosphatidylinositol (PIP), phosphatidylcholine, and phosphatidylethanolamine, for example, are membrane phospholipids and are polar.

STRUCTURE AND NOMENCLATURE

Simple Lipids

Fatty Acids

Fatty acids are carboxylic acids. They have a polar group (the carboxyl group) at one end and a methyl group at the other. A hydrocarbon chain is in the middle. Fatty acids can have a few carbon atoms or more than 20; however, chain lengths of 16 and 18 carbons are the most prevalent. There is usually an even number of carbon atoms (with no branching) in the chain. The chain may be saturated (containing no double bonds) or unsaturated (containing one or more double bonds). Monounsaturated acids have one double bond; polyunsaturated acids have two or more.

The nomenclature of fatty acids is frequently confusing because the same fatty acid can have more than one name: its common (or trivial) name and its systematic name. The common name is rarely, if ever, related to the structure of the molecule. It is sometimes derived from the plant or animal source from which the acid was first isolated. The student has no choice but to memorize these names. Common names for nutritionally important fatty acids are given in Table 10.1.

The systematic method of naming fatty acids is based on a modification of the name of the straight chain hydrocarbon having the same number of carbon atoms. The final -e from the hydrocarbon name is removed and -oic is added. This is followed by the word acid. To name the salt

TABLE 10.1
Structure and Names of Fatty Acids Found in Food

Structure	# Carbons: Double Bonds	Systematic Name	Trivial Name	Source
Saturated fatty acids				
$CH_3(CH_2)_2COOH$	4:0	*n*-Butanoic	Butyric	Butter
$CH_3(CH_2)_4COOH$	6:0	*n*-Hexanoic	Caproic	Butter
$CH_3(CH_2)_6COOH$	8:0	*n*-Octanoic	Caprylic	Coconut oil
$CH_3(CH_2)_8COOH$	10:0	*n*-Decanoic	Capric	Palm oil
$CH_3(CH_2)_{10}COOH$	12:0	*n*-Dodecanoic	Lauric	Coconut oil, nutmeg, butter
$CH_3(CH_2)_{12}COOH$	14:0	*n*-Tetradecanoic	Myristic	Coconut oil
$CH_3(CH_2)_{14}COOH$	16:0	*n*-Hexadecanoic	Palmitic	Most fats and oils
$CH_3(CH_2)_{16}COOH$	18:0	*n*-Octadecanoic	Stearic	Most fats and oils
$CH_3(CH_2)_{18}COOH$	20:0	*n*-Eicosanoic	Arachidic	Peanut oil, lard
Unsaturated fatty acids				
$CH_3(CH_2)_5CH{=}CH(CH_2)_7COOH$	16:1	9-Hexadecenoic	Palmitoleic	Butter and seed oils
$CH_3(CH_2)_7CH{=}CH(CH_2)_7COOH$	18:1	9-Octadecenoic	Oleic	Most fats and oils
$CH_3(CH_2)_5CH{=}CH(CH_2)_9COOH$	20:1	11-Octadecenoic, *trans*-vaccenic	Hydrogenated	Vegetable oils
$CH_3(CH_2)_4CH{=}CHCH_2CH{=}CH(CH_2)_7COOH$	18:2	9,12-Octadecadienoic	Linoleic acid	Linseed oil, corn oil, cottonseed oil
$CH_3CH_2(CH{=}CHCH_2)_3(CH_2)_7COOH$	18:3	9,12,15-Octadecatrienoic	Linolenic acid	Soybean oil, marine oils
$CH_3(CH_2)_4(CH{=}CHCH_2)_4(CH_2)_2COOH$	20:4	5,8,11,14-Eicosatetraenoic	Arachidonic acid	Cottonseed oil

of the acid, the -e from the hydrocarbon base is replaced with -ate. For example, the saturated, 18-carbon hydrocarbon, $C_{18}H_{38}$, has as its systematic name *n*-octadecane (the *n* means normal or no branching); its saturated fatty acid counterpart is *n*-octadecanoic acid (its common name is stearic acid); the salt is *n*-octadecanoate. The monounsaturated 18-carbon is 9-octadecene; one form of the unsaturated acid is *cis*-9-octadecenoic acid (common name, oleic acid). The salt is *cis*-9-octadecenate.

In the systematic name, it is possible to address each carbon atom as was done in the last example just cited. There are two ways of doing this: with lower-case Greek letters or with Arabic numerals. With Greek letters, the carbon adjacent to the carboxyl group is α (alpha); the next one is β (beta); the last in the molecule is ω (omega). The carboxyl carbon is not given a designation. With Arabic numerals, the carboxyl carbon is 1; the next carbon, 2; the next, 3; and so on. The number 9 in the example discussed means that a double bond exists between carbons 9 and 10.

Other conventions are also used to indicate the position of the double bond. In one of them, Δ 9 indicates a double bond between carbons 9 and 10. In another, the number of carbon atoms, the number of double bonds, and the position of each double bond are all clearly shown. For example, oleic acid is 18:1Δ9 or 18 carbons with one double bond between the ninth and tenth carbons. Similarly, the 18-carbon acid with two double bonds is linoleic acid; in this system, it would be referred to as 18:2Δ9, 12. In yet another convention, the position of the double bond from the terminal carbon (the methyl group) is indicated. The number of carbon atoms and the number of double bonds are shown as in the previous convention. The position of the double bond from the terminal carbon is then shown. For instance, oleic acid is 18:1ω9; linoleic acid is 18:2ω6. This convention is particularly useful in discussions about the interconversion of fatty acids; if carbon atoms are added between this double bond and the carboxyl group, it remains the terminal carbon.

As mentioned, fatty acids are either saturated or unsaturated. These two forms of fatty acids differ significantly in their structural considerations. In the saturated fatty acid, the hydrocarbon tail can exist in an infinite number of conformations because each carbon atom can rotate freely.

Unsaturated fatty acids, on the other hand, have a rigid feature to their structure because the carbons in the double bonds are not free to rotate; they exist as the *cis* or *trans* geometrical isomers. The *cis* configuration produces a bond in the hydrocarbon chain so that it resembles the shape of the letter U. Each *cis* configuration in the tail will add another bend. The *trans* configuration has nearly the same shape as the extended conformation of the saturated fatty acid. These structural features of the unsaturated fatty acids have a biological significance, as will be discussed in later sections.

In polyunsaturated fatty acids (PUFAs), the double bonds are not conjugated; that is, the double bonds will be separated by more than one single bond as in $-CH_2-CH=CH-CH_2-CH=CH-CH_2-$. The unsaturated fatty acids of higher plants and animals are usually palmitoleic, oleic, linoleic, and linolenic acids; the first double bond will be between atoms 9 and 10; others, if present, will be at carbon 12 or greater. Most of these unsaturated fatty acids will exist in the *cis* configuration. When vegetable oils are solidified to make margarine, some of the double bonds will be converted to single bonds through the addition of hydrogen. The process is called hydrogenation and the oils must be heated before hydrogenation will take place. When this occurs, some of the residual unsaturated fatty acids will change from the *cis* to the *trans* residual form. Margarine and vegetable shortening are thus sources of industrial-made *trans*–fatty acids in the human diet. Some fatty acids exist naturally in the *trans* configuration. Eight percent of the unsaturated fatty acids in cows' milk is in the *trans* form. In this instance, the presence of *trans*–fatty acids is due to their production by the rumen flora. Unlike the *trans*–fatty acids produced when unsaturated fatty acids are hydrogenated industrially, the *trans*–fatty acids in milk do not have atherogenic potential.[1]

Fatty acids with an odd number of carbon atoms are found in limited amounts in natural products. Less than 0.4% of the total fatty acids in olive oil and 0.8% of those in lard contain an odd number of carbon atoms. In contrast, 60% of olive oil and 40% of lard consist of the even-numbered monounsaturated fatty acid, oleic acid. Few oils or waxes contain significant amounts of odd-numbered fatty acids. Odd-numbered fatty acids can be found in vitamin B_{12}-deficient individuals because B_{12} is an essential coenzyme in the conversion of methylmalonyl CoA to succinyl CoA.[2,3] When this conversion is impaired, methylmalonic acid accumulates and some of this is used to synthesize odd-numbered fatty acids.

Of the PUFAs, linoleic and linolenic are designated as the essential fatty acids (EFA).[4–6] Linoleic is an 18-carbon fatty acid with two double bonds (ω6, 18:2, $\Delta^{9,12}$). Linolenic acid is also an 18-carbon fatty acid but with three double bonds (ω3, 18:3, $\Delta^{9,12,15}$). Both are in the *cis* configuration. Food oils of plant origin are good sources of linoleic acid, while the marine oils are good sources of linolenic acid. A few oils of plant origin contain linolenic acid (i.e., primrose oil). Most mammals require these fatty acids and cannot synthesize them. Felines, in addition, cannot convert linoleic acid to arachidonic acid (ω6, 20:4, $\Delta^{5,8,11,14}$). Hence, for these animals, arachidonic acid is an EFA. It is estimated that 1%–2% of the lipid intake as EFA should meet the needs for normal individuals. The Food and Nutrition Board of the National Academy of Science has provided figures for an acceptable macronutrient intake for the EFA as a percentage of the energy intake. For children age 1–3 years, the range for the n-6 PUFAs is 5%–10% with an energy intake from fat of 30%–40%. For children age 4–18, the range for polyunsaturated n-6 fatty acids is the same but the energy intake from fat is 25%–35%. For adults, the range for polyunsaturated n-6 fatty acids likewise is unchanged but the recommended fat intake as a percentage of energy is 20%–35%. The suggested range for the n-3 PUFAs for these population groups is 0.6%–1.2% of energy.

Triacylglycerol (Oils and Fats or Triglycerides, TGs)

Fats are formed when one or more fatty acids react with the hydroxyl group(s) of glycerol to make an ester. They are called neutral fats, glycerides, or acylglycerols. The fat most frequently found in nature has all three hydroxyl positions esterified; it is known as TG. TGs that contain the same fatty acid residue on all three carbons are simple TGs. An example would be tripalmitin. In nature, the TGs usually contain more than one fatty acid and thus are called mixed TGs or triglycerides. Most fats in nature are complex mixtures of simple and mixed TGs. Many oils and fats contain between six and ten different saturated and unsaturated fatty acids. The number of possible combinations with this many fatty acid residues is very large.

The ratio of unsaturated to saturated fatty acids is defined as the P/S ratio. A high ratio of 3:1 means that there are three molecules of unsaturated fatty acids to every saturated fatty acid present. Animal fats and the foods rich in saturated fats usually have a low P/S ratio. Most vegetable oils have a high P/S ratio. However, there are some exceptions to this. The tropical plant oils (palm and coconut) provide a solid fat with a low P/S ratio. These fats, although called *oils* are rich in medium-chain (chain lengths of 8–14 carbons) saturated fatty acids. By convention, these lipids are called oils because they are fluid at much lower temperatures (the ambient temperature of the tropics) than are the fats of animal origin. Thus, we have coconut oil, palm oil, and palm kernel oil as solids at temperatures of 18°C–22°C but liquid at 26°C–30°C. The P/S ratio of the fat in the adipose tissue of humans reflects the P/S ratio of the food these humans consumed. In order to assess the P/S ratio of the fat intake of populations, only a small sample of adipose tissue would need to be obtained and analyzed for its P/S ratio. Because the body metabolizes the fat it consumes, both lengthening and shortening the food fatty acids, an exact copy of the food lipid fatty acids will not be obtained, but some general trends will be observed.

SOURCES OF LIPIDS

Food sources of lipids primarily mean food TGs because they are the lipids that occur in foods in large quantities. Lipids are found in almost every natural food. Fruits and vegetables have small amounts of lipid while meat, whole milk, cheese, eggs, and table spreads have larger amounts. A few plant foods—olives and avocados—contain as much as 20% (by weight) fat. Nuts are rich sources of fat: pecans are 71% fat and walnuts are 60% fat. Table 10.2 shows the total fat content of several foods and also gives some values for the saturated fatty acid content and the amount of two common unsaturated fatty acids, oleic and linoleic. A more complete list of foods and their lipid content can be found on the USDA website (www.nal.usda.gov/foodcomposition).

More than one-half of dietary fat is contributed from invisible sources: the fat in whole milk and eggs, whole grain cereals, baked products, and convenience foods. The other fraction of dietary fat is visible. The marbling in meat, butter on bread or vegetables, and salad oil on lettuce are examples of the latter. The fatty acid composition of several fats and oils is given in Table 10.2. Of the saturated fatty acids, palmitic (16:0) and stearic (18:0) are the most prevalent in nature. Of the

TABLE 10.2
Percent Fat in 100 g Portions of Common Food

Item	Total Fat (% by Weight)	Total Saturated Fatty Acids (% of the Total Fatty Acids in the Fat)	Unsaturated Fatty Acids	
			Oleic	Linoleic
Animal sources				
Bacon	53	20	27	7
Butter	81	45	27	3
Chicken, broiled	3.5	1	1	1
Egg, whole	12	4	5	Trace
Hamburger	12	6	4.7	Trace
Ice cream, 10% fat	10	6	4	Trace
Lamb, leg, roasted	19	10	7	Trace
Milk, whole	3.5	2	1.2	Trace
Milk, 2%	2	1.2	0.8	Trace
Milk, skim	Trace	Trace	Trace	Trace
Pork chops	21	8	9	2
Salmon, pink	6	1	1	Trace
Nonmeat sources				
Avocados	13	2.3	6	1.8
Bread, whole wheat	2.6	0.4	1.3	0.4
Bread, white enriched	3.3	0.7	1.8	0.4
Broccoli	0.6	Trace	Trace	Trace
Cereal, 40% bran	2.8	Trace	Trace	Trace
Cereal, oatmeal	0.8	Trace	Trace	Trace
Orange juice, fresh	0.4	Trace	Trace	Trace
Peanut butter	50	12.5	25	12.5
Pecans	71	4.6	44	14
Potato, baked	Trace	Trace	Trace	Trace
Strawberries, raw	0.7	Trace	Trace	Trace
Walnuts	60	3	24	33

Source: www.nal.usda.gov/foodcomposition; accessed November 22, 2013.

unsaturated fatty acids, oleic (18:1) and linoleic (18:2) are the most abundant. Together, these two fatty acids make up 90% of the unsaturated fatty acids in the American diet. As mentioned earlier, fats of plant origin tend to be less saturated than fats of animal origin. Fats from marine creatures are usually more unsaturated than either plant fats or land animal fats. Beef fat contains a lot of stearic acid. Mutton fat and cocoa butter contain a similar array of fatty acids but not in the same amounts. Mutton fat has as much as 27% saturated fatty acids by weight, whereas cocoa butter has 2.5%. This accounts for the marked difference in the physical properties of these two fats. Milk fat is similar to lard (pig fat) because it contains large amounts of palmitic and oleic acid. Fish, on the other hand, tend to have much more PUFA in its glycerides. Freshwater fish contain more unsaturated C18 and less unsaturated C20 and C22 than do marine fish. Fatty marine fish such as mackerel contain long-chain PUFAs of the omega ω-3 or n-3 type.

Cholesterol, cholesterol esters, free fatty acids, phospholipids, and sphingolipids are also present in the foods humans consume. These compounds represent only a small fraction of the total fat consumed. Because of the population studies linking heart disease to cholesterol levels in the blood, nutritionists are frequently interested in the levels of this lipid in the food. Listed in Table 10.3 are

TABLE 10.3
Total Lipid and Cholesterol Content of 100 g Portions of Several Common Foods[a]

Food	% Fat	% Cholesterol
Codfish	0.67	0.043
Halibut	2.94	0.041
Mackerel	6.30	0.076
Salmon	3.45	0.052
Beef steak, cooked	31.8	0.36
Hamburger, cooked	12.8	0.10
Stew meat	18.8	1
Lamb chops, cooked	36.0	1.11
Pork chops, cooked	21.1	1.03
Pork sausage	46.2	1.35
Bologna	28.6	1.04
Chicken, white meat	3.5	0.64
Eggs, whole	12	4.2
Egg white	<3	—
Whole milk	3.3	0.32
Skim milk	Trace	Trace
Cheddar cheese	32	1.0
Cottage cheese (4%)	4.29	0.21
Mozzarella cheese, skim milk	17.9	4.5
Butter	81.4	2.4
Margarine	81.4	—
Fruits, all kinds	<1	—
Avocado	13	—
Leafy vegetables	<1	—
Legumes (except peanuts)	1	—
Root vegetables	<1	—
Cereals and grains	1–2	0
Crackers	1	0
Bread, white, enriched	4	<0.1

[a] Foods were selected from the vast array of foods found in the USDA data bank: www.nal.usda.gov/foodcomposition.

some human foods and their percentage fat and cholesterol content. Greater detail on the composition of the tremendous variety of foods that humans consume may be found in the USDA website: www.nal.usda.gov/foodcomposition. Other handbooks and computer programs have been developed to assess the nutrient intakes of not only man but other species as well. The data provided in these sources are averages of several different analyses, but are not absolute. Variation in the source of the food, how it is prepared, and how much fat is removed prior to preparation and consumption contributes to the uncertainty associated with these values.

Interest in the sphingolipids in food has emerged as reports have appeared suggesting that these lipids might have an anticancer or antilipemia function.[7] Sphingolipids are complex lipids having a sphingosine backbone. There are more than 60 variants of these compounds. There are various alkyl chain lengths (4–22 carbons) and varying degrees of saturation as well as varying positions for their component double bonds, chain branching, and presence of a hydroxyl group. The amino group of the sphingoid base can be substituted with a long-chain fatty acid to produce a ceramide. There are so many variants of these compounds that this group is the largest group of complex dietary lipids, yet their nutritional significance has not been well studied.

DIGESTION AND ABSORPTION

The digestion and absorption of the various food lipids involves the mouth, stomach, and intestine (Figure 10.1). The digestion of lipid is begun in the mouth with the mastication of food and the mixing with the acid-stable lingual lipase. Digestion can proceed only when the large particles of food are made smaller through chewing. The action of the tongue and teeth mixes the food with the lingual lipase. Later, the churning action of the stomach mixes the food particles with hydrochloric acid. These actions separate the lipid particles, exposing more surface area for enzyme action and emulsion formation. The changes in physical state, illustrated in Figure 10.2, are essential steps that precede absorption. In the stomach, lipid–protein complexes are cleaved, releasing lipid when the proteins of these complexes are denatured by gastric hydrochloric acid and attacked by the proteases (pepsin, parapepsin I, and parapepsin II) of the gastric juice. The remaining lipid components of the diet are mixed with other diet ingredients by the churning action of the stomach. Little degradation of fat occurs in this organ except that catalyzed by lingual lipase, which is thought to originate from the salivary glands in the back of the mouth and under the tongue. This lipase is active in the acid environment of the stomach. However, because of the tendency of

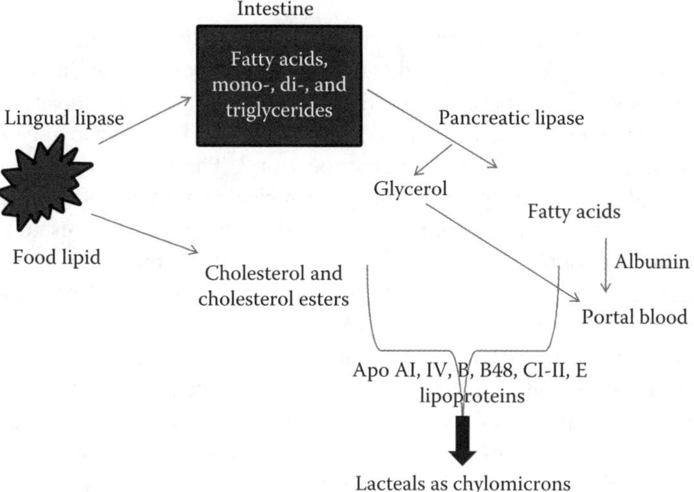

FIGURE 10.1 Overview of digestion and absorption of food lipid.

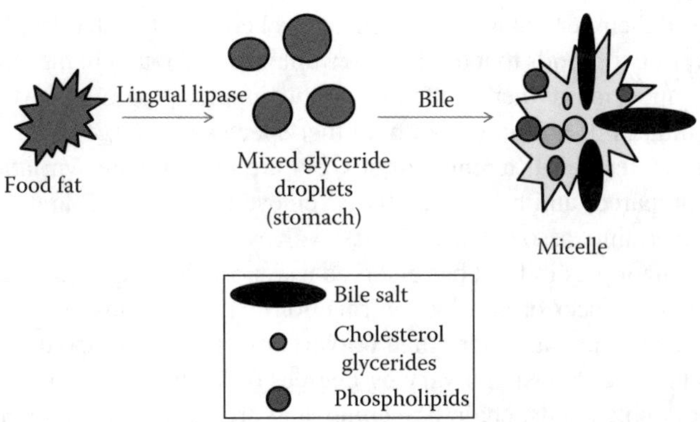

FIGURE 10.2 Changes in the physical state of food lipid as it is prepared for absorption.

lipid to coalesce and form a separate phase, lingual lipase has limited opportunity to attack the TGs. Those that are attacked release a single fatty acid, usually a short- or medium-chain one. The remaining diacylglycerol is subsequently hydrolyzed in the duodenum. In adults consuming a mixed diet, lingual lipase is relatively unimportant. However, in infants having an immature duodenal lipase, lingual lipase is quite important. In addition, this lipase has its greatest activity on the TGs commonly present in whole milk. Milk fat has more short- and medium-chain fatty acids than fats from other food sources.

Although the action of lingual lipase is slow relative to the lipases found in the duodenum, its action to release diacylglycerol and short- and medium-chain fatty acids serves another function: these fatty acids serve as surfactants. Surfactants spontaneously adsorb to the water–lipid interface, stabilizing emulsions as they form. Other dietary surfactants are the lecithins and the phospholipids. Altogether, these surfactants plus the churning action of the stomach produce an emulsion that is then expelled into the duodenum as chyme.

The entry of chyme into the duodenum stimulates the release of the gut hormones pancreozymin and cholecystokinin into the blood stream. Cholecystokinin stimulates the gall bladder to contract and release bile. Bile salts serve as emulsifying agents and to further disperse the lipid droplets at the lipid–aqueous interface facilitating the hydrolysis of the glycerides by the pancreatic lipases. The bile salts impart a negative charge to the lipids, which in turn attracts the pancreatic enzyme colipase.

Pancreozymin (secretin) stimulates the exocrine pancreas to release pancreatic juice, which contains three lipases (lipase, lipid esterase, and colipase). These lipases act at the water–lipid interface of the emulsion particles. One lipase acts on the fatty acids esterified at positions 1 and 3 of the glycerol backbone, leaving a fatty acid esterified at carbon 2. This 2-monoacylglyceride can isomerize and the remaining fatty acid can move to carbon 1 or 3. The pancreatic juice contains another less specific lipase (also called a lipid esterase), which cleaves fatty acids from cholesterol esters, monoglycerides, or esters such as vitamin A ester. Its action requires the presence of the bile salts. The lipase that is specific for the ester linkage at carbons 1 and 3 of the TGs does not have a requirement for the bile salts and, in fact, is inhibited by them. The inhibition of pancreatic lipase by the bile salts is relieved by the third pancreatic enzyme, colipase.

Colipase is a small protein (mol. wt. 12,000 Da) that binds to both the water–lipid interface and to lipase, thereby anchoring and activating the lipase. The products of the lipase-catalyzed reaction, a reaction that favors the release of fatty acids having 10 or more carbons, are these fatty acids and monoacylglyceride. The products of the lipid esterase-catalyzed reaction are cholesterol, vitamins, fatty acids, and glycerol. The phospholipids present in food are attacked by phospholipases specific to each of the phospholipids. The pancreatic juice contains these lipases as prephospholipases, which are activated by the enzyme trypsin.

As mentioned, the release of bile from the gall bladder is essential to the digestion of dietary fat. Bile contains the bile acids, cholic acid and chenodeoxycholic acid. These are emulsifying agents. At physiological pH, these acids are present as anions, so they are frequently referred to as bile salts. At pH values above the physiological range, they form aggregates with fats at concentrations above 2–5 mM. These aggregates are called micelles. The micelles are much smaller in size than the emulsified lipid droplets. Micelle sizes vary depending on the ratio of lipids to bile acids but typically range from 40 to 600 Å.

Micelles (Figure 10.2) are structured such that the hydrophobic portions (triglycerols, cholesterol esters, etc.) are toward the center of the structure, while the hydrophilic portions (phospholipids, short-chain fatty acids, bile salts) surround this center. Micelles contain many different lipids. Mixed micelles have a disc-like shape where the lipids form a bilayer and the bile acids occupy edge positions, rendering the edge of the disc hydrophilic. During the process of lipase and esterase digestion of the lipids in the chyme, the water-insoluble lipids are rendered soluble and transferred from the lipid emulsion of the chyme to the micelle. In turn, these micelles transfer the products of digestion (free fatty acids, glycerol, cholesterol, etc.) from the intestinal lumen to the surface of the epithelial cells, where absorption takes place. The micellar fluid layer next to this cell surface is homogenous, yet the products of lipid digestion are presented to the cell surface and, by passive diffusion, these products are transported into the absorptive cell. Thus, the degree to which dietary lipid, once digested, is absorbed depends largely on the amount of lipid to be absorbed relative to the amount of bile acid available to make the micelle. This, in turn, is dependent on the rate of bile acid synthesis by the liver and bile release by the gall bladder. People who have had their gall bladder removed still have their bile acids. Instead of stockpiling them in the gall bladder to be released upon the cholecystokinin signal, surgeons simply remove the gall bladder and make a direct connection between the liver and the duodenum. Once the fat has been absorbed, the bile acids pass on through the intestine, where they are either reabsorbed or conjugated and excreted in the feces.

The bile acids, cholic and chenodeoxycholic acids, are produced from cholesterol by the liver. They are secreted into the intestine, and, if not reabsorbed, the intestinal flora convert them to their conjugated forms by dehydroxylating carbon 7. Further metabolism occurs at the far end of the intestinal tract where lithocholate is sulfated. While the dehydroxylated acids can be reabsorbed and sent back to the liver via the portal blood, the sulfated lithocholate is not. It appears in the feces. All of the bile acids, the primary and dehydroxylated forms, are recirculated via the enterohepatic system so that very little of the bile acid is lost. It has been estimated that the bile acid lost in the feces (~ 0.8 g/day) equals that newly synthesized by the liver so that the total pool remains between 3 and 5 g. The amount secreted per day is on the order of 16–70 g. Since the pool size is only 3–5 g, this means that these acids are recirculated as often as 14 times a day.

The function of the bile acids is quite similar to that of enzymes. Neither are *used up* by the processes they facilitate. In the instance of fat absorption, the bile acids facilitate the formation of micelles, which, in turn, facilitate the uptake of the dietary fatty acids, monoglycerides, sterols, phospholipids, and other fat-soluble nutrients by the enterocyte of the small intestine. Not only do these bile acids recirculate, so too does cholesterol. Gallstones develop when the resecreted material is supersaturated with cholesterol, and this cholesterol-laden bile is stored in the gall bladder. With time, the cholesterol precipitates out, providing a crystalline structure for the stone. Since the bile also contains a variety of minerals, these minerals form salts with the bile acids and are deposited within and around the cholesterol matrix. Eventually, these stones irritate the lining of the gall bladder or may lodge themselves in the duct connecting the bladder to the duodenum. When this happens, the bladder becomes inflamed, the duct may be blocked, and the patient becomes unable to process the food lipid. In some cases, treatment consists of reducing the irritation and inflammation through drugs, but often the patient has the gall bladder and its offending stones removed. This surgery is called a cholecystectomy.

Virtually all of the fatty acids, as part of the mono-, di-, and TGs, and glycerol are absorbed by the enterocyte. Only 30%–40% of the dietary cholesterol is absorbed. The percent cholesterol absorbed depends on a number of factors, including the fiber content of the diet, the gut passage time, and the total amount of cholesterol present for absorption. At higher intake levels, less is absorbed and vice versa at lower intake levels. Compared with fatty acids and the acylglycerides, the rate of cholesterol absorption is very slow. It is estimated that the half-life of cholesterol in the enterocyte is 12 h. The presence of plant sterols lowers the absorption of cholesterol such that serum low-density lipoprotein (LDL) cholesterol levels are reduced. With high fiber intakes, less cholesterol is absorbed because the fiber acts as an adsorbent, reducing cholesterol availability. Chapter 9 discusses the different fibers and their biological activity. Cellulose and lignins are good adsorbents of cholesterol, while transit through the intestine can be hastened by cellulose and hemicellulose. Pectins and gums increase transit time, yet they lower serum cholesterol levels by creating a gel-like consistency of the chyme, rendering the cholesterol in the chyme less available for absorption. High-fiber diets reduce gut passage time, which, in turn, results in less time for cholesterol absorption.

The fate of the absorbed fatty acids depends on chain length. Those fatty acids having 10 or fewer carbons are quickly passed into the portal blood stream without further modification. They are carried to the liver bound to albumin in concentrations varying between 0.1 and 2.0 meq/mL. Those fatty acids remaining are bound to a fatty acid-binding protein and transported through the cytosol to the endoplasmic reticulum, whereupon they are converted to their CoA derivatives and reesterified to glycerol or residual monoacylglycerides to reform TGs. These reformed TGs adhere to phospholipids and fat-transporting proteins that are members of the lipoprotein family of proteins. This relatively large lipid–protein complex migrates to the Golgi complex in the basolateral basement membrane of the enterocyte. The lipid-rich vesicles fuse with the Golgi surface membrane, whereupon the lipid–protein complex is exocytosed or secreted into the intercellular space that, in turn, drains into the lymphatic system. The lymphatic system contributes these lipids to the circulation as the thoracic duct enters the jugular vein prior to its entry into the heart.

TRANSPORT

Blood lipid values vary depending on the age, sex, lifestyle, genetics, and diet of the population. Typical values for the different lipids are shown in Table 10.4. After a meal, the blood lipids rise. The time it takes for the peak value to appear depends on a variety of factors but, most notably, on the proximate composition of the meal. A high-fat meal leaves the stomach at a slower rate than does a low-fat meal. A high-fat meal will result in more total lipid entering the blood than a low-fat meal, but this lipid will enter the blood at a slower rate.

TABLE 10.4
Average Blood Lipid Levels for Normal Fasting Humans

	Range of Values[a]	
Fraction	**mmol/L**	**mg/dL**
Cholesterol		
Males	3.95–5.56	152–214
Females	4.08–5.88	157–226
Phospholipids		9–16 (as lipid P)
Triacyglycerides (TG)		
Males	0.77–1.30	68–115
Females	0.72–1.24	64–110
Free fatty acids		6–16

[a] Selected from a table of usual clinical findings as published by Feldman, E.B. and Cooper, G.R., Assessment of lipids and lipoproteins, in: *Handbook of Nutrition and Food*, Berdanier, C.D., Dwyer, J., Feldman, E.B., eds., CRC Press, Boca Raton, FL, 2007, pp. 683–692.

Exogenous Lipid Transport

As fat digestion and absorption proceed, TG and cholesterol are processed in the intestinal epithelial cells into lipid-rich particles containing about 1% protein. The lipid associates with amphipathic protein and together the molecule is known as a lipoprotein. Lipoproteins carry not only the absorbed food lipids but also the lipids synthesized or mobilized from organs and fat depots. Nine different lipid-carrying proteins have been identified, and each plays a specific role in the lipid-transport process. In addition, there are several minor proteins that may be involved in some aspects of lipid cycling and uptake. The proteins involved in lipid transport are listed in Table 10.5 and their characteristics are listed in Table 10.6. Mutations in the genes that encode these proteins can lead to aberrant lipid transport and the individual may have either abnormally high or low blood lipid values.[11–15] The hepatic and intestinal apolipoproteins (apos) can be distinguished using electrophoresis, a technique of separating proteins based on their electrophoretic mobility. Typically, these lipid-carrying proteins contain protein, TGs, phospholipids, and cholesterol. When separated, they have distinct characteristics of protein and lipid content, as shown in Table 10.6.

TABLE 10.5
Proteins Involved in Lipid Transport

Protein	Function
Apo A-II	Transport protein in HDL.
Apo B-48	Transport protein for chylomicrons; synthesized in the enterocyte in the human.
Apo B-100	Ligand for LDL receptor; synthesized in the liver and is secreted into the circulation as part of the VLDL.
HDLBP	Binds HDL and functions in the removal of excess cellular cholesterol.
Apo D	Transport protein similar to retinol-binding protein.
Apo (a)	Abnormal transport protein for LDL.
Apo A-I	Transport protein for chylomicrons and HDL; synthesized in the liver and its synthesis is induced by retinoic acid; antiatherogenic.
Apo C-III	Transport protein for VLDL; impairs TAG hydrolysis by inhibiting LPL.
Apo A-IV	Transport protein for chylomicrons; antiatherogenic.
Apo A-V	Reduces plasma TG by lowering VLDL production and enhancing lipolysis.
CETP	Participates in the transport of cholesterol from peripheral tissue to liver; reduces HDL size.
LCAT	Synthesized in the liver and is secreted into the plasma where it resides on the HDL. Participates in the reverse transport of cholesterol from peripheral tissues to the liver; esterifies the HDL cholesterol.
Apo E	Mediates high affinity binding of LDL's to LDL receptor and the putative chylomicron receptor. Required for clearance of chylomicron remnant. Synthesized primarily in the liver.
Apo C-I	Blocks apo E binding to receptors; transport protein for VLDL.
Apo C-II	Chylomicron transport protein required cofactor for LPL activity.
Apo H	Antiatherogenic; ligand for LDL receptor.
LPL	Catalyzes the hydrolysis of plasma triglycerides into free fatty acids.
Hepatic lipase	Catalyzes the hydrolysis of triglycerides and phospholipids of the LDL and HDL. It is bound to the surfaces of both hepatic and non hepatic tissues.
Diacylglycerol acyltransferase (DGAT 1 and 2)	Acyltransferase required for synthesis of TAG molecule.
LCAT	Catalyzes the esterification of free cholesterol to cholesterol ester on the lipoproteins.
Acyl CoA–cholesterol acyltransferase	Catalyzes cholesterol esterification.

Source: Feldman, E.B. et al., Hyperlipidemias: Major gene and diet effects, in: *Handbook of Nutrition and Food*, Berdanier, C.D. et al. (eds.), 2nd edn., CRC Press, Boca Raton, FL, 2007, pp. 715–726.

TABLE 10.6
Characteristics of the Various Lipoproteins

Fraction	% Protein	Density	TG	% Lipid (as Phospholipid)	Cholesterol
Chylomicrons	1.5–2.5	<0.95	84–89	7–9	1–5
VLDL	5–10	0.95–1.006	50–65	15–20	5–15
LDL[a]	20–25	1.006–1.019	7–10	15–20	35–401
LDL[b]	20–25	1.019–1.063	7–10	15–20	7–102
HDL	40–55	1.068–1.210	5	20–35	4–12

[a] Primarily esterified cholesterol.
[b] Primarily unesterified cholesterol.

The intestinal cell has three apos, called A-1, A-IV, and B-48. Apo B-48 is unique to the enterocyte and is essential for chylomicron release by the intestinal cell. A-1 is synthesized in the liver. Apo B-48 is actually an edited version of the hepatic apo B-100. It is the result of an apo B mRNA editing process that converts codon 2153 to a translational stop codon. Apo B-48 is, thus, an edited form of apo B-100 and this editing is unique to the intestinal cell. Failure to appropriately edit the apo B 100 gene in the intestinal cell will result in a disorder called familial hypobetalipoproteinemia. In this disorder, there will be a total or partial (depending on the genetic mutation) absence of lipoproteins in the blood. Hypobetalipoproteinemia can also develop should there be base substitutions in the gene for the apo B 100 protein. In addition to very low blood lipids, patients with this disorder also have fat malabsorption (steatorrhea). The feces contain an abnormally large amount of fat and have a characteristic peculiar odor. In this disorder, not only is the TG absorption affected, but so too are the fat-soluble vitamins. Without the ability to absorb these energy-rich food components and the vital fat-soluble vitamins, the patient does not thrive and survive. Fortunately, this genetic mutation is not very common. It is inherited as an autosomal recessive trait.

The particles of absorbed lipid and transport proteins are called chylomicrons. They are present in the blood of feeding animals but are usually absent in starving animals. As the chylomicrons circulate, they acquire an additional protein, apo C-II. This additional protein is an essential cofactor for the recognition and hydrolysis of the chylomicron by the capillary endothelial enzyme, lipoprotein lipase (LPL). The LPL hydrolyzes most of the core triglycerides in the chylomicron leaving a remnant that is rich in cholesterol and cholesterol esters. During the LPL-catalyzed hydrolytic process, the excess surface compounds, that is, the phospholipids and apos B, A-I, and A-IV are transferred to high-density lipoproteins (HDL) and, in exchange, apo E is transferred from the HDL to the cholesterol ester-rich chylomicron remnant. These remnants are then cleared from the blood by the liver. On the hepatocyte is a lipoprotein receptor that recognizes apo E, and this receptor plays an important role in remnant clearance. Figure 10.3 illustrates the process of exogenous lipid absorption, transport, and clearance.

The chylomicron is a relatively stable way of ensuring the movement, in an aqueous medium (blood), of hydrophobic molecules such as cholesterol and TGs from their point of origin, the intestine, to their point of use or storage. As mentioned, there are several unique proteins that facilitate this movement. These lipid-transporting proteins determine which cells of the body receive which lipids. At the target cell, the particles lose their lipid through hydrolysis facilitated by an interstitial LPL, which is found in the capillary beds of muscle, fat cells, and other tissues using lipid as a fuel. LPL is synthesized by these target cells but is anchored on the outside of the cells by a polysaccharide chain on the endothelial wall of the surrounding capillaries. Should this lipoprotein lipase be missing or genetically aberrant (type I lipemia or chylomicronemia) so that the chylomicrons cannot be hydrolyzed, these chylomicrons accumulate and the individual develops a lipemia characterized by elevated levels of TG and cholesterol-containing chylomicons. Also characteristic of this

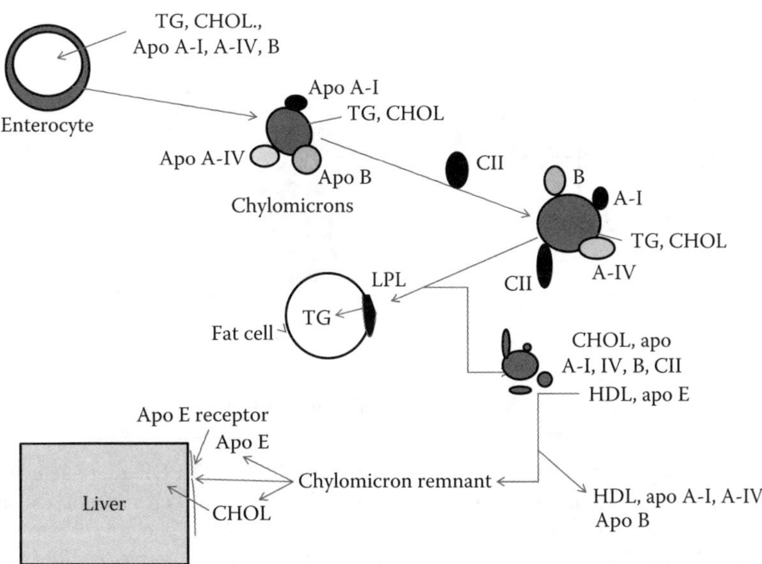

FIGURE 10.3 Schematic representation of the uptake, transport, and disposal of dietary lipids. TG, triacylglycerides; CHOL, cholesterol and cholesterol esters; apo A-I, apo B, apo E, polypeptide lipid carriers; HDL, high-density lipoprotein.

condition is considerable abdominal discomfort and the presence of an enlarged liver and spleen and of subcutaneous xanthomas (clusters of hard, saturated fatty acid and cholesterol-rich nodules). Like familial hypolipoproteinemia, this condition is rare. Of interest is the observation that, despite the very high blood lipid levels of these people, few die of coronary-vessel disease. Their shortened life span is due to an inappropriate lipid deposition in all of the vital organs, which, in turn, has a negative effect on organ function and life span.

Endogenous Lipid Transport

Fatty acids, TG, cholesterol, cholesterol esters, and phospholipids are synthesized in the body and are transported from sites of synthesis to sites of use and storage. While the transport of these lipids is, in many instances, similar to that of the dietary lipids, there are differences in the processing and in some of the proteins involved. Endogenous fat transport (Figure 10.4) involves the production and secretion of very-low-density lipoproteins (VLDL) by the liver. These lipid–protein complexes are rich in TG and also contain cholesterol. The polypeptides that transport these lipids make up approximately 10% of the weight of the VLDL. They include the polypeptides apo-B, B-100, apo C-I, apo C-II, apo C-III, and apo E. As mentioned, several of these polypeptides are also involved in exogenous lipid transport. Once the VLDLs are released by the hepatocyte, they are hydrolyzed by the interstitial LPL, and intermediate-density lipoproteins (IDL) are formed. These are cleared from the circulation as they are recognized and bound to hepatic IDL receptors. The hepatic receptors recognize the apo E that is part of the IDL. Any of the IDL that escapes hydrolysis at this step is available for hydrolysis by the hepatic LPL. This hydrolysis leaves a cholesterol-rich particle of low density (LDL). The LDL has apo B-100 as its polypeptide carrier and both hepatic and extrahepatic cells have receptors that recognize this polypeptide. Normally, about 70% of LDL is cleared by the LDL receptors and most of this is cleared by the liver. The endogenous fat transport and disposal system is diagrammed in Figure 10.4. From the foregoing, it is apparent that considerable lipid recycling occurs in the liver. The VLDLs originate in the liver, which is the primary site for LDL disposal. Other organs and tissues also participate in disposal, but their participation is minor compared with that of the liver.

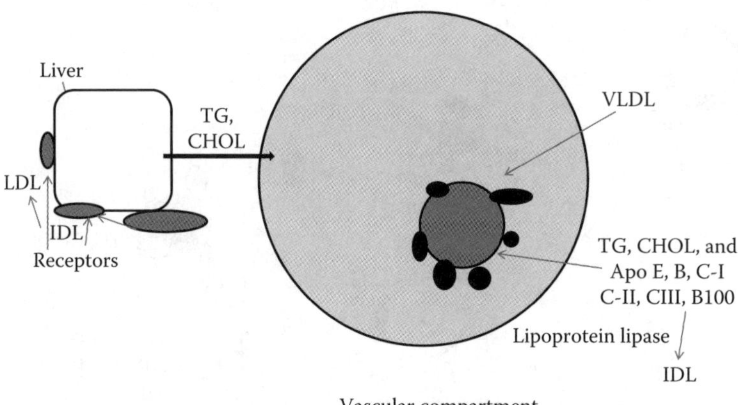

FIGURE 10.4 Lipid recycling: endogenous lipid transport and disposal. VLDL are secreted by the liver and circulated back to it, where various receptors (shown as a half-moon on the cell surface) bind and remove the lipid in a stepwise sequence. TG, triacylglycerides; CHOL, cholesterol and cholesterol esters; apo E, apo B, apo B-100, apo C-III, apo C-II, apo C-I, polypeptide lipid carriers; IDL, intermediate-density lipoproteins; LDL, low-density lipoproteins.

GENETIC BASIS FOR LIPOPROTEINEMIA

As mentioned, there are a number of proteins involved in the uptake, synthesis, and disposal of lipid. The genes for the transport proteins, apo A-I, apo A-II, apo A-IV, apo (a), apo B, apo D, apo C-I, apo C-II, apo C-III, apo D, and apo E have been identified, as have mutations that result in lipid transport abnormalities (Table 10.7). In addition to these transport proteins, we have the proteins that are important rate-limiting enzymes and receptors involved in lipoprotein processing. These include the peripheral LPL and the hepatic LPL, the lipoprotein receptors on the plasma membrane of the cells that receive and oxidize or store the transported lipids, and the rate-limiting enzymes of lipid synthesis and use.[11] These enzymes are the fatty acid synthase complex, acetyl CoA carboxylase, HMG CoA reductase, HMG CoA synthase, cholesterol ester transfer protein (CETP), fatty acid-binding protein (FABP), lecithin–cholesterol acyltransferase (LCAT), cholesterol 7-hydroxylase, and the high-density lipoprotein-binding protein (HDLBP). Many of these proteins have been isolated and studied in detail. Several of their cognate genes have been identified and mapped.[15] Listed in Table 10.7 are the chromosomal locations and mutation frequencies of these genes. With this many genes involved in the uptake, synthesis, transport, and degradation of the circulating lipids, it is not surprising to find mutations that phenotype as either lipemia or fat malabsorption. Not all of these mutations in the gene products needed for lipid transport are associated with atherosclerosis.

DEFECTS IN EXOGENOUS FAT TRANSPORT

Defects in exogenous fat transport are manifested in several ways. As described earlier, defective chylomicron formation due to mutations in either the apo B gene or its editing leads to and is characterized by fat malabsorption. This includes the malabsorption of fat-soluble vitamins as well. Many different mutations have been identified in the gene for the apo B protein.[16–22] These mutations are inherited via an autosomal recessive mode. Those that affect fat absorption are characterized not only by fat malabsorption but also by acanthocytes, retinitis pigmentosa, and muscular neuropathies. Some of the symptoms can be attributed to a relative deficiency of the fat-soluble vitamins because the absorption of fat soluble vitamins is dependent on normal fat absorption. Some of the apo B mutations phenotype as lipemia where there is a defective binding to the LDL receptor. Approximately 400 mutations have been reported in 5 classes of the LDL gene and these mutations phenotype as familial hypercholesterolemia. While a defect in the apo B gene can

TABLE 10.7
Location of Genes Involved in Lipoprotein Metabolism

Gene	Chromosome Location	Characteristics of Mutation	Frequency of Mutation
Apo A-II	1	Transport protein in HDL	?
Apo B 48	2p23–24	Hypobetalipoproteinemia	1:1,000,000
HDLBP	2q37		?
Apo D	3	Transport protein similar to retinol-binding protein	?
Apo (a)	6	Abnormal transport protein for LDL	?
LPL	8p22	Defective chylomicron clearance	1:1,000,000 40 known mutations
Apo A-I	11	Defective HDL production (Tangier's disease)	1:1,000,000
Apo C-III	11		?
Apo A-IV	11		?
Hepatic LPL (HTGL)	15q21	Defective IDL clearance	?
CETP	16q22.1		?
LCAT	16q22.1	Familial lecithin–cholesterol transferase deficiency. two types.	Rare
LDL receptor	19	Familial hypercholesterolemia	1:500
Apo B 100	2	Familial defective apo B 100	1:500–1:1,000 3,500 mutations
Apo E	19	Type III hyperlipoproteinemia	1:5,000
Apo C-I	19	Transport protein for VLDL	?
Apo C-II	19	Defective chylomicron clearance	1:1,000,000

Note: "?" indicates unknown.

account for defective fat absorption in some cases, there may be another mutation in the microsomal triglyceride transfer protein that also results in fat malabsorption.[23,24] This transfer protein is essential for apo B translocation and subsequent synthesis of chylomicrons. Defects in this transfer protein would impair apo B availability and chylomicron formation. In these defects, very low levels of chylomicrons are found in the blood. Persons with this disorder are rare (one in a million). In this circumstance, the severity of the disease is related to the size of the mutated gene product and whether it can associate with the lipids it must carry. The size of the truncated apo B can vary from apo B-9 (41 residues) to apo B-89 (4487 residues). Except in the case of the apo B-25, the result of a deletion of the entire exon 21, all the truncated forms reported to date are C-T transitions or base deletions.[23] These deletions can involve misaligned pairing deletion mechanisms.[21] Frameshift mutation can be compensated by a reading frame restoration of the apo B gene.[22]

Familial hyperchylomicronemia is characterized by elevations in chylomicrons having both triglycerides and cholesterol. Hyperchylomicronemia was found to be due to mutations in the genes that encode the enzyme LPL needed for the hydrolysis and clearance of the chylomicrons from the blood.[25] This enzyme is a glycoprotein having an apparent monomeric molecular weight of about 60,000 Da on SDS gel electrophoresis and 48,300 Da by sedimentation-equilibrium ultracentrifugation. The enzyme is linked to the endothelial cells of the capillary system. LPL is quite similar to hepatic triglyceride lipase, an enzyme found in the hepatic sinusoids. The main difference between the two lipases is that the interstitial lipase has a requirement for the lipid-carrying protein, apo C-II, for full activity, whereas hepatic LPL does not. Mutations in the gene for apo C-II can result in aberrant lipase activity because apo C-II serves as a cofactor in the LPL-catalyzed reaction.[24] Hepatic triglyceride lipase has no such requirement. Aberrations in the hepatic triglyceride lipase result in an accumulation of VLDL rather than accumulations of chylomicrons. Mutations in the genes for LPL and apo C-II are very rare, occurring at a frequency of one in a million. The gene for LPL has been mapped to chromosome 8, while that for apo C-II has been mapped to chromosome 19 and the hepatic LPL to chromosome 15.[27–32] Other features of these disorders include an inflammation of the exocrine pancreas and eruptive xanthomas. Chylomicronemia does not appear to be atherogenic. The mutations in the LPL gene appear to be insertions or deletions or due to aberrant splicing, while those in the apo C-II gene seem to be due to splice site mutations or small deletions. Twenty-two mutations in the apo C-II gene have been reported. With respect to the aberrant splicing of the LPL gene in three unrelated humans, Holzl et al.[33] reported a C→A mutation in position 3 of the acceptor splice site of intron 6, which caused aberrant splicing. The major transcript showed a deletion of exons 6 through 9 and amounted to about 3% of normal. Trace amounts of both a normally spliced LPL mRNA and a second aberrant transcript devoid of exon 7 were found. In one of these patients, Holzl et al.[33] found a 3′ splice mutation on one allele, while on the other allele, they found a missense mutation resulting in Gly 188→Glu substitution. All three subjects were classed as hyperchylomicronemic due to LPL deficiency.

The absence of LPL activity in certain tissues or in certain individuals can be attributed to mutations in LPL promoter region. Studies of tissue-specific expression of LPL in a variety of murine tissues by Gimble et al.[13] showed that *cis*-acting elements located within the –1824 bp of the 5′ flanking region were required for the expression of LPL. These include nuclear factors recognizing both the CCAAT box and the octamer sequence immediately flanking the transcriptional start site. Those tissues that have no LPL activity lack this promoter region. Since humans and mice have identical CCAAT and octamer sequences, one could suppose that humans having an intact LPL gene of normal sequence but lacking LPL activity might have a deficient or mutated promoter region. Although such has been suggested by Sparkes et al.[27], proof that this might occur is presently lacking.

Mutations in the gene for hepatic LPL result in elevated blood levels of triglycerides and cholesterol and these elevations are related to an increased risk for atherosclerosis. Hepatic LPL must be secreted by the hepatocyte into the sinusoids to function as a catalyst for the hydrolysis of core TG and surface phospholipids of chylomicron remnants, HDL, and IDL. Through its activity, it augments the uptake of HDL cholesterol by the liver (reverse cholesterol transport) and is involved in the reduction of HDL size from HDL2 to HDL3. Hepatic LPL aids in the clearance of chylomicron remnants by exposing the apo E epitopes for enzymatic action. Missense mutations in the hepatic LPL gene include substitutions of serine for phenylalanine at amino acid position 267, threonine for methionine at position 383, and asparagine for serine at position 291.[33,34] These mutations result in poorly secreted enzyme and thus the phenotypic expression of the mutation is low hepatic lipase activity. The frequency of the Asn 291 Ser mutation in a population having premature CVD has been reported as 5.2%.

Defects in chylomicron remnant clearance are much more common than any of the previous mutations.[35–41] Defective clearance due to mutations in the apo E gene results in a lipemia known as type III hyperlipoproteinemia. It is associated with premature atherosclerosis. Patients with these defects have high serum triglyceride levels as well as high serum cholesterol levels. Xanthomas are found in nearly three-quarters of the population with these defects. The lipemia is responsive to energy restriction using diets that have 40% of energy from carbohydrate, 40% from fat, and 20% from protein. Weight loss is efficacious for most people with this defect. The apo E gene codes for the protein on the surface of the chylomicron remnant that is the ligand for receptor-mediated clearance of this particle.

A number of mutations in the apo E gene have been reported, and the phenotypes of these mutations are grouped into three general groups labeled E2, E3, and E4.[42] Those of the E2 groups fail to bind the particles to the cell surface receptor for the chylomicron remnant. Those of the E3 and E4 groups have generally low remnant clearance rates. The apo E allele and phenotype frequency varies. The E2 frequency is about 8%, the E3 about 77%, and the E4 about 15% of the total population with an apo E mutation. The incidence of apo E gene mutations is about 1% of the population. Since apo E is involved in both endogenous and exogenous lipid transport and clearance, a faulty apo E gene is devastating. Mature human apo E is a 299 amino acid polypeptide. Apo E as well as other apos contains 11 or 22 amino acid repeated sequences as one of their key features. These appear to encode largely amphipathic helices, which are needed for lipid binding. There is a high degree of conservation among species of nucleotide sequences in the gene fragment that encodes the amino acid repeats. The gene for apo E has been mapped to chromosome 19, as have the genes for apo C-I, apo C-II, and LDLR. There appears to be a tight linkage among these genes that coordinates their expression. Among the common mutations are amino acid substitutions at positions 112 and 158, while less-frequent substitutions occur at other positions in the polypeptide chain. Several of these involve the exchange of neutral amino acids for acidic amino acids with the net result of alterations in polypeptide charge and subsequent inadequate binding to the appropriate cell surface receptors.

In a rare form of the disorder, the mutation is such that no useful apo E is formed. Transgenic mice have been constructed with an apo E mutation that mimics apo E deficiency in humans.[38–41] These mice, like humans, develop hypercholesterolemia and increased susceptibility to atherosclerosis. When these mice were fed low- (5%) or high-fat (16%) diets, a differential serum cholesterol pattern was observed: those fed the high-fat diet had significantly higher levels of cholesterol and VLDL and LDL than those fed a low-fat or stock diet. The transgenic mice, even when fed the stock diet, had significantly higher levels of cholesterol and VLDL and LDL than the normal control mice. There was a gender difference as well. Male transgenic mice were less diet responsive in terms of their cholesterol levels than female transgenic mice. As mentioned, there is some sequence homology between humans and mice in the apo E DNA, and it could be inferred that these responses to dietary fat intake in mice could be observed in humans as well.

While this transgenic approach used the gene-knockout paradigm (an extreme in the variants of apo E mutants), it nonetheless suggests that variation in the apo E genes could determine the responsiveness of humans with apo E defects to dietary manipulation. Indeed, such nutrient–gene interactions have been reported.[16,40–43] The dietary fat clearance in normal subjects appears to be regulated by the genetic variance in apo E sequence, and this, in turn, is related to fat intake. Not only is TG clearance affected, but so too is cholesterol clearance. One study reported that the apo E genotype determines the response to cholesterol intake with respect to blood cholesterol levels and that this genotype influences cholesterol synthesis. Those subjects who respond poorly to an oral cholesterol challenge vis-à-vis blood cholesterol clearance had higher rates of cholesterol synthesis than those who could rapidly clear their blood of cholesterol after an oral challenge. Defective HDL metabolism due to a mutation in the apo A-I gene results in a rare autosomal dominant disorder described in a small group of villagers in Italy. Affected individuals have reduced levels of HDL cholesterol and apo A-I levels, but have no increased risk of CVD. The disorder, named Apo A-I Milano, is due to a point mutation in the apo A-I gene, changing codon 173 so that cysteine is used instead of arginine. Normal apo A-I has no cysteine, so this change has an effect on the apo A-I structure.

Cholesterol traffic is also controlled by the LDL receptor and the transport protein apo B-10. Mutations in the gene for the LDL receptor or in the gene for apo B-100, the ligand for the LDL receptor, results in high serum levels of cholesterol. The former results in the disorder called familial hypercholesterolemia and occur with a frequency of about 1 in 500. Familial hypercholesterolemia is associated with early death from atherosclerosis in man and related primates. Dietary fat saturation affects transcription of LDL receptor mRNA, in that feeding a diet containing saturated fat results in decreased LDL receptor mRNA, compared with feeding an unsaturated-fat diet.[44] These results suggest that unsaturated fatty acids may interact with proteins that in turn serve as either *cis*- or *trans*-acting elements for this gene in much the same way as PUFAs affect fatty acid synthetase gene expression.[45]

Familial defective apo B-100 hypercholesterolemia is due to a mutation in the coding sequence of the apo B gene at bp 3500 that changes the base sequence such that glutamine is substituted for arginine. This is in the LDL receptor-binding region of the apo B protein and results in a binding affinity of less than 4% of normal. Polymorphic variation in the genes for both the LDL receptor and the apo B-100 have been reported for mice, and this variation has provided the opportunity to identify the genetic and molecular constraints of lipoprotein gene expression.

Both apo B and apo E serve as ligands for the LDL receptor. In contrast to apo E, apo B has little homology with the other apos. Apo B in mice is quite variable, and this variation imparts or confers a diet-responsive characteristic in inbred mouse strains vis-à-vis polypeptide sequence and activity. That is, some mouse strains have reduced levels of plasma apo B when fed a high-fat diet compared with controls fed a stock diet, while other mouse strains are unresponsive to diet vis-à-vis their plasma apo B-100 levels.

Such polymorphism also exists in humans. Apo B has been mapped to chromosome 2 and produces two gene products, apo B-100 and B-48. In the intestine, the apo B primary transcript is co- or posttranscriptionally modified. This modification converts codon 2153 from a glutamine (CAA) to an in-frame, premature termination codon (UAA), thereby causing translation to terminate after amino acid 2152. This mRNA editing thus explains the difference in size of these two proteins. If more of the apo B gene is deleted, hypocholesterolemia is observed. This is because apo B-48 is required for the transport of the chylomicrons from the intestine. If lacking, chylomicron formation is impaired and low serum cholesterol levels are observed. Both familial defective apo B-100 and familial hypercholesterolemia are characterized by high levels of LDL. Both are associated with CVD, but only the familial hypercholesterolemia is characterized by tendon xanthomas. Both are inherited as autosomal dominant disorders. Collectively, these mutations have a cumulative frequency of 1 in 250. However, because polymorphism in the apo B gene can and does occur, there is the possibility that, collectively, the frequency is much greater. It may be as high as one in five. If this is the case, then the population variation in plasma cholesterol levels could be explained on the basis of these genetic differences alone, apart from those mutations that are associated with the rest of the genes that encode components of the lipid transport system.

Genetically determined abnormalities in LDL metabolism may also be due to mutation in the large glycoprotein, apo (a). Apo (a) is a highly variable disulfide protein bonded to the apo B-100. It is thought to resemble plasminogen. In fact, the genes that encode Lp(a) and plasminogen are very close to each other on the long arm of chromosome 6. In general, LDLs containing apo (a) do not bind well to the LPL receptor, and people having significant amounts of apo (a) have a two- to threefold increase in cardiovascular disease (CVD) risk. Many individuals have little or no apo (a) and it has been suggested that those who have it are abnormal with respect to LPL activity.

Several mutations in the genes that encode the endogenous lipid transport have been reported.[46,47] The reverse cholesterol transport pathway is part of this endogenous lipid-transport system. It involves the movement of cholesterol from peripheral tissues to the liver. The peripheral tissues cannot oxidize cholesterol and so must send it to the liver, where it is prepared for excretion, via cholesterol 7 α hydroxylase, as bile acids. This pathway uses the HDL to shuttle the cholesterol in this direction. HDL consists primarily of apo A-1 and cholesterol, which is esterified by the enzyme LCAT. Mutations in the LCAT gene have been reported. One of these is called familial LCAT deficiency. Thirteen different mutations have been identified, and in one, a single T→A transversion in codon 252 in exon 6, converting met (ATG) to Lys (AAG), was observed. Three unrelated families were found to have this mutation; however, the severity of their disease varied. In these families, no other mutation in LCAT was observed. Of the remaining 12 LCAT mutations, 10 were point mutations, three were frameshifts, and one consisted of a three-base insertion that maintained its reading frame. For fish-eye disease, three mutations have been reported. This disorder is less serious than familial LCAT deficiency and is characterized by dyslipoproteinemia and corneal opacity. LCAT activity is 15% of normal and there is a reduced level of HDL in the plasma. In contrast, familial LCAT deficiency is characterized by a variety of symptoms, including lipoprotein abnormalities, renal failure, premature atherosclerosis, reduced levels of plasma cholesterol esters, and high plasma levels of cholesterol and lecithin.

The LCAT enzyme requires apo A-I as a cofactor. If there is a mutation in the gene for apo A-I, defective HDL production results. This is a rare mutation and its frequency is estimated as one in a million. Individuals with this defect have premature CVD, corneal clouding, and very low HDL levels. Plasma apo A-I has a variety of charge isoforms with similar antigenicity and amino acid composition. Humans, baboons, African green monkeys, and cynomolgus monkeys have been studied, and there are species differences in hepatic and intestinal apo A-I production. In all instances, the differences in apo A-I were reported between intestine and liver. In the liver, there was a twofold higher level of apo A-I mRNA than in the intestine, and the abundance of this mRNA was species specific. The apo A-I gene is regulated at the level of transcription and a portion of the species-specific difference in apo A-I gene expression is due to a sequence divergence in the 5′ regulatory region, including the exon/intron 1 of the apo A-I gene. The capacity to produce HDLs is both genetically controlled and tissue specific and probably explains why some genotypes respond normally to a high-fat diet by producing more HDL while other genotypes become hypercholesterolemic under these same conditions. Attempts to create a transgenic mouse expressing a human apo A-I gene have not been fully successful, but have provided additional information about the relationship of apo A-I to HDL size. The human apo A-I gene was inserted into the mouse, and in these mice, both the mouse and the human genes were expressed. This dual expression suggests a species difference in the control of this expression. In other words, the control points differed and this resulted in a broader spectrum of HDL particles.

Defective lipoprotein processing has already been discussed with respect to LDP, LCAP, and apo C-II deficiencies. A deficient CETP has been reported due to a mutation of the gene for this protein located on chromosome 16. A mutation in this gene has been used to explain the atherogenicity of high-fat diets in primates, but, to date, no evidence of such a mutation in humans has been put forward.

The majority of the cholesterol in the circulation is synthesized de novo by the body. This synthesis can be suppressed pharmacologically. The statin drugs are very effective cholesterol-lowering agents because they specifically target the rate-limiting enzyme, HMG CoA reductase enzyme. Some of the statin drugs are more effective inhibitors than are others. The fibrate drugs also lower serum cholesterol levels and TGs but are not as effective as the statin drugs in inhibiting cholesterol synthesis.

There are a few people (1 in 20,000) who cannot make cholesterol. They have a genetic disorder known as the Smith–Lemli–Opitz syndrome, abbreviated as SLO disease.[46,47] This disease is sometimes called the RSH syndrome. It is an autosomal recessive disorder characterized by an accumulation of 7-dehydrocholesterol due to a mutation in the gene that encodes Δ7 cholesterol reductase. This enzyme catalyzes an intermediate step in the synthesis of cholesterol. This metabolite accumulates in many tissues, especially the eye. In doing so, it causes cataracts to form. Children with this disorder fail to grow and develop normally (failure to thrive) because cholesterol is a vital ingredient to so many important biological structures. This is especially true with respect to the cell membranes and the lipids in the central nervous system. Some investigators have tried to provide dietary supplements of cholesterol to these children in an effort to improve their development; however, another feature of these children is their great number of food intolerances. Many are intolerant of cholesterol-rich foods such as eggs.

DIET EFFECTS ON SERUM LIPIDS

Dietary lipids, even in the absence of direct effects on transcription and translation, influence the phenotypic expression of specific genotypes either because of overconsumption or because they have effects on certain of the hormones, that is, insulin or the steroid hormones, or the catabolic hormones that regulate or influence lipid synthesis, oxidation, and storage.[50,51] For example, Chen et al.[12] showed that, in diabetic mice, insulin regulated the transcription of the apo C-III gene and that this regulation in turn affected serum triglyceride levels. Triglyceride levels fell in the insulin-treated diabetic mice subsequent to an insulin-induced increase in apo

C-III mRNA level. In turn, Chen et al. showed (in mice) that this mRNA increase was due to a specific effect of insulin on apo C-III gene transcription.

The level of cholesterol in the blood depends on the diet consumed and how much cholesterol is being synthesized.[50,51] The cholesterol content of the gut LDL of a person on a low-cholesterol diet might run as low as 7%–10% of the total lipid in the lipoprotein, while the hepatic LPL of this same individual might be as high as 58% of total lipid. People consuming a low-cholesterol, low-saturated-fat diet may reduce the contribution of the diet to the blood cholesterol while increasing the hepatic de novo cholesterol synthesis.

Persons having an LPL receptor deficiency are characterized by high serum cholesterol levels and, in some cases, by high serum TGs. The reason these blood lipids are elevated is that the individuals cannot utilize the lipids carried by the LPL due to the error(s) in the receptor molecule. Further, because these circulating lipids do not enter into the adipose and hepatic cell in normal amounts, the synthesis of TGs and cholesterol is not appropriately downregulated. Hence, this individual has elevated serum lipids not only because the LPL lipid is not appropriately cleared from the blood but also because of high rates of endogenous lipid synthesis. Individuals with this disorder have lipid deposits in unusual places such as immediately under the skin, around the eyes, on the tendons, and in the vascular tree. It is this last feature that probably accounts for the shortened life span of these people, with the cause of death being CVD. As can be seen from the metabolic characteristics of this disorder, low-cholesterol diets are probably useless in reducing serum cholesterol levels because de novo synthesis of cholesterol from nonlipid precursors can and does occur.[48,49] Treatment with lipid adsorbents (high-fiber diets and drugs such as cholestyramine that block lipid absorption) will help reduce the cholesterol (but not TGs) coming from the intestine, and there are drugs (the statins) that can safely lower de novo cholesterol synthesis as well as increase intracellular lipid oxidation. All of these therapies may help reduce the serum lipid levels, but even doing this only treats the symptoms, not the genetic disorder. Gene therapy is needed to correct the genetic disorder that is the basic underlying cause of the symptoms.

Heart disease in its various forms is also associated with elevated levels of the VLDL. A specific genetic error has not been identified; however, the disorders have been subdivided into three general categories. In one, type III lipemia, the patients are characterized by elevated serum cholesterol, phospholipid, and TG levels, elevated VLDL levels (and sometimes LDL levels), fatty deposits on the tendons and in areas on the arms just under the skin, vascular atheromas, and ischemic heart disease. This type of lipemia is inherited as an autosomal dominant trait in one person in 5000. Another lipemia (type IV) having a normal cholesterol level but an elevated TG level and elevated VLDL levels is also associated with ischemic heart disease and premature atherosclerosis. It is frequently seen in obese patients with type 2 diabetes. People with diabetes mellitus have five to six times the risk of normal people of developing premature atherosclerosis and its associated coronary events. A combination of CVD that is followed by renal disease is the leading cause of death for people with diabetes mellitus.

Those people with type 1 diabetes mellitus are more likely to develop a lipemia (type V lipemia) that is slightly different from the aforementioned type 2 diabetes-related lipemia. While the incidence of both is 2 in 1000, those with the latter problem inherited their trait in an autosomal recessive manner, while those with the type 2 diabetes-related lipemia inherited their trait as an autosomal dominant trait. Elevated chylomicron and VLDL levels and reduced dietary fat tolerance characterize this type of lipemia. Patients with this disorder are usually of normal body weight. Patients with type 2 diabetes benefit from the inclusion of n-3 fatty acids in their diet with respect to their levels of lipoprotein and with an improvement in their insulin sensitivity.[52]

Specific effects of lipids on a variety of systems have been reported. Increased consumption of PUFAs is related to a decrease in the rate of aging of the brain, eye disease, and in cognitive function.[53–57] PUFA intake also stimulates cholecystokinin release and satiety.[58] PUFAs reduced TG uptake by skeletal muscle and improved insulin sensitivity of that muscle.[59] In fructose-fed rats,

TABLE 10.8
Diet/Polymorphism Interactions

Diet Variable	Polymorphism	Outcome
Saturated fat	STAT3	↑ Saturated fat X G alleles had more obesity than controls.[64]
Saturated fat	APOA1 and APOA4	↑ Saturated fat X A alleles had smaller LDL size and ↑ susceptibilty to auto oxidation.[65]
Fat intake	APOA5, 1131T > C	↑ Fat intake → ↑ obesity, ↑ TG rich lipoproteins.[66,74,76]
PUFA intake	FADS 1	↑ PUFA → ↑ High total and non-HDL cholesterol.[69,72]
PUFA intake	PLA2G4A A→G	Myocardial infarction risk was lower in AG/GC subjects consuming PUFA than in AA subjects.[70]
Fat intake	FABP2 A→T	T genotypes have lower glucoregulatory function, greater post prandial lipemia and greater lipid oxidation rates than do A genotypes after a high fat meal.[71]

PUFAs prevented the development of the metabolic and vascular responses to fructose ingestion.[60] Increased cholesterol intake has been shown to accelerate age-related hearing loss.[61] Administering a statin drug prevented this hearing loss. Concurrent iron and EFA deficiency exacerbates the development of cognitive deficits in malnourished children.[62] It also disrupts brain monoamine metabolism and produces greater memory loss.[63]

Polymorphisms interact with dietary lipids and modulate the effects of particular lipids on such conditions as obesity and lipemia.[64–76] Some of these are listed in Table 10.8.

A polymorphism in the LPL gene has been reported to interact with the consumption of alcohol and unsaturated fat such that serum HDL-cholesterol levels are modulated.[75] Polymorphisms in the hepatic lipase (C > T) are related to insulin resistance as well as the level of liver fat.[73] Other polymorphisms interact with dietary carbohydrate to modulate the HDL-cholesterol concentration.[77] The expression of the gene for intestinal FABP was more responsive to dietary fat in the AA homozygotes than in the AB heterogyzotes.[78] This gene may also be a component of the food intake regulatory system.

NUTRIENT–GENE INTERACTIONS IN LIPID TRANSPORT

The observations of diet and genetic factors described so far suggest that lipemia and CVD could develop as a result of a nutrient–gene interaction. There are a number of genes involved in the regulation of blood lipid levels. Further, the diet influence involves not only the amount of fat consumed but also the type of fat and the amount and type of carbohydrate.[16,43,77] For example, the editing of the apo B gene is enhanced by dietary carbohydrate. A number of genes have carbohydrate-response elements and it is possible that this gene has this element in its promoter region. A carbohydrate-response element has been identified in the apo E gene. Carbohydrate influences mRNA stability and RNA processing of this gene. Similarly, the gene that encodes the seven-enzyme complex of mammalian fatty acid synthetase has a fatty acid response unit in its promoter. The expression of this gene is downregulated by dietary PUFAs. The lipid transport genes might also have a lipid-response element.

Overtranscription of the fatty acid synthase gene (which has a lipid-response element) has been shown to occur in genetically obese Zucker rats. Mouse apo A-IV gene expression in C57BL/6 mice, which was shown by Paigen et al.[41] to develop atherosclerosis, is induced by high-fat feeding. In normal mice, this does not occur. The apo A-IV gene consists of three exons and two introns. The introns separate the evolutionarily conserved and functional polypeptide domains. Intron 1 divides most of the apo A-IV signal peptide from the amino terminus of the mature plasma protein. The second intron separates a highly conserved variant amphipathic peptide repeat from the remainder of the mature apo A-IV protein. The 5′ flanking region has several features: variant

TATA- and CAT-box sequences (TTTAAA and CCAACG), 5 G-rich direct repeats of 10 nucleotides, and a short inverted repeat. The variants found in this region may determine whether dietary fat can induce apo A-IV gene expression. Some may constitute a lipid-response element, while other sequence variants may not be lipid responsive. Further studies showed that the genetic control of apo A-IV mRNA levels involves both *cis*-acting elements and genetically distinct *trans*-acting factors. The *cis*-acting elements (nucleic acid sequences) and the *trans*-acting factors (specific proteins) determine both the rate of mRNA transcription and its turnover. Transcription requires the recognition of promoter sequences by protein transcription factors. These factors may bind lipid and be part of the lipid response unit or the lipid response unit may be entirely separate. This has not been determined, merely speculated.

FUNCTION

Once the dietary lipids are transferred to the target tissues, one of several processes occurs. The fatty acids of the TGs are oxidized for energy, stored as energy in the form of resynthesized TGs, converted to eicosanoids, or are incorporated into the membranes within and around the cells. An overview of these processes is shown in Figure 10.5. Certain of the fatty acids, the EFA, linoleic and linolenic, have a special role as precursors for the 20 carbon compounds called eicosanoids. Diet can affect all of these processes and, as well, stimulate lipid synthesis. The essentiality of certain of the fatty acids, the synthesis of eicosanoids from the 20 carbon fatty acids, the auto-oxidation of fatty acids and free radical formation, and the roles these 2 processes have in the inflammatory response follow. Membrane function as a process involving lipid is also addressed.

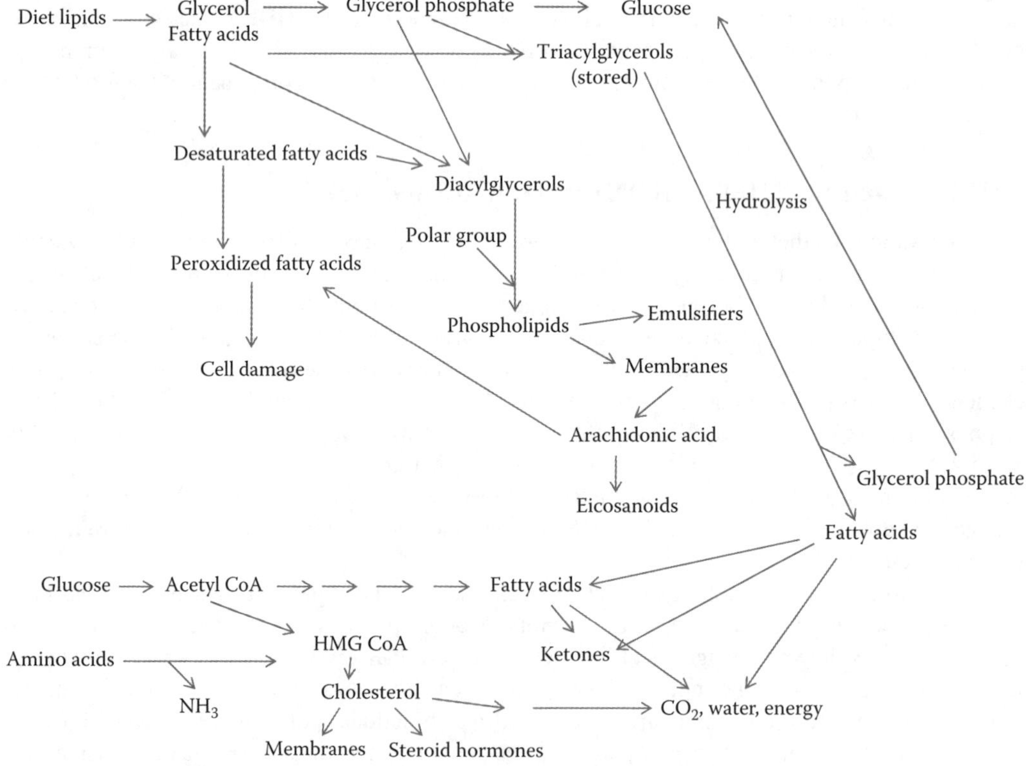

FIGURE 10.5 Overview of lipid metabolism.

lnoleic acid [18:2 (9, 12)]

$CH_3(CH_2)_3CH{=}CH\ CH_2CH{=}CH(CH_2)_7COOH$

18 12 9

γ-Linolenic acid [18:3 (6, 9, 12)]

$CH_3(CH_2)_4CH{=}CHCH_2CH{=}CHCH_2CH{=}CH(CH_2)_4COOH$

18 12 9 6

Linolenic acid [18:3 (9, 12, 15)]

$CH_3CH_2CH{=}CHCH_2CH{=}CHCH_2CH{=}CH(CH_2)_7COOH$

18 15 12 9

FIGURE 10.6 EFA showing the positions of the double bonds.

Essential Fatty Acids

EFA are deemed essential because the body cannot synthesize them. They are important precursors to longer fatty acids, especially arachidonic acid that, in turn, serves as precursor to the eicosanoids. They are also important components of membrane phospholipids contributing to the maintenance of appropriate fluidity. The EFA are shown in Figure 10.6. Although linoleic and linolenic are the stipulated EFA, γ-linolenic is included in Figure 10.6 because it can be found in certain plant oils such as primrose oil.

Animals fed diets deficient in these EFA exhibit a variety of symptoms as listed in Table 10.9. Detailed studies of cells from deficient rats have revealed diet-induced changes in energetic efficiency that include a partial loss of the ability of mitochondria to trap energy in the high-energy bond of ATP. Myocardial arrhythmias are more frequent in deficient rats and this may be due to

TABLE 10.9
Major Effects of EFA Deficiency in the Rat

1. Skin symptoms: scaly, dry skin
2. Weight: decreased weight gain in growing rats
3. Circulation: heart enlargement; decreased capillary resistance (lower blood pressure at periphery); increased permeability
4. Kidney enlargement; intertubular hemorrhage
5. Lung: cholesterol accumulation
6. Endocrine glands:
   a. Adrenals: decreased weight in females and increased in males
   b. Thyroid: reduced weight
7. Reproduction:
   a. Females: irregular estrus and impaired reproduction and lactation
   b. Males: degeneration of seminiferrous tubules
8. Metabolism:
   a. Changes in fatty acid composition of most organs.
   b. Increase in cholesterol levels in liver, adrenals, and skin.
   c. Decrease in plasma cholesterol.
   d. Changes in swelling of heart and liver mitochondria and uncoupling of oxidative phosphorylation
   e. Increased triglyceride synthesis and release by the liver.

Source: Burr, G.O. and Burr, M.M., *J. Biol. Chem.*, 82, 345, 1929; Innis, S., *Prog. Lipid Res.*, 30, 39, 1991.

the deficiency symptom of dysfunctional mitochondria. EFA deficiency also results in an impairment in the glucose transporter activity in selected cells and an alteration in insulin receptor number. Although none of these effects are especially dramatic, collectively they help explain why animals fed such a deficient diet are growth impaired and have poor food efficiency. Some of the effects shown in Table 10.9 can be due to an effect on membranes per se while other effects are attributable to a lack of arachidonic acid to serve as a precursor for eicosanoid synthesis.

Dietary fat composition can affect both membrane fatty acid composition as well as the fatty acid distribution of the stored lipids.[79] Shown in Table 10.10 are some data giving the phospholipid fatty acid composition of livers from rats fed either a 6% corn oil or hydrogenated coconut oil diet.[80] Recall that coconut oil is devoid of EFA while corn oil is a good source of the unsaturated fatty acids, linoleic, oleic, and palmitoleic, and of the saturated fatty acid, palmitic acid. Note that the corn-oil-fed rats had a phospholipid fatty acid profile that reflected their corn-oil intake. Note, too, that rats fed the hydrogenated

TABLE 10.10
Effect of 6% Corn or Coconut Oil Diets on the Phospholipid Fatty Acid Composition of Rat Liver

	Diet (% of the Total)	
Fatty Acids[a]	**Corn Oil**	**Coconut Oil**
14:0	0.09 ± 0.03	0.30 ± 0.03[b]
14:1	0.10 ± 0.02	0.05 ± 0.01
15:0	0.17 ± 0.03	0.20 ± 0.03
16:0	15.2 ± 0.03	15.4 ± 0.03
16:1	0.70 ± 0.08	2.26 ± 0.07[b]
17:0	0.38 ± 0.04	0.13 ± 0.02[b]
17:1	0.09 ± 0.02	0.11 ± 0.02
18:0	20.8 ± 0.82	2.0 ± 0.4
18:1	7.17 ± 0.61	2.0 ± 0.5[b]
18:2	14.4 ± 0.4	7.98 ± 0.27[b]
20:0	0.01 ± 0.01	0.16 ± 0.04[b]
18:3	0.41 ± 0.06	0.35 ± 0.04
20:1	ND	0.18 ± 0.04
20:2	0.89 ± 0.17	6.44 ± 0.50[b]
20:3	0.82 ± 0.16	2.20 ± 0.13[b]
20:4	29.4 ± 0.5	18.0 ± 0.7[b]
22:1	0.34 ± 0.02	0.35 ± 0.03
22:2	0.14 ± 0.02	0.48 ± 0.03[b]
24:0	0.96 ± 0.01	0.95 ± 0.03
22:4	1.37 ± 0.09	0.54 ± 0.02[b]
22:5	2.14 ± 0.25	2.24 ± 0.12
22:6	3.53 ± 0.31	6.64 ± 0.30[b]
20:5	ND	0.41 ± 0.04

Source: Berdanier, C.D., *Nutrition*, 4, 295, 1988.

Note: Hydrogenated coconut oil is deficient in EFA but is a good source for 8, 10, 12, and 14 carbon fatty acids. ND indicates nondetectable.

[a] Designations used: number of carbons in chain followed by number of double bonds.

[b] Indicates a significantly different value from that of the corn-oil-fed rats.

coconut oil, which has no linoleic or arachidonic acid, likewise had less of these fatty acids in their profile. These rats tried to compensate for their EFA-deficient diet by increasing their desaturase and elongase activity so as to preserve (as much as possible) the fluidity of their plasma and mitochondrial membranes. Thus, compared with the corn-oil-fed rats, increases in unsaturated fatty acids (16:1, 18:1, 20:2, 20:3, 22:2, 22:6) were found. Hydrogenated coconut oil contains the medium-chain saturated fatty acids, and these account for the fact that hydrogenated coconut oil is a solid at room temperature (20°C). It would be logical to assume that animals consuming this fat would have more rigid (less fluid) membranes, but Mother Nature has designed a fairly competent compensatory system that can partially overcome the diet fat effect on the membrane, thus, the increases in the unsaturated fatty acids as noted earlier. When the fatty acid unsaturation to saturation ratios (P:S) in these two groups of rats were calculated, these ratios were nearly the same. Despite this compensation, the consumption of the diet lacking the EFA resulted in some profound effects on metabolism and bodily function. Their mitochondrial OXPHOS system was compromised as was the use of glucose by both hepatocytes and adipocytes. The animals had other symptoms as well: poor food efficiency, poor coats, and so forth.[81–85] Needless to say, a fatty acid-deficient diet (the hydrogenated coconut oil diet) lacked sufficient linoleic acid for conversion to arachidonic acid that is then used for the synthesis of the eicosanoids.

Eicosanoid Synthesis

Eicosanoids are derived primarily from plasma membrane arachidonic acid but other 20 carbon polyunsaturated acids can also serve as substrates (Figure 10.7). Arachidonic acid is released from the plasma membrane phospholipids through the action of phospholipase A_2.[86–88] Membrane phospholipid arachidonate release is merely part of the constant remodeling process that membranes undergo.[87] Eicosanoids serve to mediate inflammation and immune cell function.[89] Eicosanoids include thromboxanes (TBXs), leukotrienes (LTs), and prostaglandins (PGs).[89–92] Specific

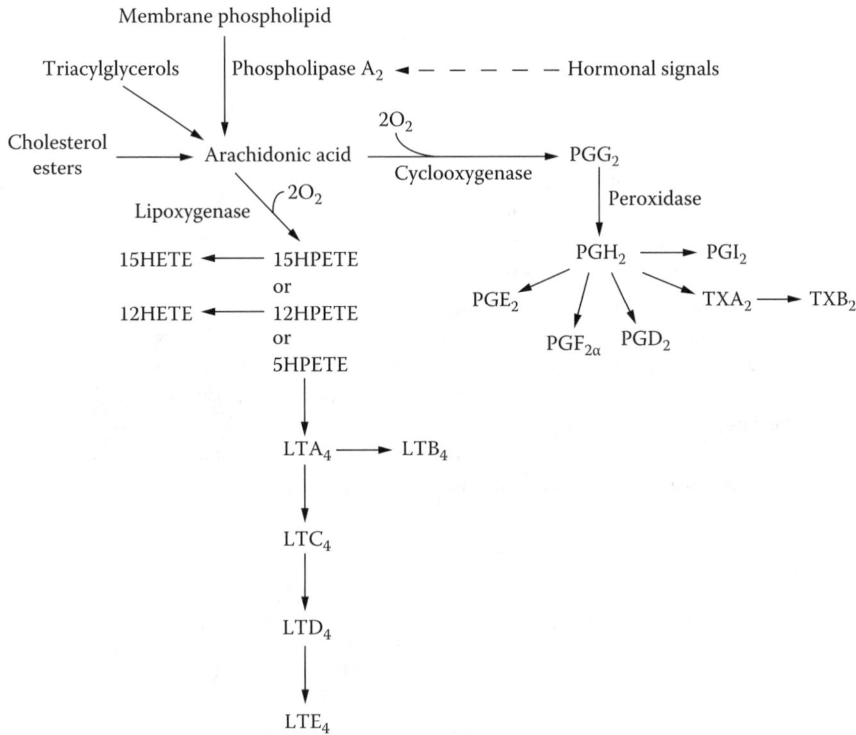

FIGURE 10.7 Overall pathway for the synthesis of the major eicosanoids.

eicosanoids have specific effects and frequently one will oppose the effect of another. PGE_2 induces cyclooxygenase 2 (COX-2) in fibroblasts and upregulates its own synthesis. It also induces the production of interleukin (IL)-6 by macrophages.

The eicosanoids fall into three general groups of compounds:

1. The PGs (compounds of the PG series)
2. The TBXs (compounds of the TBX series)
3. LTs (compounds of the LKT series)

All of these compounds arise from a 20-carbon PUFA. This fatty acid is usually arachidonic acid (20 carbons, 4 double bonds at 5, 8, 11, 14). However, in instances where the diet is rich in omega-3 (n-3) fatty acids, the precursor may be a 20-carbon, 5-double-bond fatty acid, eicosapentaenoic acid (double bonds at 5, 8, 11, 14, 17). Other eicosanoids can be synthesized from a 20-carbon fatty acid, dihomo-γ-linoleic acid, which has three double bonds at carbons 8, 11, and 14. Each of these precursors yields a particular set of eicosanoids. The functions of the various eicosanoids are listed in Table 10.11.

The 20 carbon fatty acids are the substrates for eicosanoid synthesis that involves the use of oxygen and cyclization (Figure 10.8). Dihomo-γ-linoleic acid is the precursor of PGE_1 and $PGE_1\alpha$ and subsequent PGs. Arachidonic acid is the precursor of PGs of the two series (PGE_2, $PGF_2\alpha$, etc.) and eicosapentaenoic acid is the precursor of PGs of the three series (PGE_3, $PGF_3\alpha$, etc.).

The cyclization of these 20-carbon fatty acids is accomplished by a complex of enzymes called the PG synthesis complex. The first step is the COX step, which involves the cyclization of C-9–C-12 of the precursor to form the cyclic 9–11 endoperoxide 15-hydroperoxide (PGG_2) shown in Figure 10.8. PGG_2 is then used to form PGH_2 through the removal of one oxygen from the

TABLE 10.11
Functions of Eicosanoids

Eicosanoids	Function
PGG_2	Precursor of PGH_2
PGH_2	Precursor of PGD_2, PGE_2, PGI_2, and $PGF_2\alpha$
PGD_2	Promotes sleeping behavior; precursor of PGF_2
PGE_2	Enhances perception of pain when histamine or bradykinin is given
	Induces signs of inflammation. Promotes wakefulness
	Precursor of $PGF_2\alpha$. Reduces gastric acid secretion
	Vasoconstrictor in some tissues. Vasodilator in other tissues
	Maintains the patency of the ductus arteriosus prior to birth
$PGF_2\alpha$	Induces parturition. Bronchial constrictor. Vasoconstrictor especially in coronary vasculature. Increases sperm motility; stimulates steroidogenesis and the corpus luteum; induces luteolysis
PGI_2	Inhibits platelet aggregation
PGE_1	Inhibits motility of nonpregnant uterus; increases motility of pregnant uterus. Bronchial dilator
TXA_2	Stimulates platelet aggregation. Potent vasoconstrictor
LTB_4	Potent chemotaxic agent

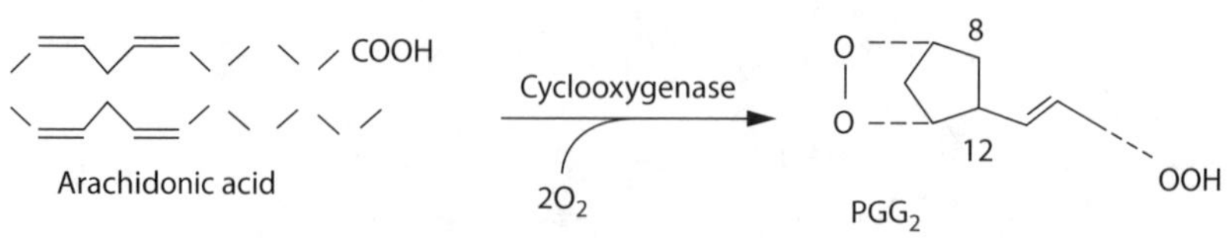

FIGURE 10.8 Cyclization and oxygenation of arachidonic acid.

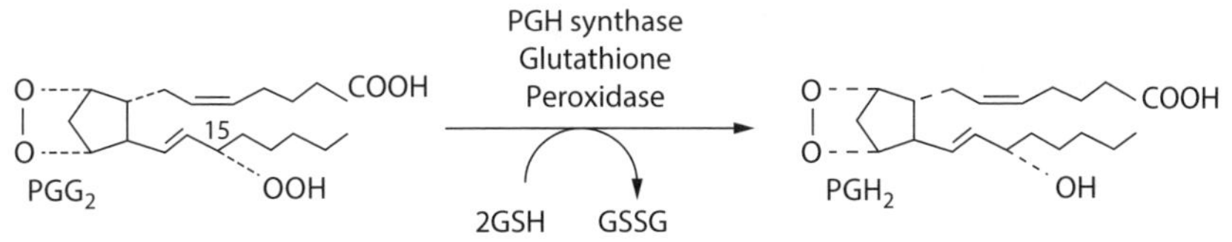

FIGURE 10.9 Formation of PGH_2.

carbonyl group at carbon 15. Glutathione peroxidase and PGH synthase catalyze the reaction shown in Figure 10.9.[88] PGH synthase is a very unstable, short-lived enzyme with a messenger RNA that is one of the shortest-lived species so far found in mammalian cells. The expression of genes for this enzyme is under the control of polypeptide growth factors such as IL-1α and colony-stimulating factor 1. Interferon-α and interferon-β inhibit expression and prostanoid production by the macrophages. Glutathione peroxidase is a selenium-containing enzyme (see Chapter 14). In animals fed a high-polyunsaturated-fat diet, one might expect to see a higher than normal requirement for selenium in the diet to accommodate the need for this enzyme in its role for eicosanoid synthesis.[90] However, such an expectation is without merit. Studies of rats fed a high-polyunsaturated-fat diet such as a marine oil-rich diet show a greater need for vitamin E to accommodate the increased need to support the antioxidation system, but not an increased need for selenium.[90] The need to make the eicosanoids is quite low compared with the need to suppress the formation of free radicals. This probably explains why the selenium requirement is not increased under these dietary conditions.

PGH_2 is then converted through the action of a variety of isomerases to PGD_2 or PGE_2 or prostacyclin I_2 (PGI_2) or $PGF_2α$.[91] These are the primary precursors of the PGs of the D, E, and F series and PGI or TBX. The conversion to subsequent PGs is mediated by enzymes that are specific to a specific cell or tissue types. Not all of these subsequent compounds are formed in all tissues. Thus, PGE_2 and $PGF_2α$ are produced in the kidney and spleen. $PGF_2α$ and PGE are also produced in the uterus only when signals from the pituitary induce their production and so stimulate parturition. PGI_2 is primarily produced by endothelial cells lining the blood vessels. This PG inhibits platelet aggregation and thus is important to maintaining a blood flow free of clots. It is counteracted by TBX A_2, which is produced by the platelets when these cells contact a foreign surface. PGE_2, $PGF_2α$, and PGI_2 are formed by the heart in about equal amounts. All of these PGs have a very short half-life. No sooner are they released than they are inactivated. The TBXs are highly active metabolites of the PGs. As mentioned previously, they are formed when PGH_2 has its cyclopentane ring replaced by a six-membered oxane ring, shown in Figure 10.9. Imidazole is a potent inhibitor of TBX A synthase and is used to block TXA2 production and platelet aggregation.

TBX A_2 has a role in clot formation and the name TBX comes from this function (thrombus means clot). The half-life of TXA_2 is less than 1 min. TXB_2 is its metabolic end product and has little biological activity. Measuring TXB_2 levels in blood and tissue can give an indication of how much TXA_2 has been produced. PGD_2 and PGE_2 are involved in the regulation of sleep–wake cycles in a variety of species.[91]

The COX reaction illustrated in Figure 10.10 can be inhibited by certain anti-inflammatory drugs such as aspirin, indomethacin, and phenylbutazone. These are the nonsteroidal anti-inflammatory drugs that are commonly available in pharmacies. These drugs block the action of COX by acetylating the enzyme. While use of these drugs for the occasional injury or headache is harmless, long-term chronic use can result in untoward effects. Long-term chronic use of aspirin, for example, can affect vascular competence and blood clotting. People consuming large amounts of aspirin over long periods of time may find an increase in bruises (subcutaneous hemorrhages). Small contact injuries that normally would not result in a bruise will do so in these people. Gastric bleeding is another possible complication with long-term chronic aspirin ingestion. Aplastic anemia can result from long-term phenylbutazone therapy. Again, the occasional use of these drugs is not likely to have these effects.

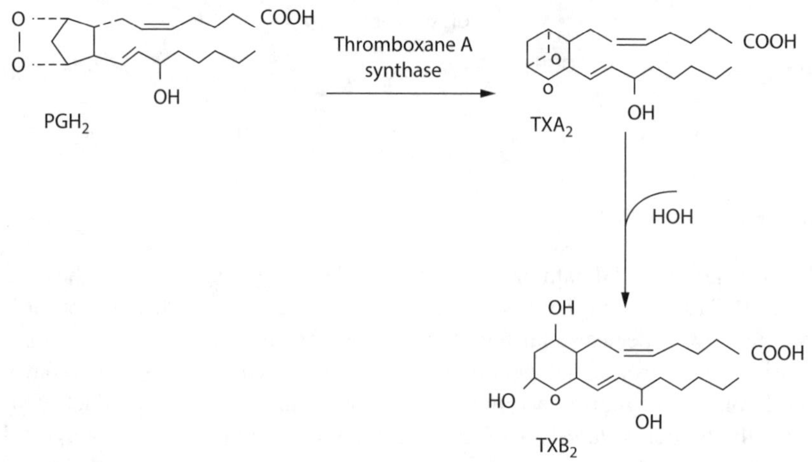

FIGURE 10.10 The reaction sequence that produces TXA_2 and TXB_2.

A second group of anti-inflammatory agents are the steroids—hydrocortisone, prednisone, and other similar compounds.[92] These drugs are prescription drugs that act by inhibiting the enzyme phospholipase A_2. Phospholipase A_2 stimulates the release of arachidonic acid from the membrane phospholipids. Hence, inhibition of this reaction will result in a decreased supply of arachidonic acid for eicosanoid synthesis. When the conversion of arachidonic acid to eicosanoid is inhibited as mentioned or when either of the other 20-carbon fatty acids are abundantly available, a different series of PGs and LTs are produced. Eicosapentaenoic acid is not as good a substrate for cyclooxygenation as is arachidonic acid. As a result, less of the arachidonic acid-related eicosanoids (even-numbered PGs and TBXs) are produced and more of the odd-numbered PGs and LTs are produced.

Although the COX pathway is quite important in the production of eicosanoids, equally important is the lipoxygenase pathway. This pathway is catalyzed by a family of enzymes called the lipoxygenase enzymes. These enzymes differ from the COX enzymes in the catalytic site for oxygen addition to the unsaturated fatty acid. One lipoxygenase is active at the double bond at carbon 5, while a second is active at carbon 11 and a third is active at carbon 15. The products of these reactions are mono-hydroperoxyeicosatetraenoic acids (HPETEs) and are numbered according to the location of the double bond to which the oxygen is added. 5-HPETE is the major lipoxygenase product in basophils, polymorphonuclear leukocytes, macrophages, mast cells, and any organ undergoing an inflammatory response. 12-HPETE is the major product in platelets, pancreatic endocrine cells, vascular smooth muscle, and glomerular cells. 15-HPETE predominates in reticulocytes, eosinophils, T lymphocytes, and tracheal epithelial cells. The HPETEs are not in themselves active hormones; rather, they serve as precursors for the LTs. The LTs are the metabolic end products of the lipoxygenase reaction. These compounds contain at least three conjugated double bonds. The unstable 5-HPETE is converted to either an analogous alcohol (hydroxy fatty acid) or is reduced by a peroxide or converted to LT. The peroxidative reduction of 5′-HPETE to the stable 5 hydroxyeicosatetraenoic acid (5-HETE) is similar to that of 12-HPETE to 12-HETE and of 15-HPETE to 15-HETE. In each instance, the carbon–carbon double bonds are unconjugated and the geometry of the double bonds is *trans*, *cis*, *cis*, respectively. In contrast to the active TBXs, which have very short half-lives, the LTs can persist as long as 4 h. These compounds make up a group of substances known as the slow-acting anaphylaxis substances. They cause slowly evolving but protracted contractions of smooth muscles in the airways and gastrointestinal tract. LT C4 is rapidly converted to LTD4, which, in turn, is slowly converted to LTE4. Enzymes in the plasma are responsible for these conversions.

The products of the lipoxygenase pathway are potent mediators of the response to allergens, tissue damage (inflammation), hormone secretion, cell movement, cell growth, and calcium flux.

Within minutes of stimulation, lipoxygenase products are produced. In an allergy attack, for example, an allergen can instigate the release of LTs, which are the immediate mediators of response. The LTs are more potent than histamine in stimulating the contraction of the bronchial nonvascular smooth muscles. In addition, LTD4 increases the permeability of the microvasculature. The mono-HETEs and LTB4 stimulate the movement of eosinophils and neutrophils, making them the first line of defense in injury resulting in inflammation.

As mentioned, when dihomo-γ-linoleic acid or eicosapentaenoic acid serves as a substrate for eicosanoid production, the products are either of the 1 series or 3 series. The products they form may be less active than those formed from arachidonic acid and this decrease in activity can be of therapeutic value. Hence, ingestion of omega-3 fatty acids leads to the decreased production of PG E_2 and its metabolites; a decrease in the production of TBX A_2, a potent platelet aggregator and vasoconstrictor; and a decrease in LT B_4, a potent inflammatory hormone and a powerful inducer of leukocyte hemotaxis and adherence. Counteracting these decreases are an increase in TBX A_3 (TXA_3), a weak platelet aggregator and vasoconstrictor; an increase in the production of PGI_3 without an increase in PGI_2, which stimulates vasodilation and inhibits platelet aggregation; and an increase in LT B_5, which is a weak inducer of inflammation and a weak chemotoxic agent. Marine oils, rich in omega-3 unsaturated fatty acids, affect (decrease) platelet aggregation because they stimulate the synthesis of TBX A_3. TBX A_3 does not have the platelet-aggregating property of the other eicosanoids. In addition, eicosapentaenoic acid is used to make the anti-aggregating PGI_3. Animals fed omega-3-rich oils produce significantly more of the eicosanoids of the LTB_5 series. LTB_4 is an important inflammatory mediator, whereas LTB_5 is not. Fish-oil consumption results in an increased neutrophil LTB_5 production, with a concomitant decrease in LTB_4 production. This diet-influenced change in LTB_4 and LTB_5 production seems to be related to a reduced incidence of autoimmune–inflammatory disorders such as asthma, psoriasis, and rheumatoid arthritis in populations consuming omega-3 fatty acids routinely. Thus, eicosanoid synthesis can be used as an explanation of the beneficial effects of fish-oil ingestion on rheumatoid arthritis. In arthritics, the joints are inflamed and painful. The PGs PGE_2 and LT are both produced from arachidonate. PGE_2 induces the signs of inflammation, which include redness and heat due to arteriolar vasodilation, swelling, and localized edema resulting from increased capillary permeability. LT prevents platelet aggregation. If there is less arachidonate available for the synthesis of these eicosanoids, then the inflammation is inhibited.

Tumorigenesis likewise can be influenced by the relative amounts of the various eicosanoids. PGG of the 2-series acts as a tumor promoter. It downregulates macrophage tumoricidal activities and inhibits IL-2 production. Increased PGE_2 levels (from omega-6 fatty acids) have been associated with aggressive growth patterns of both basal and squamous cell skin carcinomas in humans. Vegetable oils are rich in these fatty acids. Products of the lipoxygenase pathway (stimulated by the omega-3 fatty acids) have the reverse effect. While the various eicosanoids have different (and sometimes conflicting) effects on inflammatory processes and on tumor promotion, it might be anticipated that susceptibility to pathogenic organisms would be similarly affected. Studies with mice exposed to a variety of pathogens and fed either a fish-oil or a control diet showed no diet-fat-related differences in susceptibility to these organisms.

FATTY ACID AUTO-OXIDATION

Fatty acids, particularly the unsaturated fatty acids, can auto-oxidize and form reactive compounds called free radicals.[93] Free radicals (reactive oxygen species, ROS) can form when the oxygen atom is excited by a variety of drugs and contaminants and by ultraviolet light. Inflammation stimulates ROS formation as does heavy exercise, ischemia–reperfusion, xanthine oxidase, arachidonic acid metabolism, transition metals (e.g., iron), smoking, environmental pollutants, UV light, ozone, and certain environmental chemicals. The excited oxygen atom is called singlet oxygen. Pollutants such as the oxides of nitrogen or carbon tetrachloride can provoke this reaction. The unsaturated fatty acids are not the only compounds that can be radicalized yet these are the ones that are most often discussed.[93–95]

In food, auto-oxidation is responsible for the deterioration of food quality. The discoloration of red meat upon exposure to air at room temperature is an indication of the auto-oxidation process. The off-odor that accompanies this discoloration is the result of the auto-oxidation of the fatty acids and some of the amino acids in the meat. In living systems, the process of auto-oxidation is suppressed to a large extent. This is essential because the products of this oxidation, amino acid and fatty acid peroxides, can be very damaging. Peroxides denature proteins, rendering them inactive. They also attack the DNA in the nucleus and mitochondria, resulting in base-pair deletions or breaks in the DNA. In the nucleus, these breaks or deletions can be repaired or misrepaired. In the aging animal, the repair mechanism loses its efficiency and one of the characteristics of aged cells is the loss of its DNA repair ability.[95] To prevent widespread damage to cellular proteins and DNA by these radicals, there is a potent antioxidation system (see Chapter 14). This system includes the selenium-containing enzyme, glutathione peroxidase, catalase, and superoxide dismutase (SOD). These enzymes are found in the peroxisomes.[96] SOD is also found in the mitochondria. All of these components serve to suppress free radical formation.

Under circumstances where mitochondrial OXPHOS efficiency is downregulated, as under stress with the release of epinephrine or the release of uncoupling proteins, more heat is released and less ATP is produced. Under this circumstance, there is a relative excess of oxygen that then can radicalize. It is for this reason that the mitochondria possess a particularly potent peroxide suppressor, SOD. SOD in the mitochondria requires manganese ion as a cofactor. The cytosol also has SOD but this enzyme requires the copper and zinc ions. Both forms of the enzyme catalyze the reaction $O_2 + O_2 + 2H^+ \rightarrow H_2O_2 + O_2$. Two superoxides and two hydrogen ions are joined to form one molecule of hydrogen peroxide and a molecule of oxygen. In turn, the peroxide is converted to water through the action of the enzyme catalase. Peroxides can be *neutralized* through the action of glutathione-S-transferase. This reaction requires 2 mol of reduced glutathione and produces two molecules of oxidized glutathione and two molecules of water. Fatty acid radicals can also be neutralized by glutathione peroxidase, producing a molecule of an alcohol with the same chain length as the fatty acid. Glutathione-S-transferase can duplicate the action of glutathione peroxidase.

With infection, partial mitochondrial uncoupling occurs and the heat so produced (fever) combats invading pathogens, which are more sensitive to heat than normal body cells. Under these conditions, the peroxides that are formed have pathogen-killing capability. This is an important body defense system.

Food components that downregulate or upregulate free radical formation are important considerations in inflammation and oxidative stress. Szeto et al.[97] compared plasma biomarkers of antioxidant status, oxidative stress, inflammation, and risk for coronary artery disease in long-term vegetarians compared to nonvegetarians (omnivores). Vegetarians had lower blood levels of triacyglycerols, uric acid, and C-reactive protein as well as lower levels of vitamin E (α-tocopherol). Sebekova et al.[98] also studied vegetarians and omnivores and reported that vegetarians had lower levels of markers of oxidative stress that included advanced glycation end products. They had higher levels of advanced oxidation proteins (including C-reactive protein) than omnivores. Surprisingly, vegetarians appeared to consume less of the antioxidant vitamins, vitamins A, E, and C. Bowen and Borthakur[99] reported that a mild pro-oxidative state accompanies meal ingestion, which results in an increase in biomarkers of inflammation, adhesion, and endothelial dysfunction, all of which are factors in the development of CVD. After a meal, there is an abundance of energy containing substrates that could provide excess substrate for superoxide formation. This may be a dominant factor in postprandial oxidative stress and a decrease in nitric oxide. It may also be related to the observation that more heart attacks occur in the postprandial condition than in the fed or starved condition. As mentioned earlier, fatty acids, especially the PUFAs, are excellent substrates for the production of ROS. In fact, the number of fatty acid ROS is a marker of oxidative stress.

On the other hand, saturated but not unsaturated fatty acids induce apoptosis of human coronary artery endothelial cells via NFκB activation.[100,101] NFκB is nuclear factor-kB, a nuclear gene signaling factor that appears to be involved in the inflammatory response. Endothelial apoptosis contributes to atherothrombosis (blood clot in a coronary vessel).

Fatty acids and various fatty acid-derived metabolites (the eicosanoids) can affect gene expression via binding to and activating the various peroxisome proliferator-activated receptors (PPARs) (α, δ, γ). All three of these PPARs act as transcription agents that in turn affect cellular differentiation and functional properties. PPARα is expressed in the T cells and the B cells, whereas γ dominates in cells of myeloid lineage (monocytes and macrophages). PUFAs bind to these PPARs and probably have their effects on the expression of some of the genes of the inflammatory cascade in addition to their direct effects on the fatty acid radical formation.[101] There are other food constituents that can form or suppress free radical formation. The mode of action of these components is described as follows:

1. *Amino acids*—Cysteine and arginine can be converted to free radicals, and when this happens, there is an increase in C-reactive protein. Cysteine will form homocysteine and hyperhomocysteinemia is associated with CVD. It is a strong independent risk factor for new cardiovascular events; however, the mechanism of its action is unclear. A proinflammatory state has been found to exist in the elderly that is associated with hyperhomocysteinemia.[102] A study of 586 men and 734 elderly women revealed that hyperhomocysteinemia was associated with elevated levels of plasma IL-1 receptor antagonist and IL-6. The sedentary state, intakes of vitamins B_6 and folacin, and serum levels of folacin, vitamin B_{12}, vitamin B_6, and α-tocopherol were significant and independent correlates of homocysteine levels.
2. *Folacin* suppresses homocysteine formation and the C-reactive protein. Folacin also reduces adhesion molecules vascular cell adhesion molecule-1 (VCAM-1) expression in the aortic endothelium.[103,104] Hyperhomocysteinemia increases the expression of intracellular adhesion molecule-1 (ICAM-1) and monocyte chemoattractant protein-1 (MCP-1). It also increases NFκB activation and consequently increases the expression of inflammatory factors in vivo. Folacin supplementation reverses these effects.[105]
3. *Vitamin E* reduces fatty acid free radical formation. It donates reducing equivalents to a peroxide converting it to an alcohol. It is a potent antioxidant with anti-inflammatory properties. Vitamin E supplementation results in decreases in lipid peroxidation and superoxide (O_2^-) production by impairing the assembly of NADP (reduced) oxidase as well as decreasing the expression of scavenger receptors (SR-A and CD 36), particularly important to the formation of foam cells. α-Tocopherol therapy at high doses decreases the release of proinflammatory cytokines, chemokine IL-8, and plasminogen activator inhibitor-1 (PAI-1) and decreases the adhesion of monocytes to the endothelium. It also decreases the release of C-reactive protein. The mechanisms that account for the nonantioxidant function of α-tocopherol include the inhibition of protein kinase C, 5-lipoxygenase, tyrosine kinase, and cycloxygenase-2.[106,107] Although diabetes can elicit an increase in free radicals, vitamin E supplementation had no effect on the risk of diabetes nor did it have any beneficial effect on any of the diabetes-related complications.[107]
4. *Vitamin D* modulates the production of inflammation markers and oxidative stress. Vitamin D exerts effects on the immune system.[108] These effects are exerted on multiple immune cell types and are predominately suppressive at pharmacological levels yet are potent enough to have therapeutic potential in the management of the immune diseases. Receptors for active vitamin D (1α25-dihydroxycholecalciferol) have been found in human thymus cells, peripheral blood leukocytes, dendritic cells, monocytes, macrophages, and T lymphocytes. The monocytes are viewed as precursors of macrophages that are phagocytic cells capable of secreting an array of proinflammatory products and intimately involved in the host

defense against bacterial infection. The dendritic cells serve to initiate T-cell-mediated immune response and, when fully mature, express high levels of class II MHC, CD80, CD86, CD40, and an array of other accessory ligands and immunostimulatory products.[109,110] Through binding to its cognate receptor, vitamin D inhibits T-cell proliferation, IL-2 secretion, and cell cycle progression from G_{1a} to G_{1b}. Thus, vitamin D serves as an anti-inflammatory nutrient. Vitamin D also serves to suppress B-cell proliferation as well as the proliferation of natural killer cells. It inhibits the production of mitogen or antigen-stimulated immunoglobulin (IgM and IgG). The evidence for this role is not as convincing as that of its role in T-cell activity. These actions of vitamin D are probably due to its role in the expression of genes encoding elements of the immune system. Nuclear vitamin D receptor proteins have been identified and bind to specific elements in the promoter regions of a number of genes. Actually, the vitamin plays a part in the NFκB signaling pathway that consists of a number of related proteins that regulate gene expression when translocated to the nucleus as heterodimers or homodimers. This pathway is central to differentiation, maturation, activation, and survival of antigen-presenting cells (APCs), lymphocytes, and other cells of the immune system. Vitamin D also modulates signaling for the nuclear factor of activated T cells (NFAT), the PIP-3-kinase, and the mitogen-activated protein kinase (MAPK) pathway. The extensive literature documenting these effects on elements of the immune system provides strong and convincing evidence of the role for this vitamin/hormone in normal immune function. In summary, it enhances innate immunity through increased macrophage recruitment and differentiation; it prevents autoimmunity through inhibition of the ability of dendritic cells to induce Th-1-type cellular immune responses; it promotes self-tolerance through permissive effects on the generation of Th-2 or T_{reg}-type cells.

5. Conjugated (*trans*-10, *cis*-12) linolenic acid (CLA) but not *cis*-9, *trans* 11 CLA is effective in reducing the fat mass in children but not adults.[111–113] It causes a drop in leptin production in pigs,[114] and in cultured human cells, a drop in adipocyte lipid content, a decrease in insulin stimulated glucose uptake (suppression of GLUT 4 transporter), fatty acid uptake, incorporation into lipid and oxidation compared to control adipocyte cultures.[115–119] In parallel, gene expression of PPARγ and many of its downstream targets were also reduced. CLA caused a robust and sustained activation of MAPK kinase/extracellular signal-related kinase (MERK/ERK) signaling. This was linked to hypersecretion of IL-6, IL-8, and NFκB. The NFκB increase preceded that of IL 6 and 8 that in turn preceded PPARγ activation. This promotes adipocyte insulin resistance and increases the IL-6 and IL-8 production response to an increased mitogen-activated kinase. In mice, feeding CLA activated AMP-activated protein kinase especially when these mice were also treated with metformin.[116] Feeding a CLA diet also attenuated a lipopolysaccharide-induced inflammation in mice through PPARγ-mediated suppression of toll-like receptor 4.[120] The sequential responses of adipocytes to CLA has helped elucidate the sequence of events (at least in adipocytes) that occur in the inflammatory process.[115–117] There was a dramatic increase in macrophage infiltration and gene expression that appeared to promote the inflammatory response. In turn, this was interpreted as contributing to adipose tissue insulin resistance. Elevated intakes of *trans*–fatty acids in general are associated with markers of inflammation in women and there may be implications of this relationship to chronic disease; however, this has not been proven.[117] Consuming a CLA-enriched diet helped postmenopausal women lose weight and adipose tissue mass.[121] In turn, consuming a CLA diet reduced the risk of breast cancer in women.[122]
6. *Iron*—Iron is one of the transition metals that, in excess, enhances the formation of ROS. Excess iron in the circulation can occur in the genetic disease called hemochromatosis (see Chapter 14). Iron is absorbed in excess, and since there is a poor excretion mechanism, it remains in the circulation causing a variety of metabolic disturbances, among these is

the excess formation of ROS. Iron may play a role in vascular inflammation since elevated levels of ferritin result in increased levels of C-reactive protein.[123]

7. *Copper*—Excess copper absorption due to a genetic error in absorption can create metabolic problems and, like iron, can result in excess ROS formation (see Chapter 14).
8. *Vitamin A*—The carotenoids, vitamin A precursors, are potent antioxidants in foods. Foods rich in these compounds are excellent foods to reduce oxidative stress (see Chapter 11). β-Carotene quenches singlet oxygen and converts it to O_2.
9. *Flavonoids, polyphenols*—The flavonoids are a diverse group of polyphenolic compounds widely distributed in the plant kingdom. There are more than 6400 known compounds that contribute flavor and pigmentation to the fruits and vegetables in the human diet. They are divided into eight classes based on their molecular structure. The biological effects of these flavonoids are contingent upon their interaction with proteins. Some foods such as cocoa products are sources of flavan-3-ols. Intakes of flavonoid-rich foods has been shown to reduce plasma levels of proinflammatory cysteinyl LTs, inhibit human 5-lipoxygenase (a key enzyme in LT synthesis), and increase the level of nitric oxide (a vasorelaxing compound). They are also associated with a reduction in the *stickiness* of platelets (platelet aggregation). A suppression of mediators of inflammation and peroxide formation has been observed.[124–128] These changes were associated with a reduction in the risk for CVD, diabetes, and stroke.[124–139] Foods that contain the flavonoids have been studied. A few studies have been reported that compare the milk protein, casein, with soy protein containing isoflavones. Crouse et al.[140] reported that soy protein lowered plasma concentrations of total and LDL cholesterol by 4% and 6%, respectively. There were no diet effects on triglyceride levels and HDL cholesterol. Nilausen and Meinertz[141] reported that casein lowered lipoprotein(a). They concluded that soy protein may have potentially damaging effects on atherogenesis because it appeared to raise the levels of the atherogenic Lp(a). In contrast, Tonstad et al.[142] reported that adding soy protein or casein to a lipid-lowering diet significantly reduced LDL cholesterol concentrations as well as homocysteine levels without having an effect of Lp(a). Campbell et al.[143] have reported that there were no differences between soy protein and casein with respect to copper-induced LDL oxidation, serum C-reactive protein, serum IL-6, serum fibrinogen, total cholesterol, HDL cholesterol, LDL cholesterol, or triglycerides. Finally, Oner et al.[144] showed that feeding whey protein suppressed markers of oxidative stress that were part of the whole body response to burn injury. Population studies of human flavonol intakes have shown that the levels of C-reactive protein is inversely related to flavonol intake.[128] Experimental feeding studies revealed that an increase in flavonol intake is associated with reduced levels of inflammation biomarkers.[125–127]
10. *Ascorbic acid*—Ascorbic acid acts as an antioxidant. It can donate reducing equivalents to a peroxide converting it to an alcohol.

FATTY ACID AUTO-OXIDATION AND THE INFLAMMATION CASCADE

Fatty acid auto-oxidation to peroxides is an important component of the immune response to trauma and injury. Both acute and chronic inflammatory states involve the use of these peroxides. The acute inflammatory response can be elicited by either an external injury or to an internal one. If external, it is typified by redness, swelling, heat, and pain. However, an initial event can also occur internally. If acute, it too is characterized by swelling and pain. With a chronic injury, the injury might not be noticeable until sufficient time has elapsed for the symptoms of a chronic disease caused by the immunologic response to this injury to be diagnosed. In each scenario an inflammation cascade is elicited. This is diagramed in Figure 10.11.

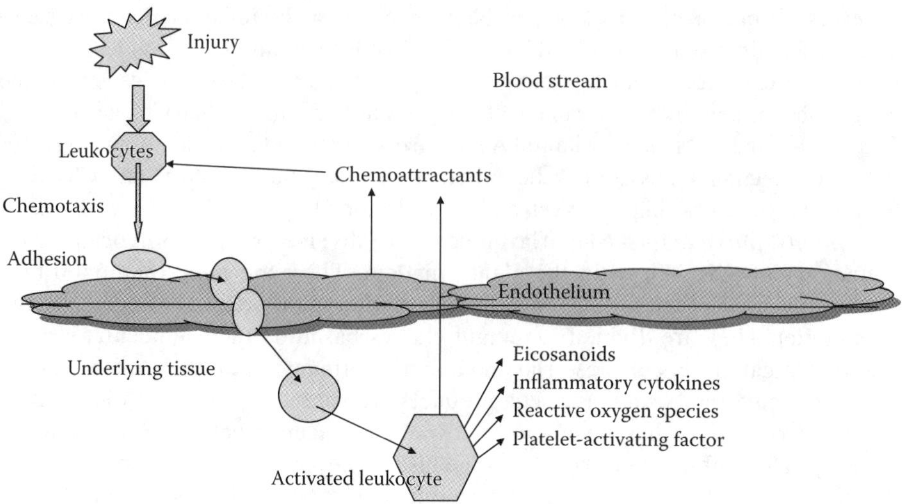

FIGURE 10.11 The injury cascade.

Injury Cycle

Following an injury, there is an increased blood flow and an increased permeability of membranes. Leukocytes are mobilized and migrate to the site of injury. Chemoattractants are released by the injured tissue and attract the leukocytes to the injury site. Adhesion molecules migrate upward from the underlying tissue and the leukocytes adhere to them. This activates the leukocytes that then release eicosanoids, inflammatory cytokines, platelet-activating factor, and ROS. Chemoattractants attract the activated leukocytes back to the endothelium and the inflammatory cycle is complete.

As noted here, injury elicits a number of almost simultaneous reactions. Included are the movement of complement, antibodies (if the injury is exogenous and involves one or more antigens), and cytokines: IL1β, IL-6, IL-8, tumor necrosis factor-α (TNFα), NFκB. The adhesion molecules include granulocytes, monocytes, macrophages, and lymphocytes.

The typical immunologic response to an external injury is a result of increased blood flow, increased permeability across blood capillaries that permits large molecules (complement, antibodies, and cytokines) to leave the bloodstream and cross the endothelial wall. This increase in blood flow and permeability also increases the movement of leukocytes from the blood stream into the surrounding tissue. Inflammation begins the immunologic process of eliminating invading pathogens and toxins and marks the beginning of the repair of the injured tissue. The movement of cells to the injury site is induced by the upregulation of adhesion molecules such as intracellular adhesion molecule-1 (ICAM-1), VCAM-1, and E-selectin on the surface of endothelial cells. This allows leukocytes to bind with the result of subsequent diapedesis (the passage of blood or any of its components through the intact walls of the blood vessels.). The earliest cells to arrive at the injury site are granulocytes followed by monocytes, macrophages, and then lymphocytes. Granulocytes, monocytes, and macrophages are involved in pathogen killing and in clearing up the cellular and tissue debris. The activity of these cells is triggered by the presence of bacterial toxins (lipopolysaccharides) that are components of the cell wall of gram-negative bacteria. This trigger induces the macrophages and monocytes to release cytokines such as TNFα, ILs (IL-1β, IL-6, and IL-8), eicosanoids, PGE_2, nitric oxide (NO), matrix metalloproteinases, and other mediators. Endotoxin also induces adhesion molecule expression on the surfaces of endothelial cells and on leukocytes. One of the more interesting aspects of this cascade is that there are genetically determined variations in the response to injury. Shen et al.[145] have shown that an individual's susceptibility to the development of metabolic syndrome is related to polymorphisms in IL1β.

Pathogens serving as antigens elicit this cascade of immunologic events since the immune system has evolved primarily to provide a rapid and effective protection against such an invasion. It has an array of potent mechanisms that can destroy invading pathogens. It is also carefully regulated to prevent self-injury (autoimmunity).

The immune system defenses are divided into two general groups: The innate group is one that is non–antigen specific; the cognate group is antigen specific. The former group is immediate in action and members of this group rapidly appear at the site of pathogen invasion. The responses are based on a fixed pattern recognition and are amplified predominantly by the production of soluble (proinflammatory) products that stimulate or attract additional cell populations. Innate immunity is defined as that which is not qualitatively and quantitatively affected by repeated contact with the same immunologic stimulus. Innate immunity is mediated by the parenchymal cells of all organs and tissues as well as by the mobile cells with specialized functions (macrophages and natural killer cells).

Cognate immunity is mediated by cells specialized for antigen presentation (dendritic cells) and antigen recognition (T lymphocytes and B lymphocytes, abbreviated as T cells and B cells). Both cell types are capable of a number of different response patterns that ultimately dictate the nature and duration of immune activity.[146] The two arms of the immune system are coordinately regulated such that invading pathogens are efficiently eliminated. With respect to nutrition, oxidative stress, and inflammatory disease, it should be noted that the endothelium lining the vasculature of the body is a key target for infectious agents.[147] A number of pathogens have been identified that target the endothelium.

Involved in the inflammatory response are the cytokines. These are protein-based regulators of inflammation and immune function.[129–148] The cytokines regulate the whole body response to infection and injury and serve to amplify the initial inflammatory signal. They are opposed by anti-inflammatory cytokines such as IL-10 and by receptor antagonists such as IL-1 receptor antagonist. The cytokines of importance to the inflammatory process are NFκB, ILs (IL-1β, IL-6, IL-8), and TNFα. The release of NFκB precedes the release of the ILs and TNFα. The link between PUFAs and inflammation is the eicosanoids that are mediators and regulators of the inflammatory process.

A fourth player in the inflammation process especially as regards to the inflammatory processes occurring in the vascular system is LDL cholesterol. When oxidized, it can injure the endothelial lining of the vessel eliciting an inflammatory response (Figure 10.12). Increased levels of oxidized

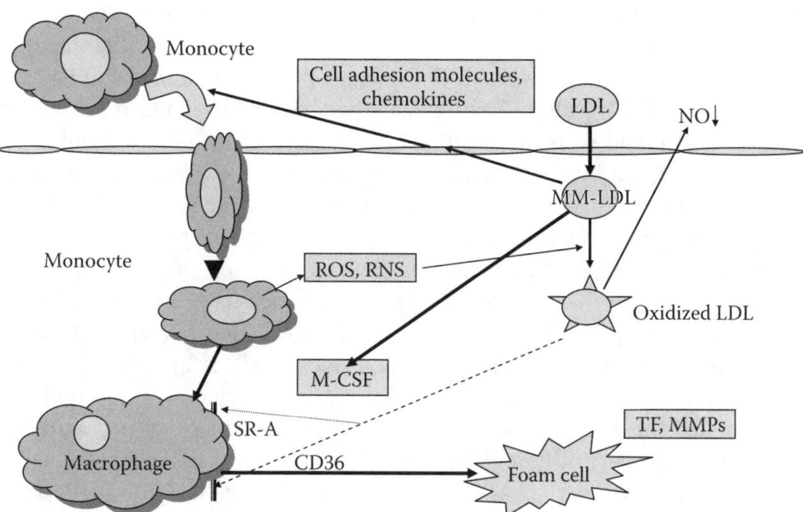

FIGURE 10.12 Oxidized LDL and injury to the vascular tissue. Scheme for the role of oxidized LDL in atherosclerosis. NO, nitric oxide (a vasodilator); LDL, low-density lipoprotein; ROS, reactive oxygen species; M-CSF, monocyte colony-stimulating factor.

LDL cholesterol result in the formation of minimally modified LDL (MM-LDL) in the subendothelial space. This stimulates the production of monocytes chemotaxic protein-1 that promotes monocytes chemotaxis. MM-LDL also stimulates production of monocyte colony-stimulating factor (M-CSF). M-CSF promotes the differentiation and proliferation of monocytes into macrophages. MM-LDL uptake by the scavenger receptor pathway of the macrophages occurs because the normal receptor for LDL does not recognize it once it is oxidized. Macrophage LDL uptake leads to appreciable cholesterol ester accumulation and foam cell formation. This is at the heart of plaque formation.

After a cholesterol-rich deposit on the endothelium develops, calcium ions are deposited within this plaque. This solidifies the plaque and, if it is rough, can attract platelets and a clot can form. The presence of a plaque narrows the passage for blood and potentiates the possibility of an outright blockage to the vessel.

C-reactive protein and LDL are both are markers of CVD risk. However, the use of C-reactive protein as a marker for CVD is no better than using LDL cholesterol as a predictor. The assay for C-reactive protein is more expensive and more complicated. Actually, any inflammation will elicit a rise in C-reactive protein so if the person has a sore throat an increase in C-reactive protein value might be obtained that has nothing to do with the development of CVD.

Relationship of Inflammation to Chronic Disease

In tissues from obese individuals, there are increases in the markers of inflammation.[149,150] Several studies have reported on the association of low-grade inflammation with metabolic syndrome. This has been reported in adolescents as well as adults.[151–159] A state of chronic inflammation has been observed in obesity and in type 2 diabetes in metabolically relevant sites such as the liver, muscle, and adipose tissue. Interference with this inflammation improves or alleviates insulin resistance. In obesity, TNFα production is elevated, and when this production is blocked, there is an improvement in insulin sensitivity. TNFα regulation of insulin sensitivity is in turn regulated by c-jun *N*-terminal kinase and by I kappa beta kinase. Since obesity and diabetes frequently are associated, a study was performed to determine whether caloric restriction of streptozotocin diabetic rats would affect oxidative stress and inflammation markers. Ugochukwu et al.[157] found that it did. Caloric restriction ameliorated the oxidative and inflammatory effects of diabetes.

Type 2 diabetes mellitus is characterized by a chronic inflammatory state associated with insulin resistance.[155–159] Hyperglycemia has been shown to induce proinflammatory cytokines and chemokine genes in monocyte cells. TNFα induces insulin resistance and has a role in obesity development as well. IL-6 alters insulin sensitivity. Hyperglycemia results in increases in the glycated hemoglobin and increases in the polyol pathway and the hexosamine pathway and activates protein kinase C activity.[158] Acidosis and nonketotic hyperglycemia induce the release of inflammatory cytokines and this can be reversed once the glycemia is normalized.[158–165] Acidosis and nonketotic hyperglycemia are associated with an elevation in proinflammatory cytokines, ROS, and cardiovascular risk in the absence of obvious infection or cardiovascular pathology. Mastorikou et al.[166] reported that people with type 2 diabetes have a defect in the metabolism of oxidized phospholipid by HDL. Park et al.[129] have shown that oxidative stress and chronic inflammation are closely related to insulin resistance, obesity, CVD, and type 2 diabetes. In these people, there appears to be an overexpression of the gene for glucose-6-phosphate dehydrogenase in adipocytes and this overexpression is linked to the expression of pro-oxidative enzymes and the activation of NFκB. Fridly and Philipson[130] have shown that glucose-dependent insulin release itself causes oxidative stress in the pancreatic islet cells. This suggests that dietary antioxidant measures might be of benefit to everyone at genetic risk to develop diabetes. Natali et al.[131] reported that type 2 diabetes clusters with inflammatory markers (cytokines), fibrinolytic markers PAI-1 and tPA, central obesity, vascular dysfunction/damage, impaired fibrinolysis, and low-grade infection.

In CVD, markers of inflammation appear to precede disease development.[132] Atherosclerosis has elements of an inflammatory disease. The process is characterized by an accumulation of cholesterol-containing LDLs in the intima of the blood vessels. Leukocyte adhesion molecules and chemokines promote the recruitment of monocytes and T cells. The monocytes differentiate into macrophages and upregulate pattern recognition receptors including scavenger receptors and toll-like receptors. The scavenger receptors internalize the LDLs that in turn lead to foam cell formation. Toll-like receptors transmit activating signals that lead to the release of cytokines, proteases, and vasoactive molecules. T cells recognize local antigens and mount T helper-1 responses with the secretion of proinflammatory cytokines that contribute to local inflammation and plaque growth. Local inflammation may lead to proteolysis, plaque rupture, and thrombus (clot) formation. This causes ischemia (reduced oxygen supply to the tissue being served by the blocked vessel) and infarction.

Likewise, in renal disease, markers of oxidative stress accompany and may even precede disease diagnosis. Kaysen and Eiserich[133] studied the role of oxidative stress-altered lipoprotein structure and function and microinflammation on cardiovascular risk in patients with minor renal dysfunction. As renal function declined, many patients became malnourished and were more likely to have deficiencies of nutrients that are anti-inflammatory. In addition, these people were also likely to have localized anoxic events that further the oxidative stress state and the inflammatory state. These patients have increased C-reactive protein levels as well as increased levels of IL-6. As renal function declines, hepatic apo A-I synthesis decreases and HDL levels fall. Inflammation causes a further structural and functional abnormal state with respect to the lipoproteins: apo C III, a competitive inhibitor of LPL, increases. Intermediate LPL increases with increases in serum triglycerides. This intermediate lipoprotein consists of VLDL and chylomicron remnants. All of these changes affect vascular relaxation. As well there is an activation of the angiotensin axis and a loss in renal mass. This in turn leads to an increase in free radical formation and a decrease in activity of the free radical suppression system. Leukocyte-derived peroxidase functions as a nitric acid oxidase in the inflamed vasculature and contributes to decreased nitric acid bioavailability and compromised vascular reactivity. All of these events are associated with hypertension and increased cardiovascular risk.

Aging may be related to an accumulation of oxidative stress events.[95,136,137,150,168] Aging is associated with a reduced ability to cope with physiological challenges. This includes a lowered ability to suppress the formation of free radicals. In turn, this is reflected in an increase in inflammatory markers, damage to important macromolecules, and impaired function. Heat shock proteins play a role in the preservation of the normal state. The heat shock proteins form a highly conserved system responsible for the preservation of the correct DNA sequence and subsequent correct protein structure. Acetyl carnitine may be another material of importance to maintain normal metabolim.[137] It plays a role in maintaining appropriate relationship of reducing equivalents between the cytosol and mitochondria thereby contributing to the maintenance of normal mitochondrial activity.

Finally, there may be some genetic influences as well with respect to free radical formation and suppression as well as in the inflammatory process. Some nutrients mediate the expression of genes encoding components of the inflammation process. These include the unsaturated fatty acids.[167] There is accumulating evidence in both humans and animal models that indicates that PUFAs of the omega three family can affect gene expression (see Chapter 7). They regulate two groups of transcription factors: sterol regulatory element-binding proteins and PPARs. There may also be polymorphisms in the codes for components of the inflammatory process that are related to the development of chronic disease and the expression of these polymorphisms may be nutrient related. Milk and dairy foods have a number of components that taken separately (as discussed earlier) could have effects on inflammatory disease as well as oxidative stress. Unfortunately, studies using whole foods are lacking in the literature. Milk fat, for example, contains ~66% of its fat as saturated fat, ~2% as linoleic, ~2% α-linolenic, and about 30% as monounsaturated fat in addition to ~0.5% cholesterol. Milk fat also contains a small amount of *trans*-fat that appears in the fat as a result of biohydrogenation of pasture and feed linoleic and linolenic acids by the rumen microorganisms.

The *trans*-fat is *trans*-11–18:1 CLA (as discussed earlier) and is found in milk fat. This *trans*-fat seems to have little relationship to any of the degenerative diseases usually associated with the consumption of *trans*-fat found in hydrogenated plant fats such as margarine.[1] Milk is also an excellent source of essential vitamins and minerals and these micronutrients play roles as described previously in suppressing free radical formation and the inflammatory response. Data are lacking as to their specific roles in these processes as components of whole foods, that is, dairy foods. Finally, as described earlier, milk contains some valuable proteins that have important nutritional functions. Calcium absorption, for example, is facilitated by the milk proteins. Integrating the functions of all of these components with respect to chronic disease that is related to oxidative stress and inflammation has been difficult and is constantly changing.

Aging and Free Radicals

Free radical attack of mitochondrial DNA (mtDNA) could be involved in the aging process. There are several reasons this occurs: (1) The mitochondria are the major producers of oxygen free radicals, (2) these radicals are in close proximity to the DNA, (3) mtDNA is naked (has no protective histone coat), and (4) mtDNA is a compact molecule and is preferentially attached to the mitochondrial inner membrane.

Free radical damage can result in large-scale deletions in the mtDNA of various tissues. A study by Wei[168] of aged humans revealed various deletion mutations in this genome. Base substitutions in this genome were found as well. With age, mitochondrial respiratory function declines in a variety of tissues coincident with rising levels of lipid peroxides and evidence of cumulative mtDNA damage. While the amount of mutated DNA is quite small, these data do support the notion that free radical damage could be involved in the aging process. Of course, there are so many mitochondria in each cell (500–25,000 depending on cell type), and each mitochondrion has 8–10 copies of its genome that the damage reported in this aging study could be rather trivial. In contrast, free radical damage to the nuclear DNA, if unrepaired, could be more serious.

Marine Oils and Health Concerns

A number of years ago, a group of Danish scientists compared the food intake and health status of Danes and Greenland Eskimos.[169,170] Both populations consumed high-protein, high-fat diets; however, where the Danish diet included a variety of milk and meat products, the Eskimo diet included primarily fish and marine creatures such as whale, walrus, and seal. These marine foods contain fat that is rich in the omega-3 fatty acids such as linolenic, eicosapentaenoic, and docosahexaenoic acids and the long-chain fatty acids having 5 or 6 double bonds. The P:S ratio of the Greenland Eskimo diet was 0.84 compared with 0.24 for the Danes. The Danish investigators observed these diet differences between Danes and Eskimos and also noticed the differences in blood lipid profiles, as well as differences in the incidence of CVD. While CVD was one of the leading causes of death among the Danes, the leading cause of death in Eskimos was cerebral hemorrhage (stroke). The Eskimos had prolonged bleeding times and a nosebleed was a serious problem. The prolonged clotting time was probably due to the omega-3 fatty acid effect on those eicosanoids involved in clot formation. These death statistics considered age-matched groups, but were not age adjusted. That is, the investigators compared the two populations using age-matched groups without correcting for total population longevity or for early death due to communicable diseases, malnutrition (in infants particularly), or the hazards of daily life. For the Eskimo, these factors could have been quite important. Furthermore, one must realize that all causes must add up to 100%. Thus, if fewer die of CVD, more may have died from communicable disease or something else. Nonetheless, the findings of the Danes regarding omega-3 fatty acid intake and CVD set off a whole flurry of animal and human studies directed toward understanding how the omega-3 fatty acids affected metabolism.

The observations on marine oils and CVD have stimulated considerable research on the responses of man and animals to the inclusion of marine oils in the diet.[171–175] Rats, mice, swine, monkeys, and rabbits have been studied in addition to normal humans and humans having a variety of diseases thought to benefit from the consumption of these oils. Whether the inclusion of omega-3 fatty acids in the diets of hyperlipidemic subjects was of benefit was tested by Phillipson et al.[173] Twenty hyperlipemic subjects were studied. Ten of these subjects had type IIb lipemia (cholesterol range, 238–411 mg/dL; triglyceride range, 198–720 mg/dL) and 10 had type V lipemia (cholesterol range, 274–840 mg/dL; triglyceride range, 896–5775 mg/dL). The subjects consumed either a corn-oil-based or a fish-oil-based diet or a control diet for 4 weeks each. In the type IIb group, fish-oil consumption resulted in a 27% decrease in plasma cholesterol and a 64% decrease in triglyceride. In the type V group, the reductions were 45% and 79%, respectively. In the type V group, the consumption of the corn-oil diet resulted in a significant rise in plasma triglyceride levels. These and other investigators reported that fish-oil consumption resulted in a decrease in VLDL levels in the blood.

Not only has there been interest in the relationship of dietary omega-3 fatty acids to CVD; there has also been interest in its relationship to diabetes. People with diabetes mellitus have five to six times the risk of people without diabetes of having CVD. Diabetes and heart disease are closely related.

With respect to marine oils and diabetes, Feldman et al.[174] studied two groups of Alaskan Eskimos. One group consumed a typical Western diet while the other consumed the traditional Alaskan Eskimo diet, which, like the Greenland Eskimo diet, is high in marine foods and low in total carbohydrates as well as sugar. As found in the Greenland Eskimos, serum lipids were very low and glucose tolerance normal, when the traditional diet was consumed. When the Eskimos consumed Western diets, which are higher in carbohydrate, particularly sugar, they had significantly higher free fatty acid and triglyceride levels, as well as minor abnormalities in their glucose tolerance. Although Alaskan Eskimos, in general, have a very low prevalence of diabetes, these findings suggest that as these Eskimos begin to include significant amounts of carbohydrate, particularly sweets, in their diet, the prevalence of diabetes may change. In addition, since the Eskimos studied by Feldman consumed significant quantities of marine foods, it might also be inferred that the development of glucose intolerance was genetically controlled and unaffected by the presence of omega-3 fatty acids in the diet.

All of the observations of the differential effects of different fatty acids on metabolism prompted nutrition scientists to investigate the possible benefits of consuming foods rich in omega-3 fatty acids. Such foods include ocean fish, marine mammals, and some plant foods. Some vegetable oils such as primrose, canola, wheat germ, linseed, and walnut also contain significant amounts of these fatty acids. Small amounts are also found in a number of other foods such as spinach, certain margarines, broccoli, and lettuce. Hens fed omega-3 fatty acid-rich fats will lay eggs containing these fatty acids in the yolks.

Fish oil in the diet easily oxidizes and forms peroxides. These peroxides are what gives these oils their peculiar and often objectionable odor. Diets containing large amounts of these oils are not as well liked by experimental animals and appetite is suppressed. Food intake may be decreased by as much as 20%. Even when the scientist takes stringent care of the diet by preventing auto-oxidation, the food intake of fat-rich diets is reduced. Despite a reduction in food intake, animals utilize their diet very well and a marine-oil diet usually is characterized by an increase in feed efficiency. That is, the animal will gain more weight per unit of food consumed than an animal consuming a diet containing some other fat source. This is not always true however. Genetically obese rats and mice gain less weight when fed a marine-oil diet than when fed a corn oil or tallow or safflower oil diet.

At any rate, a decrease in food consumption despite an increase in feed efficiency means that there is less food fat for the liver to metabolize and convert to VLDL. This also means that less VLDL food fat is transported to the peripheral fat depots for storage, and, in part, this explains the effect of the marine oils on serum lipid levels. Dietary marine oils have two other equally important effects that can also explain their serum-lipid-lowering action. The first of these is an inhibition of hepatic fatty acid, phospholipid, and cholesterol synthesis. In part, this attenuation of lipid synthesis by marine oils occurs at the level of specific genes that encode for the lipogenic enzymes. The transcription of genes encoded for enzymes necessary for lipogenesis is suppressed in hepatic tissue from rats fed the marine oils. While we realize that enzymes are never fully active in vivo and that the amount of enzyme may not fully predict the amount of product (in this case lipid) produced, these findings do contribute to our understanding of how dietary marine oils can lower serum lipid levels.

Added to the decrease in lipogenic enzyme amount and activity and decreased rates of lipid synthesis observed in animals fed marine oils is the observation that marine-oil-fed animals also have a reduced hepatic lipid output. This means that lipids formed in the liver are not as readily exported and the liver of the animal fed the marine oils contains more fat than the liver of the rat fed a control diet. Reduced hepatic lipid output by humans consuming fish oil supplements has been reported. This too results in a lowering of serum triglycerides and serum cholesterol. Accumulated lipids in the liver may be an additional reason that lipid synthesis is downregulated. Product inhibition, in this case newly synthesized lipid, is a well-recognized metabolic control mechanism.

Consumption of omega-3 fatty acids nonetheless does result in lower blood lipid levels and this effect is presumed to explain the lower incidence of CVD in the Eskimos. Whether this presumption is correct cannot be taken for granted. CVD has a complicated pathophysiology that is not well understood. Genetic factors as well as lifestyle choices can influence its development and can determine whether it is a life-threatening condition.

Lipids and Membrane Function

Biological membranes contain a large number of lipids, proteins, lipid–protein complexes, glycolipids, and glycoproteins. The arrangement of these many compounds within the membrane structure has been studied extensively. The membranes exist as a lipid bilayer because the phospholipids have amphipathic characteristics. They have both polar (the phosphorylated substituent at carbon 3) and nonpolar (the fatty acids) regions. The polar region is hydrophilic and is positioned such that it is in contact with the aqueous media around and within the cells. The nonpolar or fatty acid region is oriented toward the center of the bilayer so that it is protected from contact with the contents of the cell and the fluids that surround it. Figure 10.13 shows the arrangements of the polar phospholipids that are oriented as described with the membrane proteins embedded in this bilayer. Some proteins sit on the exterior aspect of the bilayer, other proteins rest on the interior aspect while additional proteins extend through the bilayer.

The ability of these amphipathic compounds to self-assemble into a bilayer can be demonstrated in vitro. Lipid vesicles can be made by the addition of these phospholipids to water. A lipid bilayer will form just as described. This feature of the phospholipids is consistent with one of the many

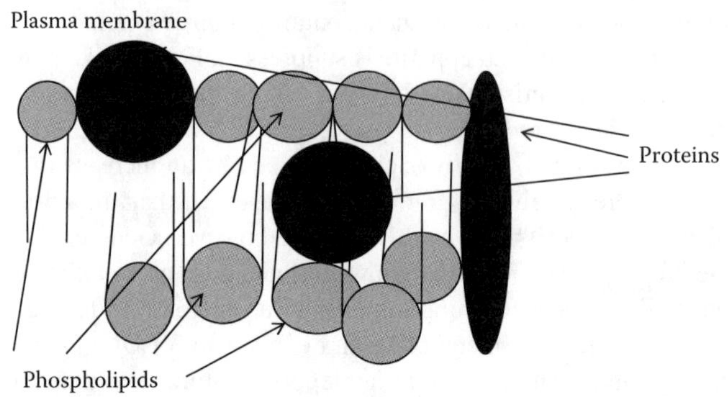

FIGURE 10.13 A schematic view of a plasma membrane.

roles a membrane serves. It is a permeability barrier for the cells and cell compartments. The lipid bilayer forms the matrix into which specific proteins are placed. Each of the individual phospholipids and the cholesterol provide specific regional characteristics that satisfy the insertion requirements of each of the many membrane proteins. The lipid bilayer serves as a seal around these membrane proteins and thus prevents nonspecific leakage. These lipids also serve to maintain the proteins in their most appropriate functional conformations. The polar position of the phospholipids satisfies the requirements for the electrostatic charge that is needed for the surface associations of specific cell surface proteins. All of these characteristics are needed and are critical to normal cell function. For example, an intact permeability barrier to sodium, potassium, calcium, and hydrogen ions is needed so that electrochemical gradients, which in turn drive other membrane transport processes, are maintained.

Cell membranes usually work best when their lipids are in the liquid crystal state. This means that there are regional differences in the physical state of the lipid. Some portions may be fairly fluid, whereas others may be fairly solid. The localized difference in physical state or fluidity has to do with the chain length and saturation of the fatty acids attached at carbons 1 and 2 of the phospholipid; it is this portion of the molecule that extends into the center of the bilayer. Membranes whose phospholipid fatty acids are saturated are less fluid than those membranes containing PUFAs in their phospholipids. Even within a membrane, there can be regional differences in fluidity due to the nature of the fatty acids in the phospholipids of that region. Differences in fluidity are due not only to the ratio of saturated fatty acids to unsaturated fatty acids but also to the ratio of cholesterol to fatty acids. This ratio varies according to the location of the membrane. Plasma membranes, for example, contain more cholesterol than do mitochondrial membranes.

Membrane Phospholipid Composition

There are three major classes of lipids in membranes: glycolipids, cholesterol, and phospholipids. The glycolipids have a role in the cell surface-associated antigens, whereas the cholesterol serves to regulate fluidity. The phospholipids have a phosphorylated compound at carbon 3 of the glycerol backbone and fatty acids attached at carbons 1 and 2. It is usual to find a saturated fatty acid attached at carbon 1 and an unsaturated fatty acid at carbon 2. In addition, phosphatidylethanolamine and phosphatidylserine usually have fatty acids that are more unsaturated than PIP and phosphatidylcholine. Less than 10% of the membrane phospholipid is PIP. Plasma membranes have no cardiolipin and the mitochondrial membranes have very little phosphatidylserine. Several of these phospholipids have important roles in the signal transduction processes that mediate the action of a variety of hormones. PIP and its role in the PIP cycle is one of the most important.[158] Phosphatidylcholine and phosphatidylethanolamine also play roles in these systems. The PIP cycle is shown in Chapter 12 ("Inositol" section). Its importance relates to the action of inositol-1,4,5-phosphate in moving the calcium ion from its intracellular store to where it can stimulate protein kinase C. PIP also serves to anchor glycoproteins to the membrane. Glycoproteins are tethered to the external aspect of the plasma membrane and play a role in the cell recognition process. Pathogens and foreign proteins are recognized by these structures.

Disease Effects on Membrane Lipids

There are numerous reviews on the effects of diet and disease on the fatty acid content of membrane fatty acids. While the primary focus has been on the abnormalities of the proteins in the membrane lipid bilayer, there is a role for the lipid in some of these disorders. Muscular dystrophy and multiple sclerosis are characterized by changes in the lipid structure of the membrane. In the former, the change consists of an increase in the amount of lysophosphatidylcholine and cardiolipin. In multiple sclerosis, there is a degeneration of the myelin of both central and peripheral nerves. The myelin is 75% lipid and 25% protein. Although the disease could be attributed to a specific abnormality in either component, there are reports that the lipid contains about 27% fatty acid (palmitate and oleate) in a covalent linkage and that multiple sclerosis is associated with a derangement in this association and a reduction in the amount of phosphatidylserine. There have been many reports of these lipid changes or a lack of change in myelin; however, it is generally agreed that the disease is not primary to the lipid portion of the membrane. Rather, it is the specific myelin protein that somehow becomes abnormal. Such other diseases as renal disease, hepatic disease, ethanol intoxication, spur cell anemia, and diabetes likewise result in secondary effects on the membrane lipids. These changes can, however, make the disease worse by compromising the functionality of the membrane and its role in metabolic regulation. In humans with cirrhotic liver disease, the erythrocyte membrane fatty acids change. In cirrhotic subjects, the membranes contain less phosphatidylethanolamine and more phosphatidylcholine than membranes from normal subjects. In these subjects, the membrane cholesterol and fatty acid content remains unchanged, but the ratio of cholesterol to phospholipid increases.

Hormonal Effects on Membrane Lipids

The hormone insulin can affect the fatty acid profile of the membrane phospholipids through its effect on glucose conversion to fatty acids and through its effect on the desaturases. Other hormones have an influence on this profile as well. Examples of this influence are shown in Table 10.12. Daily injections of the synthetic glucocorticoid, dexamethasone, resulted in an increase in the mole percent of linoleic (18:2) acid and a decrease in arachidonic acid (20:4). Thyroidectomy resulted in a small increase in rat liver mitochondrial levels of 18:2 and 20:4. This is probably due to the reduction in fatty acid turnover that occurs in the absence of the thyroid gland. Hypophysectomy, which causes a decrease in growth-hormone levels, resulted in an increase in 18:2 and a decrease in 20:4 in hepatic mitochondria. Studies on the influence of all the many hormones that affect fatty acid synthesis, phospholipid synthesis, and membrane phospholipid fatty acid levels are not as readily available as are reports on the dietary fat effects on these parameters. However, they are of interest because these hormones may also have a considerable influence on the function of the protein components that are embedded in the various membranes. These hormones may act directly on the synthesis and activation of these proteins, which in turn may affect their conformation and hence their activity. Thyroxine, for

TABLE 10.12
Effects of Glucocorticoid or Thyroid Deficiency or Diabetes on Fatty Acid Profiles of Liver or Isolated Liver Mitochondria

	Fatty Acids (mol%)						
Treatment	**16:0**	**18:0**	**18:1**	**18:2**	**20:4**	**22:6**	**Tissue**
1 mg GC/day	14.6	22.7	6.6	28.5	19.0	3.5	Liver
Control	17.0	20.3	7.61	5.12	7.4	1.5	Liver
Thyroidectomy	12.5	21	8.6	19.5	19.0	8.1	RLM
Control	13.0	20	9.0	17.4	15.7	7.0	RLM
Hypophysectomy	27.1	21.5	13.5	17.0	14.5	2.0	RLM
Control	27.4	22	12.2	12.1	17.4	2.8	RLM
Diabetes[b]	24.5	23.3	7.02	2.4	15.2	4.2	RLM
Control	16.9	23.2	9.3	22.7	22.2	3.1	RLM

Notes: GC, synthetic glucocorticoid, dexamethasone; RLM, rat liver mitochondria.
[a] Streptozotocin-induced diabetes.

example, negatively affects the activity of the Δ9 desaturase, which, because it is less active, results in fewer unsaturated fatty acids in the membrane. In turn, microsomal cytochrome b_5 activity is less dependent on the lipid environment. That is, it must be surrounded by a very fluid lipid, and this lipid must have a number of unsaturated fatty acids in it. Just as thyroidectomy results in a decrease in membrane phospholipid fatty acid unsaturation, hyperthyroidism has the reverse effect. The thyroid hormones also affect fatty acid elongation by inducing an increase in the activity of the microsomal fatty acid elongation system while having little effect on mitochondrial elongation. It has been reported that the incorporation of labeled choline into brain and liver phosphatidylcholine was less in thyrotoxic rats than in normal rats.

Age Effects on Membrane Lipids

As animals age, their hormonal status changes, as does the lipid component of their membranes. With age, there is a decrease in growth-hormone production, an increase followed by a decrease in the hormones for reproduction, and, as the animal ages, larger fat stores. Larger fat cells are resistant to insulin and insulin levels may rise as a result of increased fat cell size (insulin resistance). As mentioned in the preceding section, these hormones can affect the lipid portion of the membranes within and around the cells and hence affect how these cells regulate their metabolism. With age, the degree of unsaturation of the membrane fatty acids decreases and the cholesterol level rises. There is also an increase in the number of superoxide radicals. This increase may be responsible for the degradation of the membrane lipids, which, in turn, might explain the age-related changes in membrane function. Membranes from aging animals are less fluid and have reduced transport capacities. As animals age, there is a decline in hepatic mitochondrial respiratory rate and a decrease in the respiratory control ratio and the ADP/O ratio. In addition, there are reports of an age-related decrease in membrane fatty acid unsaturation coupled with a decrease in membrane fluidity and a decrease in the exchange of ATP for ADP across the mitochondrial membrane, a decrease in ATP synthesis, and an amelioration of these age-related decreases in mitochondrial function by restricted feeding.

Membrane Function

In the previous section, the importance of diet, age, and hormonal status was described in terms of their influence on the composition of the membrane lipids. Although not emphasized, these compositional differences have important effects on metabolic regulation. This regulation consists of the control of the flux of nutrients, substrates, and/or products into, out of, and between the various compartments of the cell.

The cellular membranes serve as the *gatekeepers* of the cells and their compartments. They regulate the influx and efflux of nutrients, substrates, hormones, and metabolic products produced or used by the cell or compartment in the course of its metabolic activity. For example, the mitochondrial membrane, through its transport of two- and four-carbon intermediates and through its exchange of ADP for ATP, regulates the activity of the respiratory chain and ATP synthesis. If too little ADP enters the mitochondria because of decreased ADP transport across the mitochondrial membrane, respiratory chain activity will decrease, less ATP will be synthesized, and there may be a decrease in other mitochondrial reactions that are either driven by ADP influx or dependent on ATP availability. Through its export of citrate from the matrix of the mitochondria, ATP regulates the availability of citrate to the cytosol for cleavage into oxaloacetate and acetyl CoA, the beginning of fatty acid synthesis. If more citrate is exported from the mitochondria than can be split to oxaloacetate and acetyl CoA, this citrate will feed back onto the phosphofructokinase reaction, and glycolysis will be inhibited. Thus, the activity of the mitochondrial membrane tricarboxylate transporter has a role in the control of cytosolic metabolism.

Other transporters such as the dicarboxylate transporter or the adenine nucleotide translocase have similar responsibilities vis-à-vis the control of cytosolic and mitochondrial metabolic activity. In the plasma membrane, receptors embedded in the membrane have a similar function. That is, they control the entry of nutrients or hormones into the cell. Further, the plasma membrane hormone receptor may bind a given hormone and, with binding, elicit a cascade of reactions characteristic of the hormone effect without permitting the entry of the hormone itself into the cytosolic compartment. An example here is the hormone insulin. Insulin binds to its receptor and, in so doing, elicits the cascade of events that include the transport and metabolism of glucose by the cell. The insulin, bound to the receptor site, is inactivated and is brought into the cell by pinocytosis for further degradation. Other hormones, notably the nonprotein steroids and the low-molecular-weight hormones such as epinephrine and thyroxine, pass through the plasma membrane and attach to receptors in the cytosol or nuclear membrane or on the endoplasmic reticulum. Once attached to their respective binding sites, they also elicit a metabolic response.

In membranes are a variety of closely packed proteins and lipids. The membrane-bound proteins have extensive hydrophobic regions and usually require lipids for the maintenance of their activity. Adenylate cyclase, cytochrome b_5, and cytochrome c oxidase have all been shown to have phospholipid affinities. Cytochrome c oxidase from mitochondria has tightly bound aldehyde lipid that cannot be removed without destroying its activity as the enzyme that transfers electrons to molecular oxygen in the final step of respiration. A number of other membrane proteins have tightly bound fatty acids as part of their structures. These fatty acids are covalently bound to their proteins as a posttranslational event and act to direct, insert, and anchor the proteins in the cell membranes. Other lipids are bound differently to membrane proteins. Some are acylated with fatty acids during their passage from their site of synthesis on the rough endoplasmic reticulum to the membrane, whereas others acquire their lipid component during their placement in the membrane. β-Hydroxybutyrate dehydrogenase, for example, requires the choline head of phosphatidylcholine for its activity. If hepatocytes are caused to increase their synthesis of phosphatidylmethylethanolamine, which substitutes for phosphatidylcholine in the membrane, β-hydroxybutyrate dehydrogenase activity is reduced.

All of these examples illustrate the importance of the cellular and intracellular membranes in the regulation of metabolism. They illustrate the fact that the gatekeeping property of the membrane is vested in the structure and function of the various transporters and receptors or binding proteins embedded in the membrane. Whereas the genetic heritage of an individual determines the amino acid sequence of the proteins and hence their function, this function can be modified by the lipid milieu in which they exist. Diet, hormonal state, and genetics in turn control the lipid milieu in terms of the kinds and amounts of the different lipids that are synthesized within the cell and incorporated into the membrane. Membranes differ in the amount of cholesterol they contain; mitochondrial membranes contain very little while plasma membranes contain somewhat more.

CANCER AND DIETARY FAT

The many different forms of cancer account for the second-largest number of deaths due to disease in developed nations. It too is probably influenced by the fat intake, but in these disorders, it is not the saturated fat that is culpable.[176] Studies on the development of mammary tumors in rats and mice have shown that high intakes of polyunsaturated fat containing the omega-6 fatty acids promote the development of the cancer. Carcinogenesis is thought to occur in two steps. The first is the initiation step. This concerns the conversion of normal DNA to the DNA typical of a cancer cell. Large segments of the gene code are deleted or so changed that the translation products are either not present or are not normal in function. This conversion can be instigated by chemicals such as 7,12-dimethylbenz(a)anthracene (DMBA), by viruses, radiation, and perhaps oxidized (free radical) food components. By itself, this initiation step will not progress to the metastatic cell unless the next step, the promotion step, also occurs. Cells whose DNA has been injured will and can repair this DNA. However, if the *right* environment is provided, this does not occur and a metastatic cell is produced and reproduced. Dietary corn oil has been shown to be a very good promoter of DMBA-induced breast cancer in rats and mice while dietary beef tallow is not. How corn oil has this effect is not known and, of course, cause-and-effect studies cannot be conducted in humans. Just as epidemiological studies cannot provide definitive proof of the role of diet in CVD development, the same is true for cancer. Both the level of intake and the type of fat have been implicated but strong proof is lacking. As with CVD and/or diabetes and/or obesity, the genetic influence is quite strong.

OTHER DISEASES

No discussion of the role of dietary fat in human disease would be complete without the mention of obesity (see Chapter 3). As discussed in the chapter on energy, this disorder has a multiplicity of causes of which the total energy intake is but a part. The excess energy consumed could easily be provided by the dietary fat since it has twice the energy value per gram as does dietary carbohydrate and protein. However, intake alone does not fully explain the obese state. Genetic factors that control energy intake, storage, and use are also important.

Gall bladder disease is frequently associated with excess body fatness (or its loss) and, as explained in the "absorption" section, may be attributable to the precipitation of cholesterol from the bile while in the gall bladder. Other genetic diseases in addition to those previously described with respect to lipid transport due to mutations in genes for specific enzymes exist. Many are associated with mental retardation and early death. None seem to be related to nutrition or dietary fat intake.

SUMMARY

1. The lipids are the third major source of energy in the human diet.
2. They are simple or compound complexes. The simple lipids are the fatty acids, acylglycerols, and sterols. All of these are found in the food supply and all except the EFA can be synthesized endogenously.
3. Saturated fatty acids and sterols are more common in foods of animal origin than in foods of plant origin. Long-chain PUFAs are found in certain plant oils and in the marine oils.
4. During digestion, the lipids are emulsified. They form micelles that are then moved through the gut absorptive layer. The short-chain fatty acids move directly into the portal systems while the other lipids enter the lymphatic system first before entering the blood stream. These lipids are joined to one or more transport proteins (lipoproteins).
5. Genetic differences have been found in these proteins and these differences can determine the subsequent disposal of the lipids.
6. Endogenously synthesized lipids also form lipoproteins as these lipids are transported from their site of origin to their site of use/storage.
7. Mutations in the protein portions of the lipoproteins can elicit a variety of abnormal characteristics. Some of these are associated with the development of CVD.
8. The functions of the lipids include serving as energy use/storage, serving as components of membranes, and serving as substrates for the synthesis of a variety of hormones including the eicosanoids.
9. Unsaturated fatty acids can auto-oxidize to form free radicals. These free radicals can cause damage to the cells. The free radical formation can be suppressed by a variety of dietary factors.

LEARNING OPPORTUNITIES

CASE STUDY 10.1

The XYZ Food company has decided to develop a new *superfood* breakfast item. They have combined oats, corn, and barley into a cereal flake and coated this flake with a combination of coconut oil, lactose, vitamin C, and B vitamins. The product is supposed to be consumed with milk. You are the consumer representative on the evaluation panel for this new product. What are the positive and negative aspects of this product? What would you change? Why? Assuming that the price was reasonable and that the product tasted good, who would benefit by consuming this product? Who would have trouble consuming this product? Why?

CASE STUDY 10.2

Shelly is a vegetarian and has been for a year. She has developed a troubling dry skin condition. In addition, her menstrual cycle has become erratic. She and her husband have been unsuccessful in achieving a pregnancy. Analyze this situation and suggest some solutions to the problem(s). Discuss the reasons why Shelly is having these problems.

CASE STUDY 10.3

Harry has very high cholesterol levels yet he has no symptoms of CVD. His vascular tree is clean as a whistle. How can that be? Everyone *knows* that high cholesterol levels are associated with heart disease; why is Harry different? Explain.

MULTIPLE-CHOICE QUESTIONS

1. Whale, seal, fish, and walrus are regular components of an Eskimo diet.
   a. This diet is rich in omega 3 fatty acids.
   b. This diet is associated with an increased risk of stroke.
   c. This diet has very little carbohydrate in it.
   d. All of the above.
2. Membranes contain
   a. Unsaturated fatty acids
   b. Cholesterol
   c. Phospholipids and proteins
   d. All of the above
3. Eicosanoids include
   a. PGs
   b. TBXs
   c. Leukotrienes
   d. All of the above
4. If arachidonic acid is absent from the cat's diet, what happens?
   a. Eicosanoid synthesis is curtailed.
   b. The cat becomes hairless.
   c. Immunocompetence is reduced.
   d. All of the above.

5. The injury cycle is associated with
   a. Depressed antibody production
   b. Depressed cytokine production
   c. Fewer adhesion molecules
   d. None of the above

REFERENCES

1. Huth, P.J. (2007) Do ruminant trans fatty acids impact coronary heart disease risk? *Lipid Tech.* 19: 59–62.
2. Peifer, J.J., Lewis, R.L. (1979) Effects of vitamin B-12 deprivation on phospholipid fatty acid patterns in liver and brain of rats fed high and low levels of linoleate in low methionine diets. *J. Nutr.* 100: 2160–2172.
3. Peifer, J.J., Lewis, R.L. (1981) Odd-numbered fatty acids in phosphatidyl choline versus phosphatidyl ethanolamine of vitamin B12 deprived rats. *Proc. Soc. Exp. Biol. Med.* 167: 212–217.
4. Burr, G.O., Burr, M.M. (1929) A new deficiency disease produced by the rigid exclusion of fat from the diet. *J. Biol. Chem.* 82: 345–367.
5. Holman, R. (1986) Nutritional and functional requirements for essential fatty acids. In: *Dietary Fat and Cancer*, (R. Holman, ed.) Alan R. Liss Inc. New York, pp. 211–228.
6. Innis, S. (1991) Essential fatty acids in growth and development. *Prog. Lipid Res.* 30: 39–103.
7. Vesper, H., Schmelz, E.-M., Nicklova-Karakasian, M.N., Dillehay, D.L., Lynch, D.V., Merrill, A.H. (1999) Sphingolipids in food and the emerging importance of sphingolipids to nutrition. *J. Nutr.* 129: 1239–1250.
8. Carr, T.P., Stanek-Krogstrand, K.L., Schlegel, V.L., Fernandez, M.L. (2009) Steareate-enriched plant sterol esters lower serum LDL cholesterol concentrations in normal and hypercholesterolemic adults. *J. Nutr.* 139: 1445–1450.
9. Myrie, S.B., Mymin, D., Triggs-Ralne, B., Johns, P.J.H. (2012) Serum lipids, plant sterols and cholesterol kinetic responses to plant sterol supplementation in phytosterolemia heterozygotes and control individuals. *Am. J. Clin. Nutr.* 95: 837–844.
10. Feldman, E.B., Cooper, G.R. (2007) Assessment of lipids and lipoproteins. In: *Handbook of Nutrition and Food* (C.D. Berdanier, J. Dwyer, E.B. Feldman, eds.). CRC Press, Boca Raton, FL, pp. 683–692.
11. Breslow, J.L. (1989) Genetic basis of lipoprotein disorders. *J. Clin. Invest.* 84: 373–383.
12. Chen, M., Breslow, J.L., Li, W., Leff, T. (1994) Transcriptional regulation of the apo C-III gene by insulin in diabetic mice: Correlation with changes in plasma triglyceride levels. *J. Lipid Res.* 35: 1918–1924.
13. Gimble, J.M., Hua, X., Wanker, F., Morgan, C., Robinson, C., Hill, M.R., Nadon, N. (1995) In vivo and in vitro analysis of murine lipoprotein lipase gene promotor: Tissue specific expression. *Am. J. Physiol.* 268: E213–E218.
14. Nishina, P.M., Johnson, J.P., Naggert, J.K., Krauss, R.M. (1992). Linkage of atherogenic lipoprotein phenotype to the low density lipoprotein receptor locus on the short arm of chromosome 19. *Proc. Natl. Acad. Sci. USA* 89: 708–712.
15. Rosseneu, M., Labeur, C. (1995) Physiological significance of apolipoprotein mutants. *FASEB J.* 9: 768–774.
16. Feldman, E.B., Siri-Tarino, P., Krauss, R.M. (2007) Hyperlipidemias: Major gene and diet effects. In: *Handbook of Nutrition and Food* (C.D. Berdanier, J. Dwyer, F.B. Feldman, eds.). 2nd edn. CRC Press, Boca Raton, FL, pp. 715–726.
17. Herbert, P.N., Assmann, G., Gotto, A.M., Fredrickson, D.S. (1983) Familial lipoprotein deficiency: A betalipoproteinemia, hypolipoproteinemia and Tangier disease. In: *The Metabolic Basis of Inherited Disease* (J.B. Stanbury, J.B. Wyngaarden, D.S. Fredrickson, J.L. Goldstein, M.D. Brown eds.). 5th edn. McGraw-Hill, New York, pp. 589–600.
18. Leppert, M., Breslow, J.L., Wu, L., Hasstedt, S., O'Connell, P., Lathrop, M., Williams, R.R., White, R., Lalouel, J.M. (1988) Inference of a molecular defect of apolipoprotein B in hyperlipoproteinemia by linkage analysis in a large kindred. *J. Clin. Invest.* 82: 847–853.
19. Huang, L.S., Ripps, M.E., Korman, S.H., Deckelbaum, R., Breslow, J.L. (1989) ApoB gene exon 21 deletion in familial hypobetalipoproteinemia (HBLP). *J. Biol. Chem.* 264: 11394–11400.
20. Talmud, P.J., Lloyd, J.K., Muller, D.P.R., Collins, D.R., Scott, J., Humphries, S. (1988) Genetic evidence from two families that the apolipoprotein B gene is not involved in apolipoproteinemia. *J. Clin. Invest.* 82: 1803–1809.

21. Groenwegen, W.A., Krul, E.S., Schonfeld, G., (1993) Apolipoprotein B-52 mutation associated with hypobetalipoproteinemia is compatible with a misaligned pairing deletion mechanism. *J. Lipid Res.* 34: 971–977.
22. Linton, M.F., Pierotti, V., Young, S.G. (1992) Reading frame restoration with an apolipoprotein B gene frameshift mutation. *Proc. Natl. Acad. Sci. USA* 89: 11431–11437.
23. Wetterau, J.R., Aggerbeck, L.P., Bouma, M.E., Eisenberg, C., Munck, A., Hermier, M., Schmitz, J., Gay, G., Rader, D.J., Gregg, R.E. (1992) Absence of microsomal triglyceride transfer protein in individuals with a betalipoproteinemia. *Science* 258: 999–1003.
24. Shoulders, C.C., Brett, D.J., Bayliss, J.D., Narcisi, T.M.E., Jarmuz, A., Grantham, T.T., Bhattacharya, S. et al. (1993) A betalipoproteinemia is caused by defects in the gene encoding the 97 kDa subunit of a microsomal triglyceride transfer protein. *Hum. Mol. Genet.* 2: 2109–2115.
25. Gretan, H., Beil, F.U. (1988) Lipase deficiencies. *J. Inherit. Dis.* 11: 1S–10S.
26. Beckinridge, W.C. (1978) Hypertriglyceridemia associated with deficiency of apolipoprotein C-II. *N. Eng. J. Med.* 298: 1265–1270.
27. Sparkes, R.S., Zollman, S., Klisak, L., Kirchgessner, T.G., Komarony, M.C., Mohandas, T., Schotz, M.C., Lusis, A.J. (1987) Human genes involved in lipolysis of plasma lipoproteins: Mapping loci for lipoprotein lipase to 8p22 and hepatic lipase to 15q21. *Genomics* 1: 138–145.
28. Langlois, S., Deeb, S., Brunzell, J.D., Kastelein, J.J., Hayden, M.R. (1989) A major insertion accounts for a significant proportion of mutations underlying human lipoprotein lipase deficiency. *Proc. Soc. Natl. Acad. Sci. USA* 86: 948–956.
29. Fojo, S.S., Beisiegel, U., Bell, U., Higuchi, K., Bojanovski, M., Gregg, R.E., Greten, H., Brewer, H.B. (1988) Donor splice site mutation in the apolipoprotein (apo) C-II gene (apo C-II Hamburg) of a patient with apo C-II deficiency. *J. Clin. Invest.* 82: 1489–1495.
30. Fogo, S.S., Statenhoef, A.F., Marr, K., Greg, R.E., Ross, R.S., Brewer, H.R. (1988) A deletion mutation in the apo C-II gene (apo C-II, Nijmegen) of a patient with a deficiency of apolipoprotein C-II. *J. Biol. Chem.* 263: 17913–17915.
31. Cox, D.W., Wills, D.E., Quan, F., Ray, P.A. (1988) A deletion of one nucleotide results in functional deficiency of lipoprotein C-II (apo C-II, Toronto). *J. Med. Genet.* 25: 649–655.
32. Durstenfeld, A., Ben-Zeev, O., Reue, K., Stahnke, G., Doolittle, M.H. (1994) Molecular characterization of human lipase deficiency: In vitro expression of two naturally occurring mutations. *Arterioscler. Thromb.* 14: 381–388.
33. Holzl, B., Haber, R., Paulweber, B., Patsch, J.R., Sandhofer, F., (1994) Lipoprotein lipase deficiency due to a 3′ splice site mutation in intron 6 of the lipoprotein lipase gene. *J. Lipid Res.* 35: 2161–2166.
34. Reymer, P., Gagne, E., Groenemeyer, B.E., Zhang, H., Forsyth, H., Jansen, H., Seidell, J.C. et al. (1995) A lipoprotein lipase mutation (Asn 291 Ser) is associated with reduced HDL cholesterol levels in premature atherosclerosis. *Nat. Genet.* 10: 28–35.
35. Morganroth, J., Levy, R.L., Fredrickson, D.S. (1975) The biochemical, clinical, and genetic features of type III hyperlipoproteinemia. *Ann. Int. Med.* 82: 158–165.
36. Lusis, A.J., Heinzmann, C., Sparkes, R.S., Scott, J., Knott, T.J., Geller, R., Sparkes, M.C., Mohandas, T. (1986) Regional mapping of human chromosome 19: Organization of genes for plasma lipid transport (APO CI, -C2, and -E and LDLR) and of the genes C3, PEPD, and GPI. *Genetics* 83: 3929–3937.
37. Weintraub, M.S., Eisenberg, S., Breslow, J.L. (1987) Dietary fat clearance in normal subjects is regulated by genetic variation in apolipoprotein E. *J. Clin. Invest.* 80: 1571–1577.
38. Lusis, A.J., Taylor, B.A., Quon, D., Zollman, S., LeBoeuf, R.C. (1987) Genetic factors controlling structure and expression of apolipoproteins B and E in mice. *J. Biol. Chem.* 262: 7594–7599.
39. Rubin, E.M., Ishida, B.Y., Clift, S.M., Krauss, R.M. (1991a) Expression of human apolipoprotein A-I in transgenic mice results in reduced plasma levels of murine apolipoprotein A-I and the appearance of two new high density lipoprotein subclasses. *Proc. Natl. Acad. Sci. USA* 88: 434–439.
40. Rubin, E.M., Krauss, R.M., Spangler, E.A., Verstuyft, J.G., Cliff, S.M. (1991) Inhibition of early atherogenesis in transgenic mice by human apolipoprotein A-I. *Nature* 353: 265–270.
41. Paigen, B., Mitchell, D., Reue, K., Morrow, A., Lusis, A.J., LeBoeuf, R.C. (1987) Ath-1 a gene determining atherosclerosis susceptibility and high density lipoprotein levels in mice. *Proc. Natl. Acad. Sci. USA* 84: 3763–3770.
42. Jones, P.J.H., Main, B.F., Frolich, J.J. (1993) Response of cholesterol synthesis in cholesterol feeding in men with different apolipoprotein E genotypes. *Metabolism* 42: 1065–1070.
43. Siri-Tarino, P., Feldman, E.B., Krauss, R.M. (2007) Effects of diet on cardiovascular disease risk. In: *Handbook of Nutrition and Food* (C.D. Berdanier, J. Dwyer, E.B. Feldman eds.). CRC Press, Boca Raton, FL, pp. 727–734.

44. Pronczuk, A., Khosla, P., Hayes, K.C. (1994) Dietary myristic, palmitic, and linolenic acids modulate cholesterolemia in gerbils. *FASEB J.* 8: 1191–1200.
45. Clarke, S.D., Jump, D.B. (1993) Regulation of hepatic gene expression by dietary fats: A unique role for polyunsaturated fatty acids. In: *Nutrition and Gene Expression* (C.D. Berdanier, J.L. Hargrove, eds.). CRC Press, Boca Raton, FL, pp. 227–246.
46. Skretting, G., Prydz, H. (1992) An amino acid exchange in exon 1 of the human lecithin: Cholesterol acyltransferase (LCAT) gene is associated with fish eye disease. *BBRC* 31: 583–587.
47. Kushwaha, R.S., Reardon, C.A., Lewis, D.S., Qi, Y., Rice, K.S., Getz, G.S., Carey, K.D., McGill, H.C. Jr. (1994) Effect of dietary lipids on plasma activity and hepatic mRNA levels of the cholesterol ester transfer protein in high and low responding baboons (Papio species). *Metabolism* 43: 1006–1012.
48. Irons, M., Elias, R., Abuelo, D. (1997) Treatment of SLO syndrome: Results of a multicenter trial. *Am. J. Med. Genet.* 68: 311–314.
49. Wassif, C.A., Maslen, C., Kachelele-Linjewele, S. (1998) Mutations in the human sterol delta-7-reductase gene at 11q 12–13 causes Smith-Lemli-Optiz syndrome. *Am. J. Hum. Genet.* 63: 55–62.
50. Rossouw, J.E., Rifkind, B.M. (1990) Does lowering serum cholesterol lower coronary heart disease risk? *Endocrinol. Metab. Clinic N.A.* 19: 279–297.
51. Hegsted, D.M., Ausman, L.M., Johnson, J.A., Dallal, G.E. (1993) Dietary fat and serum lipids: An evaluation of the experimental data. *Am. J. Clin. Nutr.* 57: 875–883.
52. Karlstrom, B.E., Jarvi, A.E., Byberg, L., Berglund, L.G., Vessby, B.O.H. (2011) Fatty fish in the diet of patients with type 2 diabetes: Comparison of the metabolic effects of food rich in N-3 and N-6 fatty acids. *Am. J. Clin. Nutr.* 94: 26–35.
53. Lukiw, W.J., Bazan, N.G. (2008) Docosahexaenoic acid and the aging brain. *J. Nutr.* 138: 2510–2515.
54. SanGiovanni, J.P., Agron, E., Meleth, A.D., Reed, G.F., Sperduto, R.D., Clemons, T.E., Chew, E.Y. (2009) ώ-3 Long chain polyunsaturated fatty acid intake and 12 y incidence of neovascular age-related macular degeneration and central geographic atrophy: AREDS report 30, a prospective cohort study from the age-related eye disease study. *Am. J. Clin. Nutr.* 90: 1601–1607.
55. Kesse-Guyot, E., Andreeva, V.A., Lassale, C., Ferry, M., Jeandel, C., Hercberg, S., Galan, P. (2013) Mediterranean diet and cognitive function: A French study. *Am. J. Clin. Nutr.* 97: 369–376.
56. Whelan, J. (2008) (n-6) and (n-3) Polyunsaturated fatty acids and the aging brain: Food for thought. *J. Nutr.* 138: 2521–2522.
57. Rapoport, S.J. (2008) Arachidonic acid and the brain. *J. Nutr.* 138: 2515–2520.
58. Maljaars, J., Romeyn, F.A., Haddeman, E., Peters, H.P.F., Masclee, A.A.M. (2009) Effect of fat saturation of satiety, hormone release and food intake. *Am. J. Clin. Nutr.* 89: 1019–1024.
59. Jans, A., Konings, E., Goossens, G.H., Bowman, F.G., Moors, C., Boekschoten, M.V., Afman, L.A., Muller, M., Mariman, E.C., Blaak, E.E. (2012) PUFAs acutely affect triacylglycerol-derived skeletal muscle fatty acid uptake and increase postprandial insulin sensitivity. *Am. J. Clin. Nutr.* 95: 825–836.
60. Masson, V.R., Lucas, A., Gueugneau, A.-M., Macaire, J.-P., Paul, J.L., Grynberg, A., Rousseau, D. (2008) Long chain(n-3) polyunsaturated fatty acids prevent metabolic and vascular disorders in fructose-fed rats. *J. Nutr.* 138: 1915–1922.
61. Gopinath, B., Flood, V.M., Teber, E., McMahon, C.M., Mitchell, P. (2011) Dietary intake of cholesterol is positively associated and use of cholesterol-lowering medication is negatively associated with prevalent age-related hearing loss. *J. Nutr.* 141: 1355–1360.
62. Baumgartner, J., Smuts, C.M., Malan, L., Arnold, M., Yee, B.K., Blanco, L.E., Boekschoten, M.V. et al. (2012) In male rats with concurrent iron and (n-3) fatty acid deficiency, provision of either iron or (n-3) fatty acids alone alters monoamine metabolism and exacerbates the cognitive deficits associated with combined deficiency. *J. Nutr.* 142: 1472–1478.
63. Baumgartner, J., Smuts, C.M., Malan, L., Arnold, M., Yee, B.J., Blanco, L.E., Boekschoten, M.V. et al. (2012) Combined deficiency of iron and (n-3) fatty acids in male rats disrupts brain monoamine metabolism and produces greater memory deficits than iron or (n-3) fatty acid deficiency alone. *J. Nutr.* 142: 1463–1471.
64. Phillips, C.M., Goumidi, L., Bertrais, S., Field, M.R., Peloso, G.M., Shen, J., McManuis, R. et al. (2011) Dietary saturated fat modulates the association between STAT3 polymorphisms and abdominal obesity in adults. *J. Nutr.* 139: 2011–2017.
65. Gomez, P., Perez-Martinez, P., Marin, C., Camargo, A., Yubero-Serrano, E.M., Garcia-Rios, A., Rodriguez, F., Delgado-Lista, J., Perez-Jimenez, F., Lopez-Miranda, J. (2010) ADOA1 and ADOP4 gene polymorphisms influence the effects of dietary fat and LDL particle size and oxidation in healthy young adults. *J. Nutr.* 140: 773–778.

66. Sanchez-Moreno, C., Ordovas, J.M., Smith, C.E., Baraza, J.C., Lee, Y.-C., Garaulet, M. (2011) APOA5 gene variation interacts with dietary fat intake to modulate obesity and circulating triglycerides in a Mediterranean population. *J. Nutr.* 141: 380–388.
67. Sanchez-Muniz, F.J., Maki, K.C., Schaefer, E.J., Ordovas, J.M. (2009) Serum lipid and antioxidant responses in hypercholesterolemic men and women receiving plant sterol esters vary by apolipoproteins E genotype. *J. Nutr.* 139: 13–19.
68. Ferguson, J.F., Phillips, C.M., Tierney, A.C., Perez-Martinez, P., Defoort, C., Helal, O., Lairon, D. et al. (2010) Gene-nutrient interactions in metabolic syndrome: Single nucleotide polymorphisms in ADIPOQ and ADIPOR1 interact with plasma saturated fatty acids to modulate insulin resistance. *Am. J. Clin. Nutr.* 91: 794–801.
69. Lu, Y., Feskins, E.J.M., Dolie, M.E.T., Imholz, S., Verschuren, W.M.M., Muler, M., Boer, J.M.A. (2010) Dietary n-3 and n-6 polyunsaturated fatty acid intake interacts with FADS1 genetic variation to affect total and HDL-cholesterol concentrations in the Doetinchem cohort study. *Am. J. Clin. Nutr.* 92: 258–265.
70. Hartiala, J., Gilliam, E., Vikman, S., Campos, H., Allayee, H. (2012) Association of PFA2G4A with myocardial infarction is modulated by dietary PUFAs. *Am. J. Clin. Nutr.* 95: 959–965.
71. Weiss, E.P., Brandauer, J., Kulaputana, O., Ghiu, I.A., Wohn, C.R., Phares, D.A., Shuldiner, A.R., Hagberg, J.M. (2007) FABP2 Ala54Thr genotype is associated with glucoregulatory function and lipid oxidation after a high-fat meal in sedentary nondiabetic men and women. *Am. J. Clin. Nutr.* 85: 102–108.
72. Gillingham, L.G., Harding, S.V., Rideout, T.C., Cunnane, S.C., Eck, P.K., Jones, J.J.H. (2013) Dietary oils and FADS1-FADS2 genetic variants modulate [^{13}C]α-linolenic acid metabolism and plasma fatty acid composition. *Am. J. Clin. Nutr.* 97: 195–207.
73. Schafer, S.N., Machann, M.F., Schick, F., Claussen, C.D., Stumvoll, M., Haring, H.U., Fritche, A. (2005) Liver fat and insulin resistance are independently associated with the—541C.T polymorphism of the hepatic lipase gene. *J. Clin. Endocrinol. Metab.* 90: 4238–4243.
74. Matei, J., Demissie, S., Tucker, K.L., Ordovas, J.M. (2009) Apolipoprotein A5 polymorphisms interact with total dietary fat intake in association with markers of metabolic syndrome in Puerto Rican older adults. *J. Nutr.* 139: 2301–2308.
75. Balk, I., Lee, S., Kim, S.H., Shin, C. (2013) A lipoprotein lipase gene polymorphism interacts with consumption of alcohol to modulate serum HDL-cholesterol concentration. *J. Nutr.* 143: 1618–1625.
76. Perez-Martinez, P., Corella, D., Shen, J., Arnett, D.K., Yiannakouris, N., Tai, E.S., Orhu-Melander, M. et al. (2009) Association between glucokinase regulatory protein (GCKR) and apolipoproteins A5 (APOA5) gene polymorphisms and triacylglycerol concentrations in fasting, postprandial and fenofibrate-treated states. *Am. J. Clin. Nutr.* 89: 391–399.
77. Junyent, M., Parnell, L.D., Lai, C-Q., Lee, Y-C., Smith, C.E., Arnett, D.K., Tsai, M.Y. et al. (2009) Novel variants at KCTD10, MVK and MMAB genes interact with dietary carbohydrates to modulate HDL-cholesterol concentrations in the genetics of lipid lowering drugs and diet network study. *Am. J. Clin. Nutr.* 90: 686–694.
78. Auinger, A., Helwig, L., Rubin, D., Herrmann, J., Jahreis, G., Pfeuffer, M., de Vrese, M., Foelsch, U.R., Schreiber, S., Doering, J. (2010) Human intestinal fatty acid binding protein 2 expression is associated with fat intake and polymorphisms. *J. Nutr.* 140: 1411–1417.
79. Field, C.J., Ryan, E.A., Thomson, A.B.R., Clandinin, M.T. (1990) Diet fat composition alters membrane phospholipid composition, insulin binding and glucose metabolism from control and diabetic animals. *J. Biol. Chem.* 265: 11143–11150.
80. Berdanier, C.D. (1988) Interaction of fat type and thyroxine on hepatic phospholipid fatty acids of BHE rats. *Nutrition* 4: 295–299.
81. Berdanier, C.D., Baltzell, J.L. (1986) Comparative studies of the responses of two strains of rats to an essential fatty acid deficient diet. *Comp. Biochem. Biophys.* 85A: 725–727.
82. Deaver, O.E. Jr, Wander, R.C., McCusker, R.H., Berdanier, C.D. (1986) Diet effects on membrane phospholipid fatty acids and mitochondrial function in BHE rats. *J. Nutr.* 116: 1148–1155.
83. Kim, M.-J.C., Pan, J.-S., Berdanier, C.D. (1990) Glucose turnover in BHE rats fed EFA deficient hydrogenated coconut oil. *Diabets Res.* 13: 43–47.
84. Pan, J.-S., Berdanier, C.D. (1991) Effect of dietary fat on adipocyte insulin binding and glucose metabolism in BHE rats. *J. Nutr.* 121: 1811–1819.
85. Pan, J.-S., Berdanier, C.D. (1991) Effect of dietary fat on hepatocyte insulin binding and glucose metabolism in BHE rats. *J. Nutr.* 121: 1820–1826.
86. Mayer, R.J., Marshall, L.A. (1993) New insights on mammalian phospholipase A2: Comparison of arachidonyl-selective and non-selective enzymes. *FASEB J.* 7: 339–348.

87. MacDonald, J.I.S., Sprechner, H. (1991) Phospholipid remodeling in mammalian cells. *Biochem. Biophys. Acta* 1084: 105–121.
88. Smith, W.L. (1992) Prostanoid synthesis and mechanisms of action. *Am. J. Physiol.* 263: F181–F191.
89. Bartolini, G., Orlandi, M., Chricolo, M., Licastro, F., Zambonelli, P., Minghetti, L., Tomasi, V. (1990) Interleukins, interferons: Yen-yang modulators of PGH synthase in human macrophages. *Biofactors* 2: 267–270.
90. Song, J., Wander, R.C. (1991) Effects of dietary selenium and fish oil (Max EPA) on arachidonic acid metabolism and hemostatic function in rats. *J. Nutr.* 121: 284–292.
91. Hayaishi, O. (1991) Molecular mechanisms of sleep-wake regulation: Roles of prostaglandins D_2 and E_2. *FASEB J.* 5: 2575–2581.
92. Duval, D., Freyss-Beguin, M. (1992) Glucocorticoids and prostaglandin synthesis: We cannot see the wood for the trees. *Prostaglandins, Leukot. Essent. Fatty Acids* 45: 85–112.
93. Esterbauer, H. (1993) Cytotoxicity and genotoxicity of lipid oxidation products. *Am. J. Clin. Nutr.* 57: 779S–786S.
94. Buettner, G.R. (1993) The pecking order of free radicals and antioxidants: Lipid peroxidation, α tocopherol and ascorbate. *Arch. Biochem. Biophys.* 300: 535–543.
95. Harman, D. (1993) Free radical involvement in aging. *Drugs Aging* 3: 60–80.
96. Just, W.W., Soto, U. (1992) Biogenesis of peroxisomes in mammals. *Cell Biochem. Funct.* 10: 159–165.
97. Szeto, Y.T., Kwok, T.C., Benzie, I.F. (2004) Effects of a long term vegetarian diet on biomarkers of antioxidant status and cardiovascular disease risk. *Nutrition* 20: 863–866.
98. Sebekova, K., Boor, P., Valachovicova, M., Blazicek, P., Parrak, V., Babinska, K., Heidland, A., Krajcovicova-Kudlackovaa, M. (2006) Association of metabolic syndrome risk factors with selected markers of oxidative status and microinflammation in healthy omnivores and vegetarians. *Mol. Nutr. Food Res.* 50: 858–868.
99. Bowen, P.E., Borthakur, G. (2004) Postprandial lipid oxidation and cardiovascular disease risk. *Curr. Atheroscler. Rep.* 6: 477–484.
100. Staiger, K., Staiger, H., Weigert, C., Haas, C., Harring, H.-U., Kellerer, M. (2006) Saturated, but not unsaturated fatty acids induce apoptosis of human coronary artery endothelial cells via nuclear factor kappa B activation. *Diabetes* 55: 3121–3126.
101. Fritsche, K. (2006) Fatty acids as modulators of the immune response. *Ann. Rev. Nutr.* 26: 45–73.
102. Gori, A.M., Corsi, A.M., Fedi, S., Gazzini, A., Sofi, F., Bartali, B., Bandinelli, S., Gensini, G.F., Abbate, R., Ferrucci, L. (2005) A proinflammatory state is associated with hyperhomocysteinemia in the elderly. *Am. J. Clin. Nutr.* 82: 335–341.
103. Li, K., Chen, J., Li, Y.S., Feng, Y.B., Gu, X., Shi, C.Z. (2006) Folic acid reduces adhesion molecules VCAM-1 expression in aortic of rats with hyperhomocysteinemia. *Int. J. Cardiol.* 106: 285–288.
104. Au-Yeung, K.K., Woo, C.W., Sung, F.L., Yip, J.C., Siow, Y.L. (2004) Hyperhomocysteinemia activates nuclear factor kappa B in endothelial cells via oxidative stress. *Circ. Res.* 94: 28–36.
105. Zhang, R., Ma, J., Xia, M., Zhu, H., Ling, W. (2004) Mild hyperhomocysteinemia induced by feeding rats diets rich in methionine or deficient in folate promotes early atherosclerotic inflammatory processes. *J. Nutr.* 134: 825–830.
106. Singh, U., Devaraj, S., Jialal, I. (2005) Vitamin E, oxidative stress and inflammation. *Annu. Rev. Nutr.* 25: 151–174.
107. Lin, S., Lee, I.-M., Song, Y., Van Denburgh, M., Cook, N.R., Manson, J.E., Burling, J.E. (2006) Vitamin E and risk of type 2 diabetes in the women's health study randomized controlled trial. *Diabetes* 55: 2856–2862.
108. Griffin, M.D., Xing, N., Kumar, R. (2003) Vitamin D and its analogs as regulators of immune activation and antigen presentation. *Annu. Rev. Nutr.* 23: 117–145.
109. Banchereau, J., Steinman, R.M. (1998) Dendritic cells and the control of immunity. *Nature* 392: 245–252.
110. Mellman, I., Steinman, R.M. (2001) Dendritic cells: Specialized and regulated antigen processing machines. *Cell* 106: 255–258.
111. Whigham, L.D., Watras, A.C., Schoeller, D.A. (2007) Efficacy of conjugated linolenic acid for reducing fat mass: A meta-analysis in humans. *Am. J. Clin. Nutr.* 85: 1203–1211.
112. Brown, J.M., Boysen, M.S., Chung, S., Fabiyi, O., Morrison, R.F., Mandrup, S., McIntosh, M.K. (2004) Conjugated linoleic acid induces human adipocyte delipidation: Autocrine/paracrine regulation of MEK/ERK signaling by adipocytokines. *J. Biol. Chem.* 279: 26735–26747.
113. Chung, S., Brown, J.M., Provo, J.N., Hopkins, R., McIntosh, M.K. (2005) Conjugated linoleic acid promotes human adipocyte insulin resistance through NFkappaB-dependent cytokine production. *J. Biol. Chem.* 280: 38445–38456.

114. Di Giancamillo, A., Rossi, R., Vitari, F., Pastorelli, G., Corino, C., Domeneghini, C. (2009) Dietary conjugated linolenic acids decrease leptin in porcine adipose tissue. *J. Nutr.* 139: 1867–1872.
115. Chung, S., Lapoint, K., Martinez, K., Kennedy, A., Boyston Sandberg, M., McIntosh, M.K. (2006) Preadipocytes mediate lipopolysaccharide-induced inflammation and insulin resistance in primary cultures of newly differentiated human adipocytes. *Endocrinology* 147: 5340–5351.
116. Poirier, H., Shapiro, J.S., Kim, R.J., Lazar, M.A. (2006) Nutritional supplementation with trans-10, cis-12-conjugated linoleic acid induces inflammation of white adipose tissue. *Diabetes* 55: 1634–1641.
117. Mozaffariaan, M., Pischen, T., Hankinson, S.E., Rifai, N., Joshipura, K., Willett, W.C., Rimm, E.B. (2004) Dietary intake of trans fatty acids and systemic inflammation in women. *Am. J. Clin. Nutr.* 79: 606–612.
118. Racine, N.M., Watras, A.C., Carrel, A.L., Allen, D.B., McVean, J.J., Clark, R.R., O'Brian, A.R., O'Shea, M., Scott, C.E., Schoeller, D.A. (2010) Effect of conjugated linolenic acid on body fat accretion in overweight or obese children. *Am. J. Clin. Nutr.* 91: 1157–1164.
119. Joseph, S.V., Jacques, H., Plourde, M., Mitchell, P.L., McLeod, R.S., Jones, P.J.H. (2011) Conjugated linolenic acid supplementation for 8 weeks does not affect body composition, lipid profile, or safety biomarkers in overweight, hyperlipidemic men. *J. Nutr.* 141: 1286–1292.
120. Jiang, S., Wang, Z., Riethoven, J.-J., Xia, Y., Miser, J., Fromm, M. (2009) Conjugated linolenic acid activates AMP-activated protein kinase and reduces adiposity more effectively when used with metformin in mice. *J. Nutr.* 139: 2244–2251.
121. Norris, L.E., Collene, A.L., Asp, M.L., Hsu, J.C., Liu, L.-F., Richardson, J.R., Li, D. et al. (2009) Comparison of dietary conjugated linolenic acid with safflower oil on body composition in obese postmenopausal women with type 2 diabetes mellitus. *Am. J. Clin. Nutr.* 90: 468–476.
122. Larsson, S.C., Bergkvist, L., Wolk, A. (2009) Conjugated linolenic acid intake and breast cancer risk in a prospective cohort of Swedish women. *Am. J. Clin. Nutr.* 90: 556–560.
123. Mainous, A.G., Wells, B.J., Everett, C.J., Gill, J.M., King, D.E. (2004) Association of ferritin and lipids with c-reactive protein. *Am. J. Cardiol.* 93: 559–562.
124. Sies, H., Schewe, T., Heiss, C., Kelm, M. (2005) Cocoa polyphenols and inflammatory mediators. *Am. J. Clin. Nutr.* 81: 304S–312S.
125. Vita, J. (2005) Polyphenols and cardiovascular disease: Effects on endothelial and platelet function. *Am. J. Clin. Nutr.* 81: 292S–297S.
126. Halliwell, B., Rafter, J., Jenner, A. (2005) Health promotion by flavonoids, tocopherols, tocotrienols and other phenols: Direct or indirect effects? Antioxidant or not? *Am. J. Clin. Nutr.* 81: 268S–276S.
127. Song, Y., Manson, J.E., Buring, J.E., Sesso, H.D., Liu, S. (2005) Association of dietary flavonoids with risk of type 2 diabetes and markers of insulin resistance and system inflammation in women: A prospective study and cross sectional analysis. *J. Am. Coll. Nutr.* 24: 376–384.
128. Collins, A.R. (2005) Assays for oxidative stress and antioxidant status: Applications for research into the biological effectiveness of polyphenols. *Am. J. Clin. Nutr.* 81: 261S–267S.
129. Park, J., Choe, S.S., Chhoi, A.H., Kim, K.H., Yoon, M.J., Suganami, T., Ogawa, Y., Kim, J.B. (2006) Increase in glucose-6-phosphate dehydrogenase in adipocytes stimulates oxidative stress and inflammatory signals. *Diabetes* 55: 2939–2949.
130 Fridly, L.E., Philipson, L.H. (2004) Does the glucose-dependent insulin secretion mechanism itself cause oxidative stress in pancreatic β-cells? *Diabetes* 53: 1942–1948.
131. Natali, A., Toschi, E., Baldeweg, S., Ciociaro, D., Favilla, S., Sacca, L., Ferranini, E. (2006) Clustering of insulin resistance with vascular dysfunction and low-grade inflammation in type 2 diabetes. *Diabetes* 55: 1133–1140.
132. Hansson, G.K., Robertson, A.-K.L., Soderberg-Naucler, C. (2006) Inflammation and atherosclerosis. *Annu. Rev. Pathol.* 1: 297–329.
133. Kaysen, G.A., Eiserich, J.P. (2004) The role of oxidative stress-altered lipoprotein structure and function and microinflammation on cardiovascular risk in patients with minor renal dysfunction. *J. Am. Soc. Nephrol.* 15: 538–548.
134. Kalantar,-Zadeh, K., Balakrishnan, V.S. (2006) The kidney disease wasting: Inflammation, oxidative stress, diet-gene interaction. *Hemodial. Int.* 10: 315–325.
135. Neuhofer, W., Beck, F.-X. (2006) Survival in hostile environments: Strategies of renal medullary cells. *Physiology* 21: 171–180.
136. Chung, H.Y., Sung, B., Jung, K.J., Zou, Y., Yu, B.P. (2006) The molecular inflammatory process in aging. *Antioxid. Redox Signal* 8: 572–581.
137. Calabrese, V., Giuffrida Stella, A.M., Calvani, M., Butterfield, D.A. (2006) Acetylcarnitine and cellular stress response: Roles in nutritional redox homeostasis and regulation of longevity genes. *J. Nutr. Biochem.* 17: 73–88.

138. Peluso, M. (2006) Flavonoids attenuate cardiovascular disease, inhibits phosphodiesterase and modulate lipid homeostasis in adipose tissue and liver. *Exp. Biol. Med.* 231: 1287–1299.
139. Zang, M., Xu, S., Maitland-Toolan, K.A., Zuccollo, A., Hou, X., Jiang, B., Wierzbicki, M., Verbeuren, T.J., Cohen, R.A. (2006) Polyphenols stimulate AMP-activated protein kinase, lower lipids, and inhibit accelerated atherosclerosis in diabetic LDL receptor deficient mice. *Diabetes* 55: 2180–2191.
140. Crouse, J.R., Morgan, T., Terry, J.G., Ellis, J., Vitolins, M., Burke, G.L. (1999) A randomized trial comparing the effect of casein with that of soy protein containing varying amounts of isoflavones on plasma concentrations of lipids and lipoproteins. *Arch. Intern Med.* 159: 2070–2076.
141. Nilausenn, K., Meinertz, H. (1999) Lipoprotein(a) and dietary proteins: Casein lowers lipoprotein(a) concentrations as compared to soy protein. *Am. J. Clin. Nutr.* 68: 419–425.
142. Tonstad, S., Smerud, K., Hoie, L. (2002) A comparison of the effects of 2 doses of soy protein or casein on serum lipids, serum lipoproteins and plasma total homocysteine in hypercholesterolemic subjects. *Am. J. Clin. Nutr.* 76: 78–84.
143. Campbell, C.G., Brown, B.D., Dufner, D., Thorland, W.G. (2006) Effects of soy or milk protein during high fat feeding challenge on oxidative stress, inflammation and lipids in healthy men. *Lipids* 41: 257–265.
144. Oner, O.Z., Ogunc, A.V., Cingi, A., Uyar, S.B., Yalcin, A.S., Aktan, A.O. (2006) Whey protein suppresses the measurement of oxidative stress in experimental burn injury. *Surg. Today* 36: 376–381.
145. Shen, J., Arnett, D.K., Peacock, J.M., Parnell, L.D., Kraja, A., Hixson, J.E., Tsai, M.Y., Lai, C.-Q., Kabagambe, E.K., Straka, R.J., Ordovas, J.M. (2007) Interleukin 1β genetic polymorphisms interact with polyunsaturated fatty acids to modulate the risk of metabolic syndrome. *J. Nutr.* 137: 1846–1851.
146. Lanzavecchia, A., Sallusto, F. (2000) Dynamics of T-lymphocyte responses: Intermediates, effectors, and memory cells. *Science* 290: 92–97.
147. Valbuena, G., Walker, D.H. (2006) The endothelium as a target for infections. *Annu. Rev. Pathol.* 1: 171–198.
148. Hill, N., Sarvetnick, N. (2002) Cytokines: Promoters and dampeners of autoimmunity. *Curr. Opin. Immunol.* 14: 791–797.
149. Horrobin, D.F. (1991) Interactions between n-3 and n-6 essential fatty acids in the regulation of cardiovascular disorders and inflammation. *Prostaglandins, Leukot. Essent. Fatty Acids* 44: 127–131.
150. Calder, P. (2006) N-3 polyunsaturated fatty acids, inflammation, and inflammatory diseases. *Am. J. Clin. Nutr.* 83: 1505S–1519S.
151. Reynolds, C.M., Drapoer, E., Keogh, B., Rahman, A., Moloney, A.P., Mills, K.H.G., Loscher, C.E., Roche, H.M. (2009) A conjugated linolenic acid enriched beef diet attenuates lipopolysaccharide-induced inflammation in mice in part through PPARg-mediated suppression of toll-like receptor 4. *J. Nutr.* 139: 2351–2357.
152. Klein-Platat, C., Drai, J., Oujaa, M., Schlienger, J.-L., Simon, C. (2005) Plasma fatty acid composition is associated with the metabolic syndrome and low grade inflammation in overweight adolescents. *Am. J. Clin. Nutr.* 82: 1178–1184.
153. Phinney, S.D. (2005) Fatty acids, inflammation, and the metabolic syndrome. *Am. J. Clin. Nutr.* 82: 1151–1152.
154. Hotamisligil, G.S. (2003) Inflammatory pathways and insulin action. *Int. J. Obes. Relat. Metab. Disord.* 3: 53S–55S.
155. Pickup, J.C., Crook, M.A. (1998) Is type II diabetes mellitus a disease of the innate immune system? *Diabetologia* 41: 1241–1248.
156. Festa, A., D'Agostino, R., Howard, G., Mykkanen, L., Tracy, R.P., Haffner, S.M. (2007) Chronic subclinical inflammation as part of the insulin resistance syndrome. *Circulation* 102: 42–47.
157 Ugochukwu, N.H., Mukes, J.D., Figgers, C.L. (2006) Ameliorative effects of caloric restriction on oxidative stress and inflammation in the brain of streptozotocin—Induced diabetic rats. *Clin. Chem. Acta* 370: 165–173.
158. Brownlee, M.B. (2002) Mechanism of hyperglycemic damage in diabetes. In: *Atlas of Diabetes* (J. Skyler ed.). 2nd edn. Lippincott Williams & Wilkins, Philadelphia, PA, pp. 125–137.
159. Stentz, F.B., Umpierrez, G.E., Cuervo, R., Kitabchi, A.E. (2004) Proinflammatory cytokines, markers of cardiovascular risks, oxidative stress and lipid peroxidation in patients with hyperglycemic crisis. *Diabetes* 53: 2079–2086.
160. Chun, O.K., Chung, S.-J., Claycombe, K.J., Song, W.G. (2008) Serum C-reactive protein concentrations are inversely associated with dietary flavonoid intake in US adults. *J. Nutr.* 138: 753–760.
161. Luke, W.M., Jenner, A.M., Proudfoot, J.M., McKinley, A.J., Hodgson, J.M., Halliwell, B., Croft, K.D. (2009) A metabolic profiling approach to identify flavonoid intake in humans. *J. Nutr.* 139: 2309–2314.

162. Landberg, R., Sun, Q., Rimm, E.R., Cassidy, A., Scalbert, A., Mantzoros, C.S., Hu, F.B., van Dam, R.M. (2011) Selected dietary flavonoids are associated with markers of inflammation and endothelial dysfunction in US women. *J. Nutr.* 141: 618–624.
163. Hollman, P.C.H., Geelen, A., Kromhout, D. (2010) Dietary flavonol intake may lower stroke risk in men and women. *J. Nutr.* 140: 600–604.
164. Wedick, N.M., Pan, A., Cassidy, A., Rimm, E.B., Sampson, L., Rosner, B., Willett, W., Hu, F.B., Sun, Q., van Dam, R.M. (2012) Dietary flavonoid intakes and risk of type 2 diabetes in US men and women. *Am. J. Clin. Nutr.* 95: 925–933.
165. Koren, E., Kohen, R., Ginsburg, I. (2010) Polyphenols enhance total oxidant-scavenging capacities of human blood by binding to red blood cells. *Exp. Biol. Med.* 235: 689–699.
166. Mastorikou, M., Mackness, M., Mackness, B. (2006) Defective metabolism of oxidized phospholipid by HDL from people with type 2 diabetes. *Diabetes* 55: 3099–3103.
167. Deckelbaum, R.J., Worgall, T.S., Seo, T. (2006) N-3 fatty acids and gene expression. *Am. J. Clin. Nutr.* 83: 1520S–1525S.
168. Wei, Y.-H., Kao, S.-H. (1996) Mitochondrial DNA mutations and lipid peroxidation in human aging. In: *Nutrients and Gene Expression, Clinical Aspects* (C.D. Berdanier, ed.). CRC Press, Boca Raton, FL, pp. 165–188.
169. Bang, H.O., Dyerberg, J. (1972) Plasma lipids and lipoproteins in Greenlandic west coast Eskimos. *Acta Med. Scand.* 192: 85–94.
170. Dyerberg, J., Bang, H.O., Stoffersen, E., Moncada, S., Vane, J.R. (1978) Eicosapentaenoic acid and prevention of thrombosis and atherosclerosis? *Lancet* 8081: 117–119.
171. Fisher, M., Levine, P.H., Leaf, A. (1989) N-3 fatty acids and cellular aspects of atherosclerosis. *Arch. Int. Med.* 149: 1726–1728.
172. DuPont, J., White, P., Feldman, E.B. (1991) Saturated and hydrogenated fats in food in relation to health. *J. Am. Coll. Nutr.* 10: 577–592.
173. Phillipson, B.E., Rothrock, D.W., Connor, W.E., Harris, W.S., Illingworth, D.R. (1985) Reduction in plasma lipids, lipoproteins and apolipoproteins by dietary fish oils in patients with hypertriglyceridemia. *N. Eng. J. Med.* 312: 1210–1216.
174. Feldman, S.A., Rubenstein, A.H., Ho, K.-J., Taylor, C.B., Lewis, L.A., Mikkelson, B. (1975) Carbohydrate and lipid metabolism in the Alaska Artic Eskimo. *Am. J. Clin. Nutr.* 28: 588–594.
175. Cockcroft, S., Thoms, G.M.H. (1992). Inositol-lipid-specific phospholipase C isoenzymes and their differential regulation by receptors. *Biochem. J.* 288: 1–14.
176. Glauert, H.P. (1993). Dietary fat, gene expression and carcinogenesis. In: *Nutrition and Gene Expression* (C.D. Berdanier, J.L. Hargrove, eds.). CRC Press, Boca Raton, FL, pp. 247–268.

11 Fat-Soluble Vitamins

There are four vitamins that are soluble only in fat solvents, not in water. As such, these vitamins are found in the lipid extracts of tissues and foods. They were named alphabetically in the order of their discovery. The A vitamers were followed by the B complex vitamins, vitamin C (ascorbic acid), and vitamins D, E, and K. Vitamins A, D, E, and K are the fat-soluble vitamins.

The National Academy of Sciences—Food and Nutrition Board has developed the daily dietary recommended intakes (DRIs) for vitamins A and E, shown in Table 11.1, and has proposed the adequate intakes (AIs*) for vitamins D and K. The vitamin A DRI is given as retinol equivalents (REs). One RE equals 1 μg retinol, 12 μg β-carotene, 24 μg α-carotene, or 24 μg β-cryptoxanthin. The DRI for vitamin E is as α-tocopherol, which includes RRR-α-tocopherol and the 2R-stereoisomeric forms of α-tocopherol that occur in fortified foods. There are recommended AIs but no DRIs for infants because there are not enough data to support DRI recommendations. This is also true for vitamins D and K. In Table 11.1, it can be seen that only AI recommendations are provided for these vitamins. Again, this is because the Food and Nutrition Board felt that there were insufficient data to support a DRI but that there were enough data to make an AI recommendation. For an updated list of the intake recommendations for these vitamins, the reader should visit the DRI website: www.nap.edu.

VITAMIN A

Vitamin A was the first vitamin identified as an essential micronutrient needed by humans.[1,2] Although it has been recognized as a chemical entity for more than 80 years, foods rich in this vitamin have been prescribed as treatment for night blindness for centuries. Ancient Egyptian physicians recommended the consumption of ox or chicken liver for people unable to see at night. In India, it was recognized that inadequate diets were related to night blindness and, in France, that diets consisting of sugar, starch, olive oil, and wheat gluten fed to animals resulted in ulcerated corneas. These diets were vitamin A deficient. Mori, in Japan, reported on the curative power of cod liver oil in the treatment of conjunctivitis and, later, Hopkins, in the United States, reported on the importance of whole milk in such treatments. During the second decade of the twentieth century, Osborne and Mendel at Yale and McCollum's group in Wisconsin identified the substance in cod liver oil, egg yolk, and butterfat, which cured night blindness and which was essential for normal growth. They called this substance *fat-soluble A*.

Structure and Nomenclature

Vitamin A is not a single compound. It exists in several forms and is found in a variety of foods such as liver and as the carotene precursor in highly colored vegetables.[1] The IUPAC-IUB Commission on Biochemical Nomenclature has proposed the following rules for naming the compounds having vitamin A activity. The parent substance, all-*trans* vitamin A alcohol, is designated *all-trans retinol*. Derivatives of this compound are named accordingly. In Table 11.2 are listed the major vitamin A compounds.

In foods of animal origin, the vitamin usually occurs as an alcohol (retinol). However, it can also occur as an aldehyde (retinal) or as an acid (retinoic acid). In foods of plant origin, the vitamin is associated with the plant pigments and is a member of the carotene family of compounds. These

TABLE 11.1
Daily Dietary Recommended Intakes (DRI) and Adequate Intake Recommendations for Fat-Soluble Vitamins

Group	Vitamin A (μg)	Vitamin E (μg)	Vitamin D (μg)	Vitamin K (μg)
Infants				
0–6 months	400*	4*	5*	2*
7–12 months	500*	5*	5*	2.5*
Children				
1–3 years	**210**	**5**	5*	30*
4–8 years	**275**	**6**	5*	55*
Males				
9–13 years	**445**	**9**	5*	60*
14–18 years	**630**	**12**	5*	75*
19–30 years	**625**	**12**	5*	120*
31–50 years	**625**	**12**	5*	120*
51–70 years	**625**	**12**	10*	120*
70+ years	**625**	**12**	15*	120*
Females				
9–13 years	**420**	**9**	5*	60*
14–18 years	**485**	**12**	5*	75*
19–30 years	**500**	**12**	5*	90*
31–50 years	**500**	**12**	5*	90*
51–70 years	**500**	**12**	10*	90*
70+ years	**500**	**12**	15*	90*
Pregnancy				
14–18 years	**530**	**12**	5*	75*
19–30 years	**550**	**12**	5*	90*
31–50 years	**550**	**12**	5*	90*
Lactation				
14–18 years	**885**	**16**	5*	75*
19–30 years	**900**	**16**	5*	90*
31–50 years	**900**	**16**	5*	90*

Source: www.nap.edu, Accessed November 22, 2013.
Note: Bold values represent DRIs; asterisks represent AIs.

compounds can be converted to vitamin A in the animal body and are known as provitamins. Of the carotenes, β-carotene is the most potent. Figure 11.1 gives the structure of vitamin A as all-*trans* retinol. Some of the biologically important compounds having vitamin A activity are shown in Figure 11.2.

Note that all of these compounds have a β-ionone ring to which an isoprenoid chain is attached. This structure is essential if a compound is to have vitamin activity. If any substitutions to the chain or ring occur, then the activity of the compound as vitamin A is reduced. For example, the substitution of methyl groups for the hydrogen on carbon 15 of the side chain results in a derivative that has no vitamin activity. However, the preparation of a methyl ester or other esters at carbon 15 results in a very stable compound with full vitamin activity. In addition to improving the chemical stability of the compound, the ester forms confer an improved solubility in food oils. These vitamin ester forms are frequently used in food products for vitamin enrichment.

TABLE 11.2
Nomenclature of Major Compounds in the Vitamin A Group

Recommended Names	Synonyms
Retinol	Vitamin A alcohol, axerophthol
Retinal	Vitamin A aldehyde, retinene, retinaldehyde
Retinoic acid	Vitamin A acid
3-Dehydroretinal	Vitamin A_2 (alcohol)
3-Dehydroretinol	Vitamin A_2 aldehyde; retinene
3-Dehydroretinoic acid	Vitamin A_2 acid
Anhydroretinol	Anhydro vitamin A
Retro retinol	Rehydrovitamin A
5,6-Epoxyretinol	5,6-Epoxyvitamin A alcohol
Retinyl palmitate	Vitamin A palmitate
Retinyl acetate	Vitamin A acetate
Retinyl β-glucuronide	Vitamin A acid β-glucuronide
11-*cis*-Retinaldehyde	11-*cis* or Neo B vitamin A aldehyde
4-Ketoretinol	4-Keto vitamin A alcohol
Retinyl phosphate	Vitamin A phosphate
β-Carotene	Provitamin A
α-Carotene	Provitamin A
γ-Carotene	Provitamin A

Source: Olson, J.A., Vitamin A, in: *Handbook of Vitamins*, L.J. Machlin, ed., Marcel Dekker, New York, 1991.

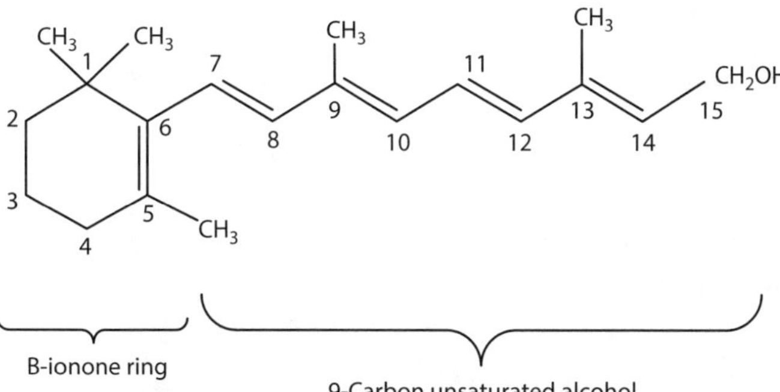

FIGURE 11.1 Structure of vitamin A.

If the side chain is lengthened or shortened, vitamin activity is lost. Activity is also reduced if the unsaturated bonds are converted to saturated bonds or if the side chain is isomerized. Oxidation of the β-ionone ring and/or removal of its methyl groups likewise reduces its vitamin activity. Some of these substituted or isomerized forms are potent therapeutic agents. For example, 13-*cis*-retinoic acid has been used in the treatment of certain kinds of cancer. Other analogs notably the fluoro and chloro derivatives have been synthesized with the hope of providing chemotherapeutic agents for the treatment of certain skin diseases and cancer.

The provitamin A group consists of members of the carotene family.[3] In plants, these compounds serve as photoprotectors of photosynthesis.[4] Shown in Figure 11.3 are the structures of some of these compounds. Also shown are structures of related compounds that, although highly colored, have little potential as a precursor of retinol.

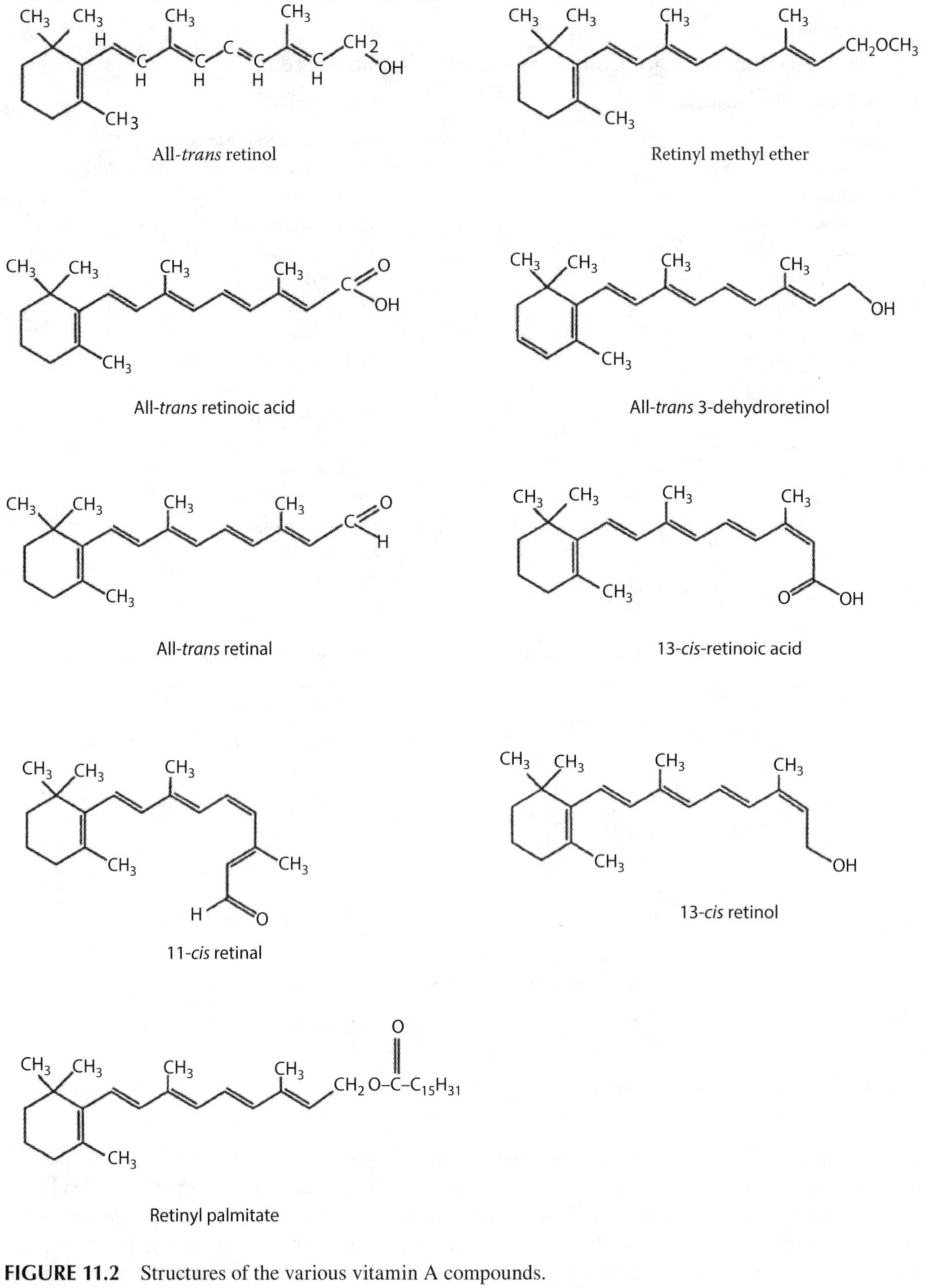

All-*trans* retinol

Retinyl methyl ether

All-*trans* retinoic acid

All-*trans* 3-dehydroretinol

All-*trans* retinal

13-*cis*-retinoic acid

11-*cis* retinal

13-*cis* retinol

Retinyl palmitate

FIGURE 11.2 Structures of the various vitamin A compounds.

More than 600 members of the carotenoid family of pigments exist. However, only 50% or about 10%[5] can be converted (or degraded) into components that have vitamin activity.[6] All these compounds have many conjugated double bonds, and thus each can form a variety of geometric isomers. β-carotene, for example, can assume a *cis* or a *trans* configuration at each of its double bonds and in theory could have 272 isomeric forms. The asymmetric carotene,

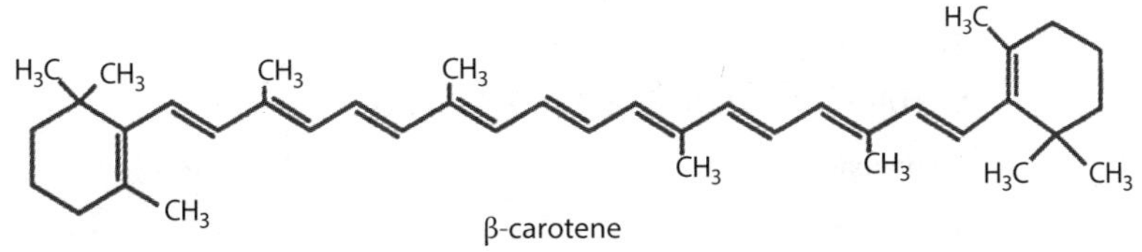

β-carotene

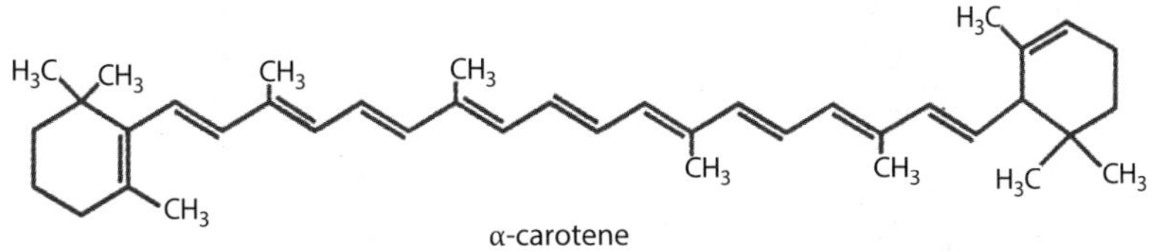

α-carotene

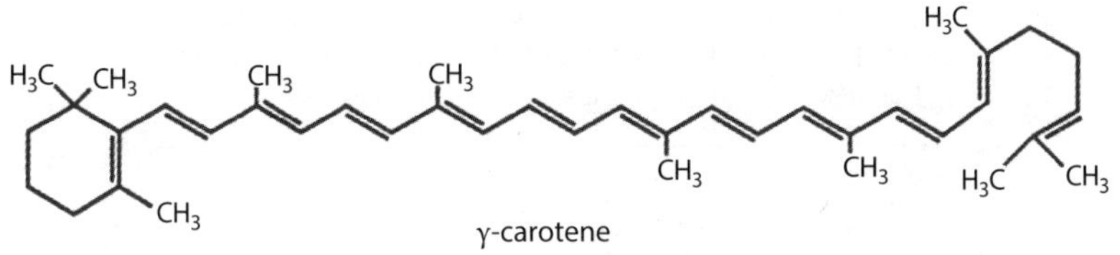

γ-carotene

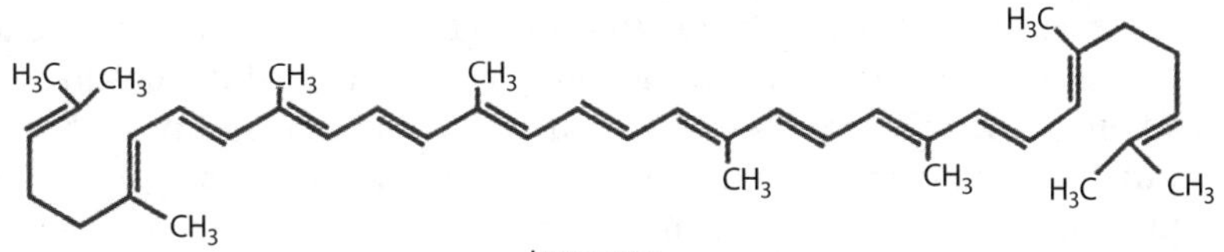

Lycopene

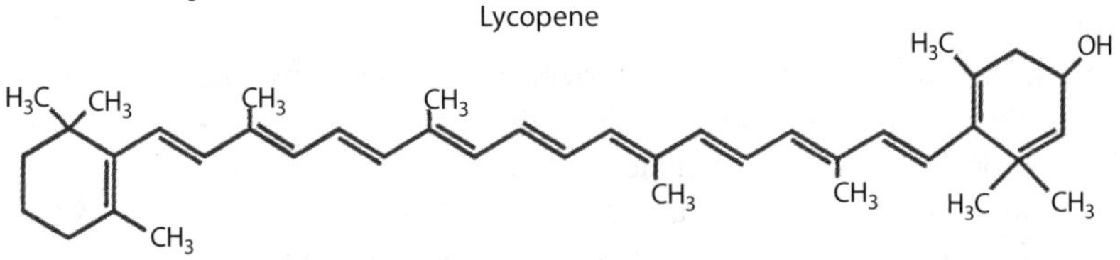

β-cryptoxanthin

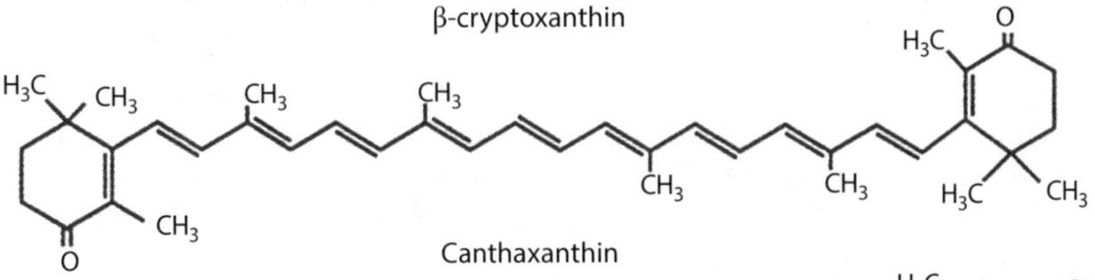

Canthaxanthin

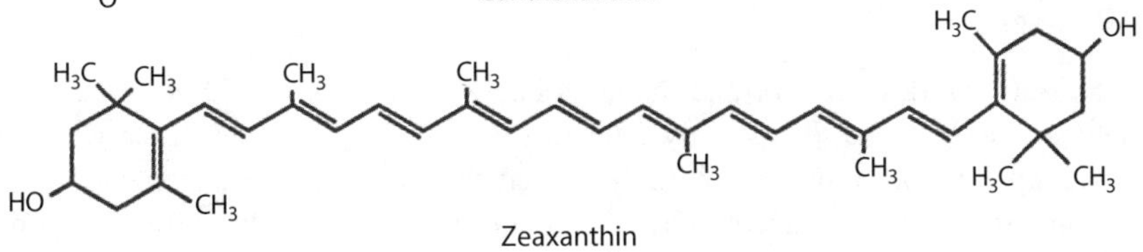

Zeaxanthin

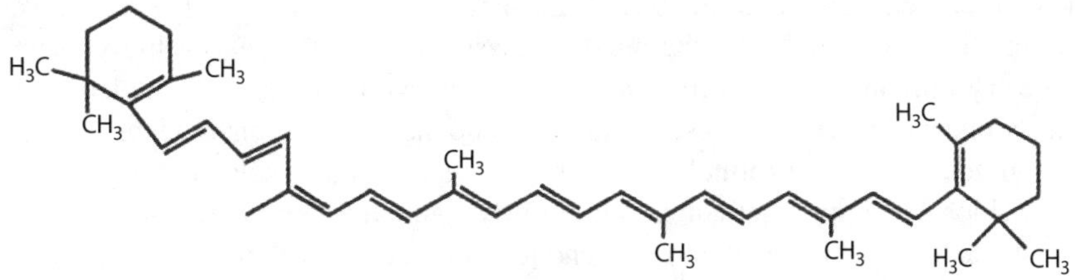

9-*cis*-β-carotene

FIGURE 11.3 Structures of carotenes having vitamin A activity.

TABLE 11.3
Carotenoids with Vitamin A Activity

Compound	Relative Potency
β-Carotene[a]	100
α-Carotene	53
γ-Carotene	43
Cryptoxanthin	57
Lycopene	0
Zeaxanthin	0
Xanthophyll	0

Note: β-carotene compared to all-*trans* retinol is only half as active.
[a] Reference compound for subsequent compounds.

α-carotene, can, in theory, appear in 512 forms. The vitamin A activity of the provitamin members of the carotene family is variable due to differences in absorption and metabolism. The β-carotene content of food varies with the growing conditions and the postharvest storage of the food. In addition, the digestibility of the food affects the availability of the vitamin. Even when fully available, β-carotene and other provitamin A compounds may not be absorbed efficiently and, further, the enzyme responsible for cleaving the β-carotene into useful vitamin A is inefficient.

In general, the β-carotene molecule will provide about 50% of its quantity as vitamin A.[7] During its cleavage by the enzyme β-carotenoid 15,15′-dioxygenase, there is some oxidative conversion of the cleavage product to retinal and some oxidation to retinoic acid. This retinoic acid is rapidly excreted in the urine. Other carotenes are less potent than β-carotene, due not only to a decrease in their absorption but also due to their chemical structures that do not meet the requirements described earlier for vitamin activity. These compounds are listed in Table 11.3. Note that some of these compounds, that is, xanthophylls and lycopenes, have no vitamin activity even though they are highly colored and are related chemically to β-carotene. They may have other functional properties, however, and may have some usefulness in the human diet.

Chemical Properties

Through the careful work of Karrer and his associates, the structures of both β-carotene and all-*trans* retinol were determined. It was only after this work was completed that it was realized that β-carotene was a precursor for retinol.[1] With the structures known, the next step was the crystallization of the compounds. This was accomplished for vitamin A from the lipid fraction of fish liver by Holmes and Corbet. Ten years later, in 1947, Arens and van Drop and also Isler et al. were able to synthesize pure all-*trans* retinol. The chemical synthesis of β-carotene was achieved shortly thereafter. With the crystallization, structure identification, and synthesis came the understanding of the physical and chemical properties of these compounds and the development of techniques to measure their presence in food. All-*trans* retinol is a nearly colorless oil and is soluble in such fat solvents as ether, ethanol, chloroform, and methanol. While fairly stable to the moderate heat needed to cook foods, it is unstable to very high heat, to light, and to oxidation by oxidizing agents. α-tocopherol or its acetate (vitamin E) through its role as an antioxidant can prevent some of the oxidative destruction of retinol.

These properties of vitamin A allow for the removal of the vitamin from foods by fat solvent extraction and its subsequent determination using agents such as antimony trichloride (the Carr-Price reaction), which produce a blue color. The intensity of the color is directly proportional to the amount of retinol in the material being analyzed. More recently, the development of high-resolution, high-pressure liquid chromatography (HPLC) has made the separation and quantification of each of the A vitamers possible.

β-carotene is also soluble in such fat solvents as acetone or ethanol. It is bright yellow in color and it, too, is stable to moderate heat but unstable to light or oxidation. The members of the large carotenoid family can be separated and quantified using HPLC. Several isomers and derivatives (Figure 11.2) of retinol have been identified. The isomerization of all-*trans* retinol to a mixture of its isomers is enhanced by high temperatures, ultraviolet (UV) light, and iodine or iron. While the isomerization of all-*trans* retinol to 11-*cis* retinol is an important in vivo reaction for the maintenance of the visual cycle, the production of isomers outside of the body through the application of high heat, light, and oxidizing agents results in a loss in biological activity of the original compounds. For example, retinyl acetate, if irradiated in hexane, forms a nonsymmetrical dimer (kitol), which has less than 1% of its original activity. This dimer has been isolated from whale liver oil, and some investigators have suggested that, in this species, the kitol could serve as a storage form of the vitamin. However, whether the kitol found in the whale liver was produced enzymatically or was consumed by the whale as a component of its food supply has not been determined. In any event, for most species, vitamin A is stored in the liver not as a kitol but as an ester with a fatty acid (usually palmitate) in a lipid–protein complex.

Retinal, the vitamin A aldehyde, combines with various amines to form Schiff bases. This reaction is important to the formation of rhodopsin within the visual cycle. If mineral oil is present with retinal and the amine, the retinal may first form a hemiacetal, which then complexes with a variety of amines to form the Schiff base. All-*trans* retinal also reacts with both the sulfhydryl and amino groups of cysteine or the amino group of tryptophan to form a five-membered thiazolidine ring. The formation of the thiazolidine ring is enhanced if formaldehyde is present. The resulting compound has a red color, which is bleached upon exposure to light. This reaction, similar to the bleaching of rhodopsin (the visual pigment in the eye) with light exposure, does not utilize the same amino acid that is used in rhodopsin. In the latter, retinal binds to the epsilon amino group of lysine rather than the amino group of tryptophan or cysteine. Bleaching occurs when the energy transmitted by the light causes a shift in the electrons within the *N*-retinyl lysine. The same principle is involved in the loss of color with light exposure of *N*-retinyl cysteine and *N*-retinyl tryptophan. Interestingly, the many retinyl–amino acid complexes possible in the laboratory apparently do not form in the body. This is probably due to the limited amounts of both the free vitamin and the free amino acids. Both are usually bound or complexed to some other compound and are not readily available for this reaction. In nature, vitamin A and carotene are bound to proteins, particularly the lipoproteins. Indeed, the vitamin is stored as an ester in those tissues (notably the liver), which synthesize the lipoproteins. Usually, retinol is covalently bound to palmitic acid as well as being associated with a protein. The vitamin also complexes with other proteins as part of its mechanism of action at the subcellular level.

Retinol and its derivatives are soluble in nonpolar solvents, but not in water. However, retinol or retinyl esters can be made miscible in water with the use of detergents such as Tween 80 (polyoxyethylene sorbitan monooleate). The resulting aqueous micellar suspension allows for the preparation of aqueous multivitamin supplements, which are then useful for infants, small children, or persons unable to swallow a capsule. Studies of the absorption of vitamin A in this form, compared to the absorption of vitamins dissolved in an oil, have shown that this form of the vitamin is readily available. This is particularly important for those persons having a fat absorption problem as in pancreatitis, celiac disease, idiopathic steatorrhea, biliary disease, or short gut syndrome. Aqueous preparations are also useful to the food processor wishing to fortify or enrich a particular food product. Some food formulations would not be compatible with an oil-based vitamin A preparation, whereas an aqueous preparation combines very well with the ingredients in the food.

TABLE 11.4
Retinol Equivalents for Humans

Compound	μg/IU	IU/μg	RE/μg
All-*trans* retinol	0.300	3.33	1.00
All-*trans* retinyl acetate	0.344	2.91	—
All-*trans* retinyl palmitate	0.549	1.82	—
All-*trans* β-carotene	1.800	0.56	0.167
Mixed carotenoids	3.600	0.28	0.083

Source: Olson, J.A., Vitamin A, in: *Handbook of Vitamins*, L.J. Machlin, ed., Marcel Dekker, New York, 1991, pp. 1–57.

Biopotency

The varying potencies of the different vitamin A compounds have, in the past, contributed confusion to the literature. This has been resolved by the establishment of a standard definition for vitamin A. One international unit (IU) of vitamin A is defined as the activity of 0.3 μg of all-*trans* retinol. Because β-carotene must be converted to retinol to be active and because this conversion is not 100% efficient, 1 μg of all-*trans* β-carotene is equivalent to 0.167 μg of all-*trans* retinol. For other members of the carotene family, appropriate (Tables 11.2 and 11.3) correction factors must be applied to determine the vitamin A activity in terms of REs. In general, however, 1 mg of retinol is roughly equivalent to 6 mg β-carotene and 12 mg of mixed dietary carotenes (Table 11.4). The use of the term REs allows for the calculation of the vitamin A activity found in a variety of foods, each containing one or more vitamin A compounds. For example, if 100 g of a given food contained 100 mg of α-carotene, which has 53% of the potency of β-carotene, the retinol equivalence would be 100 × 53 × 0.167 or 8.851. Thus, this food would provide 8.851 REs or 29.5 IU of vitamin A (8.851/0.3) per 100 g. Most tables of food composition give the vitamin A content in terms of IU; however, the reader should be aware of how these units are derived and realize that corrections must be made to allow for availability and efficiency of conversion of the provitamin to the active vitamin form, all-*trans* retinol. Table 11.4 lists the REs for major A vitamin sources. A more complete list of foods and their vitamin A content can be found on the web at www.nal.usda.gov/foodcomposition.

Sources

Vitamin A and its carotene precursors are present in a variety of foods. Red meat, liver, whole milk, cheese, butter, and fortified margarine are but a few of the foods containing retinol. Carotene-rich foods include the highly colored fruits and vegetables such as squash, carrots, rich green vegetables (peas, beans, etc.), yellow fruits (peaches, apricots), and vegetable oils. See www.nal.usda.gov/foodcomposition for the vitamin content of a wide variety of foods.

Metabolism

Absorption

The availability of the vitamin depends largely on the form ingested and on the presence and activity of the system responsible for its uptake. Figure 11.4 schematically shows the route of retinol absorption. Absorption is not as rapid as the absorption of the water-soluble vitamins because it must traverse the lymphatic system before it enters the circulation. It is generally accepted that all-*trans* retinol is the preferred form for absorption. Retinal and retinoic acid are less well absorbed, although both will disappear from the intestinal contents at a rate

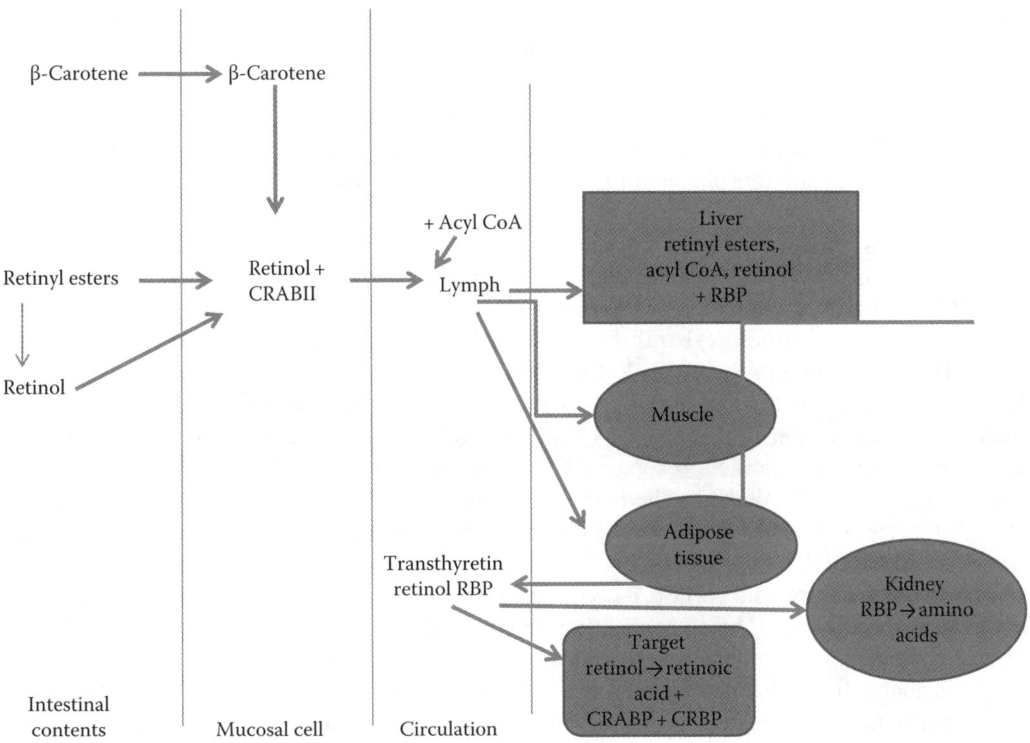

FIGURE 11.4 Uptake and transport of retinol and β-carotene.

commensurate with a rate associated with an active transport system. Absorption requires the presence of food lipid and bile salts. The vitamin appears in the lymphatic system along with the absorbed lipids.[8] The vitamin is bound to the retinol-binding protein CRABII in the mucosal cell. From the absorptive cell, it changes carriers to another RBP and then passes into the lymph with the addition of acyl CoA. From the lymph, it travels to the liver, muscle, and adipose tissue as well as to other targets. Carotenoids are absorbed less efficiently, via diffusion. There is no active carrier for carotene within the mucosal cell of the lumen. Carotene is oxidatively cleaved to retinal and to small amounts of longer chain β-apocarotenoids. Two enzymes are involved in the cleavage: The first, β-carotene-15,15′-dioxygenase, catalyzes the cleavage of the central double bond to yield two molecules of retinaldehyde. The second, retinaldehyde reductase, catalyzes the reduction of retinaldehyde to retinol. This reaction is shown in Figure 11.5. The major cleavage products are retinol and retinoic acid. Both central and eccentric cleavages are possible. The cleavage enzymes are very unstable. They are rapidly inactivated. In order for the first enzyme to work, the β-carotene must be solubilized. This means that bile salts and some lipids must be present. Oxygen is also required since this is a dioxygenase type of reaction. Carotene dioxygenase is present in the soluble cell fraction and has been isolated from rat, hog, and rabbit intestinal tissue and characterized. The enzyme of the second reaction,

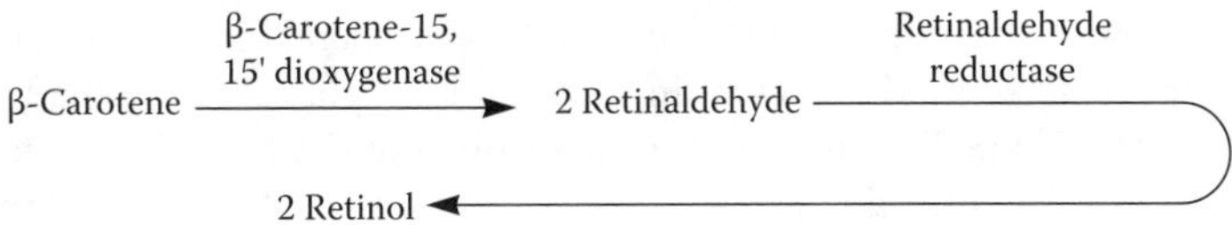

FIGURE 11.5 Breakdown of β-carotene in theory. Actually, 2-retinaldehyde and 2-retinol do not result from one β-carotene because of the inefficiency of the enzymes involved.

retinaldehyde reductase, is also a soluble mucosal cell enzyme. It requires the presence of either NADPH or NADH as donors of reducing equivalents. It is not particularly specific for the resulting retinaldehyde for it will catalyze the reduction of several short- and medium-chain aliphatic aldehydes in addition to retinaldehyde. Intestinal carotene absorption and conversion to the retinoids are under negative feedback control that adapts to the actual requirement for retinol.[9] There are polymorphisms in the genes that encode the transport proteins that determine how much carotene is absorbed.[10]

There are two pathways for retinol esterification. In the first, an acyl CoA–independent reaction is used. This involves a complex between retinol and type II cellular retinol–binding protein (CRBP II). As retinol intake increases, there is a corresponding increase in the activity of the enzyme (acyl CoA retinol acyl transferase), which catalyzes the formation of this complex. CRBP II is found only in the cytosol of the intestinal mucosal cell, and, interestingly, its synthesis is influenced by the intake of particular fatty acids. Unsaturated fatty acids, particularly linoleic and α-linolenic acid, enhance CRBP II mRNA transcription. These fatty acids also enhance S14 and retinoic acid receptor (RAR) transcription in the adipocyte. Thus, it would appear that vitamin A uptake by the mucosal cell is dependent on dietary fat not only because of its influence on its absorption but also because of its role in enhancing the synthesis of the mucosal cell CRBP II.

The second pathway is an acyl CoA–dependent pathway whereby retinol is bound to any protein, not just the specific CRBP mentioned earlier. In both pathways, the retinol is protein bound prior to ester formation. As mentioned in the section on vitamin A structure, the esterification of retinol results in a more lipophilic material readily soluble in the lipids of the cell. This, in turn, facilitates its movement into the cell and its metabolic function as well as its storage.

Retinoic acid, like retinal and retinol, is rapidly absorbed by the mucosal cells. However, it is also rapidly excreted (rather than stored as are the other vitamin forms) in the urine; thus, this form is not as useful as the alcohol or aldehyde forms.

The all-*trans* retinol esterified to palmitic acid has its ester linkage cleaved in the intestine by a specific esterase that, in some species, is activated by the bile salt sodium taurocholate. After the ester has been hydrolyzed, the resulting retinol is transported into the mucosal cell where it is then reesterified to palmitic acid and incorporated into lymph chylomicrons. The absorption of vitamin A thus follows the same route as that of the long-chain fatty acids of the dietary triacylglycerides cholesterol and cholesterol esters. The chylomicrons are absorbed by the lacteals of the lymphatic system and enter the circulation when the thoracic duct joins the circulatory system at the vena cava. Once in the vascular compartment, the triacylglyceride of the retinol-containing chylomicron is removed, leaving the protein carrier, retinol, and cholesterol. Whereas the triacylglycerides are removed from the chylomicrons primarily by the extrahepatic tissues, retinol is removed primarily by the liver. In the liver, hydrolysis and reesterification occur once again as the vitamin enters the hepatocyte and is stored within the cell associated with droplets of lipid. Interestingly, retinoic acid is absorbed not via the lymphatic system but by the portal system and does not accumulate in the liver. Retinoic acid, because it is not stored, represents only a very small percentage of the body's vitamin A content.

Transport

As mentioned, specific proteins are needed for the subsequent transport of the vitamin. The transport protein that transports the retinol from the liver to the peripheral target tissues is called RBP.[11–13] This protein was first isolated by Kanai et al. in 1968. RBP is synthesized in the liver. It is a single polypeptide chain (MW 21,000) and possesses a single binding site for retinol. The mobilization of vitamin A from the liver requires this protein. In plasma, vitamin A circulates bound to the RBP that in turn forms a protein–protein complex with transthyretin, a tetramer that also binds thyroxine in a 1:1 complex. Because this complex contains the vitamin and thyroxine, there is an association of thyroid status and vitamin A status.

The RBP of the serum has been isolated from a number of different species including man. The usual level of binding protein in plasma is about 40–50 μg/mL. However, the level of this protein is responsive to nutritional status. In protein-malnourished children, it is depressed, while in vitamin A–deficient individuals, it is elevated. When protein intakes are low, the synthesis of the binding protein is low, thus explaining the simultaneous observations of symptoms of protein and retinol deficiency in malnourished children. Once protein is restored to the diet, symptoms of both protein malnutrition and vitamin A deficiency disappear. If dietary retinol (or its precursors) is lacking, serum RBP levels will fall, while hepatic levels rise. Within minutes after retinol is given to a deficient individual, these changes are reversed: serum levels rise, while hepatic levels fall. These observations thus provide clear evidence of the importance of this binding protein in the utilization of retinol. Compounds that influence the levels of this binding protein influence the mobilization and excretion of retinol. Estrogens increase the levels of this protein, whereas cadmium poisoning, because it increases excretion, reduces the level of this protein. Patients with renal disease have elevated levels of RBP[14,15] and may be at risk of developing vitamin A toxicity if the vitamin A intake is above normal. In the patient with renal disease, the increase in the binding protein is probably due to the decreased capacity of the kidney to remove the protein. The kidney is the main catabolic site for RBP.

Once the RBP complex arrives at the target tissue, it must then bind to its receptor site on the cell membrane. Receptors for retinol and retinoic acid have been identified on the cell membranes of a variety of cells. The retinol is then released from the RBP and transferred into the cell where it is then bound to intracellular binding proteins. Of interest are the observations that these binding proteins, while similar to the binding protein in the serum, are highly specific for the different vitamin A forms. The cytosolic retinol–binding protein (CRBP) is the cellular RBP (molecular weight 14,600), while the cytosolic retinoic acid–binding protein (CRABP) is the cellular retinoic acid–binding protein. The cytosolic retinal binding protein (CRLBP) is the retinal binding protein (molecular weight 33,000) and the interstitial retinol–binding protein (IRBP) is the interphotoreceptor or interstitial RBP (molecular weight 144,000). The latter is found only in the extracellular space of the retina. As described earlier, CRBP is the RBP found in the mucosal cells of the small intestine. The presence of these binding proteins in different tissues is highly variable. Shown in Table 11.5 are the features and functions of these binding proteins.

While the bulk transport of the various A vitamers occurs via the chylomicrons that are released into the lymph, there seems to be no specific protein within the chylomicron that has a special affinity for this vitamin. However, once the chylomicron remnants (the remains of the chylomicrons that have lost some of its lipid to the muscle and the adipose tissue) are taken up by the liver, the special binding proteins have their effects. The chylomicron remnant retains most of its original vitamin A content as vitamin A esters. These esters are stored in the hepatocyte or are released following hydrolysis into the circulation bound to RBP.

Functions

Protein Synthesis

Some of the earliest reports of retinol deficiency included observations on the changes in epithelial cells of animals fed vitamin A–deficient diets. Normal columnar epithelial cells were replaced by squamous keratinizing epithelium. These changes were reversed when vitamin A was restored to the diet. Epithelial cells, particularly those lining the gastrointestinal tract, have very short half-lives (in the order of 3–7 days) and as such are replaced frequently. In vitamin A deficiency, changes in these cells, as well as other cells having a rapid turnover time, indicate that the vitamin functions at the level of protein synthesis, cellular differentiation, and turnover. Studies of protein synthesis by mucosal cells from deficient and control animals indicated that the vitamin is involved directly in protein synthesis both at the transcriptional and translational level. A variety

TABLE 11.5
Retinol Binding Proteins

Acronym	Protein	Molecular Weight	Location	Function
RBP	Retinol-binding protein	21,000	Plasma	Transports all-*trans* retinol from intestinal absorption site to target tissues
CRBP	Cellular retinol–binding protein	14,600	Cells of target tissue	Transports all-*trans* retinol from plasma membrane to organelles within the cell
CRBP II	Cellular retinol–binding protein type II	16,000	Absorptive cells of small intestine	Transports all-*trans* retinol from absorptive sites on plasma membrane of mucosal cells
CRABP	Cellular retinoic acid–binding protein	14,600	Cells of target tissue	Transports all-*trans* retinoic acid to the nucleus
CRBP	Cellular retinal–binding protein	33,000	Specific cells in the eye	Transports 11-*cis* retinal and 11-*cis* retinol as part of the visual cycle
IRBP	Interphotoreceptor or interstitial retinol–binding protein	144,000	Retina	Transports all-*trans* retinol and 11-*cis* retinal in the retina extracellular space
RAR	DNA-binding protein (retinoic acid receptor; three main forms: α, β, γ)		All cells α—liver β—brain γ—liver, kidneys, lungs	Binds retinoic acid and regions of DNA
RXR	DNA-binding protein (retinoic acid receptors, multiple forms)			Binds retinoic acid and DNA

of gene products are subject to retinoic acid influence.[16] Retinoic acid is bound to a RAR on nuclear and mitochondrial DNA and as such enhances the transcription of a large number of mRNAs that encode a large number of gene products. Such a role for retinol is supported by observations of an alteration in messenger RNA synthesis in vitamin A–deficient animals. Table 11.6 lists a number of genes for cellular proteins whose expression are regulated by retinoic acid. Two distinct families of DNA-binding proteins (RAR and RXR) have been identified, and three genes for each of these receptors have been found.[17–28] Each gene has several isoforms that arise from either different promoter usage or alternative splicing.[23–35] The differences between the receptors occur at the *N*-terminal region. In addition, they have different expression patterns in the embryo and adult. Their synthesis and activation are regulated differently by vitamin A.[29,30]

The RAR and RXR are structurally similar to the receptor that binds the steroid and thyroid hormones. The RARs are activated by the all-*trans* or 9-*cis* isomers of retinoic acid, while the RXRs are activated only by the 9-*cis* retinoic acid. These receptors function as ligand-activated transcription factors (see Table 11.6) that regulate mRNA transcription. Both nuclear and mitochondrial DNA are responsive to retinoic acid. Each compartment has its preferred form. The mitochondrial DNA has RARγ 1 and 2 as its preferred form, while the nucleus has RARα as its preferred form.[36] Both compartments will use the β-form. In some instances, these factors stimulate transcription and in other instances they suppress the process. These receptors bind to DNA as dimers, which is reflected in the paired nature of the DNA response elements RARE and RXRE, respectively, for

TABLE 11.6
Retinoic Acid–Responsive Proteins

I. Proteins that have their synthesis increased due to RA–receptor effect on the transcription of their mRNA	
Growth hormone	Neuronal cell
Transforming growth factor β_2	Calcium-binding protein
Transglutaminase	Calbindin DZ8K
Phosphoenolpyruvate carboxykinase	ODC
Gsα	Osteocalcin
Alcohol dehydrogenase	Glycerophosphate dehydrogenase
t-plasminogen activator	
II. Retinoic acid proteins that function in mRNA transcription	
1,25-$(OH)_2D_3$ receptors	MSH receptors
Interleukin-6 receptors[a]	RARs α
cfos[a]	Interleukin 2-receptors
Progesterone receptors[a]	EGF receptors (corneal epithelium)[a]
Zif 268 transcription factor	EGF receptors (corneal endothelium)
Peroxisomal proliferator-activated receptors	AP-2 transcription factor

[a] The activity of these proteins is suppressed when the RA–receptor is bound to it.

RAR and RXR. The nucleotide sequence archetype upon which the RARE and RXREs are based is in accordance with a direct repeat (DR) 1–5 rule. This pattern, suggested by Umesono et al.,[34] has a DR of the sequence AGGTCA separated by 3–5 nucleotides. The original 3–4–5 rule was extended to include a separation of one or two nucleotides depending on whether the element was for RAR or RXR. RAREs were DR2 and DR5; the RXREs, DR1, and the response elements for vitamin D and thyroid hormone were DR3 and DR4, respectively. The guideline worked well to describe several of the strongest RA-response elements, including the DR5 type that is the most prevalent of the simple DRs. The DR1–5 rule is only a framework, however, and a series of additional factors also influences the effectiveness of each response element. More than 40 genes contain these elements as part of their promoter regions.

The differences between RAR and RXR response elements go beyond simple binding preference or ligand specificity. They have separate functions. The RARs are ligand-regulated receptors that function similarly to the vitamin D and thyroid hormone–receptors; once ligand bound, they become transcription activators. The RXRs can also do this but they have another function as well. They serve as accessory factors for many members of the nuclear family of superreceptors, the so-called steroid superfamily of receptors. The RXRs can heterodimerize with these receptors without having 9-*cis* retinoic acid as a ligand.

There is also an interaction of vitamin A with other vitamins. For example, the synthesis of the calcium-binding protein calbindin is usually regulated by vitamin D. This protein, found in the intestinal mucosal cells and the kidney, is also found in the brain. In the brain, its synthesis is regulated by retinoic acid rather than vitamin D. In vitamin A–deficient brain cells, additions of retinoic acids increased the mRNA for calbindin and calbindin synthesis. Additions of vitamin D were without effect. The RARs contain zinc finger protein sequence motifs that mediate its binding to DNA. The carboxyl terminal end of the receptor functions in this ligand binding. Retinoic acid binding to nuclear receptors sets in motion a sequence of events that culminate in a change in transcription of the *cis*-linked gene. That is, proteins are synthesized and these proteins bind to regions of the promoter adjacent to the start site of the DNA that is to be transcribed. Such binding either activates or suppresses transcription and, as a result, there are corresponding increases or decreases in the mRNA coding for specific proteins, which, in turn, lead to changes in cell function. Table 11.7 lists a number of enzymes that have been reported to be affected by the deficient state. In each of these

TABLE 11.7
Enzymes That Are Affected by Vitamin A Deficiency

Enzyme	Reaction	Effect
ATPase	ATP ↔ ADP + Pi	Increase
Arginase	L-arginine → Ornithine + urea	Increase
Xanthine oxidase	Hypoxanthine → Uric acid	Increase
25,3-hydroxysteroid dehydrogenase 11-steroid hydroxylase	Progesterone, glucocorticoid, estrogen, testosterone; removal of H synthesis of steroid hormones	Decrease
ATP sulfurylase sulfotransferase	ATP + SO_4 → Adenyl sulfate + PPi^{-3} that transfers sulfuryl groups to –O and –N of suitable groups; synthesis of mucopolysaccharides	Decrease
L-γ-gulonolactone oxidase	L-gulonolactone → L-ascorbic acid	Decrease
p-Hydroxyphenol pyruvate oxidase	*p*-Hydroxyphenyl pyruvate → Homogentisic acid	Decrease

instances, it could be assumed that the reason for the change in activity could be explained by the effect of vitamin A on the expression of the genes that encode these enzymes.

There is another aspect of vitamin A nutriture that is of importance when the function of this vitamin is considered. This concerns the structure and function of the nuclear retinoic acid–binding protein, the RA–receptor. Should this receptor not be synthesized as can occur in the absence of retinoic acid, the whole cascade of events dependent on the binding of the RA–receptor complex will not occur. Further, should the receptor itself be aberrant in amino acid sequence, both its capacity to bind retinoic acid and its affinity for specific regions of the DNA will be affected. In this instance, it is easy to understand how cellular differentiation would be affected. Indeed, several investigators have suggested that this could explain the occurrence of congenital defects in a number of species where early embryonic development of the spinal column and the heart might be due to abnormal RA–receptor binding with the subsequent result of defective differentiation, organ formation, and organ function. This role for the vitamin although lacking biochemical mechanistic detail was among the first functions recognized by early investigators. Several excellent papers on retinoid signaling and the generation of cellular diversity in the embryonic mouse spinal cord have been published as has a paper on retinoid signaling in the developing heart.[20,26–31,35,36] In addition, there is a need for retinoic acid by the insulin-secreting cells of the pancreas.[18] The need probably relates to its function in stimulating mitochondrial DNA transcription. The islet cell requires large quantities of ATP for both the synthesis of insulin (and other hormones) and its release. In fact, the pancreas, brain, and kidney require more ATP than other tissues and organs in the body. Retinoic acid bound to its receptor binds to the promoter of the mitochondrial DNA to stimulate the synthesis of the 13 essential oxidative phosphorylation (OXPHOS) proteins.[33,37] This is turn stimulates OXPHOS and ATP production without which the islet cell cannot synthesize or release sufficient insulin to meet the need.

Reproduction and Growth

The role of vitamin A in the growth process is related to its function in RNA synthesis as described earlier. Animals fed vitamin A–deficient diets do not eat well, and their poor growth may stem from their inadequate intakes of the other essential nutrients. As mentioned previously, vitamin A is responsible for the maintenance of the integrity of the epithelial tissues. Since the taste buds are specialized epithelial tissues, feeding a deficient diet probably results in a change in the structure and function of these taste buds resulting in a loss in appetite. As well, other epithelial cells are also affected, particularly those cells that secrete lubricating and digestive fluids in the mouth, stomach, and intestinal tract. The lack of lubrication due to atrophy of these important cells would certainly affect food intake and, hence, result in poor growth. Reduction in food intake itself imposes a stress on the growing animal. Stress, with its attendant hormonal responses such as an increase in thyroid hormone release, and an increase in adrenal activity, would have profound influences on protein turnover and energy utilization and, of course, growth.

As mentioned, the role of the vitamin in reproduction relates to its role in RNA and protein synthesis. Ornithine decarboxylase (ODC), an enzyme that closely correlates to cell division and tissue growth, has recently been identified as a protooncogene. ODC is the first rate-limiting enzyme in the biosynthesis of polyamines, which are essential for cell growth. Retinoic acid suppresses ODC mRNA synthesis and by doing so serves as a *brake* on uncontrolled cell growth. This function of retinoic acid on ODC transcription is counterbalanced by retinoic acid–estrogen receptor binding. The latter enhances ODC mRNA transcription. Not only would the growth of a fertilized egg be affected in this manner, but also, through its effects on protein synthesis, vitamin A could affect the synthesis of enzymes needed to produce the steroid hormones that regulate and orchestrate the reproduction process. Several of the enzymes listed in Table 11.7 are involved in the synthesis of these hormones. Of the other enzymes listed, three (ATPase, arginase, xanthine oxidase) relate primarily to energy or protein wastage, as would be expected in a deficient animal, and are increased in the deficient animal. The transferase and the enzymes of retinol metabolism are unchanged, while enzymes for the synthesis of mucopolysaccharides are decreased. Observations of increases in the phospholipid content of a variety of cellular and subcellular membranes in vitamin A–deficient rats suggest that enzymes of lipid metabolism are also affected. Cholesterol absorption is increased in the deficient rat and this increase may in turn affect phospholipid synthesis and membrane phospholipid content since mammalian plasma membranes consist largely of cholesterol and phospholipids. Changes in membrane composition conceivably could explain the increased susceptibility of deficient animals to infection but equally likely is the reduction in the protective effect of a normal intact epithelium that acts as a physical barrier to the pathogenic organisms and the reduction in the synthesis of antibodies and antibody-forming cells in the spleen of vitamin A–deficient animals. Vitamin A supplementation of deficient animals has been shown to increase antibody production in response to tetanus toxoid[38] as well as exposure to a variety of other infectious materials.[39] Retinoic acid plays a key role in the differentiation of T-cell subsets, the migration of T cells into tissues, and the appropriate development of T-cell-dependent antibody responses.[39] The secondary characteristics of vitamin A deficiency again are probably related to the role of the vitamin in protein synthesis as described earlier. The primary characteristics of decreased dark adaptation, poor growth, reduced reproductive capacity, xerophthalmia, keratomalacia, and anemia are all related.

Vision

Of the various functions vitamin A serves, its role in the maintenance of dark adaptation was the first to be fully described on a molecular basis.[40] When animals are deprived of vitamin A, the amount of rhodopsin declines. This is followed by a decrease in the amount of the protein opsin. Rhodopsin is present in the rod cells of the retina of most animals. The synthesis of rhodopsin and its subsequent bleaching has been elucidated primarily through the work of Wald and others. The role of retinol in the visual cycle is illustrated in Figure 11.6. All-*trans* retinol is transported to the retina cell, transferred into the cell, and converted to all-*trans* retinal. All-*trans* retinal is isomerized to 11-*cis* retinal, which combines with opsin to form rhodopsin. Rhodopsin is an asymmetric protein with a molecular weight of about 38,000. It has both a hydrophilic and a hydrophobic region with a folded length of about 70 Å. It spans the membrane of the retina via seven helical segments that cross back and forth. It comprises about 60% of the membrane protein. The light-sensitive portion of the molecule resides in its hydrophobic region. When rhodopsin is exposed to light, it changes its shape. The primary photochemical event is the very rapid isomerization of 11-*cis* retinal to a highly strained transold form, bathorhodopsin. Note that the alcohol (retinol) and the aldehyde (retinal) are interchangeable with respect to the maintenance of the visual function. Retinoic acid is ineffective primarily because there are no enzymes in the eye to convert the retinoic acid to the active 11-*cis* retinal needed for the formation of rhodopsin. 11-*cis* retinol is also involved in the formation of iodopsin in the cones, and the photochemical isomerization of

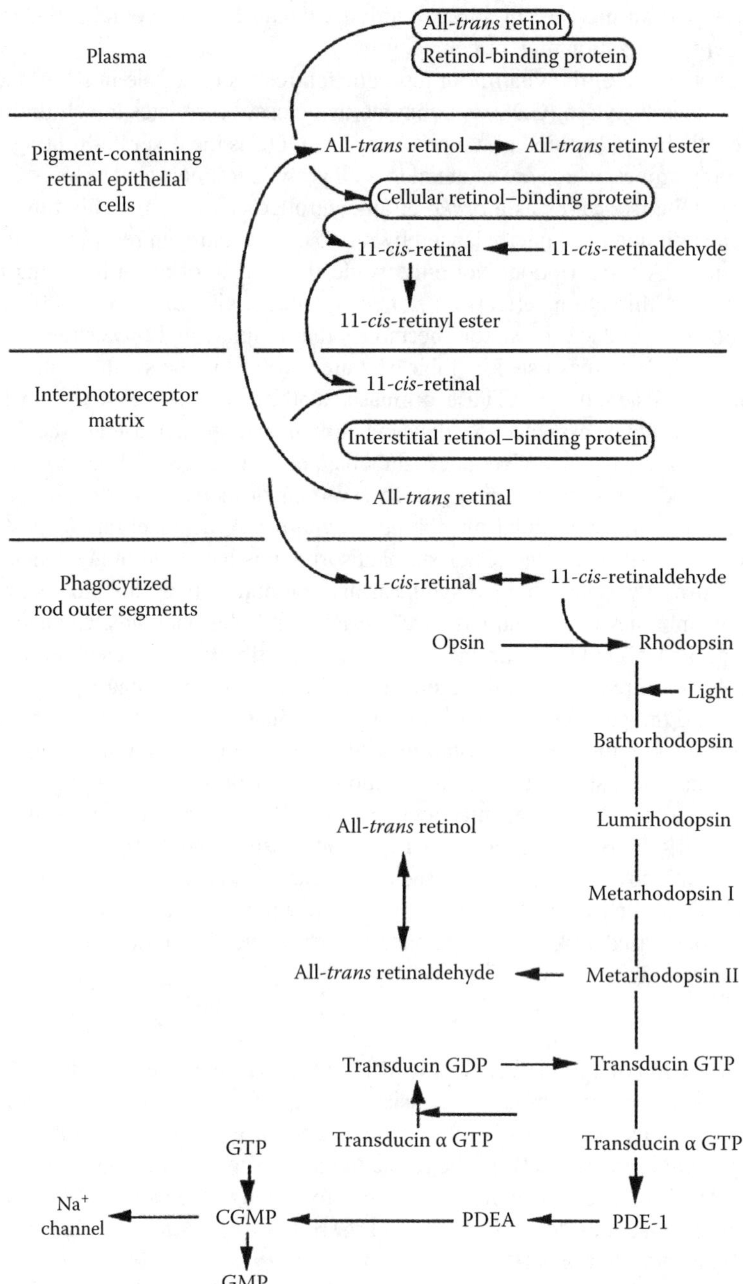

FIGURE 11.6 Vitamin A and the visual cycle.

the 11-*cis* isomer triggers the visual process. In the rhodopsin breakdown process, an electrical potential arises and generates an electrical impulse that is transmitted via the optic nerve to the brain. That 11-*cis* retinal is also involved in color vision (the responsibility of the cones) has been suggested; however, the mechanism of this involvement has not been fully explored. Three major cone pigments have been identified having absorption maxima of 450, 525, and 550 nm, respectively. Whether these are single pigments or a mixture and whether one or more contain 11-*cis* retinal has not been determined.

Hypervitaminosis A

Because the vitamin is stored in the liver, it is possible to develop a toxic condition when very high (10 times the normal intake) levels of the vitamin are consumed over a period of time.[1,41] Instances of acute vitaminosis A have been documented.[42,43] Because of the limitation in the conversion of the carotenes to retinol, vitamin A intoxication is less likely with large intakes of carotene; however, reports of yellowing of the skin of persons consuming large amounts of carrot juice have appeared. This yellowing is likely due to the deposition of carotene in the subcutaneous fat.

In humans, hypervitaminosis A is characterized by increased intracranial pressure resulting in headaches, blurring vision, vomiting, lack of muscular coordination, abnormal liver function, and pain in the weight-bearing bones and joints. In young children, a bulging fontanel has been observed. Alterations in the bone lipids have been reported.[44] There have also been reports of an interaction between hypervitaminosis A and D.[44–51] Excess vitamin A inhibits the excess vitamin D effect on renal calcification[45] and in general antagonizes the calcium response to vitamin D.[40–51] Excess vitamin D reduces the retinol bound to the erythrocyte membrane.[46,47]

There is no treatment except for discontinuance of vitamin A consumption for the hypervitaminosis state. Elevated tissue levels fall slowly after intake has stopped as the body has a tendency to conserve its vitamin store. Intakes of retinol that are higher than normal but not overtly toxic may have adverse consequences. Data from population studies have suggested that intakes in excess of the DRI for retinol may reduce bone mineralization and contribute to the development of osteoporosis. The relative risk of hip fracture, for example, appears to increase relative to the excess of retinol consumed but not with the increase in carotene consumption. The Institute of Medicine has recommended an upper limit for retinol intake based on life stage.[52] For infants, the upper limit is 600 μg/day. An upper limit based on the infant's energy intake has been suggested to be between 750 and 1000 IUs/100 kcal/day.[53] For children, it is 600–900 μg/day; for adolescents, 1700–3000 μg/day; and for pregnant and lactating women, 2800–3000 μg/day. These upper limits are two to three times the recommended intake levels for these life stage groups. See Table 11.1 for vitamin A DRI recommendations.

Vitamin Degradation and Excretion

The early Nobel Prize–winning work of Wald et al. that showed that retinol must be converted to retinal before the vitamin can function in vision led the way for other workers to investigate the further metabolism of the various active forms. Since vitamin A not only maintains the visual cycle but is also necessary for growth, epithelial cell differentiation, skeletal tissue development, spermatogenesis, and the development and maintenance of the placenta, and because each of these functions requires a specific form of the vitamin, it appears that each of these tissues has specific structural requirements. Retinal for vision has been demonstrated (see the discussion on the visual cycle). It appears that retinol but not retinal or retinoic acid is required for the support of reproduction and that all three forms support growth and cell differentiation. That the three forms are interchangeable in the latter function suggests that retinoic acid is the active form for this function. Both retinol and retinal can be converted to retinoic acid but the reverse reactions are not possible, and only in specific tissues such as the retina are retinol and retinal interconvertible. From studies using radioactively labeled retinal, retinol, and retinoic acid, it is apparent that retinoic acid is the common metabolic intermediate of the vitamin A group. Once retinol is mobilized from hepatic stores, transported to its target tissue via the RBP, and transferred to its intracellular active site via the intracellular RBPs, it is then utilized as either retinol or retinal or converted to retinoic acid. Studies of the excretion patterns of labeled retinol and retinoic acid revealed that retinol was used more slowly than retinoic acid. Label from retinoic acid was almost completely recovered within 48 h of administration, whereas more than 7 days were required to recover even half of the label from the retinol.

The use of retinoic acid labeled in several different locations allowed for the determination of the metabolic pathway of retinoic acid. The labeled retinoic acid was recovered as $^{14}CO_2$ from the expired air as well as from ^{14}C labeled decarboxylated metabolites and the β-ionone ring lacking part of its isoprenoid side chain. The structures of all the metabolites that appear in the urine and feces are not known.

Need

Adult requirements for retinol have been estimated using a variety of techniques. Reports in the literature indicate that requirements may be increased by fever, infection, cold, hyperthyroidism, chemical toxicants, and excessive exposure to sunlight. Excess alcohol consumption likewise compromises vitamin A status.[54,55] There is an interaction between alcohol vitamin A and β-carotene that is characterized by the development of hepatotoxicity and carcinogenicity.[54] Ethanol elevates the level of all-*trans* retinoic acid, and it has been suggested that fetal alcohol syndrome may be due to this alcohol effect.[42,55] People with renal disease, especially those in acute renal failure, release their hepatic stores of retinol and this affects vitamin A status.[14,15] Ultimately, this means that their vitamin need is increased since serum retinol is a positive feedback mechanism that indicates that more is needed by the peripheral tissues. Malnutrition not just due to renal disease and other diseases but also due to inadequate food supply leads to multiple nutrient deficiency. Vitamin A deficiency among children in developing nations remains the leading cause of impaired vision and blindness. It is a significant contributor to infectious disease in these children.[20] Undernutrition and malnutrition affect an estimated 254 million children and are a leading concern of the World Health Organization. It is preventable through food supplementation programs that include vitamin supplementation as well as protein and energy supplements. In addition to an inadequate food supply, there are some individuals whose genetic heritage introduces an additional measure of variability in the need for vitamin A. This variability is not easily identified but the DRIs allow for such in the recommended intakes for vitamin A. The DRIs are periodically examined and updates provided. The reader should visit the website www.nap.edu for these updates.

VITAMIN D

Just as night blindness was recognized as a disease treatable by dietary vitamin A, the classical disease of vitamin D deficiency, rickets, has been evident since ancient times. Historians do not agree as to when the first symptoms of vitamin D deficiency were reported. Some suggest that the stooped appearance of the Neanderthals (circa 50000 BC) was due to an inadequate vitamin D intake rather than being characteristic of a low evolutionary status. Evidence of rickets in skeletons from humans of the Neolithic age, the first settlers of Greenland, and the ancient Egyptians, Greeks, and Romans has been reported.

The first detailed descriptions of the disease are found in the writings of Dr. Daniel Whistler of Leiden, the Netherlands, and Professor Francis Glisson in the mid-1600s. Beyond these descriptions and the acceptance of rickets as a disease entity, little progress was made until the late 1800s when it was suggested that the lack of sunlight and perhaps a poor diet were related to the appearance of bone malformation. It was frequently reported that infants born in the spring and dying the following winter did not have any symptoms of rickets, whereas infants born in the fall and dying the next spring had rickets. Funk, in 1914, suggested that rickets was a nutrient deficiency disorder. This was verified by the brilliant work of Sir Edward Mellanby. Mellanby constructed a grain diet that produced rickets in puppies. When he gave cod liver oil, the disease did not develop. At that time, Mellanby did not know that there were two fat-soluble vitamins (A and D) in cod liver oil, and he thought that he was studying the antirachitic properties of vitamin A. Not until the two vitamins were separated and identified was it realized that Mellanby's antirachitic factor was vitamin D. The recognition of vitamin D as a separate entity from vitamin A came from the work of McCollum and associates in 1922. In a landmark paper, McCollum reported the results of his work on the characterization of vitamin A. He described the vulnerability of the vitamin to oxidation and the fact that the antirachitic factor remained even after the cod liver oil was aerated and heated and the antixerophthalmic factor (vitamin A) was destroyed.

Although the importance of sunlight had been recognized in the prevention and treatment of rickets, the relationship of UV light to the dietary intake of vitamin D was not appreciated until Steenbeck and also Goldblatt et al. demonstrated that UV light gave antirachitic properties to sterol-containing foods if these foods were incorporated into diets previously shown to produce rickets. From this point on, the research concerning vitamin D, as it was so named by McCollum and associates, became largely chemical in nature.

Structure and Nomenclature

Like vitamin A, vitamin D is not a single compound. The D vitamins listed in Table 11.8 are a family of 9, 10 secosteroids that differ only in the structures of their side chains. Figure 11.7 shows some of these different structures. There is no D_1 because when the vitamins were originally isolated and identified, the compound identified as D_1 turned out to be a mixture of the other D vitamins rather than a separate entity.

Since the other D vitamins were already described and named, the D_1 designation was deleted from the list. All the D vitamin forms are related structurally to the four-ring compounds cyclopentanoperhydrophenanthrenes from which they were derived by a photochemical reaction. The official nomenclature proposed for vitamin D by IUPAC-IUB Commission on Biochemical Nomenclature relates the vitamin to its steroid nucleus. Each carbon is numbered using the same system as is used for other sterols such as cholesterol. This is illustrated in Figure 11.8. The numbering system of the four-ring structure is retained even though the compound loses its B ring during its conversion to the vitamin.

The chief structural prerequisite of compounds serving as D provitamins is the sterol structure that has an opened B ring that contains a $D_{5,6}$ conjugated double bond. No vitamin activity is possessed by the compound until the B ring is opened. This occurs as a result of exposure to UV light. In addition, vitamin activity is dependent on the presence of a hydroxyl group at carbon 3 and upon the presence of conjugated double bonds at the 10–19, 5–6, 7–8 positions. If the location of these double bonds is shifted, vitamin activity is substantially reduced. A side chain of a length at least equivalent to that of cholesterol is also a prerequisite for vitamin activity. If the side chain is replaced by a hydroxyl group, for example, the vitamin activity is lost. The potency of the various D vitamins is determined by the side chain. D_5, for example, with its branched 10-carbon side chain, is much less active with respect to the calcification of bone cartilage than is D_3 with its 9-member side chain.

TABLE 11.8
D Vitamers Produced from Provitamin Forms When These Precursor Forms Are Exposed to UV Light

Precursor	D Vitamer
Ergosterol	D_2 (ergocalciferol)
7-Dehydrocholesterol	D_3 (cholecalciferol)
22,23-Dihydroergosterol	D_4
7-Dehydrositosterol	D_5
7-Dehydrostigmasterol	D_6
7-Dehydrocompesterol	D_7

Note: These are not active until they are hydroxylated at carbons 1 and 25.

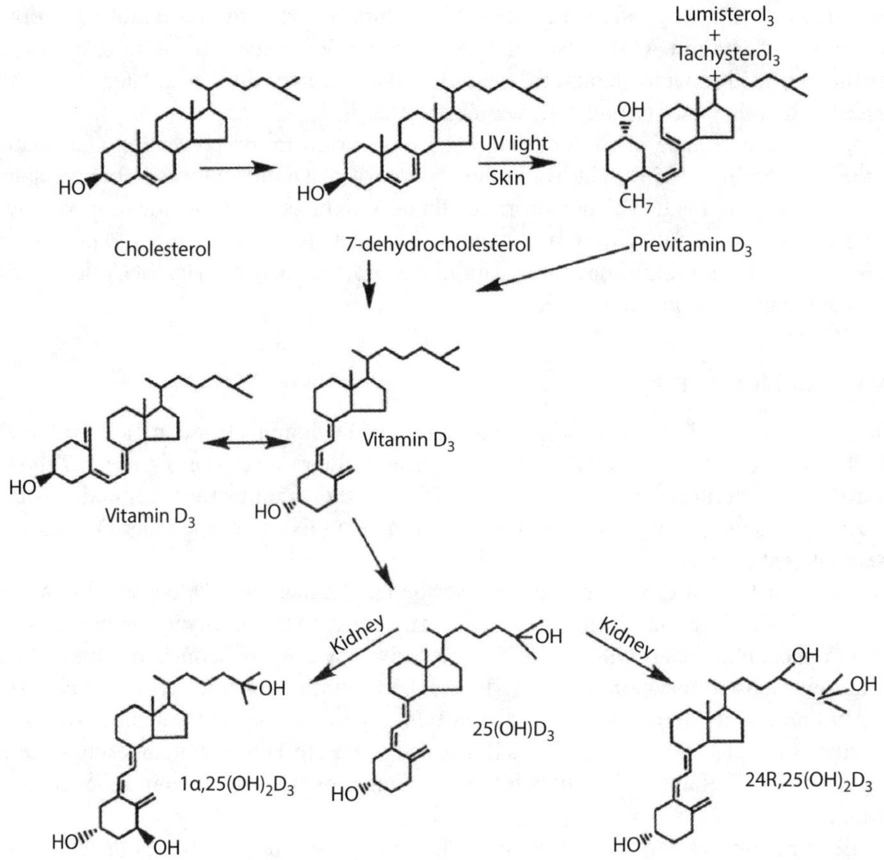

FIGURE 11.7 Compounds that have vitamin D activity. Not all of these compounds have identical activities.

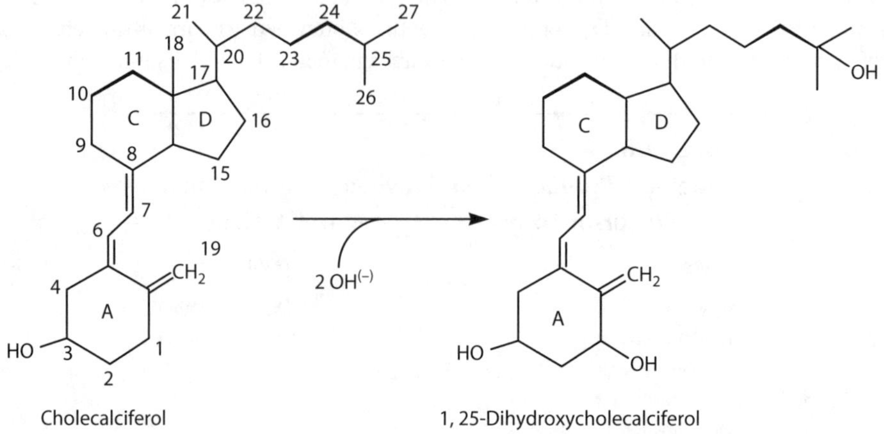

FIGURE 11.8 Conversion of cholecalciferol to 1,25-dihydroxycholecalciferol. The carbons in the structures are numbered and the rings are given letter designations. When activated, a hydroxyl group is added to carbon 25.

Of the compounds shown in Figure 11.7, the most common form is that of D_2, ergocalciferol, so-called because its parent compound is ergosterol. Ergosterol can be prepared from plant materials and, thus, serves as a commercially important source of the vitamin. Vitamin D_3, cholecalciferol, is the only form that can be generated in vivo. Cholesterol, from which cholecalciferol takes its name, serves as the precursor. The 7-dehydrocholesterol at the skin's surface is acted upon by UV light and is converted to vitamin D_3. Here, then, is the connection between diet, sunshine, and rickets sought many years ago when rickets was prevalent in young children. In the absence of sunshine, this conversion does not take place. Recall the dress patterns of the people of the eighteenth and nineteenth centuries. Children (as well as adults) wore many layers of clothing that shielded the skin from UV light. This practice severely restricted UV light–induced vitamin D synthesis.

While most mammals can convert D_2 to D_3 and use it to make the active principle (1,25-dihydroxycholecalciferol) responsible for D's biological function, birds cannot do this. Birds must be supplied with D_3 rather than D_2 as the vitamin of choice. It has been estimated that for birds, D_2 has only 1/10th the biological activity of D_3 on a molar basis.

Physical/Chemical Properties

The history of vitamin D would not be complete without mentioning the careful work of a Frenchman, Charles Tanret, who isolated and characterized a sterol from fungus-infected rye, which he called ergosterol. The melting point, optical rotation, and elemental composition of ergosterol reported by Tanret in 1889 were identical to those reported by Windaus more than 30 years later. Windaus and his associates were able to elucidate the structure of ergosterol and ergocalciferol. The structures of these compounds were verified later using x-ray analysis and infrared spectroscopy.

The precursors and the vitamins are sterols, which are members of the nonsaponifiable lipid class. At room temperature, they are white to yellowish solids with relatively low melting points. The various structural and physical characteristics of D_2 and D_3 are listed in Table 11.9. Under normal conditions, D_3 is more stable than D_2; however, both compounds undergo oxidation when exposed to air for periods of 24–72 h. When protected from air and moisture and stored under refrigeration, oxidation of the vitamin is minimized. In acid solutions, the D vitamins are unstable. However, in alkaline solutions, they are stable. All the D vitamins are moderately soluble in fats, oils, and ethanol and very soluble in fat solvents such as chloroform, methanol, and ether. All of the vitamers are unstable to light. In the dry form, the vitamers are more stable than when in solution. Stability in solution can be enhanced by the presence of such antioxidants as α-tocopherol and carotene.

Although the D vitamins are not soluble in water, they, like the A vitamins, can be made miscible with water through the use of detergents or surfactants. However, because of the vitamins' vulnerability to oxidation, such solutions are very unstable. This is due to the wide dispersion of the vitamin molecules in water which has oxygen dissolved in it. Thus, each vitamin molecule is available to the dissolved oxygen for oxidation with the resultant loss in vitamin activity. Some protection against this oxidation can be provided if α-tocopherol is added to the solution. In addition to the loss of vitamin activity through oxidation, other chemical alterations can result in decreased

TABLE 11.9
Physical Characteristics of Vitamins D_2 and D_3

Vitamin	Number of Double Bonds	Melting Point (°C)	UV Absorption Maximum (mm)	Molar Extinction Coefficient	Optical Rotation
D_2	4	121	265	19,400	$\alpha\frac{20}{D}+106°C$
D_3	3	83–85	264–265	18,300	$\alpha\frac{20}{D}+84.8°C$

vitamin potency. Saturation of any of the double bonds or the substitution of a chloride, bromide, or mercaptan residue for the hydroxyl group attached to carbon 3 results in a loss of vitamin activity.

Biopotency

The comparative potency of the D vitamers depends on the species consuming the vitamers and the particular function assessed. With respect to species specificity, in mammalian species, both the D_2 and D_3 are equivalent, and both would be given a value of 100 if rickets prevention was used as the functional criteria. However, should these two vitamers be compared in chicks as preventers of rickets, D_2 would be given a value of perhaps 10, while D_3 would be 100. In this instance, it is clear that species differ in their use of these two vitamers. A related sterol, dihydrotachysterol, a product of irradiated ergosterol, would have only 5%–10% of the activity of ergocalciferol. In contrast, the activated forms of D_3 (25-hydroxy and 1,25-dihydroxycholecalciferol) are far more potent (2–5Xs and 5–10Xs, respectively) than their parent vitamer, D_3. The synthetic analog of D_3, 1α hydroxy-cholecalciferol, likewise has 5–10 times the potency of cholecalciferol. The analog 3-deoxy-1, 25-dihydroxycholecalciferol is far more active as an agent to promote intestinal calcium uptake than as an agent to promote bone calcium mobilization. This is also true for the analog 25-hydroxy 5,6-cholecalciferol.

The reverse effects, increased bone calcium mobilization rather than increased intestinal calcium absorption, have been shown for analogs having a longer carbon chain at carbon 20 and/or having a fluorine attached at carbon 3 (see Figure 11.8). Cell differentiation, another vitamin D function, is markedly enhanced by the addition of a hydroxyl group at carbon 3, an unsaturation between carbons 16 and 17, and a triple bond between carbons 22 and 23. This analog has a greater activity with respect to cell differentiation than for intestinal calcium uptake and bone calcium mobilization.

Methods of Assay

Because mammals require so little vitamin D and because so few foods contain the vitamin, methods for its determination have to be sensitive, reliable, and accurate. A wide variety of assays have been developed that are capable of quantifying fairly well the amount of vitamin D in a test substance. These assays can be divided into two groups: chemical and biological. Biological assays with few exceptions are usually more sensitive than chemical assays because so little of the vitamin is required by animals. The least amount of vitamin detectable by the biological methods is 120 ng or 0.3 nmol, whereas, with the chemical methods, the least amount detectable is approximately nine times that of the bioassay of 2.6 nmol. The exception to this comparison is the technique that utilizes HPLC followed by UV absorption analysis. This technique can measure as little as 5 ng or 1/24th that of the bioassay techniques. Gas chromatography is also very sensitive, especially if the chromatograph is equipped with an electron capture detector. Using this technique, as little as 50 pg of the vitamin can be detected. This degree of sensitivity is needed for the detection of tissue vitamin levels, for aside from vitamin B_{12}, vitamin D is the most potent of the vitamins. Only small amounts are needed and so only small amounts will be found in those tissues requiring the vitamin. Table 11.10 summarizes the main methods that have been used for the detection of biological levels of vitamin D. Under the chemical assay techniques, note that a variety of color reactions can be used in vitamin D quantification. These color reactions are possible because the vitamin contains several rings that can react with a variety of compounds in solution and produce a color. The intensity of the color is directly related to the quantity of the vitamin in solution. While these colorimetric methods are relatively easy to perform, they have several drawbacks. First, and most important, the color reaction is possible because of the ring structure; other sterols have this same ring structure but have little vitamin activity. Thus, colorimetric methods are not specific enough to permit true vitamin quantification. The second drawback is that there must be sufficient vitamin in the test substance to react with the color reagent to produce a measurable color change. This requires instrumentation

TABLE 11.10
Summary of Methods Used in Determining Vitamin D Content of Tissues and Foods

Method	Sensitivity[a] (nmol)	Usual Working Range (nmol)	Comments
Chemical Methods			
Colorimetric[b]			
Antimony chloride	3.2	3.2–6.5	Used primarily to assess pharmaceutical preparations.
Trifluoroacetic	2.6	1–80	
UV absorption	2.6	2.6–52	A solution with 5.47 nmol of vitamin D will have an absorbance of 0.10 at 264 nm.
UV fluorescence	2.6	2.6–26	Based on the property of acetic anhydride–sulfuric acid induced fluorescence of the vitamin.
Gas chromatography	0.1 pmol	0.01–10	Based on the use of electron capture detector.
HPLC	0.01	0.05–100	Sensitive.
Gas chromatography—mass spectrometry	0.01	0.01–50	The method can separate and quantify individual vitamers in a mixture.
Biological Methods			
Rat line test	0.03	0.03–0.07	Time consuming.
Chick test	0.13	0.006–15	Time consuming.

[a] Defined as the least amount of vitamin detectable by the method.
[b] Other color reagents have also been used.

that is able to measure these changes. In general, this degree of sensitivity is missing in most instruments designed to measure colorimetric changes. Thus, the colorimetric methods lack sensitivity as well as specificity.

The ring structure of vitamin D, although common to many different sterols, can be utilized very well in assay techniques where the sterols are first separated and then assayed. The vitamin D sterol ring structure has a characteristic UV absorption spectra. At 264–265 mm, the intensity of the light absorbed is directly proportional to the quantity of vitamin D present. Sterols can be separated from the lipid component of a sample by saponification. The nonsaponifiable lipids (the sterols) can be further separated by digitonin precipitation. Vitamin D and its related sterols will not precipitate out, whereas cholesterol and the other four-ring sterols will. If the remaining supernatant containing the vitamin D components is then fractionated using chromatographic techniques, the resulting fractions can be assayed according to the amount of UV light absorbed.

The UV light absorption characteristic can also be used to determine the extent of conversion of provitamin D to D_2 or D_3. Ergosterol or cholesterol can be irradiated until the resultant compound exhibits the typical absorption spectra characteristic of the vitamin. Of course, just as UV light is needed for this conversion, one must remember that light in excess will destroy the vitamin and its usefulness will be lost.

Just as there are a number of chemical assay techniques useful for the determination of vitamin D activity in biological samples, there are also a number of biological assay techniques that can be used. The advantages of the bioassay are those of sensitivity and specificity. The disadvantages are those of time, expense, and accuracy. The basis of the bioassay is that the physiological effect is quantifiable and, theoretically, the magnitude of this effect is in direct proportion to the amount of vitamin D in the test substance. For many years, the standard bioassay for vitamin D was the rat line test first devised by McCollum in 1922. This test consisted of preparing rats and then treating them with graded amounts of the test substance for 1 week. The rats are then killed and the bones of the forepaws excised and cleaned of adhering tissue, sliced longitudinally, and placed in a solution of silver nitrate. The silver nitrate is absorbed by the areas of the bone where calcium has recently been deposited. These regions will turn black upon exposure to light. The resultant black line is then measured and compared to lines obtained from rats fed known amounts of vitamin D. Thus, the line test is based on the activity of the vitamin in promoting calcium uptake by the bone. While this is probably a good method to estimate vitamin activity in a given substance, it has the pitfall of not distinguishing between the various D forms. The user of this method also must assume that bone calcium deposition is the vitamin's most important function; this is not always true.

The use of the line test to assess vitamin content of human foods is probably acceptable since rats and humans can use all forms of vitamin D similarly. However, the use of the rat line test to assess the D content of feeds for chickens would present problems due to the fact that the chickens do not use D_2 and D_3 equally well. As pointed out earlier, chickens need D_3 in their diets rather than D_2. Other bioassays listed in Table 11.9 also are based on a physiological/metabolic parameter that assumes that the quantity of the vitamin in a test substance is proportional to the activity of the system being assessed. Tests such as the intestinal calcium uptake test, the bone calcium mobilization test, the body growth test, and the calcium-binding protein assay all have been devised and published. They all have the advantage of assessing the biological potency of the vitamin D contained in the test substance, and all are sensitive to quantities of D likely to be present in biological (as opposed to pharmacological) preparations.

International Units

Active vitamin D is given in IUs. One IU uses cholecalciferol, D_3, as the reference standard where 1.0 g of a cottonseed oil solution of D_3 contains 10 mg of the vitamin or 400 USP units. Thus, 1.0 IU of vitamin is 0.025 μg, which is equivalent to 65.0 pmol. The recommendation is that all of the various forms of the vitamin be stated in relation to their equivalent molar unit of the parent vitamin D_3. The current recommended intake for infants and children, adolescents, adults, and pregnant and lactating women is 200 IU/day (5 μg/day). For adults over the age of 51, the recommendation is for twice that amount or 400 IU/day (10 μg/day). After the age of 70, the intake recommendation is further increased to 600 IU/day (15 μg/day). This further increase in recommended intake with age is based on the observations that there is an age-related decrease in the activity of the conversion of previtamin D to 25-hydroxy vitamin D in the skin.

Metabolism

Absorption

Prior to the understanding and elucidation of the conversion of cholesterol to ergosterol and then to its activation as 1,25-dihydroxycholecalciferol, considerable attention was given to the mechanisms for the intestinal absorption of vitamin D. It was found that dietary vitamin D was absorbed with the food fats and was dependent on the presence of the bile salts. Any disease that affects fat absorption results in an impairment of vitamin D absorption. Absorption of the vitamin is a passive process that is influenced by the composition of the gut contents. Vitamin D is absorbed with the long-chain fatty acids and is present in the chylomicrons of the lymphatic system. Absorption takes place primarily in the jejunum and ileum. This has a protective effect on vitamin D stores since the bile, released into the duodenum, is the chief excretory pathway of the vitamin; reabsorption in times of vitamin need can protect the body from undue loss. However, in times of vitamin intake excess, this reabsorptive mechanism may be a detriment rather than a benefit. The vitamin is absorbed in either the hydroxylated or the unhydroxylated form.

While many of the other essential nutrients are absorbed via an active transport system, there is little reason to believe that absorption of vitamin D is by any mechanism other than by passive diffusion. The body, if exposed to sunlight, can convert the 7-dehydrocholesterol at the skin's surface to cholecalciferol, and this compound is then further metabolized in the kidney producing the active principle 1,25-dihydroxycholecalciferol. Because the body, under the right conditions, can synthesize in toto its vitamin needs, and because it needs so little of the vitamin, there appears to be little reason for the body to develop an active transport system for its absorption. However, in the person with renal disease or in persons using excessive amounts of sun blocker, the synthesis of 1,25-dihydroxycholecalciferol is impaired, and in this individual, intestinal uptake of the active form is quite important.

Because the body can completely synthesize dehydrocholesterol and ergosterol, convert it to D_2 or D_3, and then hydroxylate it to form the active form, an argument against its essentiality as a nutrient can be developed. In point of fact, because the active form is synthesized in the kidney and from there distributed by the blood to all parts of the body, this active form meets the definition of a hormone and the kidney, its site of synthesis, and meets the definition of an endocrine organ. Thus, whether vitamin D is a nutrient or a hormone is dependent on the degree of exposure to UV light. Lacking exposure, vitamin D must be provided in the diet and thus is an essential nutrient.

Transport

Once absorbed, vitamin D is transported in a nonesterified form bound to a specific vitamin D–binding protein (DBP). This protein (DBP) is nearly identical to the α2-globulins and albumins with respect to its electrophoretic mobility. All of the forms of vitamin D (25-hydroxy D_3; 24,25-dihydroxy D_3; and 1,25-dihydroxy D_3) are carried by this protein, which is a globulin with a molecular weight of 58,000 DA. Its binding affinity varies with the vitamin form. DNA sequence analysis of DBP shows homology with a fetoprotein and serum albumin. DBP also has a high affinity for actin but the physiological significance for this cross-reactivity is unknown.

Use

Once absorbed or synthesized at the body surface, vitamin D is transported via DBP to the liver. Here, it is hydroxylated via the enzyme vitamin D hydroxylase at carbon 25 to form 25-hydroxycholecalciferol. Figure 11.7 illustrates the pathway from cholesterol to 1,25-dihydroxycholecalciferol. With the first hydroxylation, a number of products are formed but the most important of these is 25-hydroxycholecalciferol. The biological function of each of these metabolites is not known completely. As mentioned, the hydroxylation occurs in the liver and is catalyzed by a cytochrome P450–dependent mixed-function monooxygenase.

Vitamin D hydroxylase has been found in both mitochondrial and microsomal compartments. It is a two-component system that involves a flavoprotein and cytochrome P450 and is regulated by the concentration of ionized calcium in serum. The hydroxylation reaction can be inhibited if D_3 analogs having modified side chains are infused into the animal fed a rachitic diet and a D_3 supplement.

The 25-hydroxy D_3 is then bound to DBP and transported from the liver to the kidney where a second hydroxyl group is added at carbon 1. This hydroxylation occurs in the kidney proximal tubule mitochondria catalyzed by the enzyme 25(OH)D_3-1α-hydroxylase. This enzyme has been characterized as a three-component enzyme involving cytochrome P450, an iron sulfur protein (ferredoxin), and ferredoxin reductase. The reductant is $NADPH_2$. Considerable evidence has shown that 1,25-dihydroxycholecalciferol is the active principle that stimulates bone mineralization, intestinal calcium uptake, and calcium mobilization.[56–65] Because this product is so active in the regulation of calcium homeostasis, its synthesis must be closely regulated. Indeed, product feedback regulation not only on the activity of this enzyme but also at the level of its transcription has been shown. In both instances, the level of 1,25-dihydroxycholecalciferol negatively affects 1α-hydroxylase activity and suppresses mRNA transcription of the hydroxylase gene product. In addition, control of the hydroxylase enzyme is also exerted by the parathyroid hormone (PTH). When plasma calcium levels fall, PTH is released, and this hormone stimulates 1α-hydroxylase activity while decreasing the activity of 25-hydroxylase. In turn, PTH release is downregulated by rising levels of 1,25-dihydroxycholecalciferol and its analog, 24,25-dihydroxycholecalciferol. Insulin, growth hormone, estrogen, and prolactin are additional hormones that stimulate the

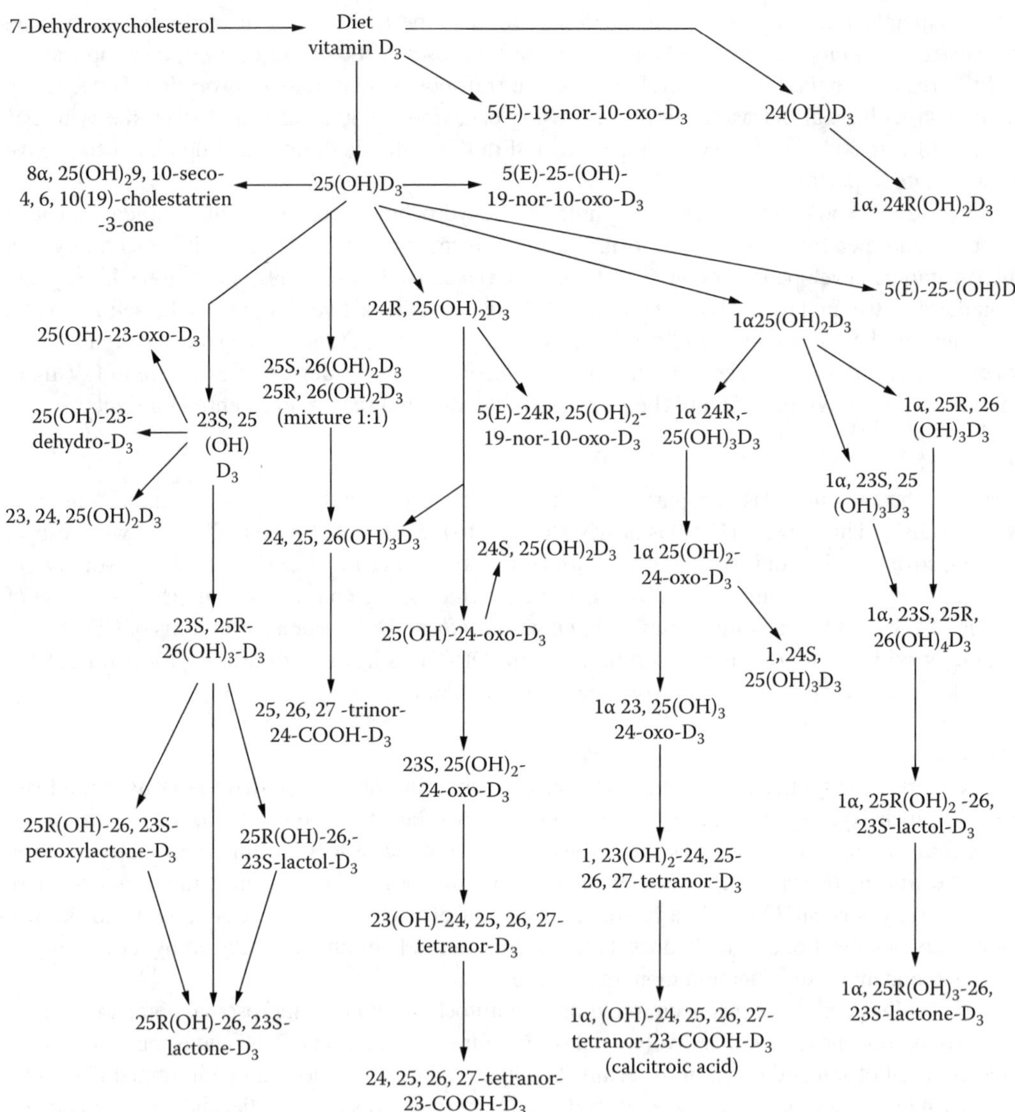

FIGURE 11.9 Pathways for vitamin D_3 synthesis and degradation.

activity of the 1α-hydroxylase. The mechanisms that explain these stimulatory effects are less well known and are probably related to their effects on bone mineralization as well as on other calcium-using processes.

Just as several metabolites are formed in the 25-hydroxylase reaction, a number of products result with the second hydroxylation. Some of these transformations are shown in Figure 11.9. Also shown are the degradative products found primarily in the feces.

D_3 is subject to other metabolic reactions as well (Figure 11.9). Whether these metabolites have specific functions with respect to mineral metabolism is not fully understood. Instead of 1,25-dihydroxy D_3, 24,25-dihydroxy D_3 may be formed and may serve to enhance bone mineralization and embryonic development and suppress PTH release. 24,25-Dihydroxy D_3 arises by hydroxylation of 25-hydroxy D_3. When 25(OH)D_3-1α-hydroxylase activity is suppressed, 24,25-hydroxylation is stimulated. This hydroxylase is substrate inducible through the mechanism of increased enzyme protein synthesis and has been found in the kidney, intestine, and cartilage.

24,25-Dihydroxy D_3 may represent a *spillover* metabolite of D_3. That is, a metabolite is formed when excess 25-hydroxy D_3 is present in the body. Other D_3 metabolites such as 25-hydroxy D_3 26,23-lactose also can be regarded as spillover metabolites since measurable quantities are observed under conditions of excess intake. While 24,25-dihydroxy D_3 does function in the bone mineralization process, it is not as active in this respect as is 1,25-dihydroxy D_3.

The question of whether the hydroxy group at carbon 25 is a requirement for vitamin activity has been posed since several D_3 metabolites lack this structural element. Studies utilizing fluoro-substituted D_3 showed conclusively that while maximal activity is shown by the 1,25-D_3, activity can also be shown by compounds lacking this structure. In part, the structural requisite for vitamin activity may relate to the role the 25-hydroxy substituents play in determining the molecular shape of the compound. This shape must conform to the receptor shape of the cellular membranes in order for the D_3 to be utilized. Specific intracellular receptors for 1,25-dihydroxy D_3 have been found in parathyroid, pancreatic, pituitary, and placental tissues. All these tissues have been shown to require D_3 for the regulation of their function. For example, in D_3 deficiency, pancreatic release of insulin is impaired. Insulin release is a calcium-dependent–D-dependent process. As can be seen in Figure 11.9, several pathways exist for the degradation of the active 1,25-dihydroxycholecalciferol. These include oxidative removal of the side chain, additional hydroxylation at carbon 24, the formation of a lactone (1,25 OH_2 D_2-26,23-lactone), and an additional hydroxylation at carbon 26. While 25-hydroxycholecalciferol can accumulate in the heart, lungs, kidneys, and liver, 1,25-dihydroxycholecalciferol does not accumulate. The active form is not stored appreciably but is found in almost every cell and tissue type.

Function

Until the recognition of the central role of the calcium ion in cellular metabolic regulation, it was thought that vitamin D's only function was to facilitate the deposition of calcium and phosphorus in bone.[59] This concept developed when it was recognized that the bowed legs of rickets was due to inadequate mineralization in the absence of adequate vitamin D intake or exposure to sunlight.[60] We now know that vitamin D plays a key role in the regulation of the glyoxylate cycle in the liver,[61] stimulates cell proliferation in the adipose tissue via reactive oxygen species,[59] and modulates adipocyte glucocorticoid function.[60]

Studies of in vivo calcium absorption by the intestine revealed that D-deficient rats absorb less calcium than D-sufficient rats and that rats fed very high levels (10,000 IU/day) absorbed more calcium than did normally fed rats. These observations of the vitamin effects on calcium uptake led to work designed to determine the mechanism of this effect. It was soon discovered that vitamin D (1,25-dihydroxy D_3) served to stimulate the synthesis of a specific protein in the gut cells that was responsible for calcium uptake.[61] This protein, called the calcium-binding protein (calbindin), was isolated from the intestine and later from the brain, bone, kidney, uterus, parotid gland, parathyroid glands, and skin. Several different calcium-binding proteins have been found, but not all of these binding proteins are vitamin D dependent. That is, once formed, their activity with respect to calcium binding is unaffected by vitamin deficiency. Many, however, are dependent on vitamin D for their synthesis.

As animals age, the levels of calcium-binding protein fall.[56] Yet when calcium intake levels fall, the synthesis and activity of the binding proteins rise. This mechanism explains how individuals can adapt to low-calcium diets. Interestingly, calcium deprivation stimulates the conversion of cholecalciferol to 25-hydroxycholecalciferol in the liver and to 1,25-dihydroxycholecalciferol in the kidney. Aging, however, seems to affect this regulatory mechanism. As humans age, they are less able to absorb calcium and may develop osteoporosis, a condition analogous to rickets in children and characterized by demineralization of the bone. In osteoporotic patients, intestinal absorption of calcium is decreased, but when 1,25-dihydroxy D_3 is administered, calcium absorption is increased. It would appear, therefore, that one of the consequences of aging is an impaired conversion of 25-hydroxy

D_3 to 1,25-dihydroxy D_3, and since less of the latter is available, less calcium-binding protein is synthesized. Measures of calcium-binding protein in aging rats, using an immunoassay technique, have shown that this is indeed the case.

Vitamin D increases the intestinal absorption of calcium by mechanisms apart from the synthesis of calcium-binding protein. It does this as part of its general tropic effect as a steroid on a variety of cellular reactions. Vitamin D elicits a change in membrane permeability to calcium at the brush border, perhaps through a change in the lipid (fatty acid) component of the membrane. It stimulates the $Ca^{++}Mg^{++}$ ATPase on the membrane of the cell wall, increases the conversion of ATP to cAMP, and increases the activity of the alkaline phosphatase enzyme. All these effects in the intestinal cell are independent of the vitamin's effect on calcium-binding protein synthesis.

In addition to its role in calcium absorption, vitamin D serves to induce the uptake of phosphate and magnesium by the brush border of the intestine. The effect on phosphate uptake is independent of its effect on calcium absorption and is due to an effect of the vitamin on the synthesis of a sodium-dependent membrane carrier for phosphate. The effect of vitamin D on magnesium absorption is incidental to its effect on calcium absorption since the calcium-binding protein has a weak affinity for magnesium. Thus, if synthesis of the calcium-binding protein results in an increase in calcium uptake, it also results in a significant increase in magnesium uptake.

Regulation of Serum Calcium Levels

Serum calcium levels are closely regulated in the body so as to maintain optimal muscle contractility and cellular function.[62] Involved are 1,25-dihydroxy D_3, produced by the kidney, PTH released by the parathyroid gland, and thyrocalcitonin released by the thyroid C cells. Each has a specific function with respect to serum calcium levels and all three are interdependent. Vitamin D_3 increases blood calcium by increasing intestinal calcium uptake and decreases blood calcium by increasing calcium deposition in the bone. In the relative absence of vitamin D, PTH increases serum calcium levels by increasing the activity of the kidney 1α,25-hydroxylase with the result of increasing blood levels of 1,25-dihydroxy D_3 and through enhancing bone mineral mobilization and phosphate diuresis. PTH in the presence of vitamin D has the reverse action on bone. When both hormones (parathormone and 1,25-D_3) are present, bone mineralization is stimulated. Even though PTH stimulates the production of 1,25-dihydroxy D_3, D_3 does not stimulate PTH release. Thyrocalcitonin serves to lower blood calcium levels through stimulating bone calcium uptake, and its effect is independent of PTH yet is dependent on the availability of calcium from the intestine. If serum calcium levels are elevated through a calcium infusion, thyrocalcitonin will be released and stimulate bone calcium uptake even in animals lacking both PTH and D_3.

Mode of Action at the Genomic Level

The process of vitamin D (1,25-dihydroxycholecalciferol) receptor binding to specific DNA sequences follows the classic model for steroid hormone action. Like vitamin A, vitamin D binds to a receptor protein in the nucleus.[65–67] The receptor protein then acquires an affinity for specific DNA sequences located upstream from the promoter sequence of the target gene.[67] These specific DNA sequences are called response elements and consist of a structure in which two zinc atoms are coordinated in two fingerlike domains. The *N*-terminal finger confers specificity to the binding, while the second finger stabilizes the complex. When bound, transcription of the cognate protein mRNA is activated. Several response elements have been identified with each being specific for a specific gene product. As shown in Figure 11.10, the response elements have in common imperfect DRs of six-base-pair half-elements separated by a three-base-pair spacer. Affinity of the nuclear receptor protein for vitamin D is modified by phosphorylation. Two sites of phosphorylation have been found on serines. One site located in the DNA-binding region at serine 51 between two zinc finger DNA-binding motifs appears to reduce DNA-binding when phosphorylated by protein kinase C (or a related enzyme). The second site is located in the N-terminal region of the

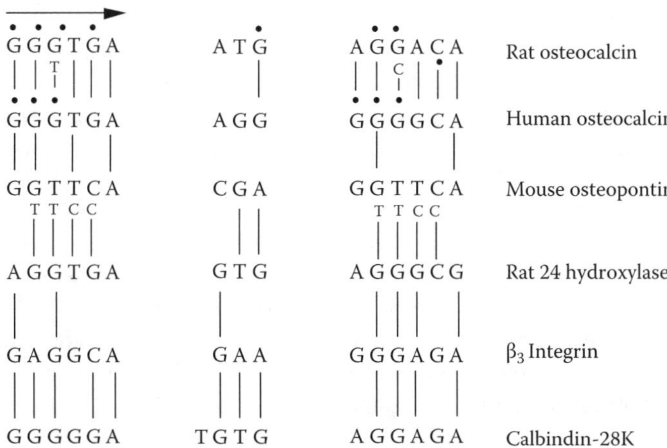

FIGURE 11.10 Vitamin D response elements for osteocalcin, osteopontin, D_3-24-hydroxylase, β_2-integrin, and calbindin 28K. Circles above bases indicate guanine residues that have shown by methylation interference experiments to be protected upon protein binding to the DRE. The small letters below the large ones indicate points at which base substitutions have been found and abolish responsiveness to vitamin D.

hormone binding region at Ser 208. It has the opposite effect. When phosphorylated, probably by casein kinase II or a related enzyme, transcription is activated.

The vitamin–protein receptor complex that binds to the DNA consists of three distinct elements: 1,25-dihydroxycholecalciferol (the hormone ligand), the vitamin receptor, and one of the retinoid X receptors (RxRα). Here is an instance where, once again, a vitamin D–vitamin A interaction can occur.[63–71] It has been reported that 9-*cis* retinoic acid can attenuate transcriptional activation by the vitamin D receptor binding to the vitamin D–responsive element (DRE). Perhaps 9-*cis* retinoic acid has this effect because when it binds to the retinoid X receptor, it blocks or partially occludes the binding site of the vitamin D–protein for DNA. Figure 11.11 illustrates the mode of vitamin D action at the genomic level. To date, the nuclear vitamin D receptor has been found in 34 different

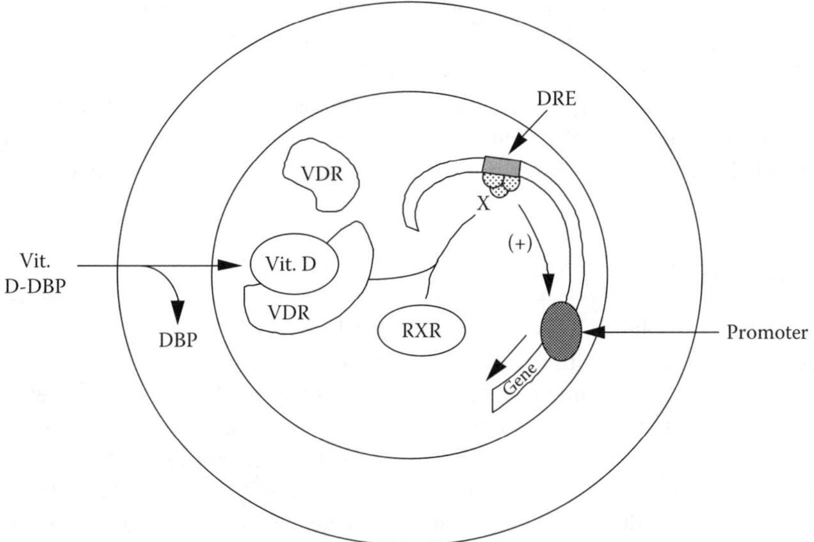

FIGURE 11.11 Schematic representation showing vitamin D bound to DBP entering the nucleus, binding to receptor (VDR), complexing with retinoid receptor (RXR), and then binding to the DREs as a transacting factor enhancing the transcription of a variety of calcium-binding proteins.

cell types, and it is quite likely that it is a universal nuclear component.[70] Probably this is because every cell has a need to move calcium into or out of its various compartments as part of its metabolic control system. Thus, the vitamin D receptor has been shown to be needed for the transcription of a wide variety of proteins such as osteocalcin, DBP osteopontin, 24-hydroxylase-β3-interferon, calbindin, prepro-PTH, calcitonin, type II collagen, fibronectin, bone matrix GLA protein, interleukin 2 and interleukin γ, transcription factors (GM-CSF, c-myc, c-fos, c-fms), vitamin D receptors calbindin D_{28x} and $_{9x}$, and prolactin.

In addition to the need for the vitamin D receptor as described earlier, it has also been shown that the gene for this receptor has several polymorphic forms. One of these is associated with the development of obesity.[68] Another polymorphism is associated with type 1 diabetes[69] and a third is associated with multiple sclerosis.[70] Sex-specific differences in the receptor polymorphisms have been shown to modify age-related cognitive decline in US adults. Males had increased declines compared to females when specific polymorphisms were compared.[71]

Deficiency

As discussed earlier, bone deformities are the hallmarks of the vitamin D–deficient child, while porous brittle bones (osteoporosis) are indications of the deficiency in the adult.[56,57,72–74] Today, with the heavy emphasis on the use of sunscreen to prevent skin cancer,[75–77] there is concern that the people who follow this recommendation may be at greater risk for developing vitamin D deficiency disorders unless they consume adequate amounts of vitamin D in the food. A recent population study of children in the northeastern part of the United States revealed low serum levels of 25(OH) D and these low levels were associated with reduced bone mass.[53] Nutrition scientists are currently discussing whether the recommended intake for the vitamin should be increased so as to prevent vitamin D deficiency.

In the child and the adult, osteoporosis can develop not only because of inadequate vitamin intake but also may be due to disease or damage to either the liver or kidney. As pointed out in the metabolism section, both these organs are essential for the conversion of cholecalciferol to 1,25-dihydroxy D_3. If either organ is nonfunctional in this respect, the deficient state will develop. On rare occasions, the deficient state will develop because of a mutation in the gene for the enzyme 1,25-hydroxylase. In the absence of the action of this enzyme, the 1,25-dihydroxy D_3 cannot be synthesized. In individuals so afflicted, 1,25-dihydroxy D_3 must be supplied to prevent the deficiency state from developing. 1,25-Dihydroxy D_3 must also be provided to the patient whose kidneys are not working or whose kidneys have been removed, since these patients cannot synthesize this hormone. Until the realization that the kidney served as the endocrine organ for 1,25-dihydroxy D_3 synthesis, renal disease was almost always accompanied by a disturbed calcium balance and osteoporosis.

Hypervitaminosis D

Since the vitamin is fat soluble, it, like vitamin A, can be stored. The storage capacity of the liver for the D precursor is much less than its capacity for A, and toxic conditions can develop if large amounts of D (in excess of need and storage capacity) are consumed over extended periods of time. Excessive amounts of vitamin D are not available from natural sources. Those individuals given supplements are those at risk for vitamin toxicity. This is a concern in the treatment of patients with hypoparathyroidism, vitamin D–resistant rickets, renal osteodystrophy, osteoporosis, psoriasis, and some cancers and those who take vitamin supplements for nonmedical reasons.[74] Because D's main function is to facilitate calcium uptake from the intestine and tissue calcium deposition, excess D in the toxic range will result in excess calcification not only of bone but of soft tissues as well. Symptoms of intoxication include hypercalcemia, hypercalciuria, anorexia, nausea, vomiting, thirst, polyuria, muscular weakness, joint pain, diffuse demineralization of bones, and disorientation. If the supplements are not stopped immediately upon recognition of the problem, death can occur. Renal stones and calcification of the heart, major vessels, muscles, and other tissues have been shown in experimental animals as well as in humans. A series of patients have been described who were unusually sensitive to vitamin D either in utero or in infancy. These patients had multiple abnormalities in soft tissues and bones and were mentally retarded. Whether excess D intakes provoke mild, moderate, or severe abnormalities is related not only to the individual's genetic background but also to his/her calcium, magnesium, and phosphorus intake. If any of these are consumed in excess of the others, vitamin D intoxication becomes more apparent. If caught early, these effects of intoxication can be reversed. Hathcock et al.[78] has suggested that upper tolerable intake limit for this vitamin is ≥250 μg/day (10,000 IU vitamin D_3). This value is higher than that suggested by the Food and Nutrition Board of the National Academy of Medicine.

Need

Because the active D_3 hormone can be synthesized in the body, an absolute requirement is difficult to determine. Few foods naturally contain sufficient preformed vitamin D. In the absence of in vivo synthesis, preformed vitamin D must be added to the diet. This is done almost to excess in the United States. Milk is fortified with 10 μg/quart and other products such as margarine are also fortified with the vitamin. Due to this fortification, infantile rickets is almost unknown today. The level of supplementation for milk was selected based on the concept that the growing child should drink one quart of milk a day, and if he/she does this, he/she will receive the recommended daily intake for growth. Adults usually do not require vitamin supplementation unless they are either pregnant or lactating. Pregnant or lactating females are also recommended to consume 10 μg vitamin D/day. There is considerable discussion today about these recommendations with respect to the relationship between sun exposure and the development of skin cancer.[75–78] Because of the fear of skin cancer, more people are using sunscreen to block the harmful actions of UV light. In blocking UV light, these people are also inadvertently blocking the synthesis of active vitamin D. One study followed 528 individuals for 5 years and examined the relationship between sun exposure and melanoma incidence and survival. Poorly nourished individuals were far more likely to die from melanoma than well-nourished individuals. One of the conclusions of this study was that individuals having an excellent vitamin D status were more likely to survive melanoma and that exposure to sunlight was the reason.[77]

VITAMIN E

While much of the excitement of the *vitamin discovery era* was devoted to the work on vitamins A and D, Evans and Bishop in 1922 discovered an unidentified factor in vegetable oil that if lacking from the diet resulted in reproductive failure. The term tocopherol was proposed by Emerson for this factor because of its role in reproduction. Rats fed diets lacking this vitamin failed to reproduce. The name tocopherol comes from the Greek words *tokos*, meaning childbirth; *pherein*, meaning to bring forth; and *ol*, the chemical suffix meaning alcohol. Vitamin E, the name suggested by Evans and Bishop, is commonly used for that group of tocol and tocotrienol derivatives having vitamin E activity. The most active of these is α-tocopherol (Figure 11.12). Much of the earlier work was devoted to tocopherol's role in reproduction such that its function as an antioxidant was ignored. However, in the last 40 years, considerable attention has been given to this role in metabolism. It is recognized that vitamin E is an essential nutrient for many animal species. The level of vitamin E in plasma lipoproteins and in the phospholipids of the membrane around and within the cell is dependent on vitamin E intake as well as on the intake of other antioxidant nutrients and on the level of dietary polyunsaturated fatty acids. Animals fed a polyunsaturated fatty acid–rich diet require more vitamin E in their diet than animals fed a low-fat or saturated fat–rich diet.[79]

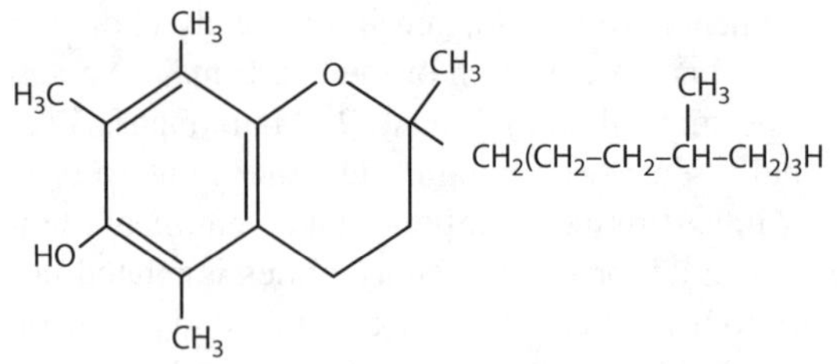

α–tocopherol (5,7,8 trimethyltocol)

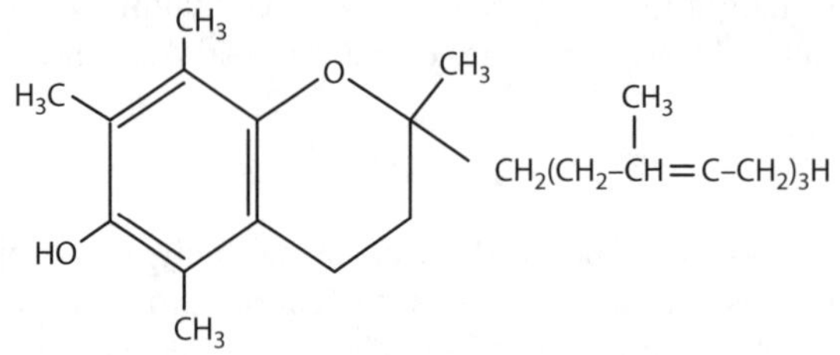

α–tocotrienol (5,7,8 trimethyltrienol)

FIGURE 11.12 Basic structures of vitamin E.

Structure and Nomenclature

The most active naturally occurring form of vitamin E is D-α-tocopherol. Other tocopherols have been isolated having varying degrees of vitamin activity. Figure 11.13 shows the other tocopherols and tocotrienols and their relationship to α-tocopherol. To have a vitamin activity, the compound must have a double-ring structure (chromane nucleus) as shown in Figures 11.12 and 11.13 and must also have a side chain attached at carbon 2 and methyl groups attached at carbons 5, 7, or 8. α-Tocopherols have methyl groups attached at all three positions and are the most active form of the vitamin. β-Tocopherols have methyl groups attached to carbons 5 and 8, γ-tocopherols have methyl groups attached at carbons 7 and 8, and δ-tocopherols have only one methyl group attached at carbon 8. If the side chain attached to carbon 2 is saturated, then the compound is a member of the tocol family of compounds; if unsaturated, it belongs to the tocotrienol family. All forms have a hydroxyl group at carbon 6 and a methyl group at carbon 2. Other forms, ε, ζ, and η, have their methyl groups at carbon 5, 5 and 7, or 7, respectively. Naturally occurring vitamin E is in the D form, whereas synthetic vitamin E preparations are mixtures of the D and L forms. Both tocols and trienols occur as a variety of isomers. There are commercially available products usually marketed as acetate or succinate esters. The ester form does not usually occur in nature. Table 11.11 lists some of these commercially available forms.

International Units and Methods of Analysis

The IU of vitamin E activity uses the activity of 1 mg of DL-α-tocopherol acetate (all-*rac*) in the rat fetal absorption assay as its reference standard. Even though D-α-tocopherol is 36% more active than the DL form, the latter was selected as the reference substance because it is readily available as a standard of comparison. This choice may be a poor one because of the lack of validation of the fetal rat absorption assay as a true test of vitamin E potency. The fetal resorption test uses female vitamin E–depleted virgin rats. These rats are mated to normal males and given the test substance. After 21 days, the number of live fetuses and the number of dead and resorbed ones are counted. The potency of the test material is compared to a known amount of DL-α-tocopherol. Other tests have also been devised and are based on other functions of vitamin E. These tests may yield more

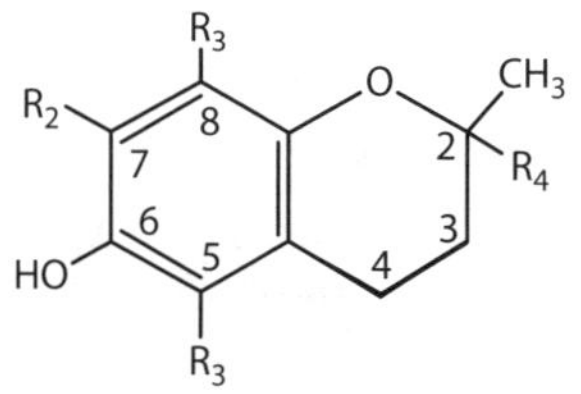

$R_1R_2R_3{=}CH_3$ or H

$R_4{=}CH_2\ (CH_2CH_2\overset{CH_3}{C}HCH_2)_3H$ (tocols)

or $CH_2(CH_2CH{=}\overset{CH_3}{C}\ CH_2)_3H$ (tocotrienols)

α-tocol or tocotrienol have $R_1R_2R_3{=}CH_3$

β-tocol or tocotrienol have $R_1R_3-CH_3$, R=H

γ-tocol or tocotrienol have $R_2R_3{=}CH_3$, $R_1{=}H$

δ-tocol or tocotrienol have $R_3{=}CH_3$, $R_1R_2{=}H$

ε-tocol or tocotrienol have $R_1{=}CH_3$ $R_2R_3{=}H$

ζ-tocol or tocotrienol have $R_1,R_2{=}CH_3$ $R_3{=}H$

η-tocol or tocotrienol have $R_2{=}C_{+3}$, $R_1R_3{=}H$

FIGURE 11.13 Structures of naturally occurring compounds having vitamin E activity.

TABLE 11.11
Commercially Available Products Having Vitamin E Activity

Form	Units of Activity (mg)
DL-α-tocopheryl acetate (all-*rac*)	1.00
DL-α-tocopherol (all-*rac*)	1.10
D-α-tocopheryl acetate (RRR)[a]	1.36
D-α-tocopheryl acid succinate (all-*rac*)	1.49
DL-α-tocopheryl acid succinate (all-*rac*)	0.89
D-α-tocopheryl acid succinate (RRR)[a]	1.21

[a] RRR, only naturally occurring stereoisomers bear this designation.

reliable comparisons and may result in a redefinition of the IU. Tests of biopotency include the red cell hemolysis test and tests designed to evaluate the potency of the test substance in preventing or curing muscular dystrophy. Using DL-α-tocopherol as the standard with a value of 100, β-tocopherol has a value of 25–40 on the fetal resorption test, 15–27 on the hemolysis test, and 12 on the preventative muscular dystrophy test using the chicken as the test animal. γ-Tocopherol is even less potent with values of 1–11, 3–20, and 5 for the same tests, respectively. The other tocopherols and tocotrienols are even less potent by comparison. Burton and Traber have reviewed the biopotency of vitamin E isomers as antioxidants.[80]

TABLE 11.12
Characteristics of the Major Tocopherols

Compound	Color	Boiling Point (°C)	Molecular Weight	Absorption Maxima (nm)	Extraction (Ethanol)
DL-α-tocopherol	Colorless to pale yellow	200–220	430.69	292–294	71–76
D-α-tocopherol	Colorless to pale yellow	—	430.69	292–294	72–76
DL-α-tocopherol acetate	Colorless to pale yellow	224	472.73	285.5	40–44
D-α-tocopheryl acetate	Colorless to pale yellow	—	472.73	285.5	40–44

Biochemical methods that utilize changes in enzyme activity rather than functional tests such as the rat fetal resorption test allow for the comparison of the different E vitamin forms. For example, plasma pyruvate kinase, hepatic glutathione peroxidase, and muscle cyclooxygenase activities are reduced in vitamin E–deficient rats. However, a true dose response curve showing intake versus changes in enzyme activity patterns that in turn precede tissue changes does not clearly provide a basis for biopotency. These enzyme activity studies are not as sensitive with respect to vitamin intake and potency as one would like.

Chemical analyses using thin-layer chromatography, gas–liquid chromatography, and HPLC are now available. These methods are very sensitive and can separate and quantify the various isomers in food, plasma, blood cells, and tissues. The HPLC method is the one of the choices because sample preparation is minimal. Amounts of the isomers in the nanogram range can be detected and quantified.

Physical and Chemical Properties

The tocopherols are slightly viscous oils that are stable to heat and alkali. They are slowly oxidized by atmospheric oxygen and rapidly oxidized by iron or silver salts. The addition of acetate or succinate to the molecule adds stability toward oxidation. The tocopherols are insoluble in water but soluble in the usual fat solvents. UV light destroys its vitamin activity. Table 11.12 gives the properties of four of the most potent tocopherols.

Sources

The tocopherols have been isolated from a number of foods. Almost all are from the plant kingdom with wheat germ oil being the richest source. European wheat germ oil contains mostly β-tocopherols, while American wheat germ oil contains mostly α-tocopherols. Corn oil contains α-tocopherols and soybean oil δ-tocopherols. Olive and peanut oil are poor sources of the vitamin. Some animal products such as egg yolk, liver, and milk contain tocopherols, but, in general, foods of animal origin are relatively poor sources of the vitamin. Table 11.13 provides values of tocopherols in a variety of foods. A more extensive list of foods and their vitamin E content can be found using the USDA website, www.nal.usda.gov/foodcomposition. Vegetable oils vary from 100 μg/g (olive oil) to nearly 1200 μg/g (wheat germ oil). Some of the foods shown in this table have a range of values given because of seasonal variations due to differences in intakes and needs of the animal from which these foods come.

Metabolism

Absorption and Transport

Because of its lipophilicity, vitamin E like the other fat-soluble vitamins, is absorbed via the formation of chylomicrons and their uptake by the lymphatic system. The tocopherols are transported as part of the lipoprotein complex.[79,80] Absorption is relatively poor. In man, studies of labeled

TABLE 11.13
Vitamin E Content of a Variety of Foods

Food	α-Tocopherol (μg/g)
Corn oil	159
Olive oil	100
Peanut oil	189
Wheat germ oil	1194
Palm oil	211
Soft margarine	139
Milk	0.2–1.1
Butter	10–33
Lard	2–38
Eggs	8–12
Fish	4–33
Beef	5–8
Pork	4–6
Chicken	2–4
Almonds	270
Peanuts	72
Oatmeal	17
Rice	1–7
Wheat germ	117
Apple	3
Peach	13
Asparagus	16
Spinach	25
Carrots	4

Source: http://www.nal.usda.gov/foodcomposition.

tocopherol absorption have shown that less than half of the labeled material appears in the lymph and up to 50% of the ingested vitamin may appear in the feces.[79] Efficiency of absorption is enhanced by the presence of food fat in the intestine. Within this macronutrient class, efficiency of absorption is enhanced by saturated fat and decreased by the presence of polyunsaturated fatty acids. The use of water-miscible preparations enhances absorption efficiency particularly in those individuals whose fat absorption is impaired, that is, persons with cystic fibrosis or biliary disease. The commercially prepared tocopherol acetate or palmitate loses the acetate or palmitate through the action of a bile-dependent mucosal cell esterase prior to absorption. The pancreatic lipases, bile acids, and mucosal cell esterases are all important components of the digestion and absorption of vitamin E from food sources. The same processes required for the digestion and absorption of food fat apply here for the tocopherols. Absorption through penetration of the apical plasma membrane of the enterocytes of the brush border is maximal in the jejunum. There are some species differences in the process in that mammals absorb the vitamin as part of a lipoprotein complex (chylomicrons) into the lymph, whereas birds have the vitamin transported directly into the portal blood. In addition, there are gender differences in absorption efficiency: females are more efficient than males. Unlike the food fats (cholesterol and the acylglycerides), hydrolysis is not followed by reesterification in the absorption process.

It appears that the tocopherols are bound to all of the lipid-carrying proteins in the blood and lymph. An excellent antioxidant, vitamin E serves this function very well as it is being transported (from enterocyte to target tissue) with those lipids that could be peroxidized and thus require protection.[79,80] Some cardiovascular researchers have suggested that one important function of vitamin E is to prevent the peroxidation of lipids in the blood, which would in turn suppress possible endothelial damage to the vascular tree and thus suppress some of the early events in plaque formation.[81–89] Whether this hypothesis about the role of vitamin E in preventing such degenerative disease is true remains to be proven.

Intracellular Transport and Storage

Although no specific transport protein has been found for the tocopherols in the blood and lymph, there appears to be such a protein within the cells.[86–88] A 30 kDa α-tocopherol-binding protein has been found in the hepatic cytosol and another 14.2 kDa in the heart and liver that specifically binds to α-tocopherol and transfers it from the liposomes to mitochondria. No doubt, we will also find that either this or another low-molecular-weight protein transfers the vitamin to the nucleus. Having the vitamin in these two organelles protects them from free radical damage. One of the targets of free radicals is the genetic material DNA, while the other is the membrane phospholipid. In either instance, damage to these vital components could be devastating. The smaller of the two binding proteins is similar in size to the intracellular fatty acid–binding protein (FABP). This protein also binds some of the eicosanoids but not α-tocopherol. The other tocopherols (β, γ, etc.) are not bound to the tocopherol-binding proteins to the same extent as α-tocopherol nor are these isomers retained as well. Tocopherols are found in all of the cells in the body with adrenal cells, pituitary cells, platelets, and testicular cells having the most per cell. The adipose tissue, muscle, and liver serve as reservoirs, and these tissues will become depleted should intake levels be inadequate to meet the need. The rate of depletion with dietary inadequacy varies considerably. Since its main function is as one of several antioxidants, other nutrients that also serve in this capacity can affect vitamin depletion. The intake of β-carotene and ascorbic acid and also the level of polyunsaturated fatty acid intake can markedly affect the rate of use of α-tocopherol as an antioxidant.[88,91–93] Increased intakes of β-carotene and ascorbic acid protect the α-tocopherol against depletion, whereas increased intakes of polyunsaturated fatty acids drive up the need for antioxidants. A further consideration is the intake of selenium.[92] This mineral is an integral part of the glutathione peroxidase system that suppresses free radical production. In selenium-deficient animals, the need for α-tocopherol is increased and vice versa. The α-tocopherol-deficient animal has a greater need for selenium. In addition, α-tocopherol protects against iron toxicity in another instance of a mineral vitamin interaction.[90] In this instance, high levels of iron drive up the potential for free radical formation and this can be overcome with increases in vitamin E intake.

Plasma vitamin E concentrations are variable and in some instances are related to polymorphisms in one or more genes.[94–96] Polymorphisms in the CD36/FAT gene can modulate blood vitamin E levels[96] as can SIRT1 polymorphisms[95] and polymorphisms in the cytokine genes.[94] Vitamin E has been shown to affect cytokine production especially TNFα. The production of this cytokine is higher in 308G than in 308A polymorphism in the gene for TNFα.[94]

Catabolism and Excretion

Upon entry into the cell, very little degradation occurs. Usually less than 1% of the ingested vitamin (or its metabolite) appears in the urine. Compounds called Simon's metabolites appear in the urine. These are glucuronates of the parent compound. The major excretory route is via the intestine. Figure 11.14 illustrates this pathway.

Function

As mentioned, the main function of vitamin E is as an antioxidant. This function is shared by β-carotene, ascorbic acid, the selenium-dependent glutathione peroxidase, and the copper–manganese- and magnesium-dependent superoxide dismutase (see fatty acid peroxidation in Chapter 10).

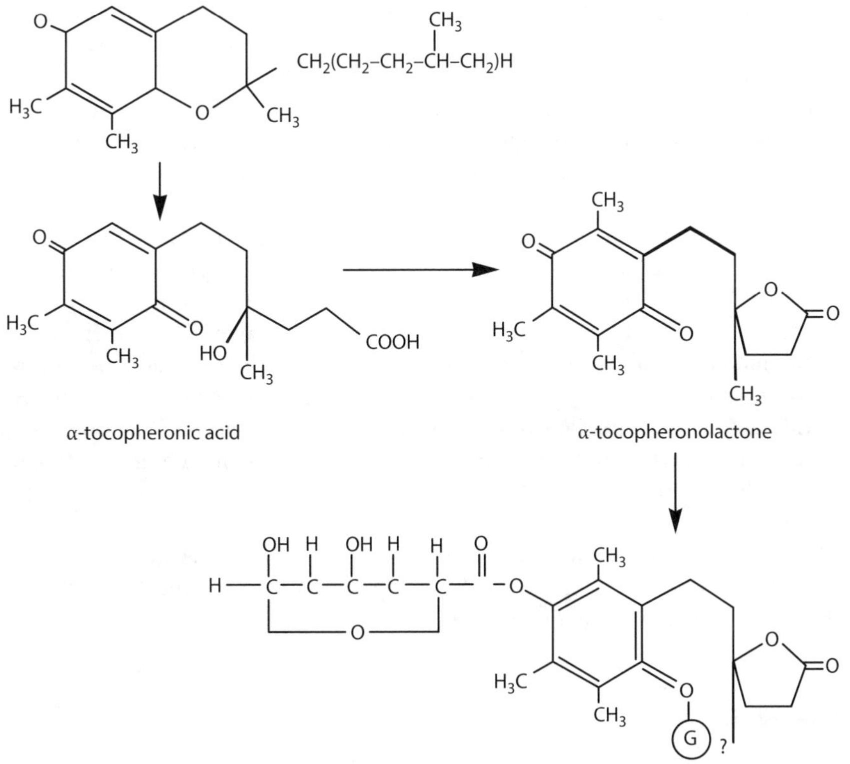

α-tocopheronic acid

α-tocopheronolactone

FIGURE 11.14 Excretory pathway for the tocopherols. These compounds are found in the feces.

In erythrocytes, the enzyme glutathione peroxidase protects hemoglobin and the cell membrane from oxidation by maintaining glutathione levels, thus regulating the redox state of the cells. This enzyme protects hemoglobin and the cell membrane by detoxifying lipid hydroperoxides to less toxic fatty acids and by preventing the initial free radical attack on the membrane lipids. Although this is a selenoenzyme, vitamin E potentiates its action by serving as a free radical scavenger to prevent lipid hydroperoxide formation.

Glutathione peroxidase has been found in other cells as well. It is present in adipose tissue, liver, muscles, and glandular tissue, and its activity is complementary to that of catalase, another enzyme that uses peroxide as a substrate. Together, these enzymes and vitamin E protect the integrity of the membranes by preventing the degradation, through oxidation, of the membrane lipids. This function of vitamin E is seen more clearly in animals fed high levels of polyunsaturated fatty acids.[97–99] As the intake of these acids increases, they are increasingly incorporated into the membrane lipids, which in turn become more vulnerable to oxidation. Unless protected against oxidation, the functionality of the membranes will be impaired and if uncorrected, the cell will die.[99] In addition, there is DNA damage by the increase in the intake of polyunsaturated fatty acid that was ameliorated by vitamin E supplementation.[96] Disturbances in the transport of materials across membranes have been shown in the liver with respect to cation flux. Liver slices from E-deficient animals lost the ability to regulate sodium/potassium exchange and calcium flux. Investigators have shown a decline in mitochondrial respiration in vitamin E–deficient rats. Damage to the mitochondrial DNA could result in aberrant mitochondrial gene products.[97] Thus, a whole cascade of responses to vitamin E insufficiency can be envisioned. Interestingly, in diseases manifested by an increased hemolysis of the red cells and a decreased ability of the hemoglobin to carry oxygen, red cell vitamin E levels are low. This has been shown in patients with sickle cell anemia and in patients with cystic fibrosis. In patients with sickle cell anemia, the low vitamin E level in the erythrocytes is accompanied by an increased level of glutathione peroxidase activity. It has been suggested that the increase in enzyme activity was compensatory to the decrease in vitamin E content.

Vitamin E and zinc have been found to have interacting effects in the protection of skin lipids. In zinc-deficient chicks, supplementation with vitamin E decreased the severity of the zinc deficiency state suggesting that zinc also may have antioxidant properties or that there may be an interacting effect of zinc with the vitamin.

In addition to this main function of vitamin E, there are other roles for this substance. One involves eicosinoid synthesis. Thromboxane (TXA_2), a platelet-aggregating factor, is synthesized from arachidonic acid (20:4) via a free radical–mediated reaction.[98] This synthesis is greater in a deficient animal than in an adequately nourished one. Vitamin E enhances prostacyclin formation and inhibits the lipoxygenase and phospholipase reactions. As mentioned, phospholipase A_2 is stimulated by lipid peroxides. Other secondary functions also are related to its antioxidant function. Oxidant damage to DNA in the bone marrow could explain red blood cell deformation as well as explain the fragility (due to membrane damage) of these cells.[99] In turn, this would explain why enhanced red cell fragility is a characteristic of the deficient state.

Steroid hormone synthesis as well as spermatogenesis, both processes that are impaired in the deficient animal, could be explained by the damaging effects of free radicals on DNA, which are corrected by the provision of this antioxidant vitamin.

Hypervitaminosis E

Even though vitamin E is a fat-soluble vitamin like A and D, there is little evidence that high intakes will result in toxicity in man. Excess is excreted in feces; however, E toxicity has been produced in chickens. It is characterized by growth failure, poor bone calcification, depressed hematocrit, and increased prothrombin times. These symptoms suggest that the excess E interfered with the absorption and/or use of the other fat-soluble vitamins since these symptoms are those of the A, D, and K deficiency states. This suggests that advocates of megadoses of vitamin E as treatment for heart disease, muscular dystrophy, and infertility (among other ailments) may unwittingly advocate the development of additional problems associated with an imbalance in fat-soluble vitamin intake due to these large E intakes.

Deficiency

One of the first deficiency symptoms recorded for the tocopherols was infertility, followed by the discovery that the white muscle disease or a peculiar muscle dystrophy could be reversed if vitamin E was provided. Later, it was recognized that selenium also played a role in the muscle symptom. Listed in Table 11.14 are the many symptoms attributed to inadequate vitamin E intake. All of these symptoms are related either primarily to the level of peroxides in the tissue or to peroxide damage to either the membranes and/or DNA.

Need

Because of the interacting effects of vitamin E with selenium and other antioxidants, the requirement for the vitamin has been difficult to ascertain. It has been estimated that the average adult consumes approximately 15 mg/day but the range of intake is very large. The DRIs are shown in Table 11.1. DRIs are periodically reviewed and updates can be found on the DRI website www.nap.edu.

TABLE 11.14
Vitamin E Deficiency Disorders

Disorder	Species Affected	Tissue Affected
Reproductive failure		
Female	Rodents, birds	Embryonic vascular tissue
Male	Rodents, dog, birds, monkey, rabbit	Male gonads
Hepatic necrosis[a]	Rat, pig	Liver
Fibrosis[a]	Chicken, mouse	Pancreas
Hemolysis[b,c]	Rat, chick, premature infant	Erythrocytes
Anemia	Monkey	Bone marrow
Encephalomalacia[b,c]	Chick	Cerebellum
Exudative diathesis[a]	Birds	Vascular system
Kidney degeneration[a,b]	Rodents, monkey, mink	Kidney tabular epithelium
Steatitis[b,c]	Mink, pig, chick	Adipose tissue
Nutritional myopathies		
Type A muscular dystrophy	Rodents, monkey, duck, mink	Skeletal muscle
Type B white muscle disease[a]	Lamb, calf, kid	Skeletal and heart muscle
Type C myopathy[a]	Turkey	Gizzard, heart
Type D myopathy	Chicken	Skeletal muscle

[a] Can be reversed by the addition of selenium to the diet.
[b] Increased intake of polyunsaturated acids potentiates deficiency.
[c] Antioxidants can be substituted for vitamin E to cure condition.

VITAMIN K

Even though vitamin K was one of the last fat-soluble vitamins discovered, its existence was suspected as early as 1929. In that year, Henrik Dam was studying cholesterol biosynthesis and observed that chickens fed a semisynthetic sterol-free diet had numerous subcutaneous hemorrhages. Hemorrhages were observed in other tissues as well, and when blood was withdrawn from these birds, it had a prolonged clotting time. At first, it was thought that these were symptoms of scurvy in birds, but the addition of vitamin C did not cure the disorder. It was then thought that the hemorrhages characterized the bird's response to a dietary toxin. This hypothesis was also disproved. Finally, it was shown that the inclusion of plant sterols prevented the disease, and thus, the disease was shown to be a nutrient deficiency.

Because the condition was characterized by a delayed blood clotting time and because it could be cured or prevented by the inclusion of the nonsaponifiable sterol fraction of a lipid extract of alfalfa, it was named the antihemorrhagic factor. Dam proposed that it be called vitamin K. The letter K was chosen from the German word *koagulation*.

Structure and Nomenclature

Subsequent to its recognition as an essential micronutrient, vitamin K was isolated from alfalfa and from fish meal. The compounds isolated from these two sources were not identical so one was named K_1 and the other K_2. Almquist was the first to show that the vitamin could be synthesized by bacteria. He discovered that putrefied fish meal contained more of the vitamin than nonputrefied fish meal. It was also learned that bacteria in the intestine of both the rat and the chicken synthesized the vitamin, thus ensuring a good supply of the vitamin if coprophagy (eating feces) were permitted.

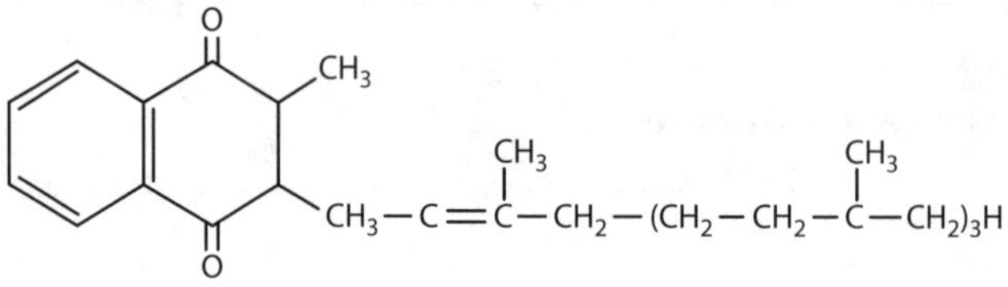

FIGURE 11.15 Structures of vitamin K_1 (phylloquinone), K_2 (menaquinone), and K_3 (menadione), a synthetic precursor that is converted to K2 by the intestinal flora.

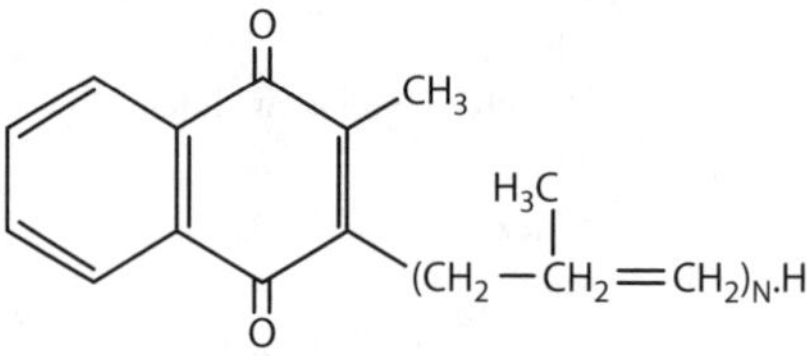

These early studies thus provided the reason to suspect that there was more than one form of the vitamin. A large number of compounds, all related to a 2-methyl-1,4-naphthoquinone, possess vitamin K activity (Figure 11.15). Compounds isolated from plants have a phytyl radical at position 3 and are members of the K_1 family of compounds. Phylloquinone (2-methyl-3-phytyl-1,4-naphthoquinone (II)) is the most important member of this family. The K vitamins are identified by their family and by the length of the side chain attached at position 3. The shorthand designation uses the letter K with a subscript to indicate family and a superscript to indicate the side chain length. Thus, K_2^{20} indicates a member of the family of compounds isolated from animal sources having a 20-carbon side chain. The character of the side chain determines whether a compound is a member of the K_1 or K_2 family. K_1 compounds have a saturated side chain, whereas K_2 compounds have an unsaturated side chain. Chain lengths of the K_1 and K_2 vitamins can vary from 5 to 35 carbons.

A third family of compounds is the K_3 family. These compounds lack the side chain at carbon 3. Menadione is the parent compound name and it is a solid crystalline material (a salt) as shown in Figure 11.15, menadione sodium bisulfite. Other salts are also available. These salts are water soluble and thus have a great use in diet formulations or mixed animal feeds. Clinically useful is menadiol sodium diphosphate. The use of this must be very carefully monitored as overdoses can result in hyperbilirubinemia and jaundice. These K_3 compounds can be synthesized in the laboratory. When consumed as a dietary ingredient, the quinone structure is converted by the intestinal flora to a member of the K_2 family.

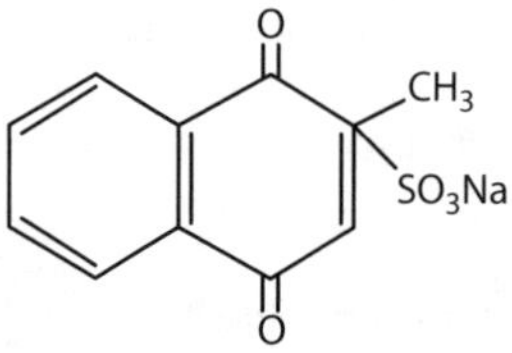

There are several structural requirements for vitamin activity: there must be a methyl group at carbon 2 and a side chain at carbon 3. The benzene ring must be unsubstituted. The chain length can vary; however, optimal activity is observed in compounds having a 20-carbon side chain. K_1 and K_2 compounds with similar chains have similar vitamin activities. The vitamin can exist in either the *cis* or *trans* configuration. All *trans*-phylloquinone is the naturally occurring form, whereas synthetic phylloquinone is a mixture of the *cis* and *trans* forms.

TABLE 11.15
Comparative Potency[a] of Various Members of the Phylloquinone and Menaquinone Families of Vitamin K

Side Chain Length (# Carbons)	Family: Phylloquinone	Family: Menaquinone
10	10	15
15	30	40
20	100	100
25	80	120
30	50	100
35	—	70

[a] Phylloquinone, K_1^{20}, is given a value of 100 and the remaining compounds are compared to this compound with reference to its biological function in promoting clot formation.

Biopotency

The various compounds with vitamin activity are not equivalent with respect to potency as a vitamin. The most potent compound of the phylloquinone series is the one with a 20-member side chain. Compounds having fewer or greater numbers of carbons are less active. Table 11.15 provides this comparison. The most potent compound in the menaquinone series is the one with a 25-member unsaturated side chain.

Physical and Chemical Properties

Phylloquinone (K_1^{20}) is a yellow viscous oil. The physical state of menaquinone (K_2^{20}) depends on its side chain length. If the side chain is 5 or 10 carbons long, it is an oil; if longer, it is a solid. Menadione (K_3) is a solid. All three families of compounds are soluble in fat solvents. Menadione can be made water soluble by converting it to a sodium salt. All the vitamin K compounds are stable to air and moisture but unstable to UV light. They are also stable in acid solutions but are destroyed by alkali and reducing agents. These compounds possess a distinctive absorption spectra because of the presence of the napthoquinone ring system.

Chemical Assays

Many different assays have been proposed for vitamin K but they all face the same problem: vitamin K is normally present in very low concentrations and numerous interfering substances, such as quinones, chlorophyll, and carotenoid pigments, are usually present.

Several colorimetric methods have been developed. One of the first, known as the Dam–Karrer reaction, is the measurement of the reddish-brown color that forms when sodium ethylate reacts with vitamin K. In another method, menadione, as the sodium sulfite, is reduced and then titrated to a green endpoint with ceric sulfate. In yet another, menadione is converted to its 2,4-dinitrophenylhydrazone when heated with 2,4-dinitrophenylhydrazine in ethanol. An excess of ammonia causes the solution to become blue-green with an absorption maxima at 635 nm.

As mentioned earlier, the K vitamins have a characteristic UV absorption spectrum. If the material is sufficiently pure, it can be identified and quantitated. Vitamin K has also been quantitated by a thin-layer and gas chromatographic technique. The menadione content of foodstuffs has been determined with HPLC. This technique has been used to determine the blood and tissue levels of the vitamin in humans. As little as 0.5 mmol/L has been detected in the blood of newborns and adults. Regardless of the assay method used, the analytical procedure should include protection of the samples from light. All of the vitamers are sensitive to UV light and will decompose if exposed. Care also should be exercised with respect to pH. The K vitamers are sensitive to alkali but are relatively stable to oxidants and heat. They can be safely extracted using vacuum distillation.

Bioassays

One of the earliest biotechniques for measuring vitamin K content of foods uses the chick. This method is sensitive to 0.1 μg phylloquinone/g diet. In this assay, newly hatched chicks are fed a K-free diet for 10 days and thus made deficient. They are then fed a supplement containing the assay food. The prothrombin level of the blood is then compared with a standard curve resulting from the feeding of known amounts of phylloquinone.

Instead of measuring prothrombin concentration, plasma prothrombin times may be measured. Prothrombin time is an indirect and inverse measurement of the amount of prothrombin in the blood: an increase in prothrombin time signifies a decrease in prothrombin concentration. The technique commonly used is a modification of the one-stage method developed by A. J. Quick. Blood removed from a patient or animal is immediately oxalated; oxalate binds the calcium and prevents prothrombin from changing into thrombin. Later, an excess of thromboplastic substance (obtained from rabbit or rat brain) and calcium is added to the plasma and the clotting time of the plasma is noted; this time is the prothrombin time. The normal prothrombin time is approximately 12 s; however, the actual time depends to a large extent on the exact procedure employed. To be valid, the prothrombin time of a vitamin K–deficient animal must be compared to that of a vitamin K–sufficient individual.

Biosynthesis

Although not too much is known about the biosynthesis of phylloquinone in plants, apparently the synthesis occurs at the same time as that of chlorophyll. The vitamin concentration is richest in that part of the plant that is photosynthetically active: carrot tops are a good source but not the root; peas sprouted in light contain more than peas sprouted in the dark; and the inner leaves of cabbage have about one-fourth less vitamin than the outer leaves.

Menaquinone is synthesized by intestinal bacteria in the distal small intestine and in the colon by intestinal bacteria. Martius and Esser found that chicks fed a vitamin K–deficient diet and then given menadione (K_3) for long periods of time will synthesize menaquinone (K_2^{20}). Apparently, this synthesis is more complete at small physiological doses than at high doses, such as are used when vitamin K is given as an antidote to dicumarol. Because of the intestinal biosynthesis, experimental animals used in K deficiency studies should be protected from coprophagy.

All of the natural forms of the K vitamins can be stored in the liver. Menadione is not stored as such but is stored as its conversion product, menaquinone. Menadione metabolism by the liver occurs at the expense of the redox state. When menadione is metabolized by Ca^{++}-loaded mitochondria, there is a rapid oxidation and loss of pyridine nucleotides and a decrease in ATP level. The effects of menadione on Ca^{++} homeostasis are probably initiated by NAD(P)H: (quinone acceptor) oxidoreductase. Large amounts of menadione have been shown to alter the surface structure and reduce the thiol content of the liver cell. Because of these changes, menadione is cytotoxic in large quantities. This may explain the induction of jaundice in the newborn of mothers given large doses of menadione just prior to delivery. This once popular obstetric practice has been discontinued. Using labeled vitamin, it was found that rats stored the vitamin in the liver. Fifty percent of the vitamin was found bound to the endoplasmic reticulum. When *cis* and *trans* forms were compared, the biologically active *trans* isomer was found in the rough membrane fraction (endoplasmic reticulum), whereas the inactive *cis* isomer was found in the mitochondria.

Antagonists, Antivitamins

Blood coagulation can be inhibited by a variety of agents that are clinically useful. Oxalates, heparin, and sodium citrate are but a few of these useful anticoagulants. These compounds work by binding one or more of the essential ingredients for clot formation. One group of anticoagulants acts by antagonizing vitamin K in its role in prothrombin compounds. The first of these is 3,3′-methyl-*bis*-(4-hydroxycoumarin) called dicumarol. It was isolated from spoiled sweet clover and was shown to cause a hemorrhagic disease in cattle. Dicumarol has been found very useful in the clinical setting as an anticoagulant in people at risk for coronary events. It is marketed as coumarin. Another use is as a rodenticide, marketed as warfarin. The structure of warfarin is also shown in Figure 11.16. A third group of antivitamin K compounds is the 2-substituted 1,3-indandiones. These are useful as rodenticides but because they can cause liver damage, they are not used in the clinical setting.

Absorption

Under normal physiologic conditions, most nutrients are absorbed before they reach the colon. In large measure, this is true of the K vitamins. However, vitamin K can be absorbed very well by the colon. This is an advantage to the individual since it ensures the uptake of K that is synthesized in the lower intestinal tract by the glut flora. The mechanism by which the K vitamins are absorbed and the rate at which this occurs is species dependent. Species such as the chicken, which have a rapid gut passage time, absorb the vitamin more rapidly than do species such as the rat, which have a long gut passage time. The absorption of K_1 and K_2 analogs is generally thought to occur via an

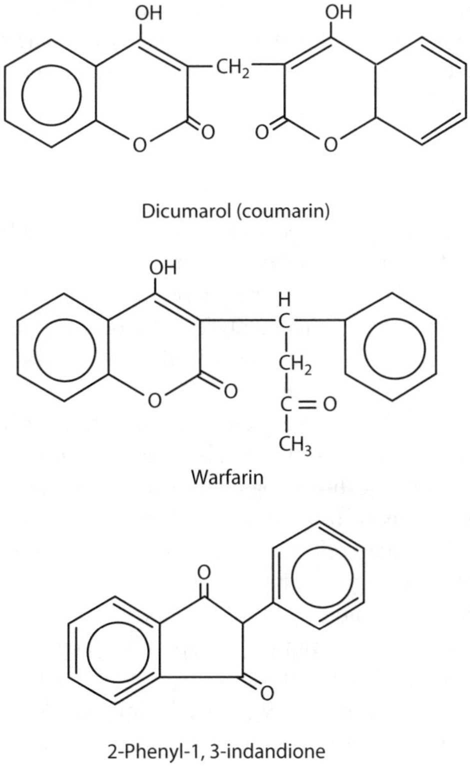

OH OH CH2 O O O O

Dicumarol (coumarin)

OH H C CH2 C=O CH3 O O

Warfarin

O O

2-Phenyl-1, 3-indandione

FIGURE 11.16 Structures of several compounds that are potent vitamin K antagonists.

active, energy-dependent, transport process, whereas K_3 (menadione) analogs are absorbed by passive diffusion.

The absorption of K_1 and K_2 requires a protein carrier and again species differ in the saturability of the carrier. In rats, the carrier is saturated at far lower vitamin concentrations than occurs in chickens. These differences in carrier saturability led early investigators to suggest that vitamin K absorption was a passive process. Subsequent studies using in vitro techniques or using labeled vitamin given in vivo showed that absorption was indeed an active process.

In contrast to the absorption of phylloquinone and the menaquinones, menadione appears to be absorbed primarily in the large intestine where the gut bacteria have converted it to a form with a side chain. Without the side chain, the absorption of K_3 is a passive process. Biosynthesis by the gut flora is an adequate source of biologically active vitamin K under normal conditions, thus making it difficult to obtain a K deficiency in humans and experimental animals. However, under conditions of stress, such as hypoprothrombinemia induced by coumarin-type anticoagulants, intestinal synthesis does not produce enough of the vitamin to overcome the effects of the drug. Proof of the importance of colonic absorption is seen in the improvement in prothrombin times in chicks and infants when given the vitamin rectally. Excessive intakes of menadione can be harmful due to their quinone structure. They can be uncouplers of OXPHOS.

Absorption of vitamin K is dependent on the presence of lipids that stimulate the release of bile and pancreatic lipases. As lipids are absorbed into the lymphatic system, so too are the K vitamers. If there is any impairment in the lipid absorption process, less vitamin K will be absorbed. For example, patients with biliary obstruction have been shown to absorb substantially less vitamin K than normal subjects.

Phylloquinone absorption shows a diurnal rhythm. In rats, the highest rate of absorption is at midnight; the lowest is at 6 am.[100] This coincides with the rats' eating pattern. The rat is a nocturnal feeder consuming most of its food between 8 p.m. and midnight. Estrogen enhances the absorption of phylloquinone for both intact and castrated males. Castrated female rats are more susceptible to uncontrolled hemorrhage due to coumarin than are intact female rats. Female rats also synthesize more prothrombin than do male rats.

Metabolism and Function

Historically, vitamin K has been regarded as a vitamin with a single function: the coagulation of blood. While the concept of this function is true, we now know that it serves as an essential cosubstrate in the posttranslational oxidative carboxylation of glutamic acid residues in a small group of specific proteins, most of which are proteins involved in blood coagulation. These proteins are the blood clotting factors II, VII, IX, and X; a calcium-binding bone protein, osteocalcin; and plasma proteins C and S.

Blood coagulation is not a single one-step phenomenon. Rather, it involves several phases that must interdigitate if a clot is to be formed. Four phases have been identified: (1) the formation of thromboplastin, (2) the activation of thromboplastin, (3) the formation of thrombin, and (4) the formation of fibrin. Following injury, a blood clot is formed when the blood protein fibrinogen is transformed into an insoluble network of fibers (fibrin) by the reaction cascade illustrated in Figure 11.17. The change of fibrinogen to fibrin (phase 4) is catalyzed by thrombin, which itself must arise from prothrombin. The synthesis of thrombin from prothrombin (phase 3) is catalyzed by prothrombinase, active proaccelerin, and the phospholipid cephalin. These factors in turn are activated by a combination of blood and tissue convertins, which represent or reflect the synthesis and activation of the thromboplastin complex (phases 1 and 2). The synthesis and activation of the thromboplastin complex requires several factors that have been named and identified. These factors, studied by different groups, were given different names, which led to considerable confusion in the understanding of the coagulation process. To clarify the literature, it was decided by the International Committee for Standardization of the Nomenclature of Blood Clotting Factors

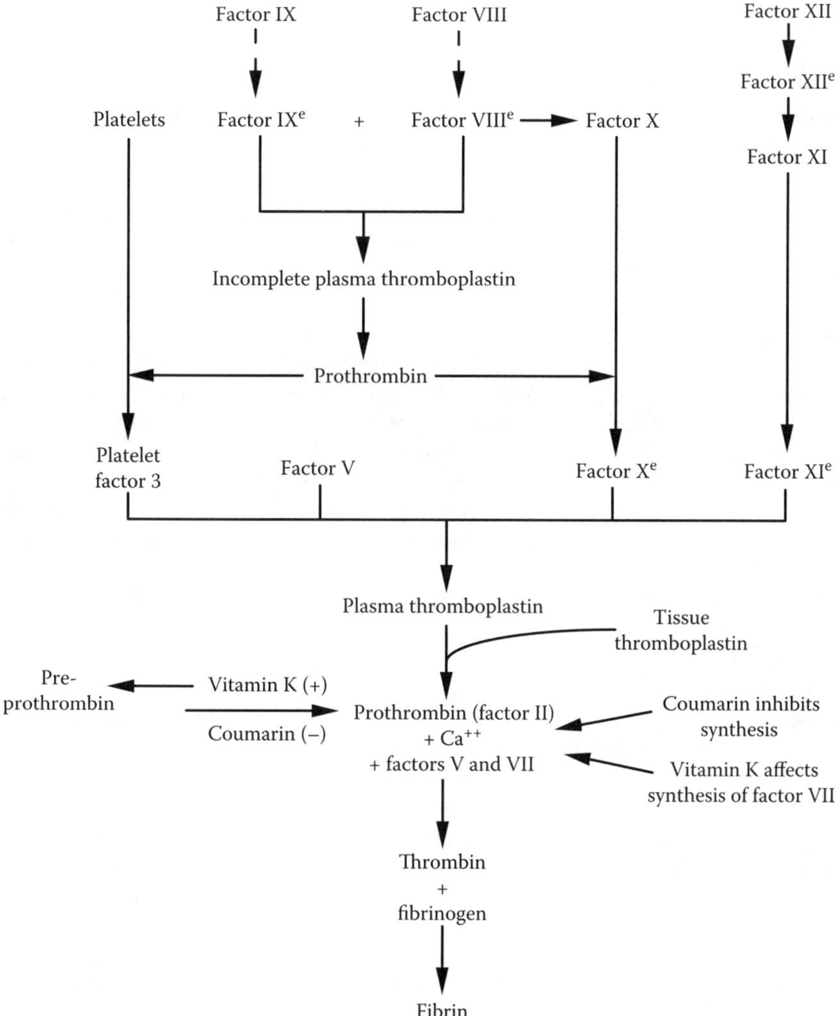

FIGURE 11.17 Formation of a clot.

to recommend the use of a numerical system for designating the various factors. This numbering system is given in Table 11.16 along with the other names in use and the function of each in the coagulation process. Note that four of the factors are proteins whose synthesis is dependent on vitamin K. These proteins, prothrombin (factor II), proconvertin (factor VII), the Christmas factor (factor IX), and the Stuart–Prower factor (factor X), are also calcium dependent. That is, calcium ions must be present for their activation and participation in the coagulation cascade (Figure 11.17). Note too that the four proteins that are vitamin K dependent are synthesized in the liver, hence the reason why the liver concentrates and stores this vitamin. One of these clotting factors, factor XIIIa, is also active in the nervous system where it may play a role in the healing of injured tissues.[101]

The function of vitamin K is as a cosubstrate in the posttranslational oxidative carboxylation of proteins at selected glutamic acid residues.[103–105] This is a cyclic process. As the vitamin serves as a cosubstrate, it is metabolized by the hepatic microsomes. Its metabolism is dependent on AIs of niacin and riboflavin, which are components of the redox systems important in the transfer of reducing equivalents. Vitamin K is reduced to the hydroquinone (vitamin KH_2)

TABLE 11.16
Blood Clotting Factors

Factor	Name	Function	Remarks
I	Fibrinogen	Provides the structural network upon which clot is formed	
II	Prothrombin	Precursor of thrombin, a proteolytic enzyme that causes fibrinogen to lose one or more peptides and polymerize	Vitamin K dependent, synthesized in liver (?).
III	Thromboplastin	Serves to stimulate prothrombin conversion to thrombin	Not a single compound; includes factors IX, XI, XII, X, and V.
IV	Calcium	Combines with prothrombin in the presence of agents	Oxalate acts as an anticoagulant by binding Ca^{++}.
V	Labile factor proaccelerin accelerator (Ac) globule	Has thromboplastic activity; released by collagen and not ADP; proceeds normally when prostaglandin synthesis is inhibited	Disappears when plasma is heated or stored with oxalate; in the activated form, may function as the Ka receptor on the platelet membrane.
VII	Proconvertin serum prothrombin conversion accelerator (SPCA) cothromboplastin, autoprothrombin I	Has thromboplastic activity	Vitamin K synthesized in liver (?).
VIII	Antihemophilic factor, antihemophilic globulin (AHG)	Activates factor X; associated with platelet membranes; may have a role in the adherence of platelets to the subendothelium	Deficiency of this factor is the cause of the classic form of hemophilia A.
IX	Plasma thromboplastic component (PTC), Christmas factor	Stimulates conversion of prothrombin to thrombin	Vitamin K–dependent deficiency results in hemophilia or Christmas disease named after the first patient to have the disease.
X	Stuart–Prower factor	Stimulates conversion of prothrombin to thrombin	Vitamin K–dependent glycoprotein; gene for human factor X is essentially identical with that for factor IX and Protein C[162a].
XI	Plasma thromboplastin antecedent (PTA)	Has thromboplastic activity	Patients with PTA are mild hemophiliacs.
XII	Hageman factor	Has thromboplastic activity	Deficiency does not result in hemophilia.
XIII	Laki–Lorand factor (LLF), fibrin-stabilizing factor	Stabilizes fibrin network; is a proenzyme in the plasma activated by thrombin and catalyzes the formation of covalent lysyl bonds between chains of fibrin monomers	
	Platelet thromboplastic factor (thromboplastin fenase)	Catalyzes formation of platelet factors	Appears when platelets disintegrate.

Source: Walsh, P.N., *Fed. Proc.*, 40, 2086, 1981.

with NADH as the coenzyme (NADH is a niacin-containing coenzyme). There are two pathways for vitamin K reduction: (1) the reduction pathway—warfarin sensitive—irreversible by coumarin and (2) DT diaphorase and microsomal dehydrogenase. This pathway is important to counteract coumarin toxicity. Upon reduction, it is then oxidized to form an epoxide. The epoxide is converted back to the quinone form by an epoxide reductase. This enzyme is a two-component cytosolic enzyme that catalyzes the reduction of the vitamin K epoxide using dithiothreitol as either a primary or secondary source of reducing equivalents. Warfarin, an antivitamin, interferes with both the reduction of vitamin K to the hydroquinone and the conversion of the epoxide back to the original compound. Warfarin is bound to a protein (likely the epoxidase and the reductase). When fed to deficient rats, the epoxide has an activity similar to that of the vitamin in inducing protein carboxylation and prothrombin synthesis. This similarity is probably due to the conversion of the epoxide to the hydroquinone. The epoxidation reaction is coupled to the carboxylation of the glutamic acid residues protruding from peptides having clusters of this amino acid. Aspartyl residues can also be carboxylated. The epoxidation reaction can be coupled to the oxidation of other peptides as well; however, only those having the clusters of glutamic acid will be oxidatively carboxylated. Unless the proteins are carboxylated, they are unable to bind calcium. For example, the precursor of prothrombin, acarboxyprothrombin, has within the first 33 amino acids at the amino-terminal end 10 tightly clustered glutamic acid residues and binds less than 1 mol of calcium per mole of protein. When carboxylated to prothrombin, the glutamic acid residues are converted to a carboxyglutamic acid residue, and now each mole of the protein can bind 10–12 mol of calcium. The carboxylated glutamic acid–rich region serves an important function in clot formation. Prior to activation by the protease factor Xa, both the prothrombin and the protease are absorbed onto the phospholipids of the damaged cells by way of calcium bridges. Without carboxylation, these bridges will not form and the adherence or absorption of the prothrombin to the phospholipids of the injured cell walls does not take place. The phospholipids are not only important to the binding of prothrombin to the injured cell wall but are also important determinants of carboxylase activity. Phosphatidyl choline has been found to be an essential component of the carboxylase enzyme system. When depleted of phospholipids, the enzyme loses activity; when repleted, its activity is restored.

Proteins other than those involved in the coagulation process have been shown to be vitamin K dependent. Carboxylated proteins have been found in the bone matrix. Up to 20% of the noncollagenous proteins (or 1%–2% of the total bone protein) is a carboxylated protein called osteocalcin. Another is called bone gla protein (BGP). Osteocalcin is synthesized in bone tissue. Bone microsomes are responsible for the posttranslational vitamin K–dependent oxidative carboxylation reaction. The synthesis of osteocalcin is highest during rapid growth periods and coincides with detectable bone mineralization.[106] The osteocalcin appears prior to mineralization and, like the blood coagulation proteins, shows a remarkable avidity for calcium. It will also bind (in order of preference after calcium) magnesium, strontium, barium, and lanthanide. In addition to its ability to bind divalent ions, osteocalcin binds hydroxyapatite, the major calcium phosphate salt of the bone. Whether osteocalcin has a direct role in bone mineralization has not been conclusively shown; however, studies of embryonic chicks treated with warfarin showed a decrease in both osteocalcin and mineralization. Warfarin-treated animals in contrast do not show this same effect; osteocalcin levels are low but bone mineralization is normal. Because the overwhelming effects of vitamin K deficiency induced through either diet or warfarin treatment result in lethal bleeding, this secondary effect on bone mineralization is difficult to study except in systems utilizing embryonic tissues.[107] Evidence of warfarin injury has been reported in humans. Mothers consuming warfarin during their first trimester of pregnancy have given birth to infants having defective bone developments such as stippled epiphyses, *saddle* nose, punctate calcifications, and frontal bossing.

BGP is a 49-residue, vitamin K–dependent protein involved in the regulation of bone calcium homeostasis rather than bone formation. It is secreted by osteosarcoma cells having an osteoblastic phenotype and appears in calcifying tissues 1–2 weeks after mineral deposition and at the approximate time that the maturation of bone mineral to hydroxyapatite is thought to occur. The synthesis and secretion of BGP from osteosarcoma cells are regulated by vitamin D. The renal cortex also contains a microsomal vitamin K–dependent oxidative carboxylation system. Its function is to produce a carboxyglutamic acid–rich protein, which serves to bind calcium. It is located in the renal tubule and may function importantly in the conservation of calcium. Unfortunately, these proteins may be entirely too active in calcium uptake and kidney stones may result. Renal stones have been found to contain a unique carboxylated peptide in addition to calcium oxalate. Whether this peptide was responsible for the stone accumulation or was attracted to it because of its high calcium content is not known.

In addition to its function as described earlier, vitamin K serves a role in the inhibition of the carcinogenic properties of benzopyrene. Menadione inhibits aryl hydrocarbon hydroxylase, thus reducing the levels of carcinogenic and mutagenic metabolites in the cell with resultant reduction in tumor formation. Vitamin K_1 and K_2 have the opposite effect. The different effects of these vitamin forms probably relate to the previously described effects of these forms on redox state, calcium ion status, and ATP production, all of which are involved in tumorigenesis.

Deficiency

Due to the fact that intestinal synthesis of vitamin K usually provides sufficient amounts of the vitamin to the body, primary vitamin K deficiency is rare. However, secondary deficiency states can develop as a result of biliary disease, which results in an impaired absorption of the vitamin. Deficiency can also occur as a result of long-term broad spectrum antibiotic therapy, which may kill the vitamin K–synthesizing intestinal flora, or as a result of anticoagulant therapy using coumadin (warfarin), which, as shown in the previous section, interferes with the metabolism and function of the vitamin. The primary characteristic of the deficiency state is a delayed or prolonged clotting time. Deficient individuals may have numerous bruises indicative of subcutaneous hemorrhaging in response to injury. Studies of human populations have shown that low intakes of vitamin K (dihydrophylloquinone) is associated with low bone mineral density.[104] Newborn infants, because they have to establish their K–synthesizing intestinal flora, have delayed coagulation times. For many years, it was common practice to give the mother an injection of menadione just prior to delivery in order to rectify the newborn's problem. However, it then became apparent that this prophylactic therapy was having no effect on the infant with respect to prothrombin time and, in addition, some infants became jaundiced with this treatment. As a result, vitamin K administration to women just prior to delivery is no longer a routine practice in obstetrics.

Sources

Phylloquinone serves as the major source of dietary vitamin K in humans. In general, studies of the vitamin K content of common foods, as determined by the chick bioassay method, reveal that green leafy vegetables contain large quantities of vitamin K, meats and dairy products intermediate quantities, and fruits and cereals small quantities. For animals, alfalfa has long been recognized as a rich source of vitamin K. The vitamin content of a variety of foods can be found on the USDA website: www.nal.usda.gov/foodcomposition.

Need

Healthy humans can usually synthesize sufficient vitamins to meet their needs. Nonetheless, there is a recommendation for vitamin K in the DRI table (see Table 11.1). Updates in the DRIs for this vitamin can be found on the NIH DRI website: www.nap.edu.

SUMMARY

1. Four vitamins are fat soluble. These are vitamins A, D, E, and K. They are needed in very small amounts.
2. All are involved in gene expression.
3. All have more than one structure.
4. Vitamins A, D, and K accumulate in the liver when consumed in excess. Vitamin E excess is excreted in the feces.
5. All of these vitamins can be bound to specific binding proteins.
6. Light blindness is a symptom of vitamin A deficiency; rickets is symptomatic of vitamin D deficiency; infertility results from vitamin E deficiency; and slow clotting times are characteristic of vitamin K deficiency.
7. Retinoic acid is the gene active form of vitamin A. It is vital to the expression of a long list of genes serving as a transcription aid that binds to a specific region of the promoter region of these genes.
8. The different forms of vitamin A are interconvertible.
9. Carotene in its many forms can be converted to retinol with varying degrees of efficiency.
10. Vitamin D functions in the synthesis of calcium-binding proteins. Calbindin is essential for calcium uptake by the intestinal cell. Other calcium-binding proteins are found in other tissues. Bone formation (mineralization) is a function of vitamin D. As well, this vitamin serves in the immunological system.
11. Vitamin E is important as an antioxidant suppressing free radical formation.
12. Vitamin K serves in the posttranslational carboxylation of several calcium-binding proteins in the coagulation cascade.

LEARNING OPPORTUNITIES

CASE STUDY 11.1 Elise Complains of Trouble Driving at Night

Elise is a 67-year-old woman who visited her eye doctor because she had trouble driving at night. She thought she needed new glasses but that was not the case. Her visual acuity had not changed. What had changed was her self-imposed fat-free, milk-free diet. She used to enjoy salads and vegetables and a good steak. But she had been reading the health food literature and was concerned that her former diet was not good for her. She now consumes lots of cereal grains, fruits, and vegetables believing that the fat in her diet was not good for her. Then she read that the chemicals used to grow fruits and vegetables were harmful so she eliminated them from her diet. Basically, she was eating only cereals, bread, and rice; she did, however, take a B vitamin supplement pill every morning. The problem she described was being unable to see the road after she passed an oncoming vehicle. This disturbed her and she was sure she would have an accident if she did not get some help. Her ophthalmologist tested her for dark adaptation and light adaptation. She definitely had a problem adjusting to differences in light intensity. What do you think was her problem? How could she fix this? If she was your friend, what would you say to her to help her out of this situation?

ANALYSIS AND PROBLEM SOLVING

1. Predict the consequences of a mutation in one of the vitamin A–binding proteins. (Itemize the protein and its gene that you are studying.)
2. What consequences would a zinc deficiency have on vitamin D and vitamin E function?

MULTIPLE-CHOICE QUESTIONS

1. A patient with undiagnosed hyperparathyroidism would probably have
   a. Low plasma phosphate and Ca^{++} levels and tetany
   b. High plasma phosphate levels and high Ca^{++} levels
   c. Increased muscle excitability and low bone mineral mass
   d. Low vitamin D levels
2. Which of the following would you expect in a person who was religious in using sunscreen and who was not a milk drinker?
   a. Osteoporosis
   b. Low levels of 1,25-dihydroxycholecalciferol
   c. Increased parathyroid secretion
   d. None of the above
3. A 25-year-old medical student spent the summer volunteering in the sub-Saharan region of Africa. He noted that the people were of short stature and had trouble with night blindness. He also realized that these people were not very fertile. There were few pregnancies and live births and few children.
   a. Their diets provided low levels of vitamins A and E
   b. They were genetically abnormal
   c. Their cultural practices limited sexual intercourse
   d. There was an abundance of UV radiation that destroyed their use

REFERENCES

1. Olson, J.A. (1991) Vitamin A. In: *Handbook of Vitamins* (L.J. Machlin, ed.). Marcel Dekker, New York, pp. 1–57.
2. Wolf, G. (1996) The history of vitamin A and retinoids. *FASEB J.* 10: 1102–1107.
3. Olson, J.A., Krinsky, N.I. (1995) The colorful fascinating world of the carotenoids: Important physiologic modulators. *FASEB J.* 9: 1547–1550.
4. Demmig-Adams, B., Gilmore, A.M., Adams, W.W. (1996) In vivo functions of carotenoids in higher plants. *FASEB J.* 10: 403–412.
5. Bendich, A, Olson, J.A. (1989) Biological actions of carotenoids. *FASEB J.* 3: 1927–1932.
6. Nagao, A., Olson, J.A. (1994) Enzymatic formation of 9-cis, 13-cis, and all-trans retinals from isomers of β-carotene. *FASEB J.* 8: 968–973.
7. Parker, R.S. (1996) Absorption, metabolism, and transport of carotenoids. *FASEB J.* 10: 542–551.
8. Chevalier, S., Ferlnad, G., Tuchweber, B. (1996) Lymphatic absorption of retinol in young, mature, and old rats: Influence of dietary restriction. *FASEB J.* 10: 1085–1090.
9. von Lintig, J. (2012) Provitamin A metabolism and functions in mammalian biology. *Am. J. Clin. Nutr.* 96: 1234S–1244S.
10. Borel, P., Lietz, G., Goncalves, A., de Edelenyi, F.S., Lecompte, S., Curtis, P., Goumidi, L. (2013) CD36 and SR-BI are involved in cellular uptake of provitamin A carotenoids by Caco-2 and HEK cells, and some of their genetic variants are associated with plasma concentrations of these micronutrients in humans. *J. Nutr.* 143: 448–456.
11. Berni, R., Clerici, M., Malpeli, G., Cleris, L., Formelli, F. (1993) Retinoids: In vitro interaction with retinol-binding protein and influence on plasma retinol. *FASEB J.* 7: 1179–1184.

12. Ross, A.C. (1993) Cellular metabolism and activation of retinoids: Roles of cellular retinol-binding proteins. *FASEB J.* 7: 317–327.
13. Newcomer, M.E. (1995) Retinol binding proteins: Structural determinants important for function. *FASEB J.* 9: 229–339.
14. Gerlach, T.H., Zile, M.H. (1991) Effect of retinoic acid and apo-RBP on serum retinol concentration in acute renal failure. *FASEB J.* 5: 86–92.
15. Gerlach, T.H., Zile, M.H. (1990) Upregulation of serum retinol in experimental acute renal failure. *FASEB J.* 4: 2511–2517.
16. Wagner, E., McCaffery, P., Mey, J., Farhangfar, F., Appleby, M.L., Drager, U.C. (1997) Retinoic acid increases arrestin mRNA levels in mouse retina. *FASEB J.* 11: 271–275.
17. Palomino, T., Sanchez-Pacheco, A., Pena, P., Aranda, A. (1998) A direct protein-protein interaction is involved in the cooperation between thyroid hormone and retinoic acid receptors and transcription factor GHF-1. *FASEB J.* 12: 1201–1209.
18. Chertow, K.R., Blanar, W.S., Rajan, N., Primerano, D.A., Meda, P., Cirulli, V., Krozowski, Z., Smith, R., Cordle, M.B. (1993) Retinoic acid receptor, cytosolic retinol binding and retinoic acid binding protein mRNA transcripts and proteins in rat insulin-secreting cells. *Diabetes* 42: 1109–1114.
19. Petkovich, M., Brand, N.J., Krust, A., Chambon, P. (1987) A human retinoic acid receptor which belongs to the family of nuclear receptors. *Nature* 220: 444–445.
20. DeLuca, L., Sandell, L.J. (1996) Retinoids and their receptors in differentiation, embryogenesis and neoplasia. *FASEB J.* 5: 2924–2933.
21. Chytil, F., Haq, R. (1990) Vitamin A mediated gene expression. *Crit. Rev. Eukaryot. Gene Expr.* 1: 61–73.
22. Jump, D.B., Lepar, G.J., MacDougald, O.A. (1993). Retinoic acid regulation of gene expression in adipocytes. In: *Nutrition and Gene Expression* (C.D. Berdanier, J.L. Hargrove, eds.). CRC Press, Inc., Boca Raton, FL, pp. 431–454.
23. Kastner, P., Krust, A., Mendelsohn, C., Garnier, J.M., Zelent, A., LeRoy, P., Staub, A., Chambon, P. (1990) Murine isoforms of retinoic acid receptor γ with specific patterns of expression. *Proc. Natl. Acad. Sci. USA* 87: 2700–2705.
24. Mangelsdorf, D.J., Borgmeyer, U., Heyman, R.A., Zhou, J.Y., Ong, E.S., Oro, A.E., Kakizuka, A., Evans, R.M. (1992) Characterization of three RXR genes that mediate the action of 9-cis retinoic acid. *Genes Dev.* 6: 329–334.
25. Mangelsdorf, D.J., Umesono, K., Kliewer, S.A., Borgmeyer, U., Ong, E.S., Evans, R.M. (1991) A direct repeat in the cellular retinol binding protein type II gene confers differential regulation by RXR and RAR. *Cell* 66: 555–560.
26. Kastner, P., Grondona, J., Mark, M., Gansmuller, A., LeMeur, M., Decimo, D., Vonesch, J.-L., Dolle, P., Chambon, P. (1994) Genetic analysis of RXRa developmental function: Convergence of RXR and RAR signaling pathways in heart and eye morphogenesis. *Cell* 78: 987–993.
27. Giguere, V., Shago, M., Zimgibl, R., Tate, P., Rossant, J., Varmuza, S. (1990) Identification of a noval isoform of the retinoic acid receptor γ expressed in mouse embryo. *Mol. Cell. Biol.* 10: 2335–2340.
28. Soprano, D.R., Harnish, D.C., Soprano, K.J., Kochhar, D.M., Jiang, H. (1993) Correlations of RAR isoforms and cellular retinoid binding protein mRNA levels with retinoid-induced teratogenesis. *J. Nutr.* 123: 367–371.
29. Chambon, P. (1994) The retinoid signaling pathway: Molecular and genetic analysis. *Cell Biol.* 5: 115–120.
30. Chien, K.R., Zhu, H., Knowlton, K.U., Miller-Hance, W., van Bilsen, M., O'Brien, T.X., Evans, S.M. (1993) Transcriptional regulation during cardiac growth and development. *Annu. Rev. Physiol.* 55: 77–95.
31. Takeyama, K., Kojima, R., Ohashi, T., Sato, T., Mano, H., Masushige, S., Kato, S. (1996) Retinoic acid differentially up-regulates the gene expression of retinoic acid receptor α and γ isoforms in embryo and adult rats. *Biochem. Biophys. Res. Commun.* 222: 395–340.
32. Suruga, K., Suzuki, R., Goda, T., Takase, S. (1995) Unsaturated fatty acids regulate gene expression of cellular retinol binding protein type II in rat jejunum. *J. Nutr.* 125: 2039–2044.
33. Everts, H.B., Berdanier, C.D. (2001) Vitamin A and mitochondrial gene expression. In: *Nutrient-Gene Interactions in Health and Disease* (N. Moustaid-Moussa, C.D. Berdanier, eds.). CRC Press, Boca Raton, FL, pp. 321–348.

34. Umesono, K., Murakami, K.K., Thompson, C.C., Evans, R.M. (1991) Direct repeats as selective response elements for the thyroid hormone, retinoic acid, and vitamin D3 receptors. *Cell* 65: 1255–1266.
35. Chien, K.R., Zhu, H., Knowlton, K.U., Miller-Hance, W., van Bilsen, M., O'Brien, T.X., Evans, S.M. (1993) Transcriptional regulation during cardiac growth and development. *Ann. Rev. Physiol.* 55: 77–95.
36. Dietz, U.H., Sandell, L.J. (1996) Cloning of a retinoic acid sensitive mRNA expressed in cartilage and during chondrogenesis. *J. Biol. Chem.* 271: 3311–3316.
37. Everts, H.B., Claassen, D.O., Hermoyian, C.L., Berdanier, C.D. (2002) Nutrient-gene interactions: Vitamin A and mitochondrial gene expression. *IUMB-Life* 53: 295–301.
38. Tan, L.,Wray, A., Ross, A.C. (2012) Oral vitamin A and retinoic acid supplementation stimulates antibody production and splenic *Strab6* expression in tetanus toxoid-immunized mice. *J. Nutr.* 142: 1590–1595.
39. Ross, A.C. (2012) Vitamin A and retinoic acid in T cell-related immunity. *Am. J. Clin. Nutr.* 96: 1166S–1172S.
40. Lolly, R.N., Lee, R.H. (1990) Cyclic GMP and photoreceptor function. *FASEB J.* 4: 3001–3008.
41. Olson, J.A. (1994) Hypervitaminosis A: Contemporary scientific issues. *J. Nutr.* 124: 14615–14665.
42. Khasru, M.R., Yaasmin, R., Salek, A.K., Khan, K.H., Nath, S.D., Selim, S. (2010) Acute hypervitaminosis in a young lady. *Mymensingh Med. J.* 19: 294–298.
43. Ramanathan, V.S., Hensley, G., French, S., Eysselein, V., Chung, D., Reicher, S., Pham, B. (2010) Hypervitaminosis A inducing intrahepatic cholestasis—A rare case report. *Exp. Mol. Pathol.* 88: 324–325.
44. Cruess, R.L., Clark, I. (1965) Alteration in the lipids of bone caused by hypervitaminosis A and D. *Biochem. J.* 96: 262–265.
45. Fu, X., Wang, X.D., Mernitz, H., Wallin, R., Shea, M.K., Booth, S.L. (2008) 9-Cis retinoic acid reduces 1alpha,25-dihydroxycholecalciferol-induced renal calcification by altering vitamin K-dependent gamma-carboxylation of matrix gamma-carboxyglutamic acid protein in A/J mice. *J. Nutr.* 138: 2337–2341.
46. Callari, D., Cicero, R., Ciancio, G., Billiteri, A. (1982) Biochemical and ultrastructural research on the antagonism between vitamins A and D at the level of the erythrocyte membrane. *Boll. Soc. Ital. Biol. Sper.* 58: 1068–1074.
47. Callari, D., Sichel, G., Billiteri, A. (1980) Role of erythrocyte membrane lipids in the antagonism between vitamins A and D. *Boll. Soc. Ital. Biol. Sper.* 56: 1726–1731.
48. Abawi, F.G., Sullivan, T.W. (1989) Interactions of vitamins A, D_3, E, and K in the diet of broiler chicks. *Poult. Sci.* 68: 1490–1496.
49. Johansson, S., Melhus, H. (2001) Vitamin A antagonizes calcium response to vitamin D in man. *J. Bone Min. Res.* 16: 1899–1905.
50. Rohde, C.M., DeLuca, H.F. (2005) All-trans retinoic acid antagonizes the action of calciferol and its active metabolite, 1,25-dihydroxycholecalciferol in rats. *J. Nutr.* 135: 1647–1652.
51. Veltmann, J.R. Jr., Jensen, L.S., Rowland, G.N. (1986) Excess dietary vitamin A in the growing chick: Effect of fat source and vitamin D. *Poult. Sci.* 65: 153–163.
52. Deltour, L., Ang, H.L., Duester, G. (1996) Ethanol inhibition of retinoic acid synthesis as a potential mechanism for fetal alcohol syndrome. *FASEB J.* 10: 1050–1057.
53. Olson, J.A. (1989) Upper limits of vitamin A in infant formulas, with some comments on vitamin K. *J. Nutr.* 119: 1820–1824.
54. Lee, M.A., Lieber, C.S. (1999) Alcohol, vitamin A and beta-carotene: Adverse interactions, including hepatotoxicity and carcinogenicity. *Am. J. Clin. Nutr.* 69: 1071–1085.
55. Kane, M.A., Folias, A.E., Wang, C., Napoli, J.L. (2010) Ethanol elevates physiological all-trans-retinoic acid levels in select loci through altering retinoid metabolism in multiple loci: A potential mechanism for ethanol toxicity. *FASEB J.* 24: 823–832.
56. Bell, N.H. (1995) Editorial: Vitamin D metabolism, aging and bone loss. *J. Clin. Endocrinol. Metab.* 80: 1051.
57. DeLuca, H.F. (1988) The vitamin D story: A collaborative effort of basic science and clinical medicine. *FASEB J.* 2: 224–236.
58. Davis, W.L., Matthews, J.L., Goodman, D.B.P. (1989) Glyoxylate cycle in the rat liver: Effect of vitamin D_3 treatment. *FASEB J.* 3: 1651–1655.

59. Sun, X., Zemel, M.B. (2005) Physiological levels of 1α, $25(OH)_2D_3$, high glucose and free fatty acid stimulate ROS production in L6 myocytes. *FASEB J.* 20: Abstract.
60. Morris, K.L., Zemel, M.K. (2005) 1,25-dihydroxyvitamin D_3 modulation of adipocyte glucocorticoid function. *Obes. Res.* 13: 670–677.
61. Gill, R.K., Christakos, S. (1993) Vitamin D dependent calcium binding protein, calbindin-D: Regulation of gene expression. In: *Nutrition and Gene Expression* (C.D. Berdanier, J.L. Hargrove, eds.). CRC Press, Boca Raton, FL, pp. 377–390.
62. Bygrave, F.L., Roberts, H.R. (1995) Regulation of cellular calcium through signaling cross-talk involves an intricate interplay between the actions of receptors, g-proteins and second messengers. *FASEB J.* 9: 1297–1303.
63. Jaaskelainen, T., Itkonen, A., Maenpaa, P.H. (1995). Retinoid X receptor α independent binding of vitamin D receptor to its response element from human osteocalcin gene. *Eur. J. Biochem.* 228: 222–228.
64. Lian, J.B., Stein, G.S. (1993) Vitamin D regulation of osteoblast growth and development. In: *Nutrition and Gene Expression* (C.D. Berdanier, J.L. Hargrove, eds.). CRC Press, Boca Raton, FL, pp. 391–430.
65. Brostrom, M.A., Brostrom, C.O. (1993) Calcium homeostasis, endoplasmic reticular function and the regulation of mRNA translation in mammalian cells. In: *Nutrition and Gene Expression* (C.D. Berdanier, J. L. Hargrove, eds.). CRC Press, Boca Raton, FL, pp. 117–142.
66. Whitfield, G.K., Hsieh, J.-C., Jurutka, P.W., Selznick, S.H., Haussler, C.A., Macdonald, P.N., Haussler, M.R. (1995) Genomic actions of 1,25 dihydroxyvitamin D_3. *J. Nutr.* 125: 1690S–1694S.
67. Minghetti, P.P., Norman, A.W. (1988) $1,25(OH)_2$-vitamin D_3 receptors: Gene regulation and genetic circuitry. *FASEB J.* 2: 3043–3053.
68. Ochs-Balcom, H.M., Chennamaneni, R., Millen, A.E., Shields, P.G., Marian, C., Trevisan, M., Freudenheim, J.L. (2011) Vitamin D receptor gene polymorphisms are associated with adiposity phenotypes. *Am. J. Clin. Nutr.* 93: 5–10.
69. Pani, M.A., Knapp, M., Donner, H., Braun, J., Baur, M.P., Usadel, K.H. (2000) Vitamin D receptor allele combinations influence genetic susceptibility to type 1 diabetes in Germans. *Diabetes* 49: 504–507.
70. Niino, M. (2010) Vitamin D and its immunoregulatory role in multiple sclerosis. *Drugs Today* 46: 279–290.
71. Beydoun, M.A., Ding, R.L.,Beydoun, H.A., Tanaka, T., Ferrucci, L., Zonderman, A.B. (2011) Vitamin D receptor and megalin gene polymorphisms and their associations with longitudinal cognitive change in US adults. *Am. J. Clin. Nutr.* 95: 163–178.
72. Weng, F.L., Shults, J., Leonard, M.B., Stallings, V.A., Zemel, B.S. (2007) Risk factors for low serum 25-hydroxyvitamin D concentrations in otherwise healthy children and adolescents. *Am. J. Clin. Nutr.* 86: 150–158.
73. McLaren, D.S. (2006) Vitamin D deficiency disorders (VDDD): A global threat to health. *Sight Life* 3: 6–15.
74. Institute of Medicine, (2002) *Dietary Reference Intakes for Vitamin A, Vitamin K, Arsenic, Boron, Chromium, Copper, Iodine, Iron, Manganese, Molybdenum, Nickel, Silicone, Vanadium, and Zinc.* National Academy Press, Washington, DC, pp. 8–9.
75. Barysch, M.J., Hofbauer, G.F., Dummer, R. (2010) Vitamin D, ultraviolet exposure, and skin cancer in the elderly. *Gerontology* 56: 410–413.
76. Reichrath, J. (2006) The challenge resulting from positive and negative effects of sunlight: How much solar UV exposure is appropriate to balance between risks of vitamin D deficiency and skin cancer. *Prog. Biophys. Mol. Biol.* 92: 9–16.
77. Berwick, M., Armstrong, B.K., Ben-Porat, L., Fine, J. (2005) Sun exposure and mortality from melanoma. *J. Nat. Cancer Inst.* 97: 195–199.
78. Hathcock, J.N., Shao, A., Vieth, R., Heaney, R. (2007) Risk assessment for vitamin D. *Am. J. Clin. Nutr.* 85: 6–18.
79. Dutta-Roy, A.K., Gordon, M.G., Campbell, F.M., Duthrie, G.G., James, W.P.T. (1994) Vitamin E requirements, transport, and metabolism: Role of α tocopherol-binding proteins. *J. Nutr. Biochem.* 5: 562–570.
80. Burton, G.W., Traber, M.G. (1990) Vitamin E: Antioxidant activity, biokinetics, bioavailability. *Annu. Rev. Nutr.* 10: 357–382.

81. Hodis, H.N., Mack, W.J., Labree, L., Cashin-Hemphill, L., Sevanian, A., Johnson, R., Azen, S.P. (1994) Serial coronary angiographic evidence that antioxidant vitamin intake reduces progression of coronary artery atherosclerosis. *JAMA* 273: 1849–1854.
82. Jialal, I., Grundy, S.M. (1992) Effect of dietary supplementation with α tocopherol on the oxidative modification of low density lipoproteins. *J. Lipid Res.* 33: 899–906.
83. Morel, D.W., Leera-Moya, M., Friday, K.E. (1994) Treatment of cholesterol fed rabbits with dietary vitamins E and C inhibits lipoprotein oxidation but not development of atherosclerosis. *J. Nutr.* 124: 2123–2130.
84. Stampfer, M.J., Hinnekins, C.H., Manson, J.E., Colditz, G.A., Rosner, B., Willett, W.C. (1993) Vitamin E consumption and the risk of coronary disease in women. *N. Eng. J. Med.* 328: 1444–1449 (see also pp. 1450–1456).
85. Upston, J.M., Terentis, A.C., Stocker, R. (1999) Tocopherol-mediated peroxidation of lipoproteins: Implications for vitamin E as a potential antiatherogenic supplement. *FASEB J.* 13: 977–994.
86. Brigelius-Flohe, R., Traber, M.G. (1999) Vitamin E: Function and metabolism. *FASEB J.* 13: 1145–1155.
87. Keaney, J.F., Simon, D.I., Freedman, J.E. (1999) Vitamin E and vascular homeostasois: Implications for atherosclerosis. *FASEB J.* 13: 965–976.
88. Buettner, G.R. (1993) The pecking order of free radicals and antioxidants: Lipid peroxidation, γ tocopherol and ascorbate. *Arch. Biochem. Biophys.* 300: 535–543.
89. Meydani, M., Meydani, S.N., Blumberg, J.B. (1993) Modulation by dietary vitamin E and selenium of clotting whole blood thromboxane A_2 and aortic prostacyclin synthesis in rats. *J. Nutr. Biochem.* 4: 322–326.
90. Omara, O.F., Blakely, B.R. (1993) Vitamin E is protective against iron toxicity and iron-induced hepatic vitamin E depletion in mice. *J. Nutr.* 123: 1649–1655.
91. Nair, P.P., Judd, J.T., Berlin, E., Taylor, P.R., Shami, S., Sainz, E., Bhagavan, H.N. (1993) Dietary fish oil-induced changes in the distribution of α tocopherol, retinol, and β carotene in plasma, red blood cells and platelets: Modulations by vitamin E. *Am. J. Clin. Nutr.* 58: 98–102.
92. Navarro, F., Navas, P., Burgess, J.R., Bello, R.I., De Cabo, R., Arroyo, A., Villalba, J.M. (1998) Vitamin E and selenium deficiency induces expression of the ubiquinone-dependent antioxidant system at the plasma membrane. *FASEB J.* 12: 1665–1673.
93. Jenkinson, A.M., Collins, A.R., Duthie, S.J., Wahle, K.W.J., Duthie, G.G. (1999) The effect of increased intakes of polyunsaturated fatty acids and vitamin E on DNA damage in human lymphocytes. *FASEB J.* 13: 2138–2142.
94. Belisle, S.E., Leka, L.S., Degado-Lista, J., Jacques, P.F., Ordovas, J.M., Meydani, S.N. (2009) Polymorphisms at cytokine genes may determine the effect of vitamin E on cytokine production in the elderly. *J. Nutr.* 139: 1855–1860.
95. Zillikins, M.C., van Meurs, J.B.J., Rivadeneira, F., Hofman, A., Oostra, B.A., Sijbrands, E.J.G., Witteman, J.C.M., Pols, H.A.P., van Duijn, C.M., Uitterlinden, A.G. (2010) Interactions between dietary vitamin E intake and SIRT1 genetic variation influence body mass index. *Am. J. Clin. Nutr.* 91: 1387–1393.
96. Lecompte, S., de Edelenyl, F.S., Goumidi, L., Maiani, A., Moschonis, G., Widhalm, K., Molnar, D. et al. (2011) Polymorphisms in the CD36/FAT gene associated with plasma vitamin E concentrations in humans. *Am. J. Clin. Nutr.* 93: 644–650.
97. Weitzman, S.A., Turk, P.W., Milkowski, D.H., Kozlowski, K. (1994) Free radical adducts induce alterations in DNA cytosine methylation. *Proc. Natl. Acad. Sci. USA* 91: 1261–1264.
98. Chen, H.W., Hendrich, S., Cook, L.R. (1994) Vitamin E deficiency increases serum thromboxane A_2, platelet arachidonate and lipid peroxidation in male Sprague-Dawley rats. *Prostag. Leukotr. EFA* 51: 11–17.
99. Paterson, P.G., Gorecke, D.K.J., Card R.T. (1994) Vitamin E deficiency and erythrocyte deformability in the rat. *J. Nutr. Biochem.* 5: 298–302.
100. Hollander, D., Kielb, M., Rim, E. (1978) Diurnal rhythmicity of absorption of a lipid compound (vitamin K-1) in vivo in the rat. *Am. J. Digest. Dis.* 23: 1125–1128.
101. Monsonego, A., Mizrahi, T., Eitan, S., Moalem, G, Bardos, H., Adany, R., Schwartz, M. (1998) Factor XIIIa as a nerve-associated transglutaminase. *FASEB J.* 12: 1163–1171.
102. Walsh, P.N. (1981) Platelets and coagulation proteins. *Fed. Proc.* 40: 2086–2092.

103. Gardill, S.L., Suttie, J.W. 1990. Vitamin K epoxide and quinone reductase activities. *Biochem. Pharmacol.* 40: 1055–1061.
104. Suttie, J.W. (1993) Synthesis of vitamin K dependent proteins. *FASEB J.* 7: 445–452.
105. Chung, A., Suttie, J.W., Bernatowicz, M. (1990) Vitamin K-dependent carboxylase: Structural requirements for propeptide activation. *Biochem. Biophys. Acta* 1039: 90–93.
106. Greer, F.R. (1995) The importance of vitamin K as a nutrient during the first year of life. *Nutr. Res.* 15: 289–310.
107. Troy, L.M., Jacques, P.F., Hannan, M.T., Kiel, D.P., Lichtenstein, A., Kennedy, E., Booth, S.L. (2007) Dihydrophylloquinone intake is associated with low bone mineral density in men and women. *Am. J. Clin. Nutr.* 86: 504–508.

12 Water-Soluble Vitamins

Water-soluble vitamins are a group of fairly small organic molecules that, for the most part, can be dissolved in water. As such, the body does not store them extensively. Compared to fat-soluble vitamins, it is relatively easy to develop a deficiency state for the water-soluble vitamins. It is therefore very important to consume each of these nutrients every day. The Food and Nutrition Board of the National Academy of Science has published the daily dietary recommended intakes (DRIs) and acceptable intakes (AIs) for water-soluble vitamins. These are shown in Table 12.1. There are periodic reviews of these recommendations, and if changes are warranted, they are made. The reader can visit the FNB website www.nap.edu to determine the latest recommendations.

ASCORBIC ACID

Historically, ascorbic acid, or vitamin C, has been recognized as a needed nutrient for centuries.[1] Although its chemical identity was unknown, foods rich in this micronutrient have long been used as treatments for the symptoms of scurvy. Ancient Egyptians, Greeks, and Romans referred to scurvy as a plague that interfered with victory in military campaigns. Accounts of the scourge of scurvy have appeared in the writings of the sixteenth, seventeenth, and eighteenth centuries. Reports (in Latin) of the efficacious effects of cloud berries on the prevention/cure of scurvy appeared in 1635.[2]

Perhaps the best known treatise on scurvy is that written by the Scottish surgeon James Lind. Dr. Lind demonstrated that the inclusion of limes, oranges, and lemons in sailors' diets would successfully prevent the development of scurvy. Other reports similar to Lind's were published, but his remains the classic paper in this field. Even though the value of citrus fruits was amply demonstrated by Lind, it took 30 years for his recommendations to be adopted. Most nutrition historians credit Captain James Cook, discoverer of the Hawaiian Islands, as the first sea captain to include citrus fruits as part of his ship's stores and part of the sailors' diets. He, thus, was able to demonstrate that long ocean voyages need not result in scurvy for the crew.

Despite the knowledge that scurvy could be avoided, many sailors and explorers continued to die from scurvy. Even as recently as 1912, Captain Scott and his team were killed by scurvy as they explored the polar regions of the southern hemisphere.

While the knowledge that certain foods prevented or cured scurvy was available in the eighteenth century, the isolation and synthesis of the antiscorbutic factor did not occur until the early twentieth century. The isolation of ascorbic acid was accomplished by two independent groups of chemists in 1928. Szent-Gyorgy isolated a compound that he called hexuronic acid from orange juice, cabbage, and adrenal glands. King likewise isolated the vitamin from lemon juice and showed that it was identical to the compound isolated by Szent-Gyorgy. The structure of the vitamin was accomplished by Haworth and its synthesis by Reichstein. While this exciting chemistry was being pursued, an interesting fact became known and that was that few species required ascorbic acid in their diets. The guinea pig, the primates (including humans), the fruit bat, and some fishes and birds were identified as being unable to synthesize the vitamin in vivo. All other species examined were found to be able to synthesize it from glucose (Figure 12.1). The reason why ascorbic acid–dependent species cannot synthesize ascorbic acid is because they lack the enzyme L-gulonolactone oxidase.

TABLE 12.1
Daily Dietary Reference Intakes (DRI) and Acceptable Intakes (AI*) for Various Age Groups

Group	Ascorbic Acid (mg)	Thiamin (mg)	Riboflavin (mg)	Niacin[a] (mg)	Vitamin B_6 (mg)	Folacin (μg)	Pantothenic Acid (mg)	Vitamin B_{12} (μg)	Biotin (μg)	Choline (mg)
Infants										
0–6 months	—	—	0.3*	2*	0.1*	65*	1.7*	0.4*	5*	125*
7–12 months	—	—	0.4*	4*	0.3*	80*	1.8*	0.5*	6*	150*
Children										
1–3 years	**13**	**0.4**	**0.5**	**6**	**0.5**	**150**	2*	**0.9**	8*	200*
4–8 years	**22**	**0.5**	**0.6**	**8**	**0.6**	**200**	3*	**1.2**	12*	250*
Males										
9–13 years	**39**	**0.7**	**0.9**	**12**	**1.0**	**300**	4*	**1.8**	20*	375*
14–18 years	**63**	**1.0**	**1.3**	**16**	**1.3**	**400**	5*	**2.4**	25*	550*
19–30 years	**75**	**1.0**	**1.3**	**16**	**1.3**	**400**	5*	**2.4**	30*	550*
31–50 years	**75**	**1.0**	**1.3**	**16**	**1.3**	**400**	5*	**2.4**	30*	550*
51–70 years	**75**	**1.0**	**1.3**	**16**	**1.7**	**400**	5*	**2.4**[c]	30*	550*
70+ years	**75**	**1.0**	**1.3**	**16**	**1.7**	**400**	5*	**2.4**[c]	30*	550*
Females										
9–13 years	**39**	**0.7**	**0.9**	**12**	**1.0**	**300**	4*	**1.8**	20*	375*
14–18 years	**56**	**0.9**	**1.0**	**14**	**1.2**	**400**	5*	**2.4**	25*	400*
19–30 years	**60**	**0.9**	**1.1**	**14**	**1.3**	**400**	5*	**2.4**	30*	425*
31–50 years	**60**	**0.9**	**1.1**	**14**	**1.3**	**400**	5*	**2.4**	30*	425*
51–70 years	**60**	**0.9**	**1.1**	**14**	**1.5**	**400**	5*	**2.4**[c]	30*	425*
70+ years	**60**	**0.9**	**1.1**	**14**	**1.5**	**400**	5*	**2.4**[c]	30*	425*
Pregnancy										
14–18 years	**66**	**1.2**	**1.4**	**18**	**1.9**	**600**[b]	6*	**2.6**	30*	450*
19–30 years	**70**	**1.2**	**1.4**	**18**	**1.9**	**600**[b]	6*	**2.6**	30*	450*
31–50 years	**70**	**1.2**	**1.4**	**18**	**1.9**	**600**	6*	**2.6**	30*	450*
Lactation										
14–18 years	**96**	**1.2**	**1.6**	**17**	**2.0**	**500**	7*	**2.8**	35*	550*
19–30 years	**100**	**1.2**	**1.6**	**17**	**2.0**	**500**	7*	**2.8**	35*	550*
31–50 years	**100**	**1.2**	**1.6**	**17**	**2.0**	**500**	7*	**2.8**	35*	550*

Source: www.nap.edu.

Note: Figures in bold are those for DRI, whereas figures with asterisks are AIs.

[a] Niacin and niacin equivalents assuming a conversion of tryptophan to niacin, 60:1.

[b] In view of the data linking birth defects to inadequate folacin intake early in pregnancy, it recommended that any woman of an age to become pregnant consume 400 μg folate/day from fortified foods and supplements.

[c] Because 10%–30% of older people may malabsorb this vitamin, it is advisable for those older than 50 years of age to meet their vitamin requirement through consuming foods rich in this vitamin and through use of a vitamin supplement.

Structure

Ascorbic acid and dehydroascorbic acid (the oxidized form) are the trivial names for vitamin C. The chemical name is 2,3-didehydro-L-threo-hexano-1,4-lactone. The compound can readily donate or accept hydrogen ions and thus exists in either state as shown in Figure 12.2. In order for the compound to have vitamin activity, it must have a 2,3-enediol structure and be a six-carbon lactone.

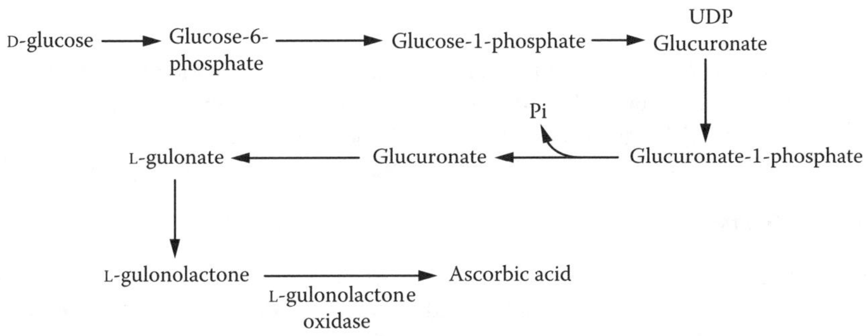

D-glucose → Glucose-6-phosphate → Glucose-1-phosphate → UDP Glucuronate

UDP Glucuronate → Glucuronate-1-phosphate → Glucuronate (Pi) → L-gulonate

L-gulonate → L-gulonolactone → Ascorbic acid (L-gulonolactone oxidase)

FIGURE 12.1 Biosynthesis of ascorbic acid.

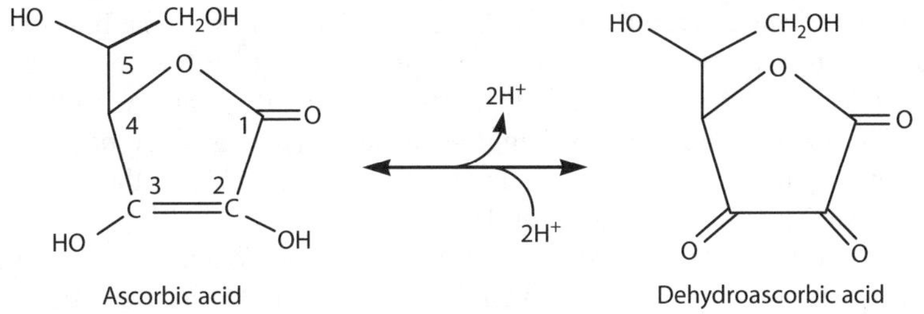

Ascorbic acid ⇌ Dehydroascorbic acid (2H+)

FIGURE 12.2 Structures of ascorbic acid and dehydroascorbic acid.

Physical and Chemical Properties

L-Ascorbic acid (Figure 12.2) is a rather simple compound chemically related to the monosaccharide glucose with an empirical formula of $C_6H_8O_6$. It is a white crystalline solid with a molecular weight of 176. It is soluble in water, glycerol, and ethanol but insoluble in such fat solvents as chloroform and ether. It exists in both D- and L-forms but the L-form is the biologically active form. This is in contrast to its related monosaccharide glucose, which is biologically active as the D-form. The vitamin is stable in the dry form but once dissolved in water, it is easily oxidized. It is relatively stable in solutions with a pH below 4.0; as the pH rises, the vitamin becomes less stable. Ascorbic acid is easily oxidized by metals such as iron or copper. While ascorbic acid is readily oxidized, it is less perishable in food mixtures. It is oxidized in alkaline environments especially when heated, exposed to air, or in contact with iron or copper salts. Fortunately, those foods rich in ascorbic acid are relatively acid and lack iron and copper. If the food is not cooked quickly with a minimum of water, significant losses will occur, which will decrease the value of the food as a source of the vitamin.

The oxidation and reduction of ascorbic acid is the basis for its biological function. Further oxidation results in the formation of diketogulonic acid, which is biologically inactive. The conversion of ascorbate to dehydroascorbate is aided by sulfhydryl compounds such as glutathione. The strong reducing power of ascorbate can be used to good advantage in its assay. Ascorbate will react with a variety of cyclic compounds to form a color that can be measured spectrophotometrically. Dyes such as dichlorophenolindophenol and 2,4-dinitrophenylhydrazine are the most commonly used compounds in the assay for vitamin C. Chromatographic techniques are also available for use. An excellent enzymatic assay has been designed using the enzyme ascorbate oxidase, which is both sensitive and specific. For the assay of the vitamin content of tissues such as liver or blood cells, the more sensitive thin-layer chromatographic technique is preferred. In animal and plant tissues, vitamin C is in milligram amounts. Human plasma, for example, contains about 10 mg/L.

Sources

Ascorbic acid is found in citrus fruits, strawberries, and melons, and some vitamin can be found in raw cabbage and related vegetables. The reader can visit the USDA website to find the ascorbic acid content of a wide variety of foods: www.nal.usda.gov/foodcomposition.

Absorption and Metabolism

The metabolic fate of ascorbic acid depends on a number of factors, including animal species, route of ingestion, quantity of material, and nutritional status. In species requiring dietary ascorbate, ascorbate is absorbed in the small intestine, primarily the ileum, by an active transport system that is sodium and energy dependent.[3] Studies in vitro have demonstrated clearly that the vitamin moves from the mucosal to the serosal sides of the lumen against a concentration gradient. The influx of the vitamin at the brush border follows saturation kinetics and is specific for the L-isomer. Influx can be inhibited by D-isoascorbate, a naturally occurring analog. If sodium is absent, influx does not occur.

The mechanism of absorption involves a carrier protein to which both Na^+ and ascorbate are attached. The carrier translocates these two through the mucosal membrane to the cytosol of the absorbing cell. The sodium disassociates from the carrier at the inner side of the mucosal membrane, the sodium is pumped out via the sodium–potassium pump, and the vitamin free of the membrane-bound carrier moves into the cytosol.

The carrier then resumes its original position in the membrane and is available to repeat the process. Although this process is similar to that for glucose and alanine, these compounds do not compete with ascorbate for absorption via the carrier described. Those species able to synthesize sufficient ascorbic acid do not possess this active transport system, and dietary ascorbate is absorbed via passive diffusion. These species differences in transport phenomena lend further evidence of a bifurcation in the evolutionary process that separates guinea pigs, primates, and other ascorbate-requiring species from those species that do not require this vitamin in their diet.

Once absorbed, there appears to be a central pathway for metabolism common to all species. In primates, the excess is excreted primarily as ascorbic acid in the urine. There is a very efficient reabsorption mechanism in the kidneys that serves to conserve ascorbic acid in times of need. In the guinea pig, the excess is oxidized to CO_2.[4] In humans, very little oxidation of ascorbate to CO_2 occurs. Over 50 metabolites of ascorbate have been identified in the urine. Most of these are excreted in very small amounts. The main metabolites are ascorbate-2-sulfate, oxalic acid, ascorbate, dehydroascorbate, and 2,3-diketogulonic acid.

Distribution

One of the earliest investigations of ascorbic acid function included studies of the distribution of the vitamin throughout the body. Table 12.2 presents some of the findings made in humans and rats. Ascorbic acid is also found in the brain uniformly distributed where it serves as a cofactor for an enzyme that converts dopamine to norepinephrine.

Ascorbic acid pool sizes and turnover have been estimated using isotopically labeled vitamin. In depleted humans consuming a vitamin C–free diet, about 3% of the total existing pool of ascorbic acid is degraded daily. When the depleted subjects were given doses of vitamin C, this vitamin did not appear in the urine until the body pool approached the size of about 1500 mg. Body pool sizes of more than 1500 mg have not been observed even when megadoses of the vitamin are consumed. These observations indicate that mega intakes are not useful with respect to the body's vitamin C content. The first signs of scurvy incidentally were observed in humans having pool sizes of 300–400 mg, and these signs did not disappear until the pool size increased to 1000 mg.[5] Vitamin C turnover has likewise been estimated for normally nourished humans to be 60 mg/day.[6] Smokers, incidentally, have higher turnover rates and require more ascorbic acid to maintain their pool sizes.[7]

TABLE 12.2
Distribution of Ascorbate in Human and Rat Tissues

	mg/100 g Tissue (Wet Weight)	
Tissue	**Human**	**Rat**
Adrenals	30–40	280–400
Pituitary	40–50	100–130
Liver	10–16	25–40
Spleen	10–15	40–50
Lungs	7	20–40
Kidneys	5–15	15–20
Testes	3	25–30
Thyroid	2	22
Heart	5–15	5–10
Plasma	0.4–1.0	1.6

Turnover is estimated by measuring the intake rate, the excretion rate, and the total body pool size. This can be accomplished by giving a dose of radioactively labeled vitamin and measuring its distribution and excretion.

In contrast to many vitamins, ascorbic acid does not need a carrier for its transport within the body. Like glucose, it is readily carried in the blood in its free form and, likewise, freely crosses the blood–brain barrier. Ascorbate rapidly travels to all cells once it has entered the body. Human skeletal muscle, for example, is highly responsive to changes in ascorbate intake.[8] It is even more responsive than leukocytes and indeed may serve as a labile pool of the vitamin that can be raided in times of need.

Function

Although we had information about the chemistry of this vitamin, its metabolic function remained elusive for many years. Because it readily converts between the free and dehydro forms, it functions in hydrogen ion transfer systems and aids in the regulation of redox states in the cells. Since it is a powerful water-soluble antioxidant, it helps to protect other naturally occurring antioxidants that may or may not be water soluble.[9,10] For example, polyunsaturated fatty acids and vitamin E are protected from peroxidation by ascorbic acid. Ascorbic acid protects the lipids of the plasma membranes from oxidative damage[5] and other labile components of the cell.[11] Ascorbic acid protects certain proteins from oxidative damage, and in addition to its role as an antioxidant, it serves to maintain the unsaturation–saturation ratio of fatty acids. Ascorbic acid aids in the conversion of folic acid to folinic acid and facilitates the absorption of iron by maintaining it in the ferrous state. Ascorbic acid plays a role in the detoxification reactions in the microsomes by virtue of its role as a cofactor in hydroxylation reactions. Table 12.3 provides a list of those enzymes in which ascorbate is a coenzyme. Many of these are dioxygenases. Again, this is due to the ascorbate–dehydroascorbate interconversion. A number of these enzymes are involved in collagen synthesis. This explains the poor wound healing found in deficient subjects. The hydroxylation of proline to hydroxyproline, an important amino acid in the synthesis of collagen, is ascorbic acid dependent. The poor wound healing typical of scurvy is related to the need to form collagen to seal the wound. The vitamin has been shown to be needed for the incorporation of iron into ferritin and for maintaining either iron or copper in the reduced state. The anemia associated with scurvy may be related to the inability of iron and copper to remain in the reduced state in hemoglobin. Ascorbic acid serves as an important cofactor in hydroxylation reactions. The hydroxylation of tryptophan to 5-hydroxytryptophan and the conversion of 3,4-dehydroxyphenylethylamine (DOPA) to norepinephrine are examples of other reactions dependent on ascorbic acid. Although these reactions will occur in the absence of the vitamin, they will occur at a very slow rate.

TABLE 12.3
Enzymes Using Ascorbate as a Coenzyme

Cytochrome P_{450} oxidases (several)
Dopamine-β-monooxygenase
Peptidyl glycine α-amidating monooxygenase
Cholesterol 7α-hydroxylase
4-Hydroxyphenylpyruvate oxidase
Homogentisate 1,2-dioxygenase
Proline hydroxylase
Procollagen-proline 2-oxoglutarate 3-dioxygenase
Lysine hydroxylase
γ-butyrobetaine, 2-oxoglutarate 4-dioxygenase
Trimethyllysine 2-oxoglutarate dioxygenase

Deficiency

As with other nutrients, there are large differences among individuals in their needs for ascorbic acid. As well then, there are large differences in the duration of time needed to develop scurvy when consuming a vitamin C–deficient diet. Hodges et al.[5] fed volunteers a diet devoid of vitamin C and described their symptoms as they developed (Table 12.4). He noted an increased fatigability, especially in the lower limbs, and a mild general malaise as the symptoms of scurvy became apparent. Mental and emotional changes occurred after 30 days of treatment with symptoms of depression and suicidal tendencies developing. After 112 days on the ascorbic acid–free diet, some subjects complained of vertigo (feeling of faintness), inappropriate temperature sensing, and profuse sweating. After 26 days of depletion, small petechial hemorrhages on the skin were observed, and after 84–91 days, small ocular hemorrhages were present. Gingival hemorrhages and swelling in various degrees appeared at different times in the subjects. Hyperkeratosis was observed after 2 months of depletion. All of these symptoms were reversed when the subjects were provided with ascorbic acid.

One of the explanations for the variability in ascorbic acid need has to do with the genetic variability of the mucosal membrane ascorbate carrier. Polymorphisms in the carrier have been reported in the gene labeled SLC23A1.[12] Variation at rs3397313 was associated with a reduction in circulating ascorbate. Several variants were found at this location. Ascorbate levels in the blood were directly related to these polymorphisms.

TABLE 12.4
Signs of Ascorbic Acid Deficiency

Hyperkeratosis
Congestion of follicles
Petechial and other skin hemorrhages
Conjunctival lesions
Sublingual hemorrhages
Gum swelling, congestion
Bleeding gums
Papillary swelling
Peripheral neuropathy with hemorrhages into nerve sheaths
Pain, bone endings are tender
Epiphyseal separations occur with subsequent bone (chest) deformities

Toxicity

Although vitamin C is a water-soluble vitamin and is not usually stored, toxic states can develop if long-term large intakes are maintained. As mentioned earlier, oxalate is an end product of ascorbate metabolism and is excreted. As the dose consumed increases, the urinary oxalate does not increase and some investigators have suggested that megadoses of vitamin C may be a risk factor in renal oxalate stores. Megadoses of vitamin C have been advocated for the treatment of cancer. However, studies of cancer patients have revealed that such treatment was of little benefit.[13] Massive doses of vitamin C have been shown to reduce serum vitamin B_{12} levels.[14] In part, this may be due to an effect of ascorbic acid on vitamin B_{12} in food. Ascorbic acid destroys B_{12} in food. Ascorbic acid also inhibits the utilization of β-carotene.[15,16]

Needs

Over the years, different countries have had widely different recommended daily allowances for ascorbic acid intake. This was due primarily to the differing standards of adequate nutritional status. In Canada, the absence of scorbutic symptoms was used as the indication of adequate nutrient intake. In the United States, adequate intake has been defined as the saturation of the white blood cell with ascorbic acid. For many years, these different definitions have meant that there was a twofold difference in the two countries' recommendations. Now, however, there is similarity in the recommendations for intake. The DRIs for ascorbic acid are shown in Table 12.1. Lactating and pregnant women should consume more (+40 and +20, respectively) and children less depending on age. Vitamin C requirements may be higher in stressed or traumatized persons. In rats, administration of ACTH or cortisone has been shown to lower plasma and hepatic levels of the vitamin. In addition, women taking contraceptive steroids may absorb less vitamin or may metabolize it more quickly and thus may require more than 60 mg/day.[17–19] Diabetes may also affect vitamin C requirements.[20] Requirements by these groups of people have not been established as yet.

THIAMIN

The discovery of the chemical structure and synthesis of thiamin marked the end of a difficult search spanning continents to identify the substance in rice polishings responsible for the cure of the disease beriberi.[21–23] One of the earliest recorded accounts of the disease was by Jacobus Bontius, a Dutch physician. He wrote, in 1630, "A certain troublesome affliction which attacks men is called by the inhabitants [of Java] beri beri. I believe those whom this disease attacks with their knees shaking and legs raised up, walk like sheep. It is a kind of paralysis or rather tremor: for it penetrates the motion and sensation of the hands and feet, indeed, sometimes the whole body…."

In 1894, Takaki, a surgeon in the Japanese Navy, suggested that the disease was diet related. By adding milk and meat to the Navy diet, he was able to decrease the incidence of the disease. He thought the problem was one of a lack of dietary protein. About the same time (1890), a Dutch physician in Java named Eijkman observed a beriberi-like condition (polyneuritis) in chickens fed a polished rice diet. He was able to cure the condition by adding rice polishings. Eijkman suggested that polished rice contained a toxin that was neutralized by rice polishings.

In 1901, another Dutch physician named Grigens gave the first correct explanation for the cure of beriberi by rice polishings. He theorized that natural foodstuffs contained an unknown factor absent in polished rice that prevented the development of the disease. Jansen and Donath in 1906 and Funk in 1912 reported the isolation of material from rice polishings that cured beriberi. Funk called the material vita amine or vitamine.

In 1926, Jansen and Donath isolated a crystalline material that cured polyneuritis in birds. Jansen gave the material the trivial name aneurine. This name was used extensively in the European literature. It is now considered an obsolete term, as are the terms vitamin B_1, oryzamin, torulin,

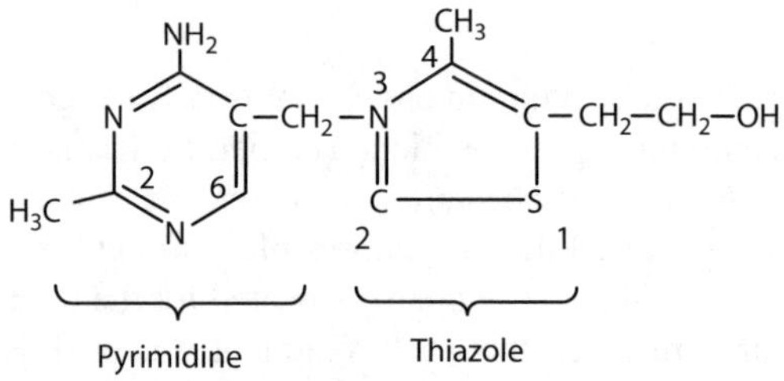

FIGURE 12.3 Structure of thiamin.

polyneuramin, vitamin F, antineuritic vitamin, and antiberiberi vitamin. All these terms arose as early nutrition scientists identified diseases associated with thiamin deficiency that were reversed when the active principle now known as thiamin was provided.

In 1934, Williams et al. isolated enough of the material to make structure elucidation possible. In 1936, thiamin was synthesized by the same group. With synthesis demonstrated, the stage was set for the commercial preparation of thiamin followed by an outburst of publications on its function and metabolism.

Structure

Thiamin is a relatively simple compound of a pyrimidine and a thiazole ring (Figure 12.3). It exists in cells as thiamin pyrophosphate (TPP). TPP used to be called cocarboxylase. The name thiamin comes from the fact that the compound contains both a sulfur group (the thiol group) and nitrogen in its structure. Its biological function depends on the conjoined pyrimidine and thiazole rings, on the presence of an amino group on carbon 4 of the pyrimidine ring, on the presence of a quaternary nitrogen at an open carbon at position 2, and a phosphorylatable alkyl group at carbon 5 of the thiazole ring. In its free form, it is unstable. For this reason, it is available commercially as either a hydrochloride or a mononitrate salt. The HCl form is a white crystalline material that is readily soluble (1 g/L mL water) in water, fairly soluble in ethanol, but relatively insoluble in other solvents. The chemical name for the HCl form is 3-(4′-amino-2′-methyl pyrimidine-5′-yl) methyl-5-(2-hydroxyethyl)-4-methylthiazolium chloride hydrochloride. It is stable to acids up to 120°C but readily decomposes in alkaline solutions especially when heated. It can be split by nitrite or sulfite at the bridge between the pyrimidine and thiazole rings. The mononitrate form is a white crystalline substance that is more stable to heat than is the hydrochloride form. This form is used more often for food processing than the HCl form. Other forms are also available. These include thiamin allyl disulfide, thiamin propyl disulfide, thiamin tetrahydrofurfuryl disulfide, and *o*-benzoyl thiamin disulfide. The molecular weight of the disulfide form is 562.7 with a melting point of 177°C. While the hydrochloride form has a molecular weight of 337.3, the mononitrate form is 327.4. The latter two are white crystalline material, whereas the disulfide form is a yellow crystal. Thiamin exhibits characteristic absorption maxima at 235 and 267 mm corresponding to the pyrimidine and thiazole moieties, respectively.

When oxidized, the bridge is attacked and thiamin is converted to thiochrome. Thiochrome is biologically inactive. These structures are shown in Figure 12.4.

Thiamin Antagonists

The two most commonly used antagonists to thiamin are oxythiamin and pyrithiamin. A pyridine ring is substituted for the thiazole ring of thiamin in pyrithiamin. A hydroxyl group is substituted for the amino group of the pyrimidine moiety of the thiamin molecule in oxythiamin. It appears that thiamin activity is decreased when the number 2 position of the pyridine ring is changed.

Both the molecules are potent thiamin antagonists but differ in the mechanism by which this is accomplished. Oxythiamin is readily converted to the pyrophosphate and competes with thiamin

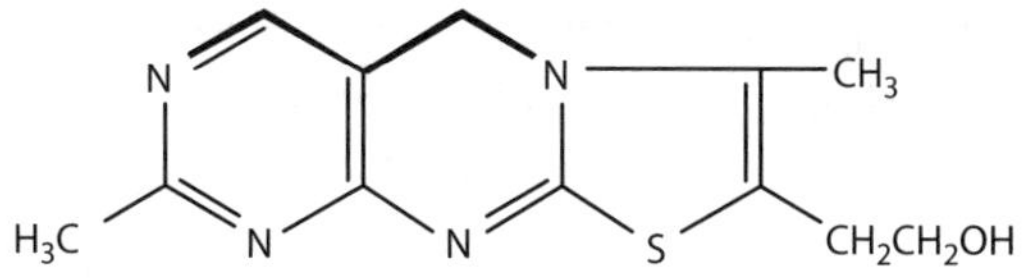

Thiochrome

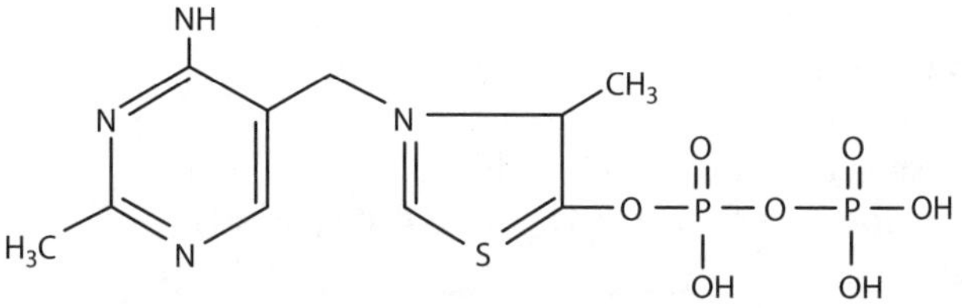

Thiamin pyrophosphate (TPP)

FIGURE 12.4 Structures of thiochrome and thiamin pyrophosphate.

for its place in the TPP-enzyme systems. Pyrithiamin prevents the conversion of thiamin to TPP by interfering with the activity of thiamin kinase.

Oxythiamin depresses appetite, growth, and weight gain and produces bradycardia, heart enlargement, and an increase in blood pyruvate, but it does not produce neurological symptoms. Pyrithiamin results in a loss of thiamin from tissues, bradycardia, and heart enlargement but does not produce an increase in blood pyruvate.

A natural antagonist is an enzyme called thiaminase. It was discovered by accident when raw fish was incorporated into a commercially available feed for foxes. Foxes fed this diet developed symptoms of thiamin deficiency. When heated, this enzyme is denatured and loses its enzymatic activity. The enzyme has several forms and has been found in fish, shellfish, ferns, betel nuts, and a variety of vegetables. Also found in tea and other plant foods are antithiamin substances that inactivate the vitamin by forming adducts. Tannic acid is one such substance; another is 3,4-dihydroxycinnamic acid (caffeic acid). Some of the flavonoids and some of the dihydroxy derivatives of tyrosine have antithiamin activity.

Assays for Thiamin

There are various chemical, microbiological, and animal assays available for thiamin. In animal tissues, thiamin occurs principally as a phosphate ester, whereas in plants, it appears in the free form. Both forms are protein bound.

The thiochrome method is a widely used chemical assay for thiamin. It depends upon the alkaline oxidation of thiamin to thiochrome. Thiochrome in turn exhibits an intense blue fluorescence, which can be measured fluorometrically. Other chemical tests for thiamin are the formaldehyde-diazotized sulfanilic acid method, the diazotized sulfanilic acid method, the diazotized *p*-aminoacetophenone method, and the bromothymol blue method. All of these assays must be preceded by extraction and removal of protein.

Lactobacillus viridescens is the microorganism often used to measure thiamin concentrations. It requires the intact thiamin molecule for growth. Other organisms are available but they are less useful.

Animal assays can be used to determine thiamin in food. The rat is the preferred animal to use. The material being tested measures the curative effect of the food source on rats that have been made thiamin deficient and compares it to the curative effect of the pure vitamin. The most sensitive chemical assay uses chromatographic techniques. Both high-performance liquid chromatography (HPLC) and thin-layer chromatography yield excellent results.

Sources

Thiamin is widely distributed in the food supply. Pork is the richest source, while highly refined foods have virtually no thiamin. Polished rice, fats, oils, refined sugar, and unenriched flours are in this group. Many products are made with enriched flour and so provide thiamin to the consumer. Enrichment means that the flour has had thiamin added to it to the level that was there prior to processing. Peas and other legumes are good sources; the amount of thiamin increases with the maturity of the seed. Cereal products contain nutritionally significant amounts of thiamin. Dried brewer's yeast and wheat germ are both rich in thiamin. The USDA website gives the thiamin content of a wide variety of foods: www.nal.usda.gov/foodcomposition.

Absorption and Metabolism

Thiamin is absorbed by a specific active transport mechanism.[24] In humans and rats, absorption is most rapid in the proximal small intestine. Studies in vivo on intact loops of rat small intestine revealed saturation kinetics for thiamin over the concentration range of 0.06–1.5 μM. At higher concentrations (2–560 μM), absorption was linearly related to the luminal B_1 concentration. In vitro studies using inverted jejunum sacs indicated an active transport mechanism, which is energy and Na^+ dependent and carrier mediated.

Thiamin undergoes phosphorylation either in the intestinal lumen or within the intestinal cells. This phosphorylation is closely related to uptake indicating that the carrier may be the enzyme thiamin pyrophosphokinase. There is some argument about this however. Figure 12.5 illustrates TPP synthesis. While thiamin can accumulate in all cells of the body, there is no single storage site per se. The body does not store the vitamin, and thus a daily supply is needed.

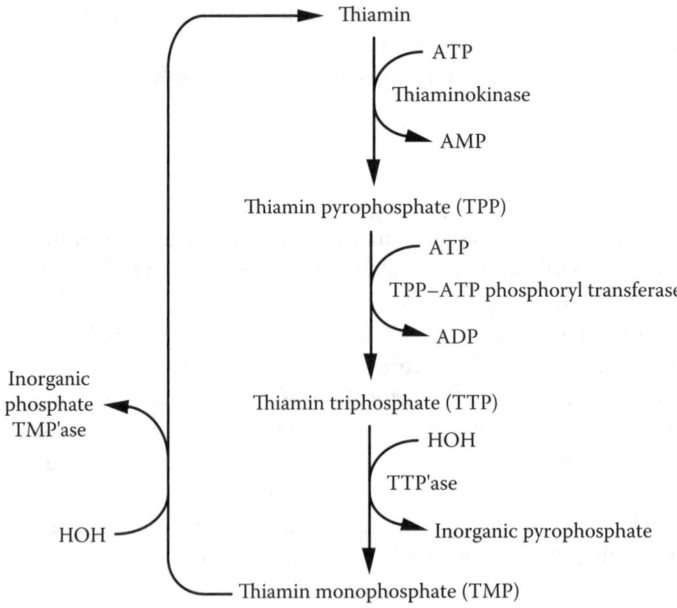

FIGURE 12.5 Formation of TPP through the phosphorylation of thiamin. About 80% of thiamin exists as TPP, 10% as TTP, and the remainder as TMP.

Biological Function

Thiamin is a part of the coenzyme TPP. This coenzyme consists of thiamin with two molecules of phosphate attached to it. It is also known as cocarboxylase. It is required in the metabolism of carbohydrates.[25] Figure 12.6 illustrates the structure of TPP. The mechanism of action for the TPP is due to the resonance possible in the thiazolium ring. The thiazolium dipslo ion, known as ylid, will form. Because of the formation of the ylid, the thiazole ring of TPP can serve as a transient carrier of a covalently bound *active* aldehyde group. Mg^{++} is required as a cofactor for these reactions.

Intermediary metabolism is slowed in thiamin deficiency. There are two oxidative decarboxylation reactions of α-keto acids: the formation or degradation of α-ketols and the decarboxylation of pyruvic acid to acetyl coenzyme A (CoA) as it is about to enter the citric acid cycle. This reaction is catalyzed by the pyruvate dehydrogenase complex, an organized assembly of three kinds of enzymes. The mechanism of this action is quite complex. TPP, lipoamide, and flavin adenine dinucleotide (FAD) serve as catalytic cofactors; nicotinamide adenine dinucleotide (NAD^+) and CoA serve as stoichiometric cofactors.[26]

As a consequence of impairment of this reaction in thiamin deficiency, the level of pyruvate will rise. When thiamin is withheld from the diet, the ability of tissues to utilize pyruvate does not decline uniformly indicating that there are tissue differences in the retention of TPP. Thiamin promotes the nonenzymatic decarboxylation of pyruvate to yield acetaldehyde and CO_2. Studies of this model revealed that the H at C-2 of the thiazole ring ionizes to yield a carbanion, which reacts with the carbonyl atom of pyruvate to yield CO_2 and a hydroxyethyl (HE) derivative of the thiazole.

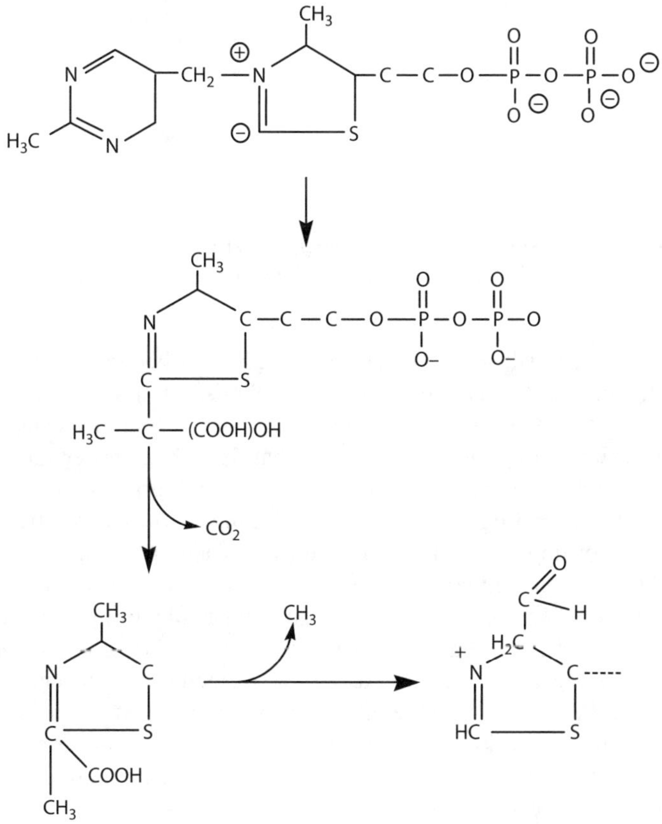

FIGURE 12.6 Structure of the coenzyme TPP.

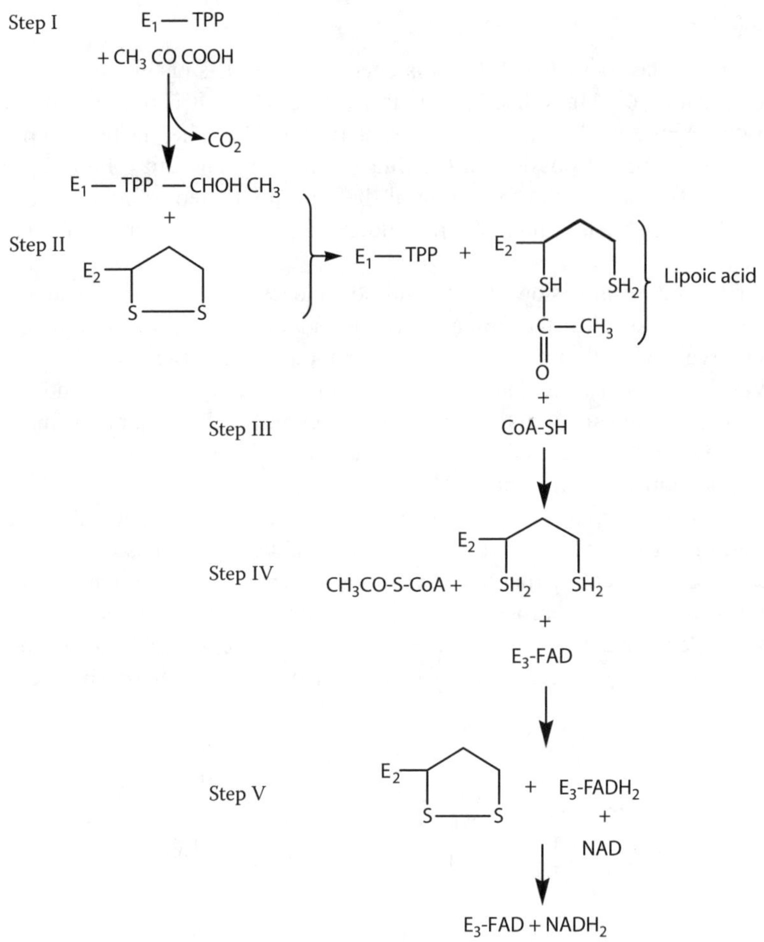

Step I E_1—TPP
+ CH_3 CO COOH
→ CO_2
E_1— TPP —CHOH CH_3
+
Step II E_2 (S—S ring) → E_1—TPP + E_2 SH SH_2 C—CH_3 =O Lipoic acid
+
Step III CoA-SH
Step IV CH_3CO-S-CoA + E_2 SH_2 SH_2
+
E_3-FAD
Step V E_2 (S—S ring) + E_3-$FADH_2$
+
NAD
E_3-FAD + $NADH_2$

FIGURE 12.7 Oxidation of the pyruvate in the mitochondrial matrix. E_1, pyruvate dehydrogenase; TPP, thiamin pyrophosphate; TPP, CHOH-CH_3–α-hydroxyethylthiamin pp; E_2, dihydrolipoyl transferase; E_3, dihydrolipoyl dehydrogenase.

The HE may then undergo hydrolysis to yield acetaldehyde or become oxidized to yield an acyl group. Figures 12.7 and 12.8 illustrate pyruvate metabolism and show where thiamin plays a role. Thiamin is active in the decarboxylation of α-ketoglutaric acid to succinyl CoA in the citric acid cycle. The mechanism of action is similar to that described earlier for pyruvate. Step I is similar to nonoxidative decarboxylation of pyruvate in alcohol fermentation. Step II involves the hydroxyethyl group. It is dehydrogenated and the remaining acetyl group is transferred to the sulfur atom at C6 (or C8) of lipoic acid. This constitutes a covalently bound prosthetic group of the second enzyme of the complex lipoate acetyltransferase. The transfer of H+ to the disulfide bond of lipoic acid converts the latter to its reduced or dithiol form dihydrolipoic acid. Step III involves the enzymatic transfer of the acetyl group to the thiol group of CoA, and a second H+ is added to form the dihydrolipoyl transacetylase. The Ac CoA so formed leaves the enzyme complex in the free form. Lastly, Step IV occurs when the dithiol form of lipoic acid is reoxidized to its disulfide form by the transfer of H+ and associated electrons to the third enzyme of the complex, dihydrolipoyl (lipoamide) dehydrogenase, whose reducible prosthetic group is FAD, $FADH_2$ which remains bound to the enzyme and transfers its electron to NAD+ to form NADH. These steps are illustrated in Figure 12.7.

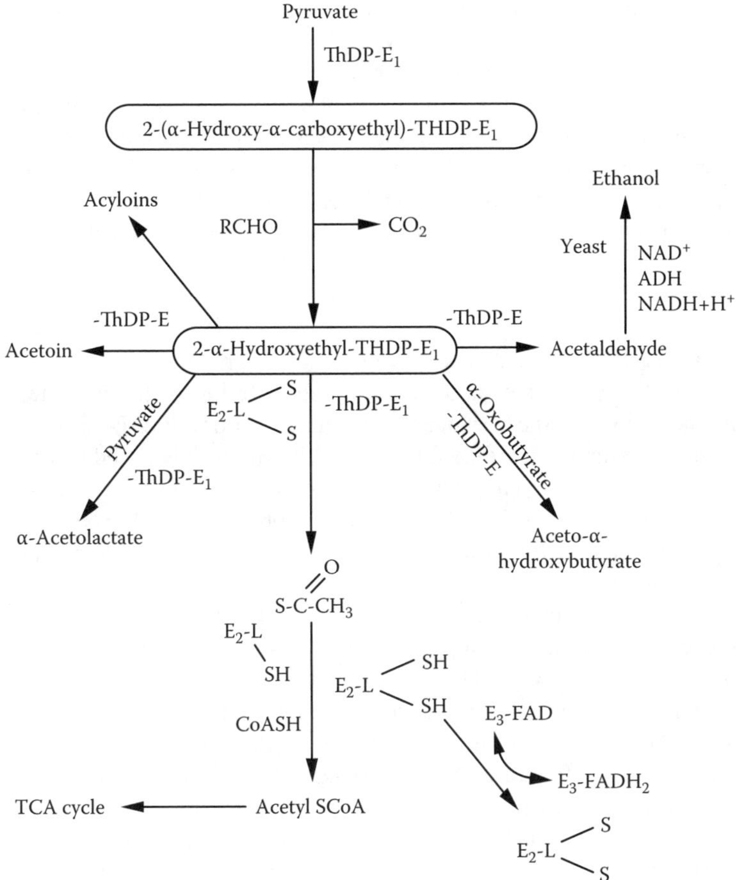

FIGURE 12.8 Summary of the metabolic pathways for pyruvate.

The oxidation of αKG to succinyl CoA is energetically irreversible and is carried out by the αKG DH complex:

$$\alpha\text{KG} + \text{NAD}^+ + \text{CoA} \Leftrightarrow \text{Succinyl CoA} + \text{CO}_2 + \text{NADH}_2 \Delta\text{G}^0 = 8.0 \text{ kcal mol}^{-1}$$

This reaction is analogous to the oxidation of pyruvate to acetyl CoA and CO_2 and occurs by the same mechanism with TPP, lipoic acid, CoA, FAD, and NAD participating as coenzymes.

The metabolism of ethanol also requires thiamin. The same pyruvate dehydrogenase complex that converts pyruvate to acetyl CoA will also metabolize acetaldehyde (the first product in the metabolism of ethanol) to acetyl CoA. This system probably accounts for only a small part of ethanol degradation.

TPP participates in the transfer of a glycolaldehyde group from D-xylulose to D ribose 5P to yield D-sedoheptulose 7P and glyceraldehyde 3P. These are reactions in the hexose monophosphate shunt. Glyceraldehyde 3P is also an intermediate of glycolysis. Transketolase contains tightly bound TPP. In this reaction, the glycolaldehyde group ($CH_2OH{\cdot}CO$) is first transferred from D-xylulose 5P to enzyme-bound TPP to form the α,β-dehydroxyethyl derivative of the latter that is analogous to the α-hydroxyethyl derivative formed during the action of PDH. The TPP acts as an intermediate carrier of this glycolaldehyde group that is transferred to the acceptor molecule D-ribose 5P. The thiamin coenzymes are involved in the oxidation of alcohol (see the Chapter 9). The rate-limiting step in alcohol oxidation is the amount of alcohol dehydrogenase present.

In addition to its role as a coenzyme, it is speculated that thiamin has an independent role in nervous tissue since it has been shown that stimulation of nerve fibers results in release of free thiamin and thiamin monophosphate. If a neurophysiologically active form of thiamin exists, it is as thiamin triphosphate. However, thiamin's role in the central nervous system (CNS) at present is viewed as an intriguing enigma. There has been a report of an inverse relationship between depressive symptoms and thiamin nutritional status,[27] but a explanation for this relationship is lacking.

Deficiency

The major symptoms of thiamin deficiency are loss of appetite (anorexia), weight loss, convulsions, slowing of the heart rate (bradycardia), and lowering of the body temperature. Loss of muscle tone and lesions of the nervous system may also develop. Because the heart muscle can be weakened, there may be cardiac failure resulting in peripheral edema and ascites in the extremities. The urine of rats with a thiamin deficit contains a higher pyruvate–lactate ratio than that of normal animals. Thiamin-deficient rats also exhibit a reduced erythrocyte transketolase activity.[28,29] Administration of thiamin to rats brings about a remarkable reversal of deficiency symptoms in less than 24 h.

The classical pathological condition arising from thiamin deficiency in humans is beriberi. This disease was quite common in the Orient prior to the discovery of its cause. Thiamin deficiency can arise not only from poor intake of food but also from its faulty utilization or absorption.

Beriberi is classified into several types: acute-mixed, wet, or dry (Table 12.5). The acute-mixed type is characterized by neural and cardiac symptoms producing neuritis and heart failure. In wet beriberi, the edema of heart failure is the most striking sign; digestive disorders and emaciation are additional symptoms. In dry beriberi, a loss of function of the lower extremities or paralysis predominates; it is often called polyneuritis. Clinical manifestations of thiamin deficiency vary depending upon the severity of the deprivation. The deficiency state is characterized by a symmetrical foot and wrist drop associated with a great deal of muscle tenderness. It may also affect cardiac muscle metabolism and may result in congestive heart failure.

TABLE 12.5
Clinical Features of Thiamin Deficiency

Wet and dry beriberi malaise	Heaviness and weakness of legs
	Calf muscle tenderness
	Pins and needles and numbness in legs
	Anesthesia of skin
	Increased pulse rate and heart palpitations
Wet beriberi	Edema of legs, face, trunk, and serous cavities
	Tense calf muscles
	Fast pulse
	Distended neck veins
	High blood pressure
	Decreased urine volume
Dry beriberi	Polyneuritis
	Difficulty walking
	Wernicke–Korsakoff syndrome
	Encephalopathy; disorientation; short-term memory loss
	Jerky movements of eyes
	Staggering gait

Thiamin deficiency is the most common vitamin deficiency seen in chronic alcoholics in the United States. It is known as alcoholic beriberi. It is seen in those individuals who consume alcohol in preference to food and thus have a minimal intake of thiamin. The most serious form of thiamin deficiency in alcoholics is the Wernicke syndrome. It is characterized by ophthalmoplegia, sixth nerve palsy, nystagmus, ptosis, ataxia, confusion, and coma, which may terminate in death. Oftentimes, the confusional state persists after treatment of the acute thiamin deficiency. This is known as Korsakoff's psychosis. The signs and symptoms of thiamin deficiency are listed in Table 12.5. All forms of thiamin deficiency respond to thiamin treatment unless the pathology is irreversible, a situation not infrequently found with pathological changes in the nerve tracts (polyneuropathy).

Red cell transketolase activity seems to be a sensitive index of thiamin nutritional status. Brin et al.[24] have suggested an in vitro test to differentiate between the enzymatic lesions caused by thiamin deficiency and those due to nonspecific causes. This test consists of the stimulation of red cell transketolase activity using glyceraldehyde-3-phosphate as the substrate in the presence of saturating amounts of TPP. This is coupled to an NADH indicator reaction. The reaction results in the so-called TPP effect (TPPE) and is claimed to be a good indicator of thiamin nutritional status.

In addition to the enzymatic test, a measure of urinary thiamin in relation to dietary intake has been the basis for balance studies to assess the adequacy of intake. When thiamin excretion is low, a larger portion of the test dose is retained, indicating a tissue need for thiamin. A high excretion indicates tissue saturation. On low intakes, excretion drops to zero.

Needs

Thiamin needs of an individual are influenced by many factors: age, caloric intake, carbohydrate intake, and body weight. The presence of infection may drive up the need for thiamin.[30] Table 12.1 gives the DRIs for humans.

Toxicity

Although thiamin produces a variety of pharmacological effects when administered in large doses, the dose required is thousands of times greater than those required for optimal nutrition. Generally, toxic effects are reported when subcutaneous, intramuscular, intraspinal, or intravenous injections are administered but not through oral administration. In rare cases, large doses of thiamin have elicited symptoms of anaphylactic shock.

RIBOFLAVIN

While thiamin and niacin were being recognized as the causative factors in beriberi and pellagra, respectively, riboflavin, the second B vitamin, was ignored. A food fraction isolated by McCollum and Kennedy in 1916 was shown by Emmett and Luros and later by Goldberger and Lillie to have several functions: one as an antiberiberi curative, one as a pellagra curative, and a third whose function was not known.[21] These fractions were all water soluble but differed in their stability toward heat and light. In 1932, Warburg and Christian isolated and described a flavoprotein that was recognized by others as having vitamin properties. This then became the vitamin riboflavin. Since it was first isolated with thiamin and niacin, it was given a letter designation in England as vitamin B_2 and in the United States as vitamin G. As our knowledge of vitamins increased, this nomenclature was dropped in favor of the name riboflavin.

Structure

Riboflavin (Figure 12.9) is a yellow-orange crystalline substance frequently associated with flavoproteins. As a solid, it is red-orange in color. In solution, the color changes to a greenish

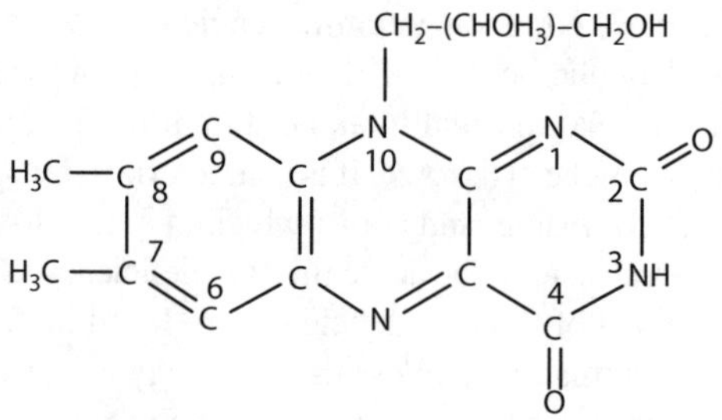

7, 8 Dimethyl-10-(1 D-ribityl) isoalloxazine
or
6, 7 Dimethyl-9-(D-1 ribityl) isolloxazine,
if only the carbons are numbered

FIGURE 12.9 Structure of riboflavin.

yellow. It was first synthesized by Kuhn and also by Karrer et al. in 1935 as a needlelike crystal with limited solubility in pure water or in acid solutions.

Physical and Chemical Properties

Solubility increases as the pH of the solvent increases; however, as the pH of the solution rises, riboflavin's stability to heat and light decreases. Milk loses 33% of its riboflavin activity in 1 h of sunlight. In solution, riboflavin is easily destroyed by light and must be protected at all times from exposure. Biochemists working with riboflavin take such precautions as using deep red glassware and darkened work areas to ensure maximal recovery or assessment of vitamin activity. Because riboflavin fluoresces due to a shifting of bonds in the isoalloxazine ring, this property can be used as a basis for its determination by spectrophotometric or photofluorometric techniques. The fluorescence is due to the presence of a free 3-imino group. If substitutions are made for this group, there is no fluorescence. Fluorescence can be measured before and after reduction by such compounds as sodium hydrosulfite. Fluorescence is pH dependent and is best measured at pH values between 4 and 8; maximal fluorescence occurs at 556 nm.

The oxidized forms of different flavoenzymes are intensely colored. They are characteristically yellow, red, or green due to strong absorption bands in the visible range. Upon reduction, they undergo bleaching with a characteristic change in the absorption spectrum as illustrated in Figure 12.10. In order to have vitamin activity, positions 7 and 8 must be substituted with more than just a hydrogen, and the amine group in position 3 must be unattached. There must be a ribityl group in position 10. If the ribityl group is lost, then vitamin activity is lost as shown in Figure 12.11. There are some antivitamins that interfere with riboflavin's usefulness. These compounds compete for the prosthetic groups or competitively inhibit its phosphorylation to form the coenzymes flavin mononucleotide (FMN) or FAD. The structures of FAD and FMN are shown in Figure 12.12.[26]

Sources

The best sources are foods of animal origin: milk, meat, and eggs. Wheat germ is also a good source. For the riboflavin content of a large variety of foods, visit the USDA website www.nal.usda.gov/foodcomposition.

Assay

The most sensitive procedure for the determination of riboflavin is that which uses HPLC. As mentioned, the vitamin must be protected from light and acid. The coenzyme forms must be separated from the free form. This can be done by differential solubility. The free form is soluble in benzyl alcohol, while the coenzymes are not.

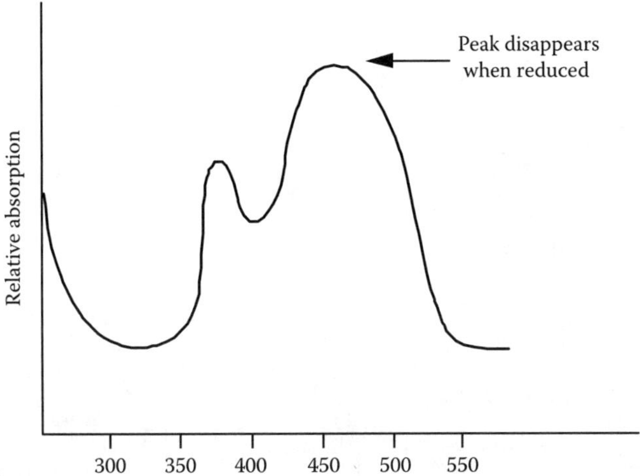

FIGURE 12.10 Absorption spectra of riboflavin.

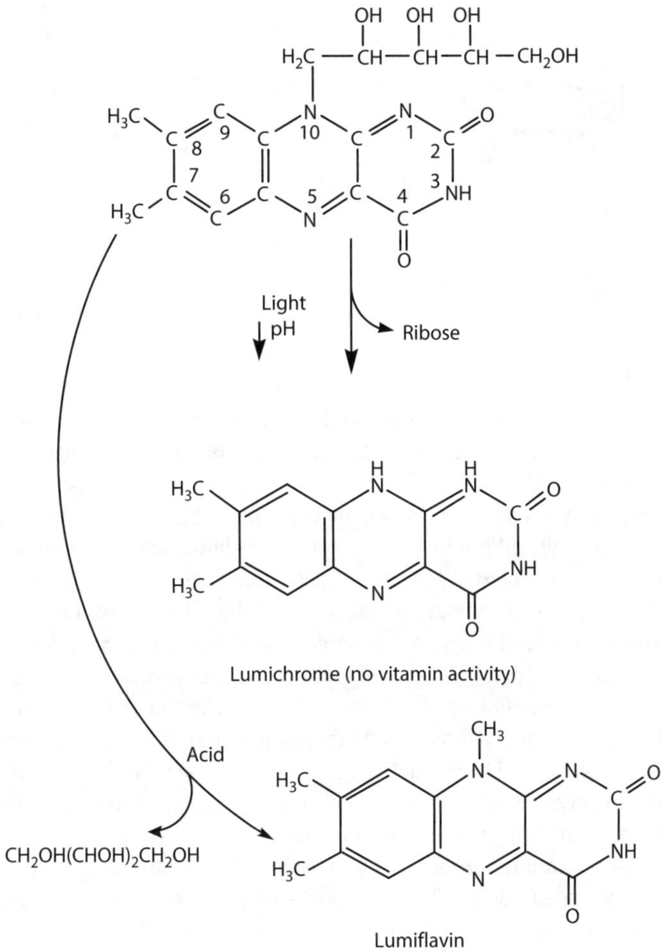

Light
pH
Ribose
Lumichrome (no vitamin activity)
Acid
$CH_2OH(CHOH)_2CH_2OH$
Lumiflavin

FIGURE 12.11 Degradation of riboflavin to lumichrome and lumiflavin. Neither of these compounds have vitamin activity.

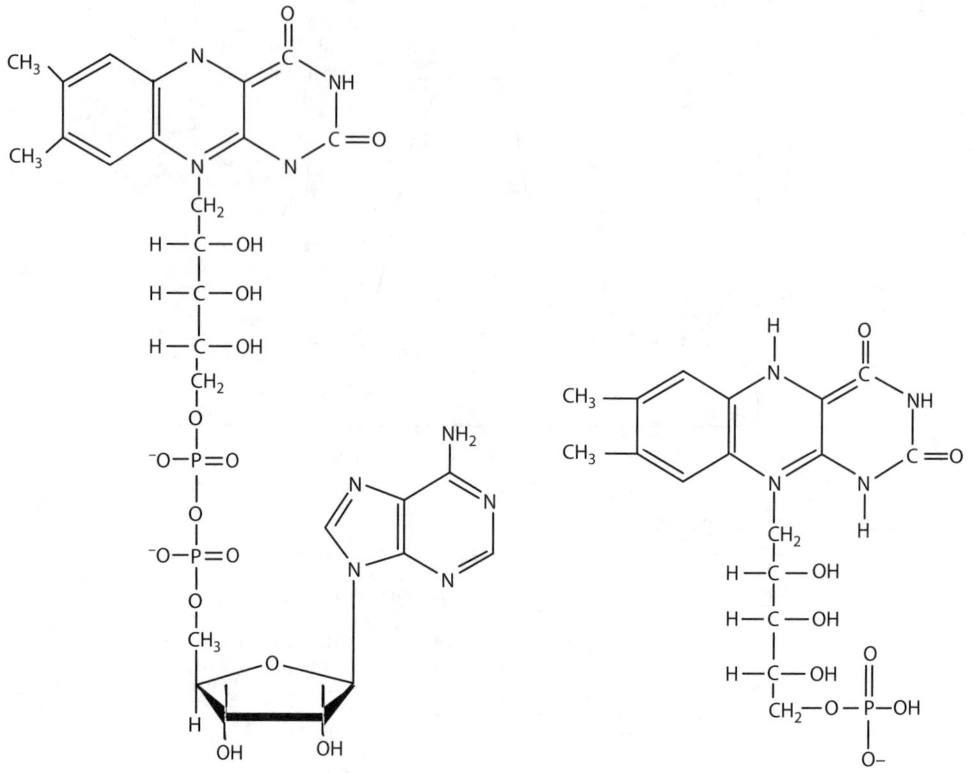

FIGURE 12.12 Structures of FAD and FMN.

Absorption and Metabolism

Absorption occurs by way of an active carrier and is energy and sodium dependent.[31,32] Maximum absorption occurs in the proximal segment (the jejunum) of the small intestine with significant uptake by the duodenum and ileum.

After a load dose, peak values in the plasma appear within 2 h. The phosphorylated forms (coenzyme forms) are dephosphorylated prior to absorption through the action of nonspecific hydrolases on the brush border membrane of the duodenum and jejunum. There is a pyrophosphatase that cleaves FAD and FMN and an alkaline phosphatase that liberates the vitamin from its coenzyme form. Bile salts appear to facilitate uptake and a small amount of the vitamin circulates via the enterohepatic system. Prior to entry into the portal blood, some of the vitamin is rephosphorylated to reform FAD and FMN. After absorption, the vitamin circulates in the blood bound to plasma proteins notably albumin. Specific riboflavin-binding proteins have been isolated and identified in several species. These proteins are of hepatic origin.[33–35] There is active uptake of the free vitamin by all of the vital organs.[36] For example, isolated liver cells will accumulate up to five times the amount of the vitamin in the fluids that surround them. Although cells will accumulate the vitamin against a concentration gradient, these cells also use the vitamin quite rapidly so there is little net storage. The usual blood levels of riboflavin are in the range of 20–50 mg/L, while 500–900 μg/day is excreted in the urine. Excretion products include 7- and 8-hydroxymethyl riboflavin, 8α-sulfonylriboflavin, riboflavin peptide esters, 10-hydroxyethylflavin, lumiflavin, 10-formylmethylflavin, 10-carboxymethylflavin, lumichrome, and of course free riboflavin. Very small amounts of riboflavin and metabolites can be found in the feces. Upon entry into the cell, riboflavin is reconverted to FMN and FAD as shown in Figure 12.13.[31]

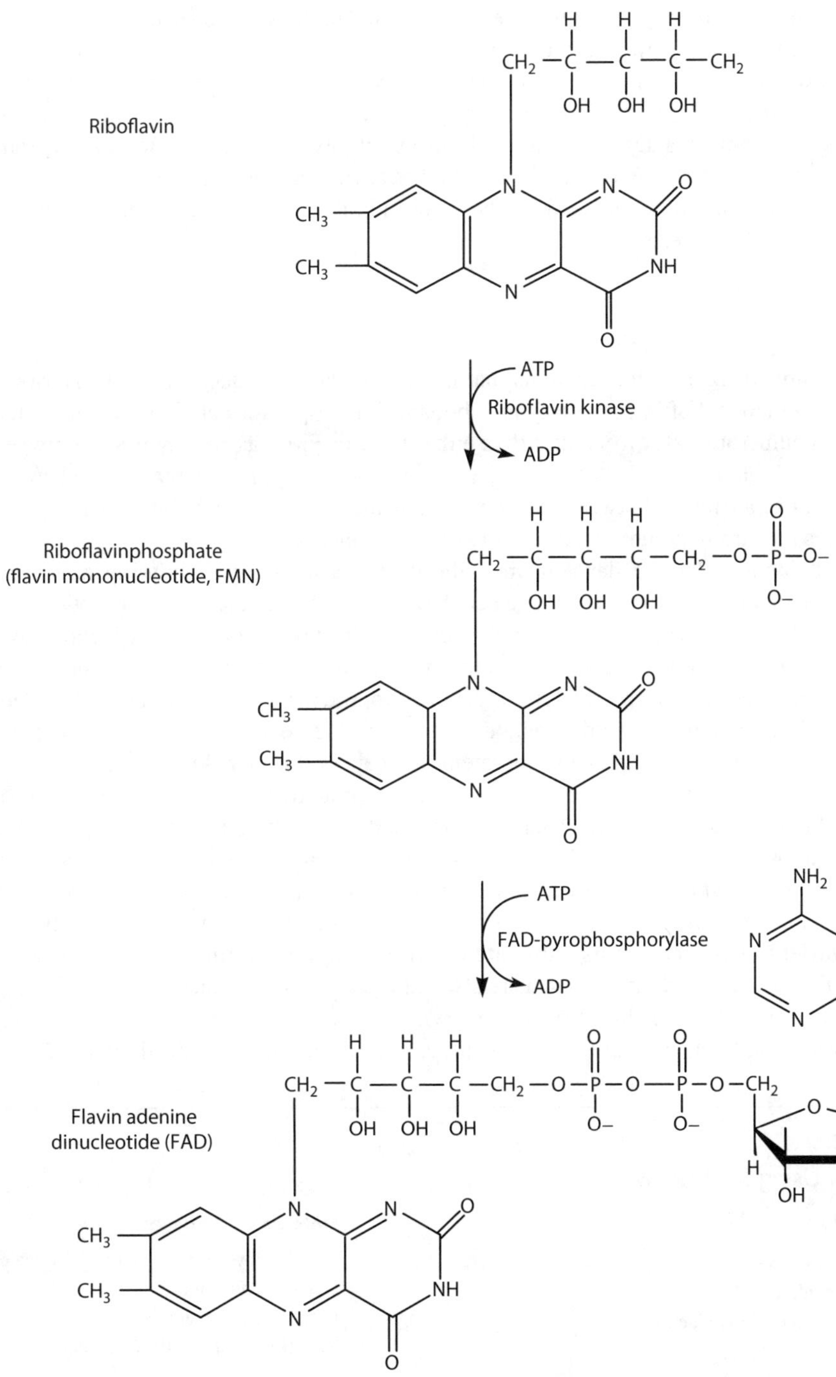

Riboflavin

ATP
Riboflavin kinase
ADP

Riboflavinphosphate
(flavin mononucleotide, FMN)

ATP
FAD-pyrophosphorylase
ADP

Flavin adenine
dinucleotide (FAD)

FIGURE 12.13 Syntheses of FMN and FAD.

The initial phosphorylation reaction is zinc dependent. Hyperthyroidism is associated with increased synthesis of FMN and FAD, whereas hypothyroidism is associated with decreased synthesis. FAD is linked to a variety of proteins via hydrogen bonding and also with purines, phenols, and indoles. Covalent bonding with certain enzymes also occurs and involves the riboflavin 8-methyl group, which forms a methylene bridge to the peptide histidyl imidazole function or to the thioether function of a former cysteinyl residue. When bound to these proteins, these coenzymes are protected from degradation. However, flavins in excess of that which are protein bound are rapidly degraded and excreted in the urine. Degradation begins with hydroxylation at positions 7 and 8 of the isoalloxazine ring by hepatic microsomal cytochrome P450 enzymes. The methyl groups at these positions are removed, and the compound loses its activity as a vitamin. Because degradation and excretion occur at a fairly rapid rate, the rate of riboflavin degradation determines the requirement for the vitamin rather than the need for the vitamin in its function as a coenzyme, that is, the rate of FMN and FAD synthesis.

Functions

FAD and FMN are coenzymes for reactions that involve oxidation–reduction.[28,29] Thus, riboflavin is an important component of intermediary metabolism. The respiratory chain in the mitochondria and reactions in numerous pathways that utilize either FAD or FMN as coenzymes require riboflavin.[38–40] Shown in Table 12.6 is a list of some of these enzymes. They include reactions where reducing equivalents are transferred between cellular compartments as part of a shuttle arrangement as well as reactions that are in a mitochondrial or cytosolic sequence.

In most glutathione reductase flavoenzymes, the flavin nucleotide is tightly but noncovalently bound to the protein; an exception is succinate dehydrogenase in which the flavin nucleotide, FAD, is covalently bound to a histidine residue of the polypeptide chain of the enzyme.[41] The metalloflavoproteins contain one or more metals as additional cofactors. Flavin nucleotides undergo reversible reduction of the isoalloxazine ring in the catalytic cycle of flavoproteins to yield the reduced nucleotides $FMNH_2$ and $FADH_2$. The mechanism of action is shown in Figure 12.14. Each of the steps in this sequence is fully reversible allowing the flavoprotein to accept or donate reducing equivalents, which in turn can be joined to oxygen. Many of the flavoproteins (proteins linked with FAD or FMN) also contain a metal ion such as iron, molybdenum, or zinc, and the combination of these metals and the flavin structure allows for its easy and rapid transition between single- and double-electron donors.

Note in Table 12.6 that a number of enzymes are members of the oxidase family of enzymes. The oxidases transfer hydrogen directly to oxygen to form hydrogen peroxide. Xanthine oxidase uses a variety of purines as its substrate converting hypoxanthine to xanthine, which is then converted to uric acid. Xanthine oxidase also catalyzes the conversion of retinal to retinoic acid (see Chapter 11). Among the important enzymes shown in Table 12.6 are those that are essential to mitochondrial respiration, ATP synthesis, and the mitochondrial citric acid cycle.

TABLE 12.6
Reactions Using FAD or FMN

FAD-Linked Enzymes	FMN-Linked Enzymes
Ubiquinone reductase	NADH dehydrogenase (respiratory chain)
Monoamine oxidase	L-amino acid oxidase
NADH-cytochrome P450 reductase	Lactate dehydrogenase
D-amino acid oxidase	NADH cytochrome P450 reductase
Acyl CoA dehydrogenase	
Dihydrolipoyl dehydrogenase (component of PDH and α-KGDH)	
Xanthine oxidase	
Cytochrome reductase	
Succinate dehydrogenase	
α-Glycerophosphate dehydrogenase	
Electron transport respiratory chain	
Glutathione reductase	

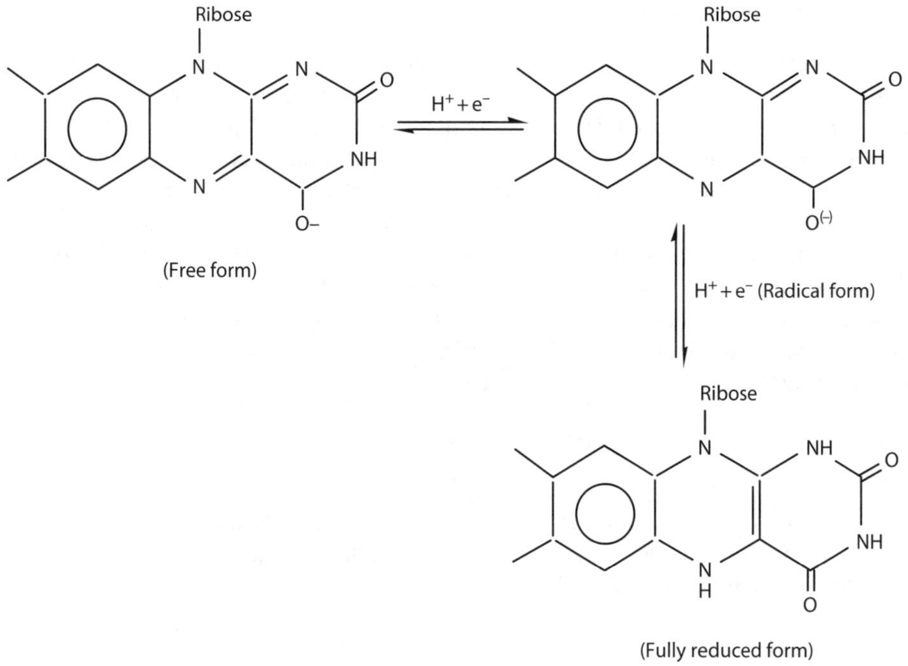

FIGURE 12.14 Mechanism of action of the riboflavin portion of the coenzyme.

Succinate dehydrogenase is one of these enzymes and its activity has been used as a biomarker of riboflavin intake sufficiency. The acyl CoA dehydrogenases catalyze another of the essential pathways that is fatty acid oxidation. These are FAD linked. Fatty acid synthesis requires the presence of FMN-linked enzymes. While the list of enzymes shown in Table 12.6 is by no means complete, it gives evidence of the intimate and essential need for riboflavin in metabolic pathways. In humans, clinical signs of deficiency appear in less than 6 weeks on intakes less than 0.6 mg/day.

Deficiency

Despite our knowledge about riboflavin's function as coenzyme, there are a few symptoms that are specific to riboflavin deficiency.[42] Poor growth, poor appetite, and certain skin lesions (cracks at the corners of the mouth, dermatitis on the scrotum) have been observed. However, these symptoms can also occur for reasons apart from inadequate riboflavin intake. This lack of a direct correlation of symptoms to intake is due to the almost universal need for FAD and FMN as coenzymes in such a wide variety of the reactions of intermediary metabolism. There is a relationship between riboflavin status and anemia. Women whose poor riboflavin status was corrected with riboflavin supplements showed an improvement in their hematological status.[43]

Nutrition assessment of adequate riboflavin intake relies upon a few reactions in readily available cells, that is, blood cells, which can predict intake adequacy. Erythrocyte FAD-linked glutathione reductase is one of these as is succinate dehydrogenase. Low enzyme activity is associated with inadequate intakes.

Needs

As mentioned, there is almost no riboflavin reserve. Thus, a daily intake of riboflavin is essential. The DRIs for humans are shown in Table 12.1.

NIACIN, OR NICOTINIC ACID

Few vitamins have as tortured a history of discovery as niacin. This vitamin has a number of names: vitamin B_3, nicotinic acid, niacin, or nicotinamide.[21,22] The synthesis of nicotinic acid was accomplished long before it was discovered to be a vitamin. Some 50 years elapsed before it was connected to the disease pellagra. Pellagra was described in the mid-1800s and called *mal de la rosa*. Its development was associated with the consumption of low-protein–high-corn diets. The disease was more prevalent in very poor populations and again associated with the consumption of corn. At one time, it was thought to be due to a toxin found in corn; however, as descriptions of pellagra arose in the literature from populations that did not consume corn, this idea was discarded. Some years later, Goldberger demonstrated that pellagra was a nutrient deficiency disease and that the nutrient in question was niacin or nicotinic acid. The term niacin is a generic term, which includes both the acid and amide forms.

STRUCTURE

Niacin occurs in two forms as shown in Figure 12.15. Nicotinic acid and nicotinamide are widely distributed in nature.[44] Nicotinic acid is the primary constituent of the coenzymes NAD^+ and nicotinamide dinucleotide phosphate ($NADP^+$).[22]

PHYSICAL AND CHEMICAL PROPERTIES

The molecular weight of nicotinic acid is 123.1 and that of nicotinamide 122.1. Nicotinamide is far more soluble in water than is nicotinic acid. Both are white crystals with an absorption maximum of 263 nm. The melting point of the acid form is 237°C, while that of the amide is 128°C–131°C. In order to have vitamin activity, there must be a pyridine ring substituted with a β-carboxylic acid or corresponding amide, and there must be open sites at pyridine carbons 2–6. Nicotinic acid is amphoteric and forms salts with acids and bases. Its carboxyl group can form esters and anhydrides and can be reduced. Both the acid and amide forms are very stable in the dry form, but when the amide form is in solution, it is readily hydrolyzed to the acid form.

Several substituted pyridines can antagonize the biological activity of niacin. These include pyridine 3-sulfonic acid, 3-acetylpyridine, isonicotinic acid hydrazide, and 6-aminonicotinamide. HPLC is the analytical method of choice for vitamin analysis. Niacin does not occur in large amounts as the free form. Most often it occurs as the coenzyme NAD^+ or $NADP^+$. Chemical analysis using the Koenig reaction, which opens up the pyridine ring with cyanogen bromide followed by reaction with an aromatic amine to form a colored product, is used. The most widely used method employs a chromophore-generating base, *p*-methylaminophenol sulfate, sulfanilic acid, or barbituric acid. The color intensity so developed is dependent on the concentration of the vitamin.

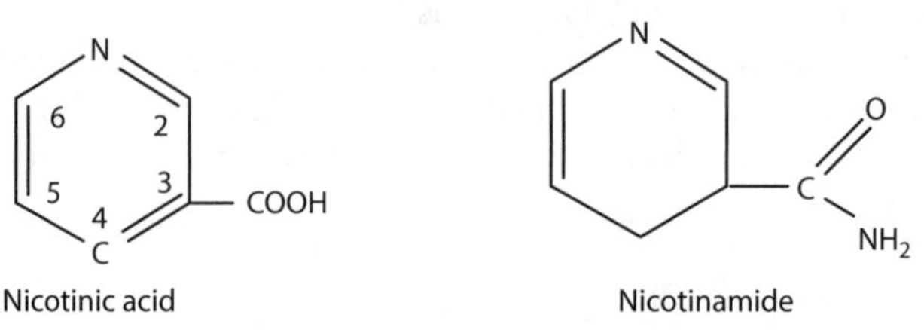

N
6
2
5
3
4
C
COOH
Nicotinic acid

N
O
C
NH_2
Nicotinamide

FIGURE 12.15 Structures of nicotinic acid (niacin) and nicotinamide.

Sources

This vitamin is widely distributed in the human food supply. Especially good sources are whole grain cereals and breads, milk, eggs, meats, and vegetables that are richly colored. Visit the USDA website www.nal.usda.gov/food-composition for the niacin content of a large variety of foods.

Absorption and Metabolism

In contrast to thiamin and riboflavin, niacin is not absorbed via an active process.[45] Rather, both nicotinic acid and nicotinamide cross the intestinal cell by way of simple diffusion and facilitated diffusion. There are species differences in the mechanism of absorption. In the bullfrog, absorption is via active transport. In the rat, there is evidence of a transporter that is saturable and sodium dependent. This suggests facilitated diffusion. After absorption, the vitamin circulates in the blood in its free form. That which is not converted to NAD^+ or $NADP^+$ is metabolized further and excreted in the urine. The excretory metabolites are *N′*-methylnicotinamide, nicotinuric acid, nicotinamide-*N′*-oxide, *N′*-methylnicotinamide-*N′*-oxide, *N*-methylnicotinamide-*N* oxide, *N*-methyl-4-pyridone-3-carboxamide, and *N* methyl-2-pyridone-5-carboxamide. Niacin can be synthesized from tryptophan in a ratio of 60 molecules of tryptophan to 1 of nicotinic acid.[46] The pathway for conversion is shown in Figure 12.16. Note the involvement of thiamin, pyridoxine, and riboflavin in this conversion.

Function

The main function of this vitamin is that of the coenzymes NAD^+ and $NADP^+$.[25] Both function in the maintenance of the redox state of the cell. These coenzymes are bound to the dehydrogenase enzyme protein relatively loosely during the catalytic cycle and therefore serve more as substrates than as prosthetic groups. They act as electron acceptors during the enzymatic removal of hydrogen atoms from specific substrates. One hydrogen atom of the substrate is transferred as a hydride ion to the nicotinamide portion of the oxidized NAD^+ or $NADP^+$. This yields the reduced coenzyme form $NADH^+$ H or $NADPH^+H^+$. The second hydrogen ion remains loosely associated. Most enzymes are specific for NAD^+ or $NADP^+$ and these enzymes are members of the oxidoreductase family of enzymes.

Most of the NAD- or NADP-linked enzymes are involved in catabolic pathways, that is, glycolysis or the pentose phosphate shunt. NAD^+ turns over quite rapidly in the cell. Its degradation is shown in Figure 12.17. However, $NADH^+H^+$ also plays an important role in covalent modifications of histones (DNA-binding proteins) as described in Chapter 7. Actually, NAD^+ is the substrate for several families of ADP-ribosylation reactions that control processes such as DNA repair, replication, transcription, the activity of the G proteins, chromatin structure, and intracellular calcium signaling.[47] $NADH^+H^+$ provides the substrate that leads to poly-ADP-ribosylation of glutamate residues in histones, mediated by poly-ADP-ribose polymerase (PARP-1). PARP-1 is the most active of the PARP enzymes and has been implicated in both prevention and aggravation of disease processes. Inhibition of poly-ADP-ribose formation can prevent many acute disease processes such as stroke, myocardial infarction, and septic shock but will tend to cause genetic instability and tumorigenesis under chronic conditions. Niacin-deficient rats give evidence of DNA strand breaks and reduced PARP activity, and this emphasizes the role of this vitamin in the maintenance of normal cell cycle.[48]

Beyond its use in biological systems as a precursor of NAD^+ or $NADP^+$, nicotinic acid has a pharmacological use. When consumed in pharmacological doses, it is degraded as though it was benzoic acid. Nicotinic acid, the drug, is used as a lipid-lowering drug.[49,50] Niacin treatment lowers the apolipoproteins (apo) B–containing lipoproteins and increases the apo A-1–containing lipoproteins (the high-density lipoproteins). Niacin treatment also inhibits triglyceride synthesis, thus lowering serum triglycerides. Large intakes (1 g/day) lower serum cholesterol. However, large doses also result in flushing due to its effect on vascular tone. The flushing involves the niacin receptor GPR109A.[51] Nicotinic acid elicits a fibrinolytic activation of very short duration. Both nicotinic acid and nicotinamide can be toxic if administered at levels greater than 10 μmol/kg.[52]

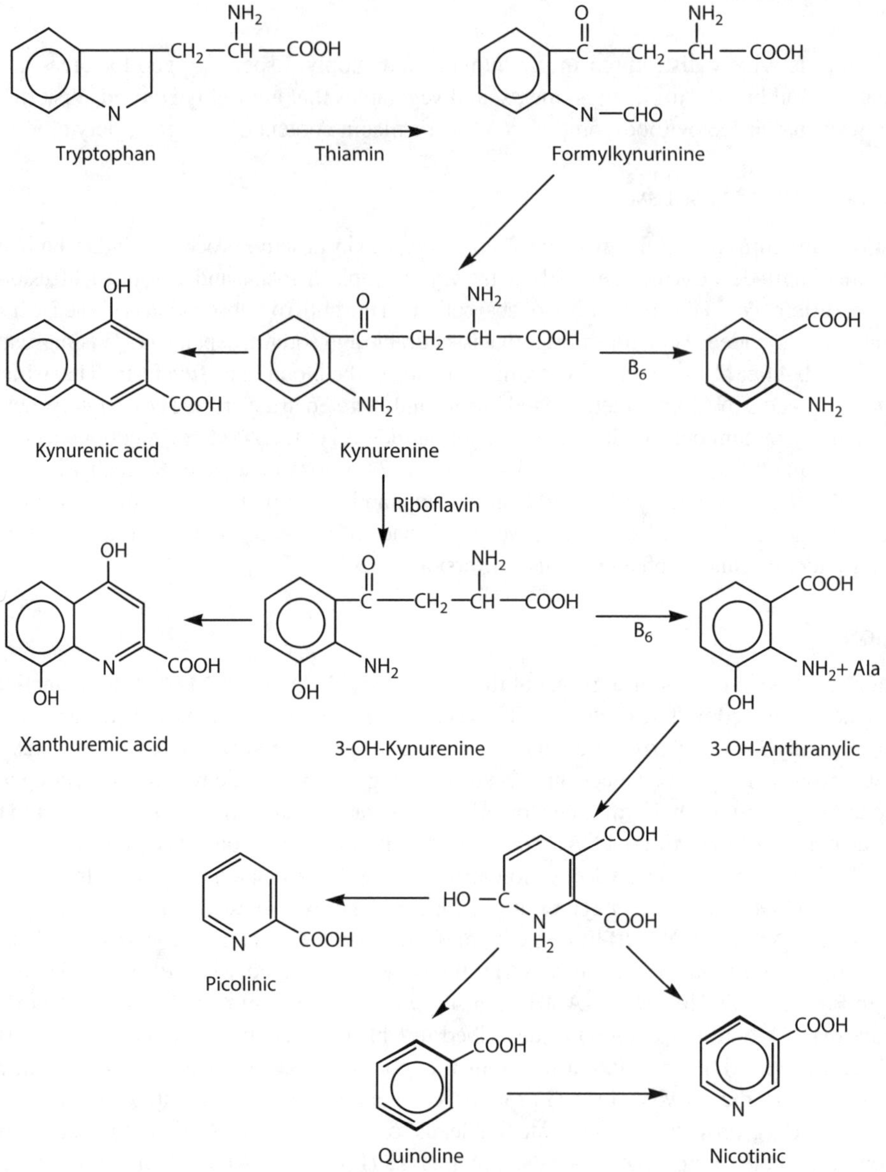

FIGURE 12.16 Synthesis of niacin from tryptophan.

Chronic administration of 3 g/day to humans results in a variety of symptoms, including headache, heartburn, nausea, hives, fatigue, sore throat, dry hair, inability to focus the eyes, and skin tautness. In experimental animals, nicotinic acid supplements result in a reduction in adipocyte free fatty acid release by streptozotocin-diabetic rats, an inhibition of adipocyte adenylate cyclase activity in normal hamsters, and degenerative changes in the heart muscle of normal rats.[53]

Deficiency

Pellagra has been well described as the niacin deficiency disease. It is characterized by skin lesions that are blackened and rough especially in areas exposed to sunlight and abraded by clothing. The typical skin lesions of pellagra are accompanied by insomnia, loss of appetite,

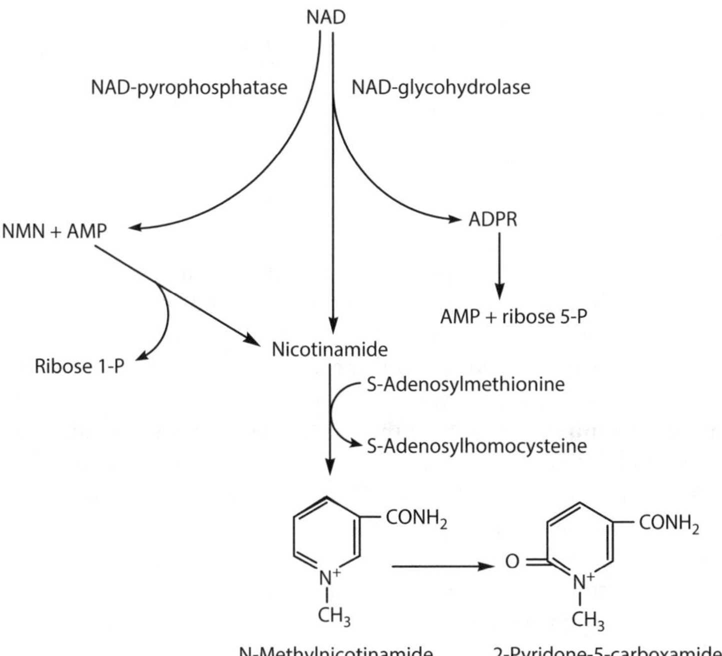

FIGURE 12.17 Degradation of NAD.

weight loss, soreness of mouth and tongue, indigestion, diarrhea, abdominal pain, burning sensations in various parts of the body, vertigo, headache, numbness, nervousness, apprehension, mental confusion, and forgetfulness. Many of these symptoms can be related to niacin deficiency–induced deficits in the metabolism of the CNS. This system has, as its choice metabolic fuel, glucose. Glycolysis with its attendant need for NAD^+ as a coenzyme is appreciably less active. As the deficient state progresses, numbness followed by a paralysis of the extremities occurs. The more advanced cases are characterized by tremor and a spastic or ataxic movement that is associated with peripheral nerve inflammation. Death from pellagra ensues if the patient remains untreated.

Early indications of niacin deficiency include reductions in the levels of urinary niacin metabolites especially those that are methylated (*N′* methylnicotinamide and *N′*-methyl-2-pyridone-5-carboxamide).[54] Since the discovery early in this century of the curative power of nicotinic acid and nicotinamide, pellagra is very rare. The exception is in the alcoholic population. This population frequently substitutes alcoholic beverages for food and thereby is at risk for multiple nutrient deficiencies, including pellagra. The metabolism of ethanol is NAD dependent. In part, the CNS symptoms of alcoholism are those of pellagra as described earlier.

There is another very small population at risk for developing niacin deficiency. This group carries a mutation in the gene for tryptophan transport and is called Hartnup's disease. Its symptoms, apart from tryptophan inadequacy effects on protein synthesis, are very similar to those of niacin deficiency. This is because of the use of tryptophan as a precursor of nicotinic acid. If niacin supplements are given to people with Hartnup's disease, the pellagra-like symptoms disappear.

Needs

Age, gender, and protein intake affect the DRI for niacin. Low-protein diets would increase the need for niacin in the diet since there would be little excess tryptophan available for conversion to niacin. Because tryptophan can be converted to nicotinic acid, the DRI is stated in terms of niacin equivalents. A niacin equivalent is equal to 1 mg of niacin or 60 mg of tryptophan. The need for niacin is related to energy intake as well, particularly the carbohydrate intake. However, the DRI takes into account varying diet compositions as well as individual differences in nutrient need. The DRI for niacin is given in Table 12.1.

PYRIDOXINE

Of all the B vitamins whose nomenclature has been changed to trivial names, one vitamin remains known by its letter designation: vitamin B_6.[55,56] This vitamin was first defined by Gyorgy in 1934 as "that part of the vitamin B complex responsible for the cure of a specific dermatitis developed by rats on a vitamin-free diet supplemented with thiamin and riboflavin." The dermatitis is unlike that seen with other deficiencies of the B complex. There is a characteristic scaliness about the paws and mouth of rats in addition to a loss of hair from the body.

The vitamin was crystallized in 1938 by three different groups of researchers and was subsequently characterized and synthesized. Even though the vitamin was identified, crystallized, and synthesized in the late 1930s, it was not realized until 1945 that there were three distinct forms of the vitamin: pyridoxamine (an amine), pyridoxal (an aldehyde), and pyridoxine (an alcohol). These forms are interconvertible. Pyridoxine was isolated primarily from plant sources, while pyridoxal and pyridoxamine were isolated from animal tissues. The latter two are more potent growth factors for bacteria and are more potent precursors for the coenzymes pyridoxal phosphate (PPS) and pyridoxamine phosphate.

STRUCTURE

The three forms are shown in Figure 12.18. Vitamin B_6 is the generic descriptor for all 2-methyl-3,5-dihydroxymethyl pyridine derivatives. To have vitamin activity, it must be phosphorylated at the 5-hydroxymethyl group, and the substituent at carbon 4 must be convertible to the aldehyde form. Pyridoxine hydrochloride is the commercially available vitamin and is also shown in Figure 12.18.

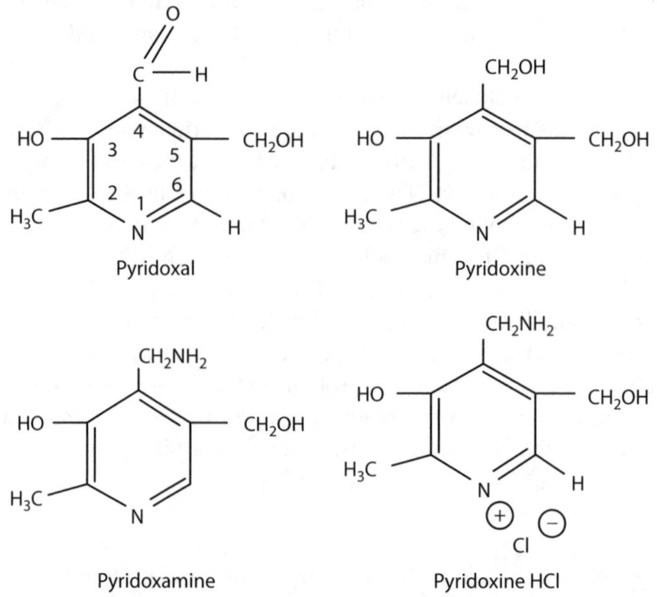

FIGURE 12.18 Structures of naturally occurring vitamin B_6.

Physical and Chemical Properties

The molecular weight of pyridoxal is 167.2. Pyridoxine HCl has a molecular weight of 205.6. Both occur as a white crystal that is readily soluble in water. Pyridoxine HCl is stable to light and heat in acid solutions. In neutral or alkaline solutions, it is unstable to light and heat. This feature was recognized in an unfortunate way: infant formulas that were autoclaved lost their vitamin content, and the infants became deficient.[57] The aldehyde form (pyridoxal) is much less stable. Its instability to heat is a major concern in food processing since foods that are rich in the vitamin are neutral to slightly alkaline. When heat treated, as is necessary to kill foodborne pathogens and prevent spoilage, vitamin activity may be lost. This is particularly true for foods that are autoclaved (i.e., infant formulas).

Pyridoxine, pyridoxal, and pyridoxamine can be assayed in a variety of techniques. Pyridoxal has an absorption maximum of 293, while pyridoxine HCl has absorption maxima of 255 and 326. Microbiological, colorimetric/spectrophotometric, and chromatographic techniques are available. The method of choice is HPLC.

Sources

Vitamin B_6 is widely distributed throughout foods from the plant and animal kingdoms. Meats, cereals, legumes, lentils, nuts, fruits, and vegetables all contain the vitamin. Thus, persons consuming a diet containing a variety of raw and cooked foods likely will not develop a deficiency of the vitamin. Visit the USDA website www.nal.usda.gov/foodcomposition for the vitamin content of a large variety of foods.

Absorption and Metabolism

Studies on rat and hamster small intestine both in vivo and in vitro have provided no evidence of an active transport mechanism for the vitamin. Uptake into everted sacs of rat jejunum over a concentration range of 0.01–10 M of pyridoxine did not show saturation kinetics, nor was uptake inhibited by anoxia, DNP, lack of sodium, ouabain, or the presence of a structural analog 4-deoxypyridoxine. Thus, pyridoxine uptake is by passive diffusion rather than by active transport (Figure 12.19). Once absorbed, it is carried by the erythrocyte to all cells in the body. Significant amounts of the vitamin may be found in liver, brain, spleen, kidney, and heart, but like the other water-soluble vitamins, there is no appreciable store and this vitamin must be present in the daily diet. It is carried in the blood tightly bound to proteins, primarily hemoglobin and albumin. The vitamin binds via the amino group of the N-terminal valine residue of the hemoglobin α-chain, and this binding has twice the strength of its binding to albumin. Pyridoxal is converted via a saturable process to PPS. The reaction shown in Figure 12.20 is catalyzed by pyridoxal kinase, an enzyme present in the cytoplasm of the mucosal cell. When pyridoxal is phosphorylated, transmural absorption decreases,

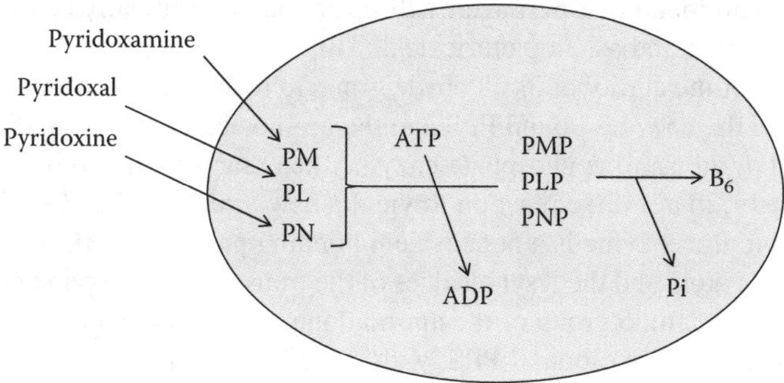

FIGURE 12.19 Absorption of the B_6 vitamins.

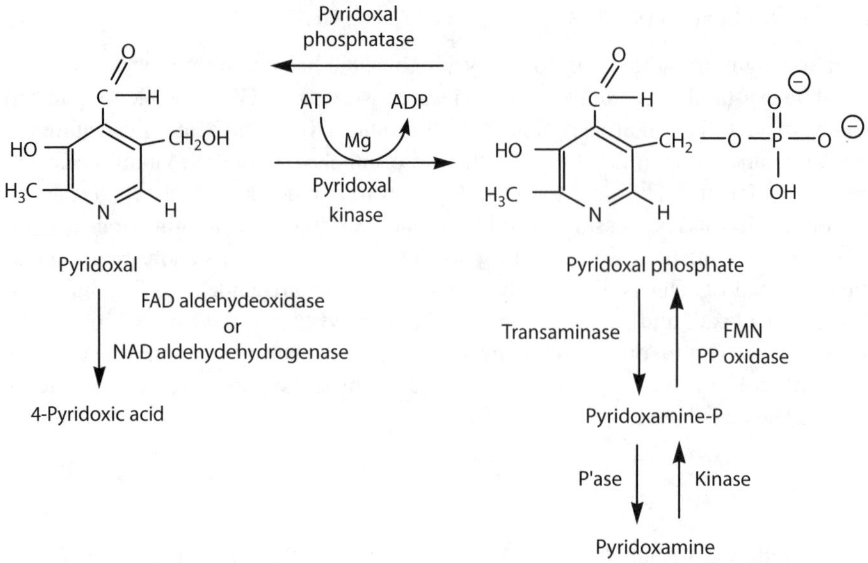

FIGURE 12.20 Phosphorylation of pyridoxal.

whereas uptake is unaffected. Phosphorylation serves as a means to control of the cellular PP level. PPS is essential to the absorption of other nutrients.

A major metabolite is 4-pyridoxic acid. It accounts for 50% of B_6 excreted in the urine. The reaction sequence is shown in Figure 12.20. Other metabolites have been found in the urine in addition to the three forms of the vitamin. Amphetamines, chlorpromazine, oral contraceptives, and reserpine all increase B_6 loss. Oral contraceptives increase tryptophan use and thus increase B_6 use.

Function

PPS serves as a coenzyme in reactions whose substrates contain nitrogen.[58] Well over 100 reactions are known that involve PPS. About 50% of these are transaminase reactions. Reactions such as transamination, racemization, decarboxylation, cleavage, synthesis, dehydration, and desulfhydration have been shown to be dependent on PPS. In transamination, the α-amino of such amino acids as alanine, arginine, asparagine, aspartic acid, cysteine, isoleucine, lysine, phenylalanine, tryptophan, tyrosine, and valine is removed and transferred to a carbon chain such as α-ketoglutarate, which in turn can transfer the amino group to the urea cycle for urea synthesis. PPS functions in transaminations in a Schiff base mechanism as shown in Figure 12.21. The binding of PPS to its apoenzyme is shown in Figure 12.22. The active coenzyme forms of vitamin B_6 are PPS and pyridoxamine phosphate. Our present understanding of the role of these coenzymes came from the work of Snell et al., who found that pyridoxal will react nonenzymatically at 100°C with glutamic acid to yield pyridoxamine and α-ketoglutaric acid. This led to the proposal that PPS functions as a coenzyme by virtue of the ability of its aldehyde group to react with the α-amino group to yield a Schiff's base between the enzyme-bound PPS and the amino acid, converting it to the α-keto acid. The resulting bound pyridoxamine phosphate enzyme then reacts with another α-keto acid, called an amino acid acceptor, in a reverse reaction to yield a new amino acid and PPS.[59] The linkage of pyridoxal phosphate to the enzyme is a noncovalent bonding presumably through the charged ring containing the nitrogen atom and the lysyl residues of the transaminase enzyme protein. In transamination, the unprotonated amino group of the amino donor is covalently bound to the carbon atom of the aldehyde group of enzyme-bound PPS, with the elimination of water, to form an aldimine that tautomerizes to the corresponding ketamine. The step involves the movement of an electron pair from the amino acid to the pyridine ring of the prosthetic group followed by tautomerization to

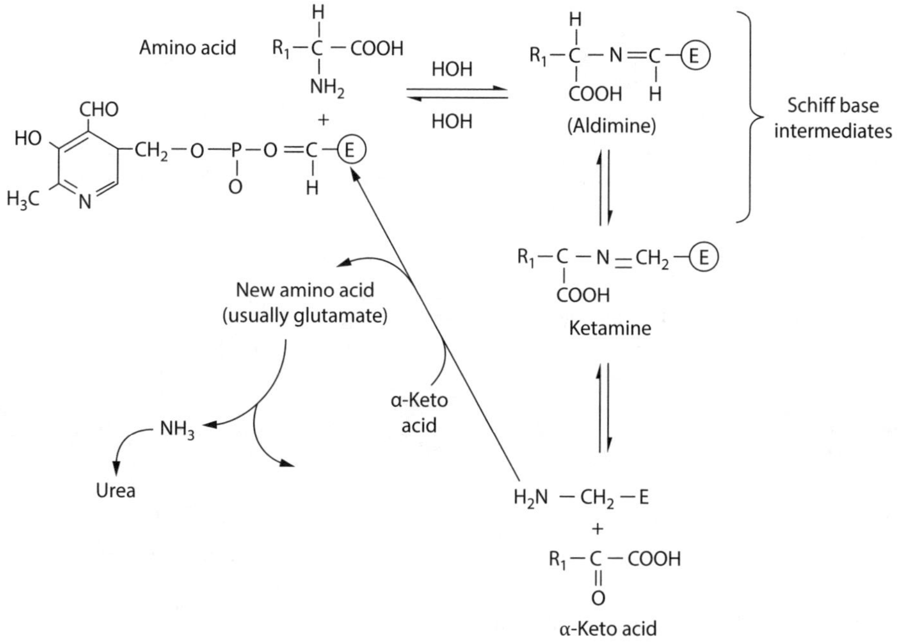

FIGURE 12.21 PPS functions in transamination reactions using a Shiff base mechanism. Symbols used are R_1, amino acid, and E, apoenzyme.

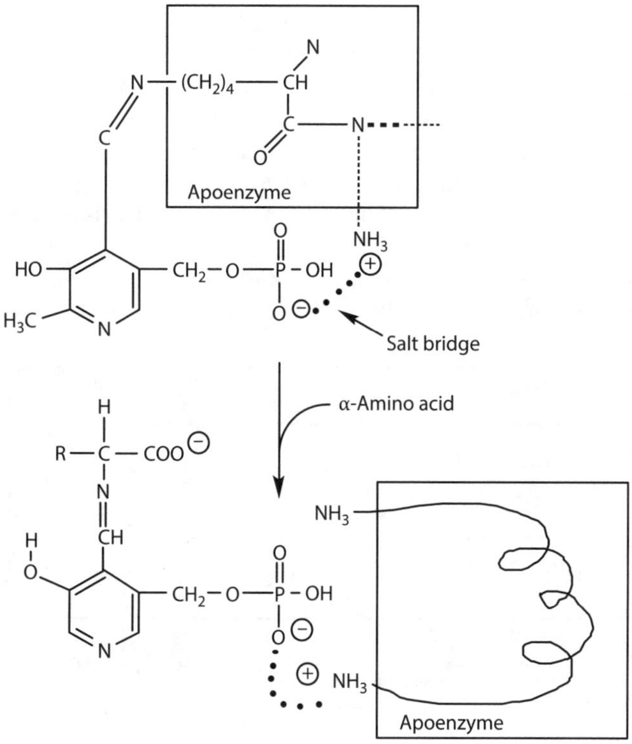

FIGURE 12.22 Binding of PPS to its apoenzyme. When an α-amino acid enters, it displaces the ε-amino group of the lysyl residue of the apoenzyme.

1. Glutamate —(Glutamate decarboxylase; P'al P)→ γ-Aminobutyric acid (GABA)

2. Tryptophan —(O_2; Hydroxylase)→ 5-Hydroxy tryp —(CO_2; P'al P)→ 5-OH-Tryptamine (serotonin)

3. Tyrosine —(O_2; Hydroxylase)→ DOPA → —(CO_2; P'al P)→ Dopamine —(O_2; Hydroxylase)→ Norepinephrine —(CH_3)→ Epinephrine

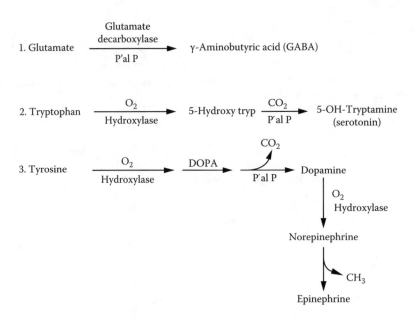

FIGURE 12.23 B_6 and the synthesis of transmitters.

the ketamine. Addition of water leads to the formation of a free α-keto acid and Enz–PP complex. By oscillating between the aldehyde and amino groups, the PP acts as an amino acid carrier. Thus, the transamination reaction is an example of a double displacement reaction.

PPS also acts with cystathionine lyase to catalyze the cleavage of cystathionine to yield free enzyme, free cysteine with α-ketobutyrate, and NH_3 as other products. PPS is important to the synthesis of the neurotransmitters γ-aminobutyric acid (GABA), serotonin, dopamine, norepinephrine, and epinephrine. Pyridoxine excess is also associated with sensory neuropathies[56] that may be related to its function in the synthesis of the listed neurotransmitters. These reactions are outlined in Figure 12.23. The role of vitamin B_6 in neurotransmitter synthesis explains the CNS symptoms associated with the deficient state. Convulsions are a common symptom together with other derangements in metabolism and anemia. The symptom of anemia arises from the role of PPS in hemoglobin synthesis as outlined in Figure 12.24.

More recently, we have come to understand a role of vitamin B_6 in steroid hormone–induced protein synthesis.[57,58] New studies have shown that B_6 has an important role as a physiological

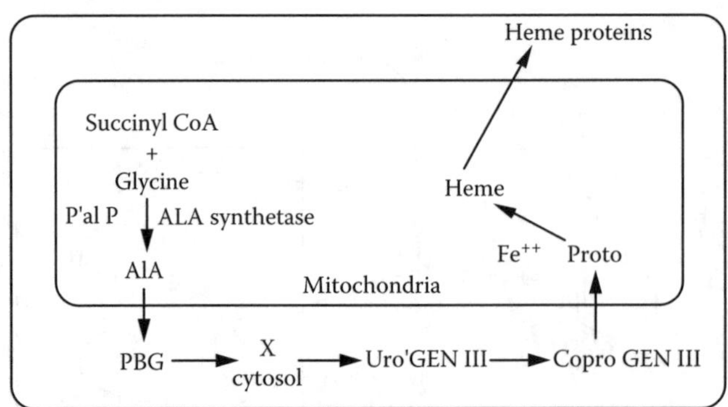

FIGURE 12.24 Role of PPS (PLP) in heme synthesis. *Abbreviations:* ALA, aminolevulinic acid; PBG, porphobilinogen; URO GEN III, uroporphyrinogen III; Copro Gen III, coproporphyrinogen III; Proto, protoporphyrin IX; and X, intermediates. Enzymes catalyzing heme biosynthesis omitted except ALA synthetase.

mediator of steroid hormone function. In this role, B_6 binds to steroid hormone–receptor and in so doing inhibits the binding of the steroid hormone–receptor complex to specific DNA sites.[58,59] In this way, B_6 acts as a negative control of steroid hormone–induced protein synthesis. Progesterone, glucocorticoids, estrogen, and testosterone effects on RNA polymerase II and RNA transcription have been shown to be inhibited by the presence of PPS. In each of these instances, the PPS binds to the receptor protein and in so doing has a negative effect on hormone–receptor binding to DNA. This role for B_6 is in addition to its role as a coenzyme in a wide variety of enzymes involved in cell growth and cell division. One of these is ornithine decarboxylase, an enzyme that plays an important role in cell division. In rapidly growing tumor cells, B_6 levels are much lower than in normal cells, and some of the major chemotherapies for cancer are based on the need for B_6 by these cells.[59,60] Antivitamin B_6 compounds are important chemotherapeutic agents in this setting.

Deficiency

In laboratory animals, dermatitis (acrodynia) is the chief symptom. Lesions occur on paws, ears, nose, chin, head, and upper thorax. This skin disorder resembles EFA deficiency. A high-fat diet protects somewhat against a B_6 deficiency. Other symptoms include poor growth; muscular weakness; fatty livers; convulsive seizures; anemia; reproductive impairment; edema; nerve degeneration; enlarged adrenal glands; increased excretion of xanthurenic acid, urea, and oxalate; decreased transaminase activity; decreased synthesis of ribosomal RNA, messenger RNA (mRNA), and DNA; and impaired immune response. High-protein intakes accelerate the development of the deficiency.

In humans, the deficiency syndrome is ill defined.[61–63] It is characterized by weakness, irritability and nervousness, insomnia, and difficulty in walking. Cheilosis (cracks at the corners of the mouth) that is not responsive to biotin or riboflavin may also be a sign of deficiency. Infants consuming B_6-deficient milk formula have convulsive seizures, which can be corrected almost immediately with intravenously administered vitamin. Behavioral changes have been described that include depression and irritability.

Tryptophan metabolism is deranged with elevated levels of kynurenine in the blood and evidence of increased excretion of xanthurenic acid.[64] In B_6 deficiency, the conversion of tryptophan to niacin is impaired, and thus skin lesions develop that resemble those of pellagra and riboflavin deficiency. Should there be a chronic systemic inflammatory state as occurs in cardiovascular disease (CVD), diabetes, or obesity, vitamin B_6 status is impaired. Such individuals require more B_6 than persons without inflammation.[64–66]

Hypochromic, sideroblastic anemia is a common finding and is due to the role B_6 plays in hemoglobin synthesis. B_6 plays an important role in glutathione synthesis, and when B_6 intakes are inadequate, red cell glutathione synthesis is reduced.[67] Marginal B_6 status has effects on the levels of n-3 and n-6 PUFA. Lower levels of these fatty acids are found in marginally deficient adults. Such changes in blood lipids might have an effect on subsequent development of CVD.[68]

While B_6 is found in a wide variety of foods, B_6 deficiency can be observed when antivitamin drugs are used. For example, isoniazid, a drug used in the treatment of tuberculosis, results in excessive B_6 loss. Penicillamine, a drug used in the treatment of Wilson's disease, has antivitamin activity. Lastly, higher than normal doses of B_6 have been prescribed for the treatment of skin disease and for neuromuscular and neurological diseases. Whether this prescription has a positive effect on the pathophysiology of these diseases remains under discussion.

There are several congenital diseases of importance to B_6 status. Homocysteinuria due to a defect in the gene for the enzyme cystathionine-β-synthase is characterized by dislocation of the lenses in the eyes, thromboses, malformation of skeletal and connective tissue, and mental retardation. PPS is a coenzyme for this synthase. Cystathioninuria due to a defect in the gene for cystathionine γ-lyase is characterized by mental retardation. This defect drives up the need for B_6. GABA deficiency due to a mutation in the gene for glutamate decarboxylase is manifested by a variety of neuropathies.

Sideroblastic anemia due to a mutation in the gene for δ-aminolevulinate synthetase is characterized by anemia, cystathioninuria, and xanthurenic aciduria. All of these genetic disorders can be ameliorated somewhat by massive doses of the vitamin. Why this is effective is not known.

Needs

The need for B_6 depends on the composition of the diet and on the age and gender of the individual. The B_6 DRIs are shown in Table 12.1. Aging and diabetes both may have effects on vitamin need. In both instances, an increase in intake is warranted.[61,62,68]

PANTOTHENIC ACID

Pantothenic acid was isolated and synthesized in the late 1940s and recognized as an essential growth factor for yeast. Its essentiality for mammalian species did not come until it was shown to prevent or cure chick dermatitis. It was subsequently recognized as essential for the rat, monkey, pig, dog, fox, turkey, fish, hamster, and human. Pantothenic acid is synthesized by plant tissues but not by mammalian tissues. It is found in a variety of tissues in the bound form. In 1946, it was discovered to be an essential part of enzyme A.

Structure

Pantothenic acid is the trivial name for the compound dihydroxy-β,β-dimethyl butyryl-β-alanine. Figure 12.25 gives the structure of this vitamin. It has two metabolically active forms: as CoA and as part of acyl carrier protein (ACP).

Physical and Chemical Properties

Pantothenic acid exists as the free acid (molecular weight, 219.2) or as a calcium salt (molecular weight, 476.5). It is the condensation product of β-alanine and a hydroxyl- and methyl-substituted butyric acid, that is, pentanoic acid. It is an unstable pale yellow oil, commercially available as a white stable, crystalline calcium or sodium salt. When dry, the salt is stable to air and light but is hygroscopic. The salt is soluble in water and glacial acetic acid. The vitamin is stable in neutral solution but is readily destroyed by heat and either alkaline or acid pH. When heated, there is hydrolytic cleavage of the molecule yielding β-alanine and 2,4-dihydroxy-3,3-dimethyl butyrate. Pantothenic acid may be assayed colorimetrically following the reaction with 1,2-naphthoquinone-4-sulfonate or ninhydrin. Radioimmunoassay also is used as are microbiological methods. The method of choice is HPLC.

Sources

Pantothenic acid is widely distributed in nature. Excellent food sources are organ meats, mushrooms, avocados, broccoli, and whole grains. Visit the USDA website for the pantothenic acid content of a large variety of foods: www.nal.usda.gov/foodcomposition.

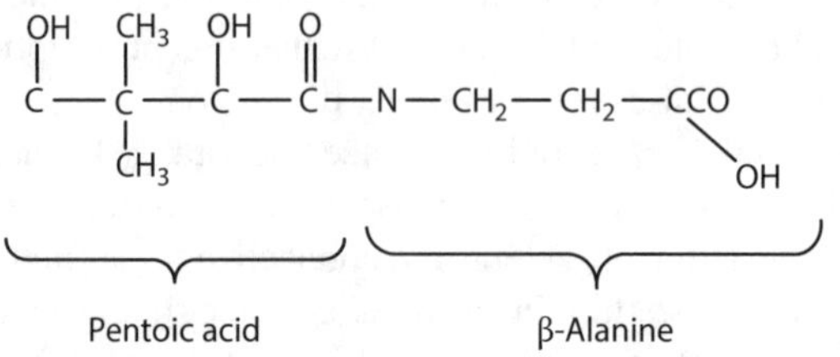

OH CH$_3$ OH O

C—C—C—C—N—CH$_2$—CH$_2$—CCO

CH$_3$ OH

Pentoic acid β-Alanine

FIGURE 12.25 Structure of pantothenic acid.

Absorption and Metabolism

Absorption occurs via facilitated diffusion[69] and travels in the blood within the erythrocytes as well as in the plasma.[72] Large doses of pantothenic acid are rapidly excreted in the urine, indicating no storage (except for a limited amount in fat cells) and little metabolism/degradation.

Function

Pantothenic acid has as its main function a role in fatty acid metabolism as a component of CoA. Pantothenic acid does not comprise the functional unit of CoA; instead, it provides the backbone for its derivative, pantetheine, whose SH group forms the reactive site. The structure of CoA is shown in Figure 12.26 and its synthesis shown in Figure 12.27. The function of CoA is to serve as a carrier of acyl groups in enzymatic reactions involving fatty acid oxidation, fatty acid synthesis, pyruvate oxidation, and biologic acetylations. It cannot cross the cell membrane and must therefore be synthesized in cells. Acetyl CoA (active acetate) is formed during the oxidation of pyruvate or fatty acids. It may also be generated from free acetate in the presence of the enzyme acetyl CoA synthetase. Acetyl CoA may then react with an acyl group acceptor such as choline to yield acetylcholine or oxaloacetate for citrate (Figure 12.28). Acetyl CoA is also an important donor of acetyl groups in the acetylation of histones (DNA-binding proteins), as described in Chapter 7. Acetylation of histones at gene promoters is an important event in the transcriptional activation of genes. The sulfhydryl group of the β-mercaptoethylamine is the site at which acyl groups are linked for transport by the coenzyme. The ability of the CoASH to form thioesters with carboxylic acids is responsible for the vital role of the coenzyme in numerous metabolic processes.

All known acyl derivatives of CoA are thiol esters. These acyl derivatives of CoA may participate in a number of metabolic reactions: condensation, addition, acyl group interchanges, and nucleophilic attack.

These reactions fall into three general categories:

1. Acetylation of choline and certain aromatic amines such as sulfonamides
2. Oxidation of fatty acids, pyruvate, α-ketoglutarate, and acetaldehyde
3. Synthesis of fatty acids, cholesterol, sphingosine, citrate, acetoacetate, porphyrin, and sterols

CoA serves as a central integrator of intermediary metabolism as illustrated in Figure 12.29. Fatty acid synthesis in the cytoplasm involves an additional role of pantothenic acid in the form of a

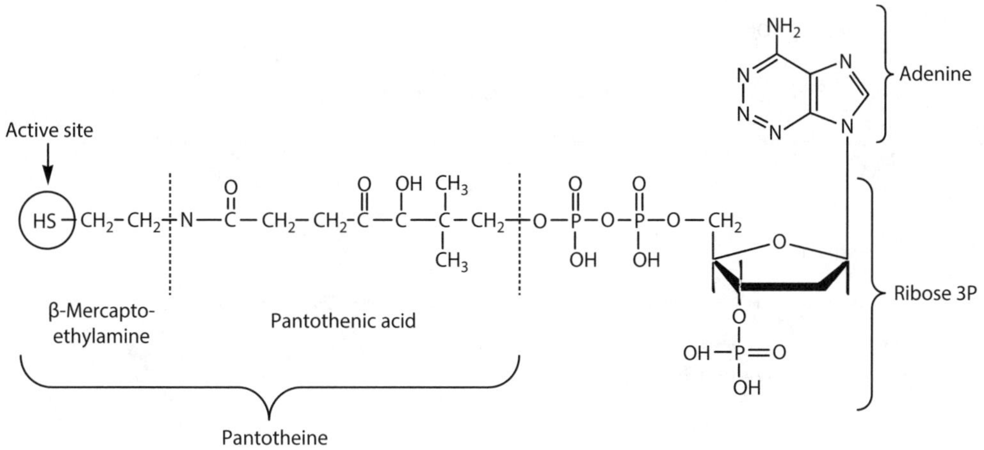

FIGURE 12.26 Structure of CoA.

cofactor 4′-phosphopantetheine. This factor is bound to a protein commonly called acyl carrier protein. ACP plus 4-phosphopantetheine appears to be involved in fatty acid synthesis. Its structure is shown in Figure 12.29. The acyl intermediates formed during fatty acid synthesis are esterified to the SH group. Phosphopantetheine is a cofactor bound to the GTP-dependent acyl CoA synthetase. Thus, 4′-phosphopantetheine serves in a capacity analogous to CoA during fatty acid oxidation. Carnitine reacts with fatty acyl CoA esters to form carnitine esters capable of crossing the mitochondrial membrane. CoA does not travel across membranes and thus must be synthesized within each cell as the need for it arises.

Deficiency Symptoms

Deficiency symptoms are species specific (Table 12.7). Pantothenic acid deficiency has not been described in humans as a single entity. If it occurs, it is accompanied by other deficiency disorders as well. The exception to this is in patients treated with the pantothenic acid antagonist

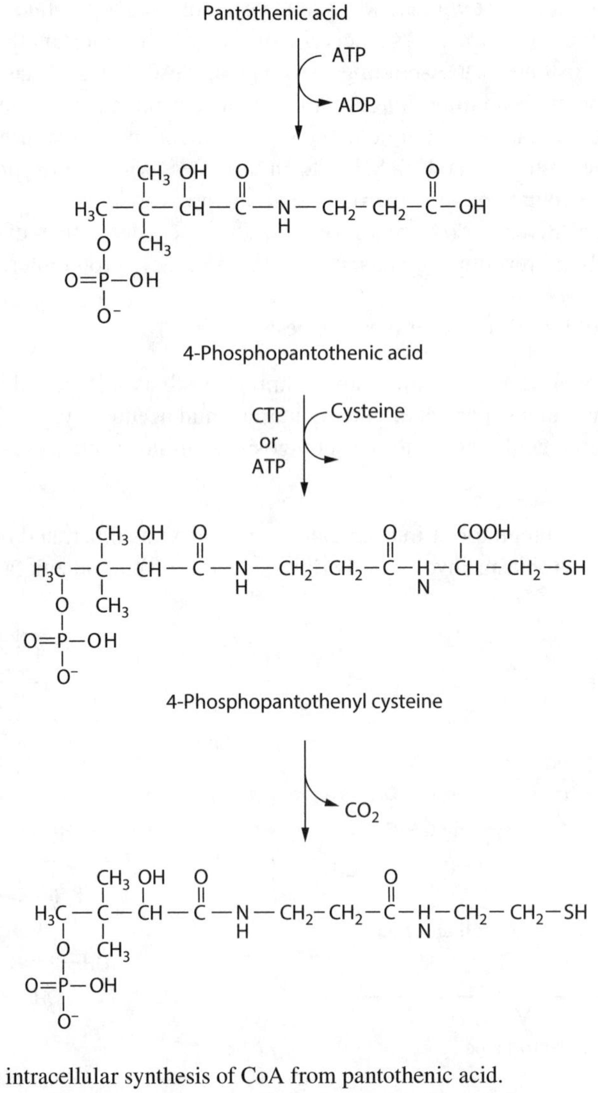

Pantothenic acid

ATP → ADP

4-Phosphopantothenic acid

CTP or ATP; Cysteine

4-Phosphopantothenyl cysteine

CO_2

FIGURE 12.27 The intracellular synthesis of CoA from pantothenic acid. *(Continued)*

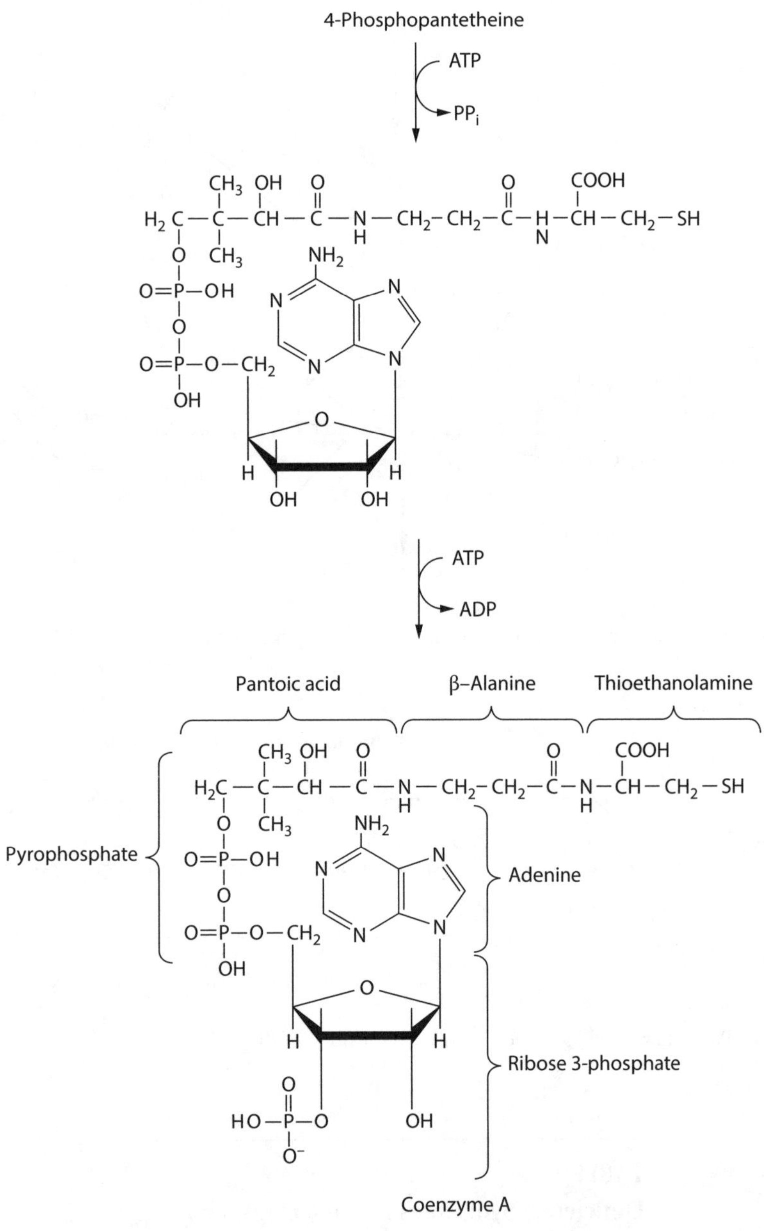

FIGURE 12.27 (CONTINUED) The intracellular synthesis of CoA from pantothenic acid.

ω-methyl pantothenic acid. In these patients, neurological symptoms (paresthesia of toes and feet) depression, fatigue, insomnia, vomiting, and muscle weakness have been reported. Changes in glucose tolerance, increased sensitivity to insulin, and decreased antibody production have also been noted.

Needs

An AI has been developed for pantothenic acid and is given in Table 12.1. Age has an effect on pantothenic need.[70,71] Check the NIH website for updates to these recommendations: www.nap.edu.

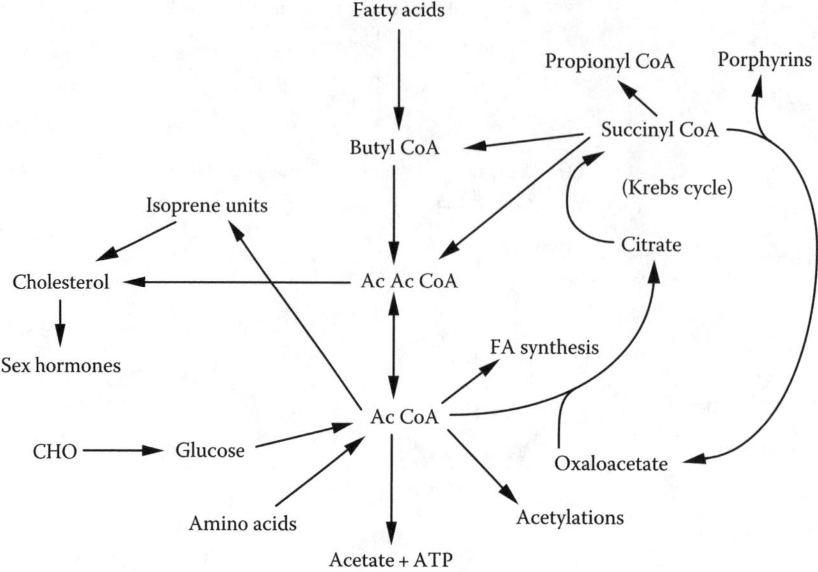

FIGURE 12.28 The central role of acetyl CoA in intermediary metabolism.

4-Phosphopantetheine

$$O{=}C\backslash CH{-}CH_2{-}O{-}\underset{OH}{\overset{O}{\overset{\|}{P}}}{-}O{-}CH_2{-}\underset{CH_3}{\overset{CH_3}{C}}{-}CHOH{-}\overset{O}{\overset{|}{C}}{-}HN{-}CH_2{-}CH_2{-}\overset{O}{\overset{\|}{C}}{-}HN{-}CH_2{-}CH_2{-}SH$$

Pantothenic acid

FIGURE 12.29 Pantothenic acid attached to the seryl residue of the ACP.

TABLE 12.7
Deficiency Symptoms in Rats, Dogs, and Pigs

Rat	*Dog*
Dermatitis	Appetite
Achromotrichia (graying)	Hair loss
Adrenal necrosis	Runny nose
Hemorrhage	Fatty liver
Spectacle eye	Irritability
Spastic gait	Hypoglycemia
Anemia	
Leukopenia	*Pig*
Infertility	Spastic gait
Impaired antibody formation	Hair loss
Gonadal atrophy	Same as above

BIOTIN

At the end of the nineteenth century, it was discovered that yeast needed a factor for growth that was not any of the already discovered essential nutrients. This factor was called *bios*. Later, scientists realized that bios was a mixture of inositol and biotin and that bios could overcome *egg-white injury*. At this point, it was named vitamin H or factor H and was found to be needed for cellular respiration. Because of its essentiality for respiration, it was named coenzyme R. In the late 1930s, Gyorgy finally integrated all these bits and pieces and together with Kšgl, du Vigneaud, and Harris realized the essential nature of a material they had isolated and synthesized. Biotin was chosen as its name.

STRUCTURE

Biotin is the trivial name for the compound cis-hexahydro-2-oxo-1H-thieno(3,4-d)imidazole-4-pentanoic acid. Its structure is shown in Figure 12.30. In order to have vitamin activity, the structure must contain a conjoined ureido and tetrahydrothiophene ring, and the ureido 3′N is sterically hindered, preventing substitution. The ureido 1′N is a poor nucleophile. Biotin occurs in eight isomeric forms, but only D-biotin has vitamin activity. Several biotin analogs have been synthesized or isolated from natural sources. Among these are oxybiotin or biotinol, biocytin, dethiobiotin, and biotin sulfoxide. The latter two are inactive as vitamins, whereas the first two have some vitamin activity.

PHYSICAL AND CHEMICAL PROPERTIES

Biotin is a white crystalline substance that in its dry form is stable to air, heat, and light. Its molecular weight is 244.3 and melting point is 167°C. It decomposes at 230°C–232°C. It has a limited solubility in water (22 mg/mL HOH) and is more soluble in ethanol. When in solution, it is unstable to oxygen, strong acid, or alkaline conditions and will be gradually destroyed by ultraviolet light. The analytical method of choice is HPLC in combination with avidin-binding assays. Microbiological methods are also available. These methods use *Lactobacillus casei*, *Lactobacillus plantarum*, *Neurospora crassa*, *Ochromonas danica*, or *Saccharomyces cerevisiae*. These microorganisms require biotin for growth and are sensitive to varying quantities of biotin in the growth media. Using avidin, a protein found in egg white that binds biotin at the ureido group, an isotope dilution assay has been developed and is sensitive in the range of 4–41 pmols. Colorimetric assays based on the reaction of biotin with *p*-(dimethylamino) cinnamaldehyde or on the absorbance of iodine

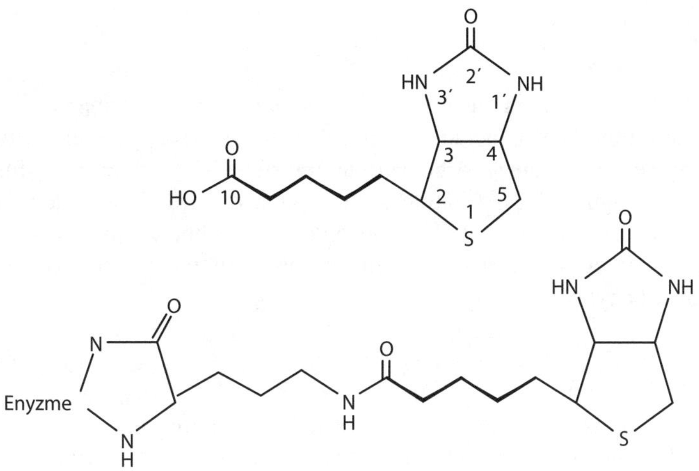

FIGURE 12.30 Structure of biotin and enzyme-bound biotin.

formed during the oxidation of biotin to its sulfone with potassium iodide have been developed. The colorimetric assays are not as sensitive as the avidin-binding assays.

Sources

There are numerous food sources for biotin. Biotin is found in every living cell in minute amounts where it exists either in its enzyme-bound form or as an amide. Rich sources include organ meats, egg yolk, brewer's yeast, and royal jelly. Soy flour or soybean, rice polishings, various ocean fish, and whole grains are good sources of the vitamin. Human milk contains biotin.[72,73]

Absorption and Metabolism

Biotin in food exists in the free and enzyme-bound form. The protein-bound form can be digested, which in turn yields biocytin, a combination of biotin and lysine. Biocytin is hydrolyzed via the action of biotinidase to its component parts.[74] The resultant biotin is then available for absorption. Biotin is absorbed via facilitated diffusion. The jejunum is the major site for this absorption. Once absorbed, it circulates as free biotin. There may be some species differences in absorptive mechanism. In addition, there is synthesis of the biotin by the gut flora.

Biotinidase is present in plasma as well, where it has a similar function, that is, to release biotin from the breakdown products of biotin-dependent carboxylases.[75,76] Biotinidase, if mutated, results in an autosomal recessive disorder that results in a secondary biotin deficiency that can be overcome with biotin supplements.[77] The clinical symptoms of this genetic disorder are the same as those of the biotin-deficient state and relate to the function of biotin as a coenzyme in intermediary metabolism, especially the carboxylase reactions.

Biotinidase has been cloned and sequenced and its distribution throughout the body has been determined.[78] Although active in the intestinal tract, its activity is not sufficient to catalyze all of the bound biotin found in food. It has been estimated that less than 50% of the bound biotin found in foods of plant origin is hydrolyzed to provide the free form. The availability of biotin in food depends on the percent that is bound. In general, protein-bound biotin is more readily available from foods of animal origin compared to those of plant origin. Biotin can be rendered unavailable by avidin, a protein found in raw egg white. Once the egg is cooked, the avidin is denatured and no longer binds the biotin. This binding is the explanation of the disorder *egg-white injury*. Other proteins, particularly membrane and transport proteins, bind biotin and are responsible for its entry into all cells that use the vitamin.

Function

Once absorbed, biotin travels to the liver where it is bound to a liver plasma membrane receptor.[77,78] Biotin has two major functions in metabolism. First, biotin serves as a mobile carboxyl carrier as it is attached to enzymes that catalyze carboxy group transfer.[77] The formation of this biotin–enzyme complex is shown in Figure 12.31. A number of enzymes require biotin as a prosthetic group for their function. These are listed in Table 12.8. Second, biotin is bound covalently to histones (DNA-binding proteins), as described in Chapter 7. Binding of biotin to both carboxylases and histones is mediated by holocarboxylase synthetase.[78]

Deficiency

In humans, the symptoms of severe deficiency include dermatitis, skin rash, hair loss (alopecia), developmental delay, seizures, conjunctivitis, visual and auditory loss, metabolic ketolactic acidosis, hyperammonemia, and organic acidemia. Biotin deficiency results in reproductive failure and impairs the growth and development of the fetus.[79] Abnormal plasma fatty acid profiles are also

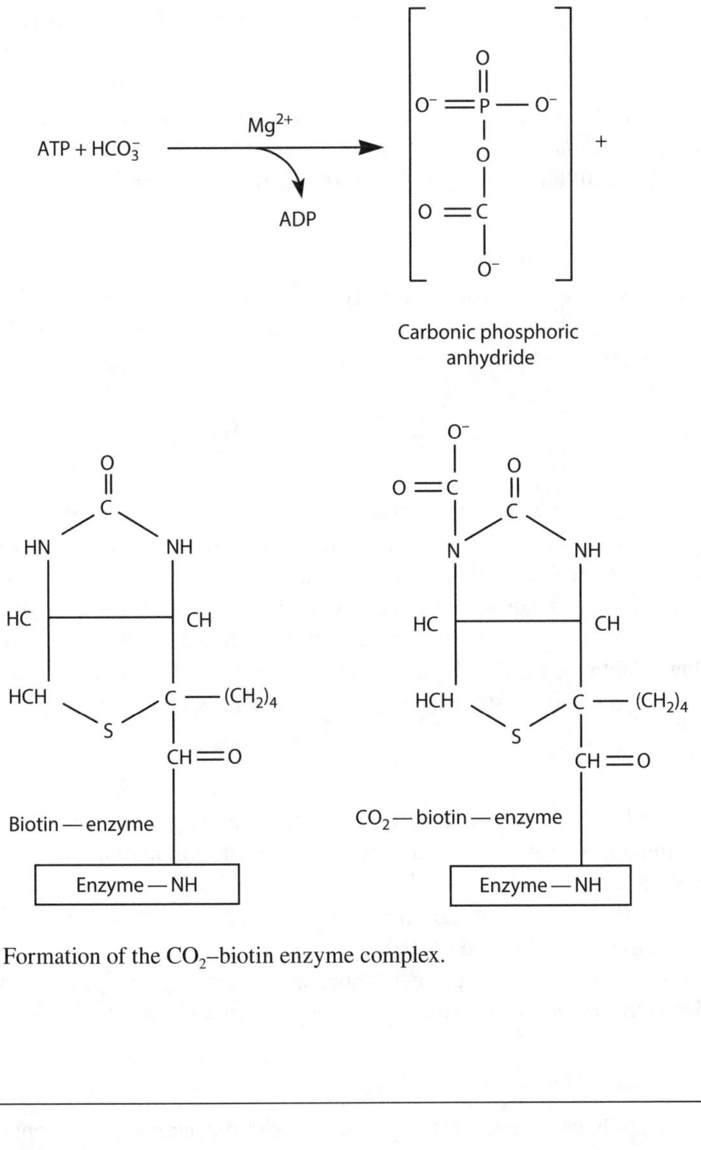

FIGURE 12.31 Formation of the CO_2–biotin enzyme complex.

TABLE 12.8
Biotin-Dependent Enzymes in Animals

Enzyme	Role	Location
Pyruvate carboxylase	First reaction in pathway that converts 3-carbon precursors to glucose (gluconeogenesis) Replenishes oxaloacetate for citric acid cycle	Mitochondria (rate-limiting step in gluconeogenesis)
Acetyl CoA carboxylase	Commits acetate units to fatty acid synthesis by forming malonyl CoA	Cytosol (rate-limiting step in fatty acid synthesis)
Acetyl CoA carboxylase-β	Synthesis of malonyl CoA, which is an inhibitor of fatty acid transport into mitochondria	Mitochondria (inhibitor of β-oxidation of fatty acids)
Propionyl-CoA carboxylase	Converts propionate to succinate, which can then enter citric acid cycle	Mitochondria
β-Methylcrotonyl-CoA carboxylase	Catabolism of leucine and certain isoprenoid compounds	Mitochondria

observed in biotin deficiency.[80] These symptoms have been reported in persons lacking normal biotinidase activity through a genetic error.[81] In a genetically normal human population, a true biotin deficiency is extremely rare. However, in persons that are suffering from protein–energy malnutrition, biotin deficiency may develop secondarily. Only a few instances of biotin deficiency have been reported. In one, the deficient state was caused by the chronic consumption of 30 raw eggs/day for several months. In this individual, the symptoms were primarily related to the skin.

Needs

Because the vitamin is present in a wide variety of foods and because it can be synthesized by the intestinal flora, a fixed intake figure has been difficult to determine. However, the National Academy of Sciences Food and Nutrition Board has published an adequate dietary intake (AI) for this vitamin (Table 12.1).

FOLIC ACID

More than 50 years ago, folate was discovered as a necessary constituent of every living cell of every organism whether plant or animal.[82] It took years of meticulous work to separate its function from that of vitamin B_{12} for both are involved in the one-carbon transfer that is so important in the synthesis of the purines and pyrimidines that are constituents of DNA and RNA. Actually, until the genetic material and its function in the cell were worked out, there was no progress in understanding the role of the folates in nucleic acid synthesis. With the advent of our growing knowledge of how genes are made and how they work, we finally have come to understand the importance of folic acid in cellular function.

Structure

Folic acid or folate or folacin is the generic term for pteroylmonoglutamic acid and its related biologically active compounds. A number of derivatives have vitamin activity (Table 12.9). The basic structure of pteroylglutamic acid is shown in Figure 12.32. The derivatives include the addition of hydrogen at N5 and N10, and only one glutamate attached to para-aminobenzoic acid (PABA). This derivative is called tetrahydrofolic acid (THF).

Other derivatives can have a methyl group attached at N5, a methyl bridge between N5 and N10 or a methylene bridge at this position, or an aldehyde group at either N5 or N10 or a HCNH group at N5.

Physical and Chemical Properties

All of these derivatives have vitamin activity because vitamin activity is dependent on the presence of a pteridine (pterin) structure with variable hydrogenation or methyl addition at N5 or N10 and the presence of at least one glutamyl residue linked via peptide bonds to *p*-amino benzoic acid. Methotrexate (4-amino-N^{10}-methyl folic acid, an antineoplastic agent) and aminopterin (4-amino folic

TABLE 12.9
Derivatives of Folic Acid

Derivative	N5	N10
Tetrahydrofolic acid	–H	–H
5-Methyfolic acid	$–CH_3$	–H
5,10-Methanylfolic acid	–CH=	$–CH_2=$
5,10-Methylenefolic acid	$–CH_2–$	$–CH_2=$
5-Formylfolic acid	–HCO	H
10-Formylfolic acid	H	–HCO

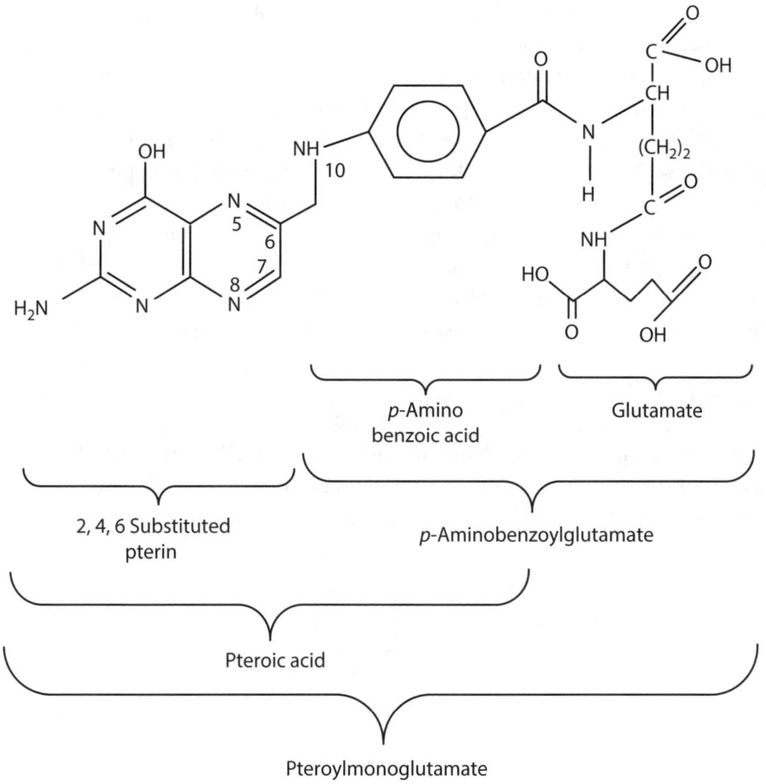

FIGURE 12.32 Structure of folic acid.

acid, a rodenticide) are folate antagonists and as such are useful pharmaceutical agents against cell growth. The pteroyl monoglutamate form has a molecular weight of 441.1 and is moderately soluble in water (0.0016 mg/L mL water). It has absorption maxima at 256, 283, and 368 mM. It is a yellow-orange crystal with a melting point of 250°C. It is unstable to ultraviolet light, heat, oxygen, acid condition, and divalent metal ions such as iron and copper. As mentioned, it is methyl addition at N5 or N10 and the presence of at least one glutamyl residue linked via peptide bonds to *p*-amino benzoic acid. Folacin is present in all living cells in small amounts. HPLC is the method of choice. In addition to the HPLC methodology,[83] there is also a radioimmunological technique that involves the binding of the vitamin to an isotopically labeled protein followed by antibody precipitation and quantification.

Sources

Folate is found in a wide variety of foods of both animal and plant origin. However, because it is so unstable, food sources may be insufficient to meet need. Good sources include meats, fruits, vegetables (especially asparagus), dry beans, peas, nuts, and whole grain cereal products. Visit the USDA website for the folacin content of a wide variety of foods: www.nal.usda.gov/foodcomposition.

Absorption and Metabolism

Folate transport in the intestine is a carrier-mediated, pH-dependent process with maximum transport occurring after glutamation in the jejunum.[84–86] There are specific folate-binding proteins that function in the absorption process.[85] One is a low-affinity folate-binding protein found in the brush border membrane of the absorptive cell. There is another high-affinity folate-binding protein that is localized to the jejunal brush border cells. Affinity is optimized at pH 5.5–6.0. The high-affinity binding protein is similar to the one found in the kidney. A number of drugs inhibit active folate transport.[88] These include ethacrynic acid, sulfinpyrazone, phenylbutazone, sulfasalazine, and furosemide. All of these are amphipathic substances. That is, they are compounds with a polar–apolar character. Absorption is also inhibited by cyanide and 2,4-dinitrophenol, drugs that poison oxidative phosphorylation and thus reduce the ATP supply. ATP is necessary for the active transport process to work. Absorption can also occur by passive diffusion, but this is a secondary means for folate uptake. Very little folate appears in the feces.

After folate is absorbed, it circulates in the plasma as pteroylmonoglutamate. That which is not used by the cells is excreted in the urine as pteroylglutamic acid, 5-methyl-pteroylglutamic acid, 10-formyl tetrahydrofolate, or acetamidobenzoylglutamate. Uptake by cells is mediated by a highly specific folate-binding protein. This protein has been isolated from the membranes of a variety of cells, and a cDNA probe has been prepared.[93] Folate appears to stimulate the transcription of the mRNA for this protein.

Function

Folate's main function is as a coenzyme in one-carbon transfer.[89–91] However, before it can do this, it must be activated. Activation consists of the reduction of folic acid to dihydrofolic acid and thence to THF as shown in Figure 12.33. Dihydrofolate reductase is a therapeutic target for a number of

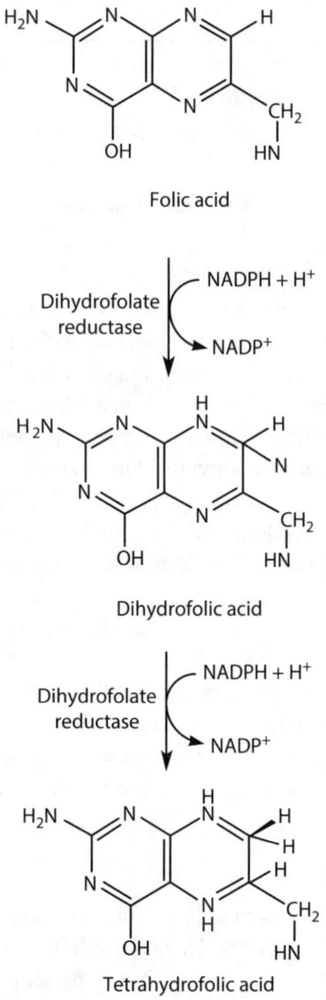

FIGURE 12.33 Activation of folic acid.

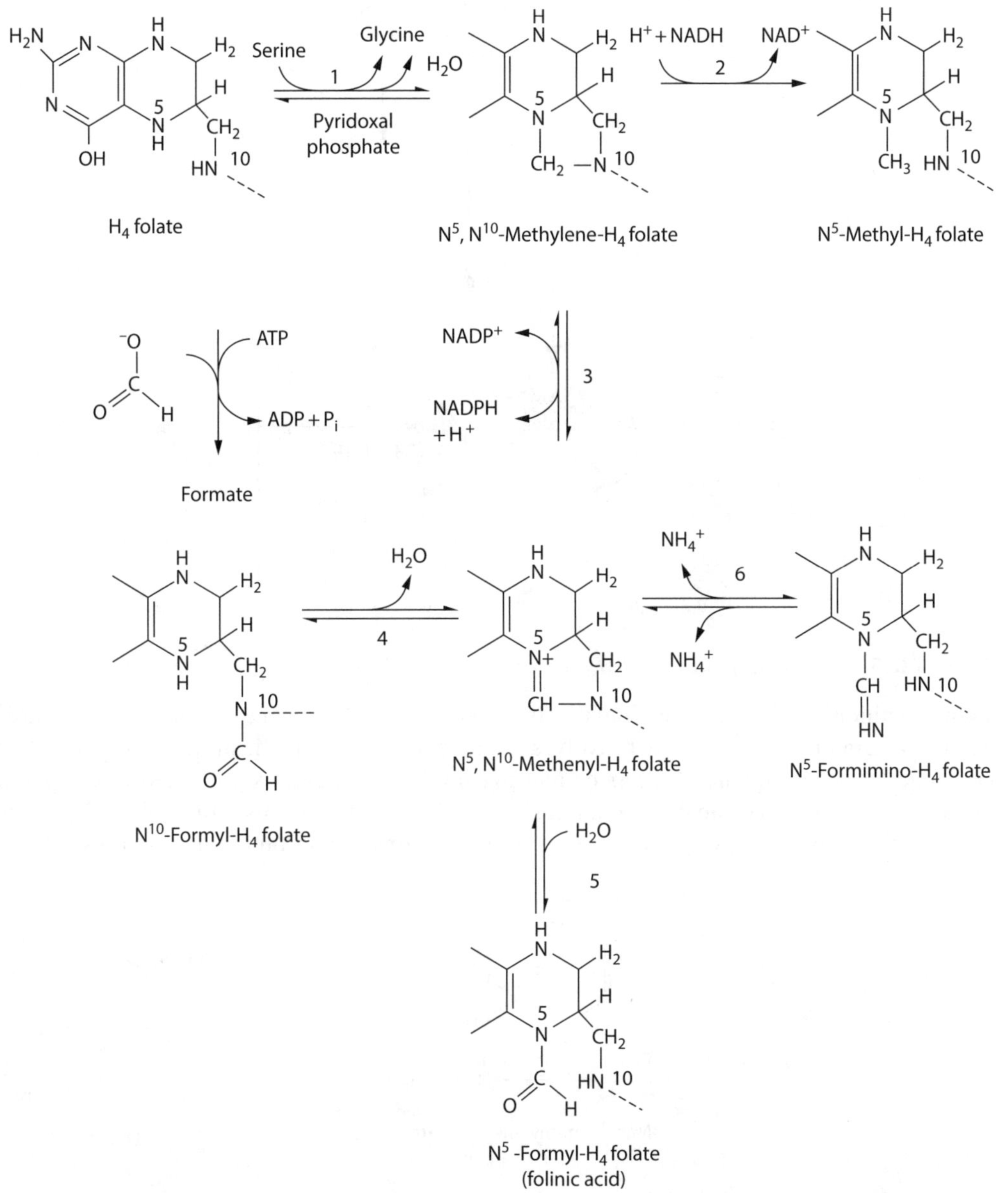

FIGURE 12.34 Interconversions of one-carbon moieties attached to tetrahydrofolate.

anticancer drugs that work through inhibiting cell cycle. A number of folate derivatives have vitamin activity, and these derivatives are interconvertible, as shown in Figure 12.34. Methyl group transfer also involves B_{12}, as illustrated in Figure 12.35.

The regulation of methyl group transfer is complex and involves a number of enzymes and substrates. While serine is a good source for the methyl group, methyl groups arise from other substrates as well. The major source of single methyl groups involves a cycle of reactions catalyzed by serine, hydroxymethyltransferase, 5,10-methylene-FH_4 reductase, and methionine synthetase. The last of these reactions is rate limiting for the cycle, whereas the second is inhibited by S-adenosylmethionine (SAM) as well as 5-methyl FH_4. As described in the next section on vitamin B_{12}, methionine metabolism depends on the transfer of labile methyl groups from 5-methyl folate to B_{12} that, as methyl B_{12}, donates this methyl group to homocysteine

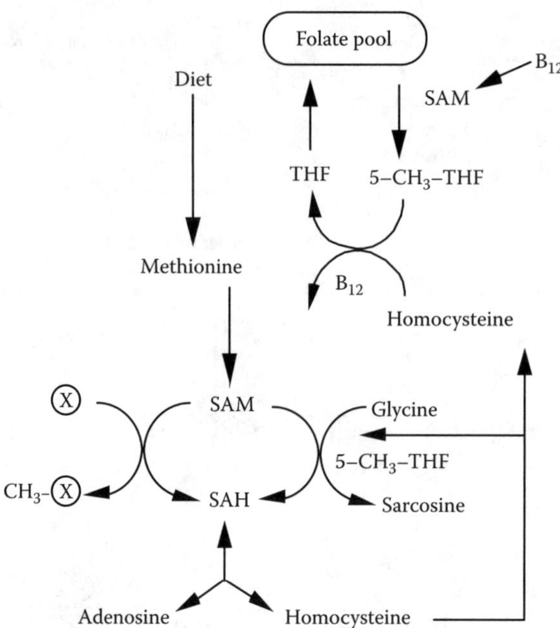

FIGURE 12.35 Involvement of B_{12} in methyl group transfer via SAM.

making methionine. One-carbon transfer is important in purine and pyrimidine syntheses. The mechanism of this transfer that involves folate (and also B_{12}) is illustrated in Figure 12.36. The whole reaction sequence for purine and pyrimidine syntheses is presented in Chapter 7. In this sequence, methyl transfer occurs at several different points (listed in Table 12.10), and it is immediately apparent why folate and vitamin B_{12} are so important to gene expression.[88–95]

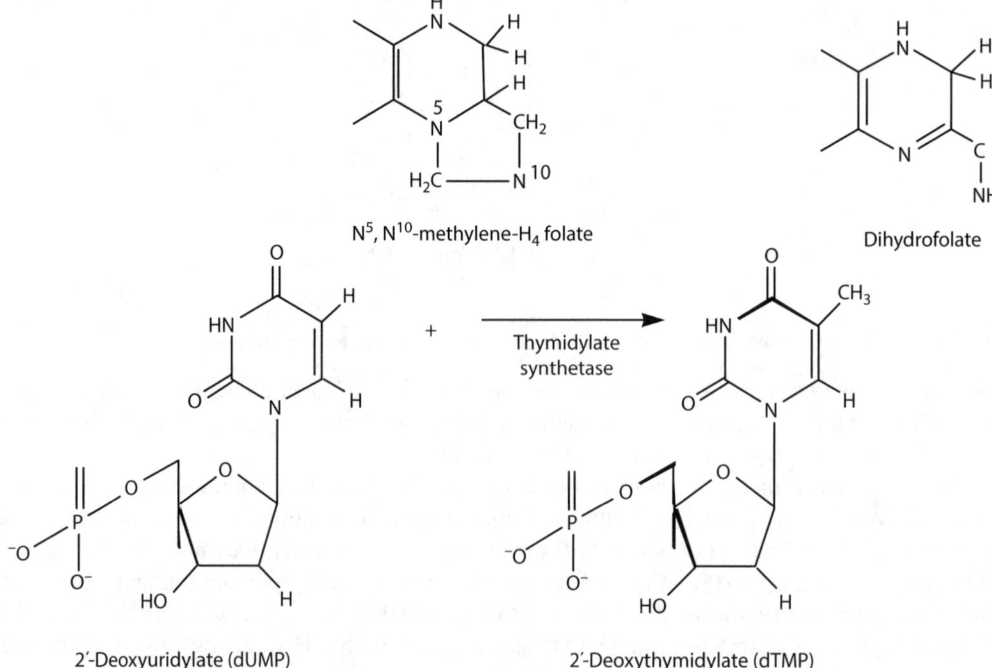

FIGURE 12.36 Addition of methyl groups to deoxyuridylate using the methyl group transfer function of folate.

TABLE 12.10
Metabolic Reactions in Which Folate Plays a Role as a Coenzyme

Enzyme	Role
Thymidylate synthetase	Transfers formaldehyde to C-5 of dUMP to form a dTMP in pyrimidine synthesis
Glycinamide ribonucleotide transformylase	Donates formate in purine synthesis
5-5-Amino-4-imidazolecarboxamide transformylase	Donates formate in purine synthesis
Serine hydroxymethyl transferase	Accepts formaldehyde in serine catabolism
10-Formyl-FH_4 synthetase	Accepts formaldehyde from tryptophan catabolism
10-Formyl-FH_4 dehydrogenase	Transfers formate for oxidation to CO_2 in histidine catabolism
Methionine synthase	Donates methyl group to homocysteine to form methionine
Formiminotransferase	Accepts formimino group from histidine

While nuclear DNA, once made, merely reproduces itself within the cell cycle, new mRNA is made every minute as new proteins are needed by the cell. While some of the purine and pyrimidine bases can be salvaged and reused, this recycling is not 100% efficient. mRNA has a very short half-life (seconds to hours) compared to the other nucleic acid species in the cell. Thus, newly synthesized purines and pyrimidines must be available. If not available, de novo protein synthesis and of course new cell formation will be adversely affected.

More recently, roles of folate-dependent methylation of DNA and histones (DNA-binding proteins) have attracted considerable attention (see Chapter 7).[93] For example, methylation of cytosine residues in cytosine-/guanosine-rich regions (*CpG islands*) in gene promoters is associated with gene silencing. Methylation of cytosine residues is mediated by DNA methyltransferases DNMT1, DNMT3a, and DNMT3b; SAM serves as a methyl donor in these reactions. DNMT1 is considered a *maintenance* methyl transferase (reestablishing methylation patterns after cell division), whereas DNMT3a and DNMT3b are de novo methyl transferases (creating new methylation marks in DNA). Moreover, methylation of lysine residues in histones may cause transcriptional silencing or activation of genes, depending on the site where the methylation mark resides. For example, folate-dependent dimethylation (binding of two methyl groups) to the ε-group of lysine-9 in histone H3 is associated with gene silencing, whereas trimethylation of lysine-4 is associated with gene activation. In these reactions, SAM serves as a donor of methyl groups, and the generation of SAM depends on folate.

Deficiency

While anemia, dermatitis, and impaired growth are the chief symptoms of folate deficiency in humans, scientists are now beginning to recognize the importance of adequate folate intake in early embryonic development. Inadequate intake by the mother prior to and/or during the early stages of development can have teratogenic effects on the embryo. Embryonic development, particularly the neural tube, is impaired in folate deficiency.[95,96] As a result, infants with spina bifida and other neural tube defects (NTDs) are born.[96] It is estimated that about 2500 infants per year are born with these defects. Available evidence indicates that women contemplating pregnancy should consume 400 μg/day as a prophylactic measure. Those women who have already had a NTD-affected birth and are planning another pregnancy should consume 4 mg/day of folic acid to prevent another NTD-affected child. Low folate intake has been suggested as a factor in the development of colon cancer as well as in the bronchial squamous metaplasia (premalignant lesions) of smokers and cervical dysplasia (another premalignant lesion) in women.[97] Folate antagonists serve important roles as anti-infective, antineoplastic, and anti-inflammatory drugs.[98–102] These antagonists work by inhibiting dihydrofolate reductase, a key enzyme in the synthesis of thymidylate and therefore DNA.[98] Low zinc intake compromises folate status by negatively affecting intestinal folate uptake. Other symptoms of deficiency are leukopenia (low white cell count), general weakness, depression, and polyneuropathy. The latter sign is probably related to the folate–B_{12} interaction.[102] Alcoholism drives up the need for folacin as well as that of vitamin B_{12}.[96,100]

In rats, folate deficiency has been shown to result in an increased rate of mitochondrial DNA deletion, decreased mitochondrial DNA content, and decreased mitogenesis.[101] These changes were accompanied by an increase in expression of nuclear encoded genes that regulate mitochondrial gene expression as well as biogenesis. Folate deprivation induced aberrant mitochondrial function via aberrations in mitochondrial DNA, and the cell tried to compensate for this by increasing the synthesis of nuclear factors that upregulate mitochondrial gene expression. Whether this decrease in expression ultimately impinged upon mitochondrial oxidative phosphorylation has not been determined. Studies have not been performed in humans to determine whether folate status affects mitochondrial DNA or mitochondrial function, yet there is every indication that folate may play an important role in mitochondrial health.

Needs

The latest DRIs are given in Table 12.1. Updates to the DRIs can be found on the NIH website www.nap.edu. However, as mentioned in the preceding section, women contemplating pregnancy should increase their intake twofold. There are racial and ethnic differences in the usual folic acid intake, and it has been suggested that despite food fortification, every woman of child-bearing age should take a folic acid supplement. Since folate is not toxic, this is probably a good idea, with the caveat that B_{12} status is normal.[106,107] The status of the vitamin B_{12} intake should be ascertained such that if additional B_{12} is needed, it can be supplied. If this is not the case, excess folate could mask a B_{12} deficiency until the irreversible neurologic features of B_{12} deficiency appear. Excess folate intake leads to specific and significant downregulation of intestinal and renal folate uptake.[109] Excess folate and vitamin B_{12} given to pregnant women has been reported to result in atopic dermatitis in their infants.[110] This suggests that the supplements provided to pregnant women be carefully prescribed to avoid excess intake of one or both vitamins.

Polymorphisms in the methylenetetrahydrofolate reductase (MTHFR) gene are associated with differences in folacin need as well as differences in susceptibility to CVD. [103–110] The CT genotype was more susceptible to CVD than the TT genotype when combined with a polymorphism in the hydroxymethyltransferase gene but not when only the TT genotype was considered alone.[103] Polymorphisms in the MTHFR gene also interact with folate intake to regulate DNA methylation. This has implications in our understanding of how such methylation affects aging, cancer, and the development of other chronic diseases.[104] The TT genotype effect on folate status is dependent on choline intake and riboflavin intake.[105] This nutrient interaction probably is a factor in the determination of whether and how much the folate intake influences NTD development. The use of riboflavin as a targeted strategy for managing hypertension in patients with the TT genotype offers another window onto the function of folate in chronic disease.[106] Other instances of an interaction between folate and the TT polymorphism have been reported in population studies of the incidence of colorectal cancer, CVD, and stroke.[107–110]

Cognitive development has been related to folacin and vitamin B_{12} status in infants and adolescents.[111,112] Cognitive decline in older adults has been studied, and supplements of these vitamins have prevented this decline. Providing supplements over the long term promoted an improvement in cognitive functioning aging subjects.[113,114]

VITAMIN B_{12}

Vitamin B_{12} is one of the more recently discovered vitamins, yet it is the most potent.[115] Very little is required to prevent the symptoms of pernicious anemia and subsequent neurological change. It was isolated in 1948 and shortly thereafter shown to be the required substance needed to prevent pernicious anemia.

Structure

Vitamin B_{12} is a very complex structure as shown in Figure 12.37. The term B_{12} is the generic descriptor for all corrinoids, those compounds that have a corrin ring. Cyanocobalamin is the trivial designation for this compound. In order to have vitamin activity, it must contain a cobalt-centered corrin ring. Below the ring, it may have a side chain heterocyclic nitrogen or may have nothing attached here. Above the ring, it may have a hydroxo, aqua, methyl, 5-deoxyadenosyl, CN^-, Cl^-, Br^-, nitro, sulfito, or sulfato group. There are a number of structural analogs that have vitamin activity. Regardless of the substituents present above or below the cobalt-centered corrin ring, unless the ring is present, there will be no vitamin function. The ring consists of four reduced pyrrole rings linked by three methylene bridges and one direct bond. The cobalt atom is in the 3^+ state and can form up to six coordinate bonds. It is tightly bound to the four pyrrole N atoms and can also bond a nucleotide and a small ligand below and above the ring, respectively. Commercially viable synthesis of this compound is very difficult although one such process has been developed using two moles of 5-aminolevulinate to form porphobilinogen, a

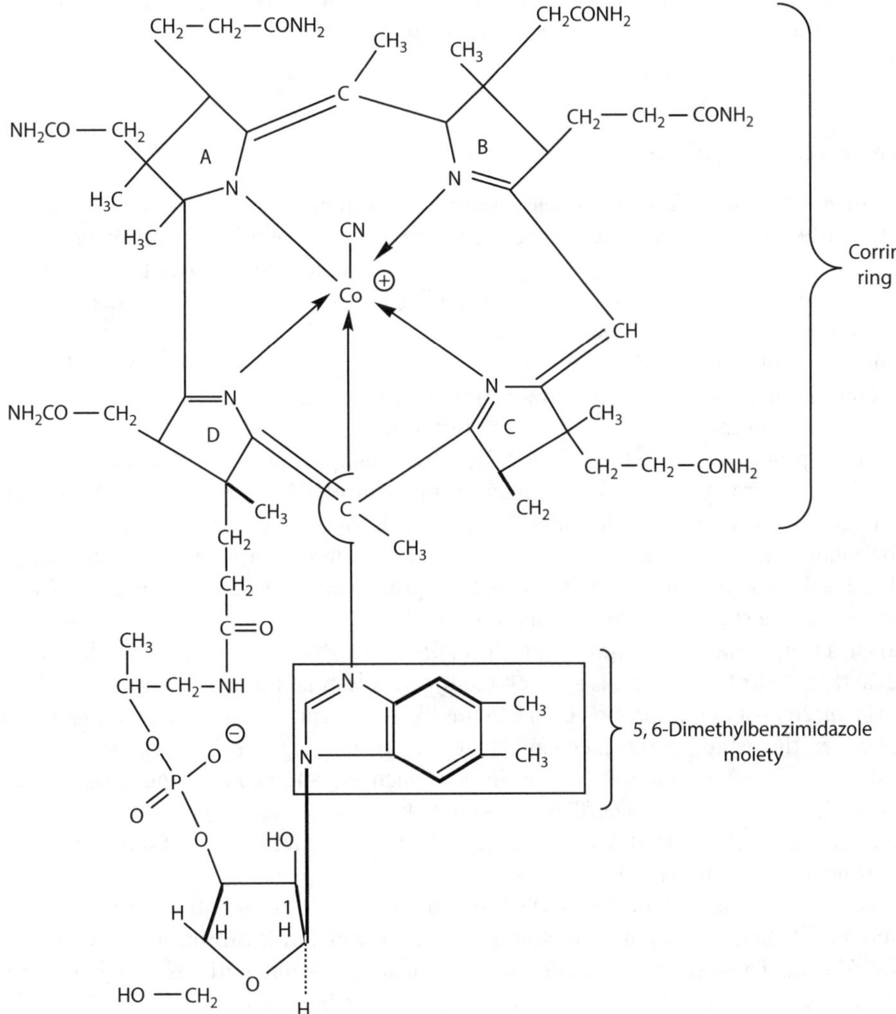

FIGURE 12.37 Structure of vitamin B_{12}.

pyrrole ring with an aminomethyl group on C-2, an acetate group on C-3, and a proprionate on C-4. Four of these are linked together to form hydroxymethylbilane, which in turn cyclizes, and then the cobalt atom is added to form the vitamin.

Physical and Chemical Properties

Vitamin B_{12} has a molecular weight of 1355.4 and is moderately soluble in water (12.5 mg/mL). It is insoluble in fat solvents. Its absorption maxima occur at 278, 361, and 550 nm. It is a heat-stable red crystal but will decompose at temperatures above 210°C. The crystal will melt at temperatures above 300°C. It is unstable to ultraviolet light, acid conditions, and the presence of metals such as iron and copper. Vitamin B_{12} is very difficult to assay. It is primarily the product of microbial synthesis and thus is not usually present in large amounts in most foods. Organ meats are good sources of B_{12}. It is synthesized in the gastrointestinal system by the resident flora. At this time, the best assay system is one that uses B_{12}-dependent microorganisms. The most responsive and specific of these is *Ochromonas malhamensis*. Although sensitive to small amounts of the vitamin, these procedures are tedious. Spectrophotometric assays that can detect as little as 25 μg/mL are also available but not practical because their sensitivity is so limited.

Absorption and Metabolism

Most mammals depend on a very complex absorptive system for vitamin B_{12}.[116–118] The process of absorption begins in the stomach where preformed B_{12} is bound to a carrier protein called intrinsic factor.[117] As B_{12} is made by the gut flora, it too is bound to a carrier protein.[126] Whether this carrier is identical to that available in the stomach is not known. It probably is. Likely, future research will show that the synthesis of this carrier is directed by the vitamin in a manner analogous to that of retinol and the retinol receptor protein (see Chapter 11). Actually, there are four structurally distinct B_{12} carrier proteins. Intrinsic factor is one of these and another, called R binder, is found in the proximal part of the intestine. R binder is degraded by the pancreatic peptidases and proteases, while the intrinsic factor–B_{12} complex proceeds intact to the distal portion of the ilium where in the presence of calcium and neutral pH, the complex binds to a receptor (called IF) on the surface of the luminal epithelial cell. Subsequent to binding of the complex to IF, the vitamin appears in the portal blood bound to a fourth protein called transcobalamin II (TCII). The blood contains an additional R-type protein called transcobalamin I (TCI), which assists in the transport of the vitamin to its target cells.

Although absorption occurs mainly in the distal ilium, it also occurs in the large intestine.[119] This takes advantage of the fact that B_{12} is synthesized by the intestinal flora in this part of the intestinal tract.[119] The mechanism of absorption by the ileum likely is an active one mediated by the intrinsic factor; however, the details of this mechanism are unknown except for the need for the carriers as described earlier. Persons with a variety of diseases such as pancreatitis, tropical sprue, fluoroacetate poisoning, and pancreatic insufficiency do not absorb B_{12} efficiently and often show signs of pernicious anemia until provided with oral B_{12} supplements or injected with B_{12}. Absorption by the large intestine likely occurs via passive diffusion.

Once absorbed, B_{12} is transported in the blood bound to one of three transport proteins: TCI, TCII, and TCIII. Small amounts are stored (as methylcobalamin) in the liver, kidney, heart, spleen, and brain. Thus, if an individual lacks intrinsic factor due perhaps to a genetic disease or surgical loss of the stomach (gastrectomy) or, as described earlier, has one of the diseases that affect B_{12} absorption, an injection of B_{12} can be given once a month and this will correct the problem of inadequate supply.

TABLE 12.11
Enzymes Requiring B_{12} as a Coenzyme

N^5-methyltetrahydrofolate homocystine methyltransferase
Acetate synthetase
Glutamate mutase
Methylmalonyl-CoA mutase
α-Methylene mutase
Dioldehydrase-α
Dioldehydrase-β
Glycerol dehydrase
Ethanolamine ammonia-lyase
L-β-lysine mutase
D-α-lysine mutase
Ornithine mutase
L-β-leucine aminomutase

Function

Vitamin B_{12} functions in one of two ways: (1) It participates as a coenzyme in reactions that utilize 5′-deoxyadenosine linked covalently to the cobalt atom (adenosylcobalamin). (2) It participates as a coenzyme in reactions that utilize the attachment of a methyl group to the central cobalt atom (methylcobalamin). The conversion of cobalamin to methylcobalamin is catalyzed by the enzyme B_{12} coenzyme synthetase. It catalyzes the reduction of the molecule, then catalyzes the reaction with deoxyadenosyl mostly derived from ATP. In addition to ATP, this reaction needs a diol or a dithiol group, a reduced flavin or a reduced ferredoxin as the biological alkylating agent. The enzymes requiring B_{12} as a coenzyme are listed in Table 12.11. The first of these is required for thymidine synthesis. This reaction removes a methyl group from methyl folate and delivers it to homocysteine, which, in turn, delivers it to deoxyuridylate converting it to thymidine. This process is also dependent on folacin. B_{12}-deficient animals show decreased methylation of tetrahydrofolate and decreased cellular folate levels despite dietary folate sufficiency. One of the characteristics of the B_{12}-deficient state is an anemia characterized by few mature red cells. Many immature nucleated cells (megaloblasts) can be found, but few mature ones. Among the other enzymes listed in Table 12.11 is methylmalonyl-CoA mutase, which participates in propionate metabolism. The overall reaction using B_{12} as a coenzyme in proprionate metabolism is shown in Figure 12.38. Proprionate metabolism, although a minor pathway in monogastric animals, is of some importance in neural tissue.[120] Loss of this metabolic activity may explain the peripheral neural loss that characterizes long-term B_{12} deficiency. Methylmalonic aciduria characterizes the

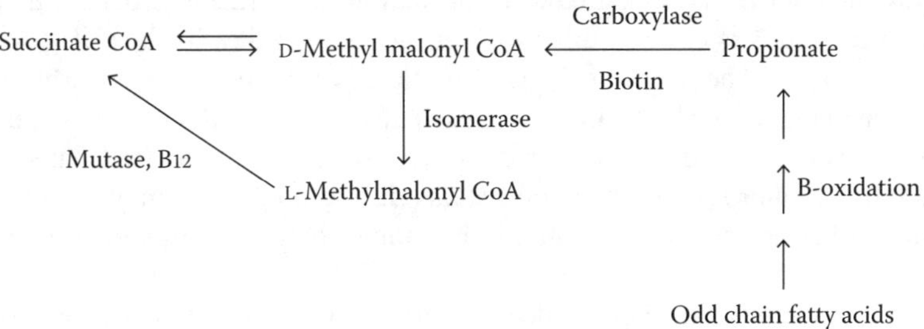

FIGURE 12.38 Vitamin B_{12} serves as a coenzyme in propionate metabolism.

B_{12}-deficient individual. Studies with rats made B_{12}-deficient show an increase in odd-numbered fatty acids in the neural and hepatic lipids and low hepatic methylmalonyl-CoA mutase activity. Replacement of B_{12} in the diet corrects both these responses.[121] The effect of B_{12} on mutase activity is such that it is likely that the vitamin not only serves as the coenzyme in the reaction but also serves a role in the synthesis of that enzyme. Several reports of B_{12} activity vis-à-vis protein synthesis have appeared in the literature in addition to the one concerning the synthesis of the mutase. Whether this relates to the role of B_{12} in DNA and RNA syntheses, that is, the synthesis of pyrimidines and purines, or whether a B_{12}–protein complex acts as a cis- or trans-acting factor in the pathway for the expression of the specific genes for these enzymes is unknown.

Methionine synthetase is another of the cobalamin-dependent enzymes.[122] Severe inhibition of this enzyme in humans results in megalobastic anemia and eventually in subacute combined degeneration of the spinal cord. It also results in an abnormal distribution of folate and folate derivatives. Epidermal growth factor appears to serve as a local mediator of the neurotrophic action of cobalamin in rat CNS and likely in humans.[123]

Deficiency

As described in the preceding section, the deficiency state has, as its main characteristic, pernicious anemia and peripheral neuropathy. While inadequate B_{12} intake can result in anemia, this is a rather unusual nutritional state because most foods of animal origin contain B_{12} and so little is needed. More common as a cause of pernicious anemia is a genetically determined deficiency of intrinsic factor. This trait is inherited as an autosomal dominant trait and occurs in about 1 in 1000. It can be treated with monthly B_{12} injections (~60–100 μg/dose). In the absence of this trait, the people most at risk for pernicious anemia are those who abstain from eating foods of animal origin. In addition to these are those who have had one of the illnesses described earlier that impair absorption. Humans who have had a gastrectomy or some disease of the gastric mucosa or some disease resulting in malabsorption are in this category.

Following the development of pernicious anemia (which is reversible) is the irreversible loss of peripheral sensation. This is due to the degenerative changes in these nerves including demyelination or loss of the lipid protective coat that surrounds the nerve tracts. Once the myelin is lost, the nerve dies. Neural loss begins in the feet and hands and progresses upward to the major nerve trunks such that a progressive neuropathy develops. Because both folate and B_{12} are interactively involved in DNA and RNA syntheses, it used to be difficult to segregate one deficiency anemia from the other. However, given the presence of methylmalonic aciduria and differential analysis of the red cell, one can determine the cause of the anemia. In addition to folacin and B_{12}, deficient intakes of iron, copper, and zinc can also explain anemia.

Needs

The daily requirement for B_{12} is very small. The normal turnover rate is about 2.5 μg/day; thus, the recommendation for adults is close to this turnover rate or 2 μg/day. Table 12.1 gives the DRI for humans of different ages. The need for B_{12} is also related to the intake of ascorbic acid, thiamin, carnitine, and fermentable fiber.[124–127] Each of these nutrients affect the production of proprionate, and in their absence or relative deficiency, proprionate production is increased. This, in turn, drives up the need for B_{12}. Compromised cobalamin status during pregnancy may put both mother and child at risk for further deterioration of vitamin B_{12} status compromising the growth and development of the infant.[128]

Biomarkers of B_{12} adequacy include the determination of the levels of methylmalonic acid, cobalamin, and holotranscobalamin.[129–134] Homocysteine levels have also been used and, when elevated, are thought to indicate B_{12} (as well as folacin) deficiency.[135,136]

CARNITINE

Carnitine can be synthesized in the body in amounts usually sufficient to meet needs. Thus, it is not considered an essential nutrient for the healthy individual. However, there are instances where the carnitine supply is insufficient. Interest in the essentiality of carnitine was stimulated by Broquist and colleagues who showed that carnitine was synthesized from lysine, an amino acid frequently in short supply in malnourished individuals. Follow-up work by Borum[137] showed that the premature infant could not synthesize sufficient carnitine to meet the needs for growth and normal metabolism. These reports stimulated the consideration of carnitine as an essential nutrient.

Structure

Carnitine is a quaternary amine, β-hydroxy-γ-*N*-trimethyl aminobutyric acid. Its structure is shown in Figure 12.39.

Physical and Chemical Properties

It is very hygroscopic with a molecular weight of 161.2. As mentioned, it is synthesized in the body (primarily the liver) from lysine. This pathway is shown in Figure 12.40. There are a number of essential nutrients involved: niacin as part of NAD, iron in the ferrous state, ascorbate to keep iron in its ferrous state, and of course lysine together with methionine as a methyl donor. As long as the diet provides these nutrients, carnitine will be synthesized to meet the needs of the normal individual. There are instances, however, where despite the provision of these essential nutrients carnitine synthesis does not take place to the extent that is needed.

In this instance, carnitine becomes an essential nutrient. This occurs in the premature infant. Due to its prematurity, its biochemical pathways, especially that for carnitine synthesis, are not well developed. The mother's carnitine status will influence that of the infant. If mothers are supplemented with carnitine, the fetal carnitine status is improved. In addition, maternal supplementation stimulates the enzymes carnitine palmitoyltransferase and pyruvate dehydrogenase.[138]

In severely traumatized individuals, the need for carnitine can exceed endogenous synthesis. The whole-body response to trauma involves a catecholamine–glucocorticoid response that greatly increases lipolysis and fatty acid oxidation. This drives up the need for carnitine and in this situation, endogenous synthesis is inadequate. The aging may also have an increased need for carnitine especially if they are obese.[139–141] Carnitine functions as an acyl group acceptor that facilitates the mitochondrial export of excess fatty acids in the form of acylcarnitines. In the obese and also the diabetic, it is not unexpected that there would be an excess of fatty acids needing export to the cytosol.[141] This might drive up the need for carnitine in excess of endogenous synthesis.

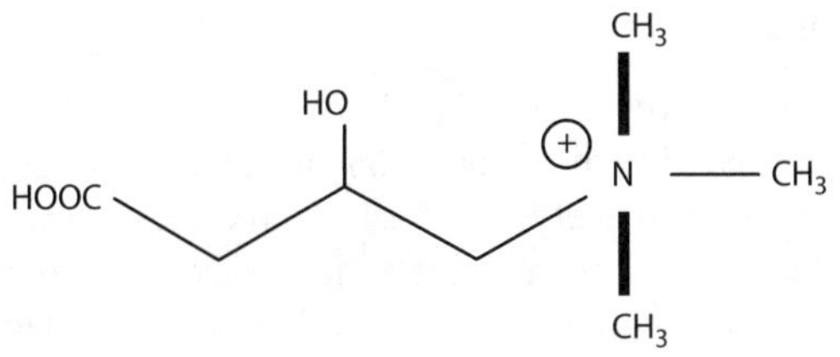

FIGURE 12.39 Structure of carnitine.

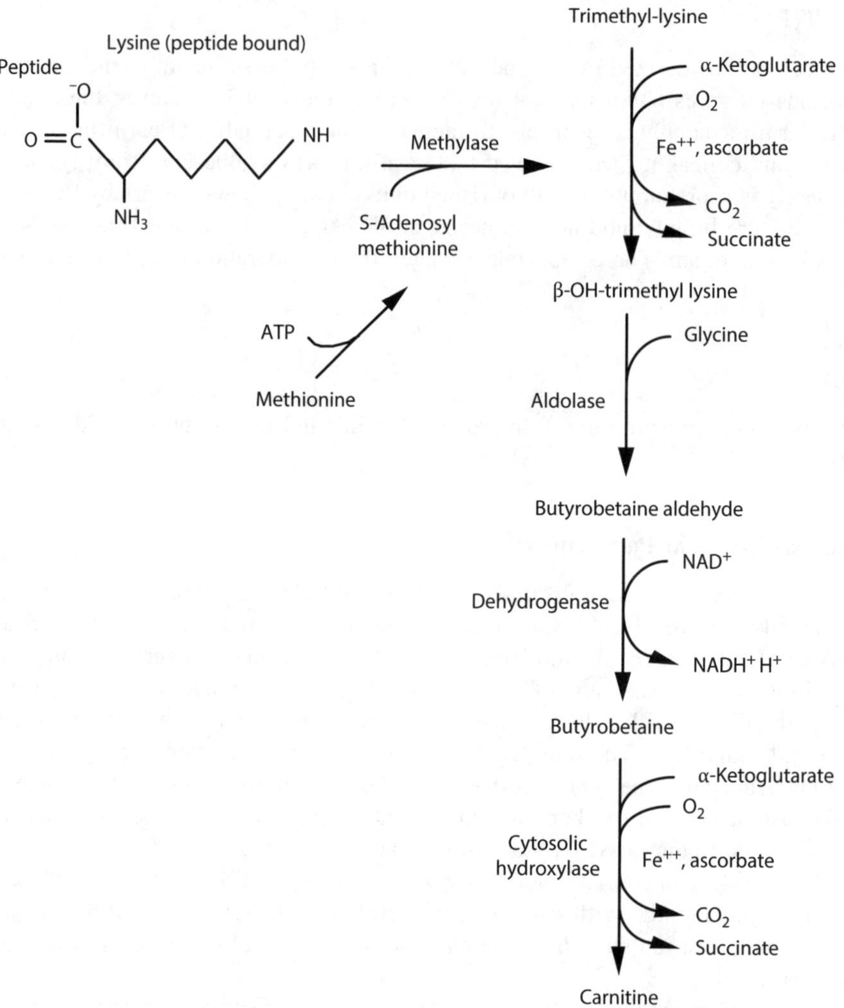

FIGURE 12.40 Synthesis of carnitine.

Sources

The techniques for food carnitine analysis are not well developed. However, despite the inadequacies of the methodology, it is safe to indicate that good sources of carnitine include red meats and some organ meats. Milk, whole grains, and some vegetables (i.e., spinach, cauliflower, avocado, and peanuts) contain modest amounts.

Absorption and Metabolism

Carnitine is absorbed via an active process involving sodium and a carrier. Carnitine in large amounts is also absorbed by passive diffusion. Concurrent with its absorption is its acetylation. It is transported in both the free and acetylated forms to the muscles where 90% of the total body carnitine may be found. The turnover of carnitine is quite slow. Although it is needed for fatty acid oxidation particularly by the working muscle, it is continuously recycled rather than degraded and excreted. The kidney plays an important role in carnitine conservation in that 90% of the carnitine that arrives at the kidney is reabsorbed by the glomerulus and returned to the circulation. In instances of kidney failure, this conservation is lost and again we have a situation where exogenous

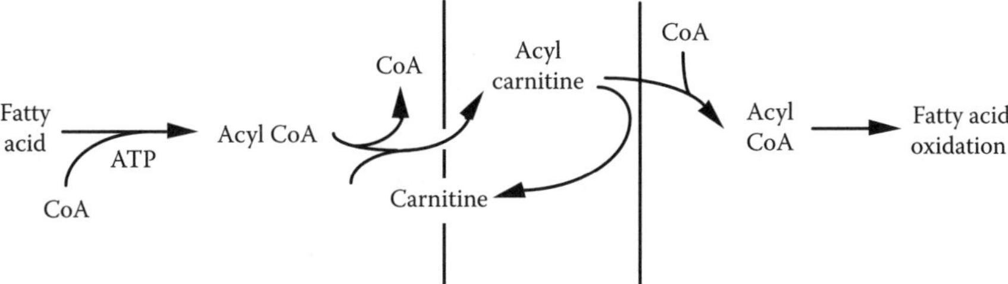

FIGURE 12.41 The carnitine acyltransferase system.

carnitine must be supplied. A small amount of acylcarnitine ester may be found in the urine of normal subjects. This probably represents less than 1% of the total body carnitine pool.

Function

Carnitine serves as part of the carnitine acyltransferase system located in the mitochondrial membrane. This system is shown in Figure 12.41. There are two transferases involved: carnitine acyltransferase I located on the outer side of the inner mitochondrial membrane and carnitine acyltransferase II located on the matrix side of the membrane. These enzymes catalyze the synthesis and hydrolysis of the fatty acylcarnitine esters as well as work with the transporter protein (acetyl translocase) that catalyzes the movement of the fatty acids into the mitochondrial matrix. There is no other known function for carnitine (Figure 12.41).

Deficiency

Low levels of carnitine in tissues and blood typify the carnitine-deficient individual in addition to hyperlipidemia, cardiomyopathy, and muscle spasm.

Because carnitine can be synthesized in the body, no recommended intake levels have been set for normal children and adults.[141] Work continues on developing intake recommendations for preterm infants and others with special needs.

CHOLINE

While many nutrition scientists have presumed that the list of required vitamins is complete, others would argue that there are certain circumstances where a dietary supply of a compound is essential for the support of normal metabolism. Choline is one of these compounds. In rats given a choline-deficient diet, one can observe a fatty liver as well as certain CNS deficits. Human cells grown in culture also have an absolute requirement for choline, and humans sustained by choline-free parenteral solutions develop symptoms similar to those of the deficient rat. It is on this basis that the inclusion of choline in a list of essential micronutrients is argued.[142–148]

Structure

Choline is the trivial name for 2-hydroxy-*N*,*N*,*N*-trimethyl-ethanaminium. The structure for this compound is shown in Figure 12.42.

Physical and Chemical Properties

Choline is freely soluble in water and ethanol but insoluble in such organic solvents as ether or chloroform. It is extremely hygroscopic. It is a strong base and readily decomposes in alkaline solutions, resulting in the production of trimethylamine. Because of its unique structure, choline serves

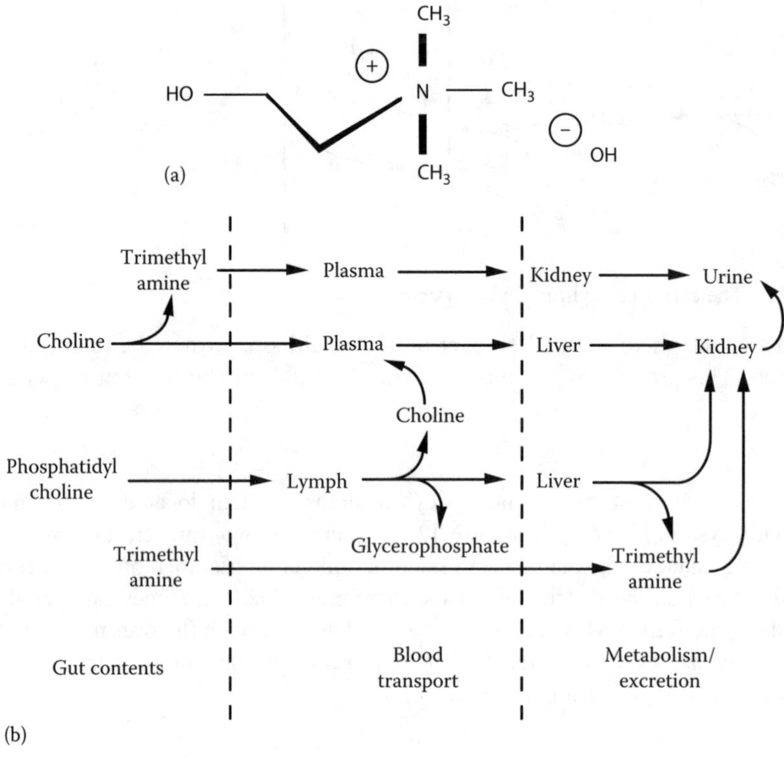

FIGURE 12.42 (a) Structure of choline. (b) Absorption and metabolism of choline.

as a donor of methyl groups. It has a molecular weight of 121.2 and belongs to a class of compounds that function either as methyl donors or as membrane constituents. Related compounds are listed in Table 12.12. Because of its instability, the determination of choline in food and biological tissues is fraught with difficulty. Commonly used is the reineckate method, which involves the precipitation of choline as a reineckate salt and the development of a characteristic color. Unfortunately, this method lacks the sensitivity and specificity provided by newer chromatographic and isotopic methods that are combined with rapid inactivation, via microwave, of choline degradative enzymes. Work is ongoing for the development of sensitive and specific methods for choline assay.

TABLE 12.12
Choline and Related Metabolites

As a methyl donor
Choline
Methionine
Folacin
Betaine
As a choline metabolite
Choline, acetylcholine
Phosphorylcholine
Betaine
Phosphatidylcholine (lecithin)
Lysophosphatidylcholine (lysolecithin)
Sphingomyelin

Sources

Choline is widely distributed in foods and is consumed mainly in the form of lecithin (phosphatidylcholine). Lecithin is not only a naturally occurring common food ingredient but also a common additive to processed foods. It serves as a food stabilizer and emulsifying agent. Choline chloride and choline bitartrate are added to infant formula to assure equivalency to breast milk, which contains 7 mg/100 kcal (7 mg/420 kJ). Seven milligrams is about 50 μmol. Recent assessments of commercial infant formulas, however, showed less choline in the preparation than shown on the label. Choline content in this report ranged from 100 to 647 μmol. In part, this discrepancy may be due to the lability of choline once in a solution (the infant formula) that is mildly alkaline and in part due to the relative difficulty in assessing choline content accurately and sensitively.

Absorption and Metabolism

There is a good bit of difficulty in assessing choline absorption. Currently, it is believed to be absorbed via a sodium-dependent carrier-mediated mechanism. If large amounts of choline are consumed, uptake of the excess is by passive diffusion. One study using labeled choline showed that about 65% of the dose was found in the urine as trimethylamine within 12 h of ingestion. When labeled choline was incorporated into lecithin and ingested, significantly less of the label was recovered in the urine as trimethylamine. About 50% of the ingested labeled lecithin entered the thoracic duct intact. The use of antibiotics to reduce the population of gut flora reduced the loss of trimethylamine in the urine. This showed that one of the major degradative steps in the loss of choline is through the action of the gut flora. The route of choline and lecithin metabolism and degradation is shown in Figure 12.42. In addition to the action of the gut flora, phosphatidylcholine is subject to enzymatic degradation. Phospholipases A_1, A_2, and B catalyze the ester bonds that link the fatty acids at the glycerol carbons 1 and 2 resulting in free fatty acids and glycerophosphocholine. Most of the lecithin that is ingested has only one of its fatty acids removed prior to absorption. Sphingomyelin, a related complex lipid containing choline, is not degraded at all in the intestinal lumen. All of the phospholipids are transported into the lymphatic circulation from the gut and appear in the plasma lipoproteins. All classes (high-density lipoproteins, low-density lipoproteins, very low-density lipoproteins and chylomicrons) contain phosphatidylcholine. The chylomicrons are the major carriers from the gut, but once into the blood, the phosphatidylcholine is redistributed among the lipoprotein classes. From the blood it is then taken up by all cell types following the lipase action and resynthesis pattern used by the transport and uptake of the triacylglycerides.

Most species can synthesize choline using methionine as the methyl donor. This synthesis is shown in Figure 12.43. Methionine is converted to SAM. The methyl groups are then joined to

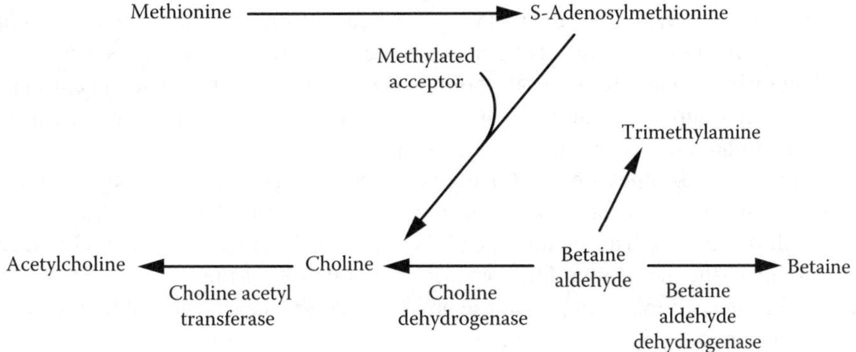

FIGURE 12.43 Use of methionine in the synthesis of choline and subsequent use of choline in betaine and acetylcholine synthesis.

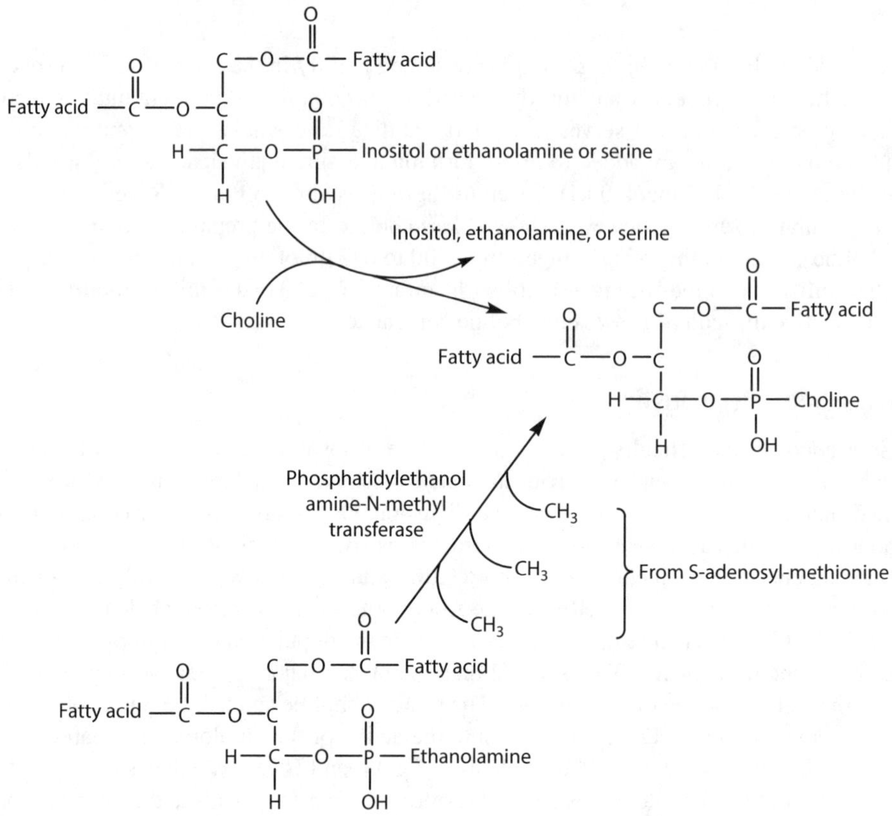

FIGURE 12.44 Biosynthesis of phosphatidylcholine.

form choline. The de novo synthesis of phosphatidylcholine usually occurs by using phosphatidylethanolamine, another phospholipid, as the starting material. Aside from the diet, this conversion of phosphatidylethanolamine to phosphatidylcholine is the only source of de novo synthesized choline in the mammalian body. This synthesis is outlined in Figure 12.44. Shown in this figure is the exchange of inositol, ethanolamine, or serine for choline.

Function

Choline serves as a precursor for the neurotransmitter acetylcholine. The intake of choline can affect brain levels of acetylcholine, and this may be a benefit to patients showing acetylcholine deficits as in tardive dyskinesia. Some benefit is also achieved with people having short-term memory loss as in Alzheimer's disease. In addition, choline plays an important role in fetal neuronal development. Dietary choline supplementation of rat diets enhances memory performance and increases the hippocampal phospholipase D activity in the offspring.[142,143]

As important as the synthesis of acetylcholine is the synthesis of the membrane phospholipid phosphatidylcholine. This phospholipid is an important structural element of the membrane and, depending on the chain length and saturation of the fatty acids attached to carbons 1 and 2, contributes to the fluidity of the membrane. The consideration of fluidity is important to the function of the membrane-embedded proteins. Many of these proteins change shape as part of their action, and the fluidity of the surrounding lipid determines the ease with which they can do this.

Phosphatidylcholine functions not only in the transport of lipids as part of the lipoproteins but also in the transmembrane lipid transport system. In this role, phosphatidylcholine serves as a lipotrope. It also plays a role in cell signaling.[142]

Lastly, because choline serves as a precursor of betaine, it serves as a methyl donor in the one-carbon metabolic pathways. These pathways include the formation of methionine from homocysteine and the formation of creatine from guanidoacetic acid.

Deficiency

Because choline can be synthesized in the body and because it is universally present in our food supply, a true deficiency in normal humans is rare indeed. Choline deficiency can occur in poultry fed a low-choline diet or one deficient in methionine and/or methyl donors. Depressed growth, fatty liver, and hemorrhagic renal disease have been reported to occur in deficient animals of a number of species. Choline deficiency induces apoptosis in SV40-immortalized CWSV-1 rat hepatocytes in culture, and it is possible that choline might have this effect in vivo.[145] However, this has not been shown. Of interest is an early report of an effect of choline deficiency on body carnitine pools.[146] A 50% reduction has been reported and due to the importance of carnitine in fatty acid oxidation, this relationship may explain the fatty liver of deficient animals. Nonalcoholic fatty liver disease in humans has been found to associate with low choline intake.[147]

In rats, choline deprivation impairs brain mitochondrial function.[148] In mice, dietary choline reverses some but not all of the effects of folate deficiency on neurogenesis and apoptosis in the brain.[149] Likely, there are genetically determined differences in choline need and function.[150,151]

Needs

There are suggested intakes (AI) for choline (Table 12.1). Rebouche has outlined these needs.[141]

INOSITOL

Until fairly recently, little attention has been paid to the role of inositol in the diet. This has occurred despite the recognition that dietary inositol has been shown to prevent the development of a fatty liver in rats and to cure alopecia in rats and mice and despite a report made over a 100 years ago that diabetic humans excreted large quantities of this substance in their urine. Inositol is an essential part of every cell.[153] It is a key ingredient for one of the membrane lipids phosphatidylinositol (PI), and it is critical to the inositol signaling system (the phosphatidyl inositol system) that plays a key role in the regulation of hormone release and cellular response to a variety of signals.[154–156] It is not considered an essential nutrient for humans.

Structure

Inositol is a six-carbon sugar that is configuratively related to D-glucose. Its structure is shown in Figure 12.45. It occurs in nature in nine possible isomeric forms. However, only one, myoinositol, is biologically important as a nutrient.

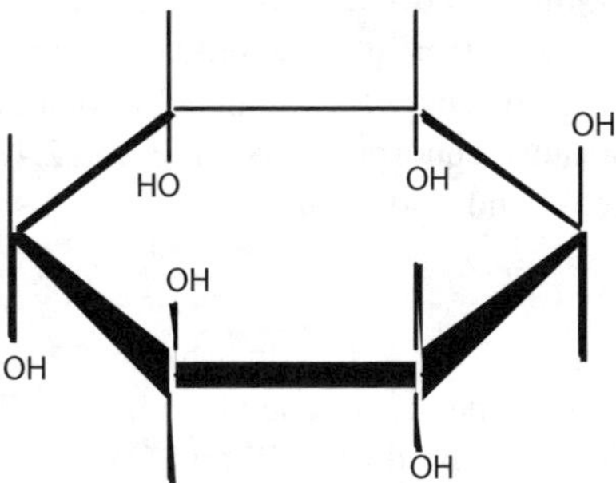

FIGURE 12.45 Myoinositol structure.

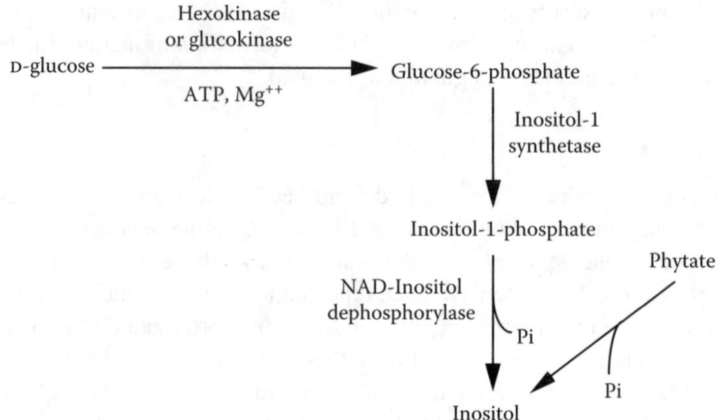

FIGURE 12.46 Synthesis of free inositol from either glucose or phytate. The conversion of glucose to inositol is an insulin-dependent pathway, whereas the dephosphorylation of phytate is not.

Physical and Chemical Properties

Myoinositol is a water-soluble, cyclic, six-carbon compound (cis-1,2,3,5 trans-4,6-cyclohexane-hexanol). Inositol is widely distributed in foods of both plant and animal origin. In plants and animals, it exists as part of the PI of the cell membranes or as free inositol. Phytic acid, a component of many grain products, can be converted to myoinositol with the removal of the phosphate groups (Figure 12.46). Phytate or phytic acid can bind calcium, magnesium, and other divalent ions[166] within the intestinal compartment making them unavailable for absorption by mucosal cells. Once the phytate is dephosphorylated through the action of phytase, the inositol residue remains. The divalent ions are released and the free inositol is absorbed. Both free inositol and cell membrane PI are found in foods of animal origin.

Absorption and Metabolism

Dietary PI is acted on by the luminal enzyme phospholipase and converted to lysophosphatidylinositol. This compound can then be further hydrolyzed to produce glycerophosphorylinositol and then free inositol or acted upon by an acyltransferase in the intestinal cell that converts it back to PI. This is then transported out of the gut absorptive cell as a component of the lipoproteins.

Free inositol in the lumen is transported into the luminal cells via an active, energy-dependent, sodium-dependent transport process quite similar to that which transports glucose. Although similar, it is not identical to it. Free inositol is then transported in the blood at a concentration of about 300 μM.

As mentioned, inositol can be synthesized from glucose by a variety of mammalian cells. Synthesis in the testes, brain, kidney, and liver has been reported. Humans can synthesize up to 4 g/day in the kidneys alone. Synthesis from glucose proceeds from glucose to glucose-6-phosphate to inositol-1-phosphate to inositol. The enzymes are glucokinase or hexokinase followed by inositol 1 synthetase and then NAD-inositol-dephosphorylase. Figure 12.46 illustrates the pathway for the production of inositol from glucose and also from phytate.

Function

Inositol functions as a constituent of the membrane phospholipid PI. Free inositol is added to diacylglycerol (DAG) via a CDP reaction producing PI and CMP. The enzyme catalyzing this reaction is CDP DAG–inositol phosphatidyltransferase, sometimes called PI synthetase. This synthesis takes place in the microsomes and the enzyme has a K_m of 4.6 mM for inositol. This reaction is

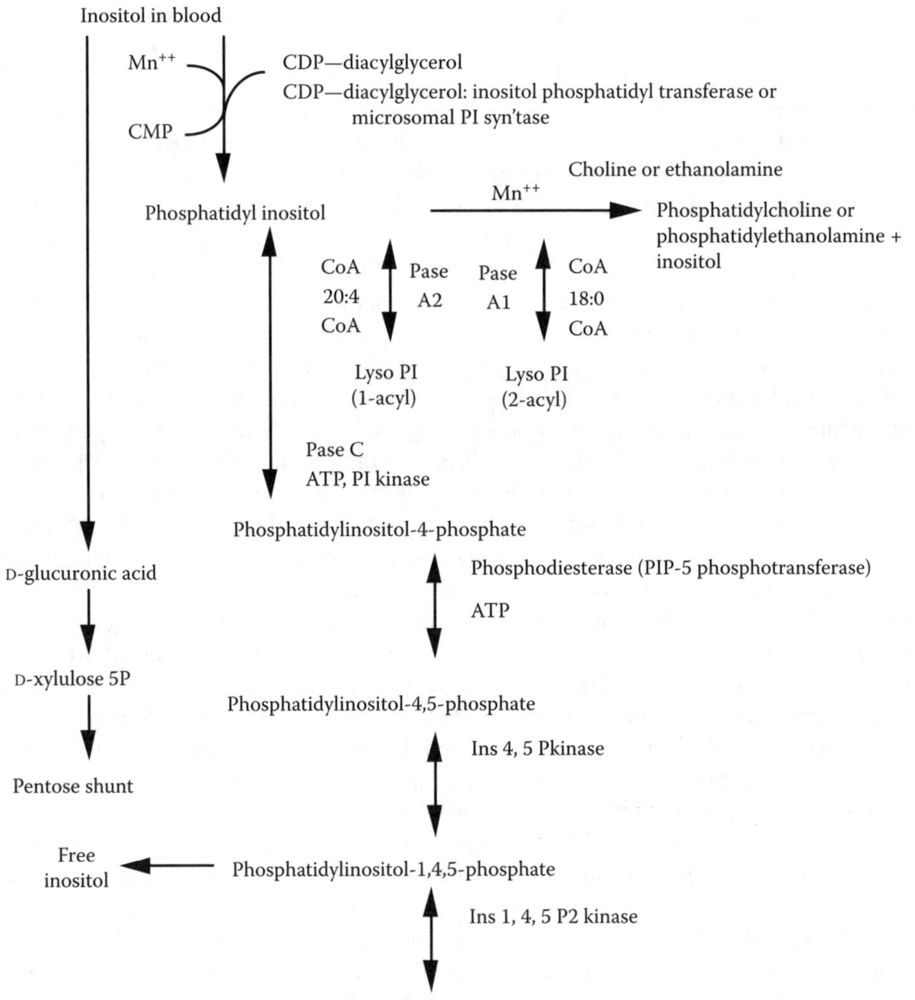

FIGURE 12.47 Inositol metabolism and the PIP cycle.

illustrated in Figure 12.47. PI can also be synthesized via an exchange reaction where free inositol can exchange for either choline or ethanolamine in either phosphatidylcholine or phosphatidylethanolamine. The K_m for the Mn^{++}-dependent reaction is 0.024 mM. Once formed, the PI migrates from the microsomes where it is formed to any one of the membranes within and around the cell. It comprises approximately 10% of the phospholipids in the cellular membranes. Recently, its function as a part of a unique cellular second messenger system (different from the cyclic AMP system) has been explored. This system, called the PIP system or PIP cycle, has been reported to function in insulin release by the pancreatic insulin producing β-cells,[157–160] in the regulation of protein kinase C, in the mobilization of intracellular calcium, and in the regulation of Na^+K^+ ATPase activity and may have a role in blood clotting, blood pressure regulation, and renal function.

Once formed, PI serves as a substrate for one of several enzymes. These reactions are shown in Figure 12.47. Phospholipase A1 acts on PI to produce lyso PI (2-acyl-PI). Phospholipase A2 acts to produce a 1-acyl-PI. Both A1 and A2 act to remove one of the fatty acids from the phospholipids; A1 removes the fatty acid (usually stearic acid, 18:0) from the glycerol carbon 1, while A2 removes the fatty acid (usually arachidonic acid, 20:4) from the glycerol carbon 2. When phospholipase A2 is activated, arachidonic acid is released and this fatty acid serves as the substrate for prostaglandin synthesis. Prostaglandins are another group of hormonelike substances that are important in the regulation of blood pressure and blood clotting. A third enzyme also has PI as its substrate. This enzyme is ATP PI kinase (phospholipase C) and initiates the PIP cycle also illustrated in Figure 12.47. Phospholipase C action is mediated by the guanine nucleotide–binding protein called the G protein. Phospholipase C cleaves the phosphorylated inositol from the glycerol backbone producing DAG and PI 1-4,5-phosphate (PIP_2). DAG serves to activate protein kinase C, an important regulatory enzyme discovered in 1979. Neutral DAG remains within the membrane, while the liberated inositol 4,5-bisphosphate migrates into the cytoplasm and, in the process, is again phosphorylated to form inositol 1,4,5-phosphate (PIP_3). This compound causes a release of calcium ion from nonmitochondrial vesicular, intracellular stores. The triphosphate inositol binds to a receptor protein associated with these stores to effect this release. Ca^{++} release from the endoplasmic reticulum is elicited via an opening of a gated channel. Cyclic AMP-dependent phosphorylation of the receptor protein seems to be involved. The magnesium ion is also involved. Inositol 1,4,5-phosphate can then either be dephosphorylated to release free inositol or be phosphorylated once again to form inositol 1,3,4,5-phosphate (PIP_4) via the enzyme D-myo-inositol 1,4,5-triphosphate 3-kinase. This kinase is stimulated by a Ca^{++} in the presence of calmodulin and protein kinase C, and thus the level of the inositol 1,4,5-phosphate is carefully regulated. Inositol 1,3,4,5-phosphate also is an active metabolic regulator in that it modulates calcium ion either through the reuptake of Ca^{++} into the intracellular stores or through control of the Ca^{++} transfer process between pools that are inositol 1,4,5-phosphate sensitive and insensitive. The kinase enzyme might be the target for the enzyme protein tyrosine kinase. All of these phosphorylations of inositol are reversible, and amounts of each of the phosphorylated intermediates depend on the hormonal status of the individual as well as on the availability of inositol for PI synthesis. Insulin, various growth factors, and PGF2α (one of the prostaglandins) have all been shown to stimulate the PI cycle. Of particular interest are the reports that inositol turnover is increased in acute diabetes. Other observations on the relationship of diabetes to inositol status include the following: anti-insulin antiserum treatment of the diabetic neutralizes the effect of the exogenous insulin on inositol turnover; insulin treatment of acute insulin deficiency reverses the effect of diabetes on inositol turnover; insulin increases the synthesis of PI, DAG, and protein kinase C activity in a variety of cells from normal animals. All of these findings suggest that there may be circumstances where the synthesis of the inositol by the body might be inadequate to meet the body's need and that this substance must be provided in the diet. Under these circumstances, inositol becomes an essential nutrient. One of these circumstances is the disease diabetes mellitus.

Diabetes, regardless of whether it is insulin dependent or noninsulin dependent, is characterized by a failure to appropriately regulate blood glucose levels. With high blood levels of glucose, the sorbitol pathway is stimulated.[159] If this pathway is stimulated, endogenous synthesis of myoinositol is reduced.[159] Further, cellular uptake of glucose is impaired in the diabetic state. If cellular glucose uptake is impaired, less inositol is synthesized from glucose and less is available for PI synthesis.[159,160] Hence, the diabetic excretes more inositol in the urine while having an intracellular deficiency because of inadequate endogenous synthesis. In turn, this means that more preformed inositol should be provided to the body via the diet. Thus, the diabetic may have a significantly greater requirement for inositol than the nondiabetic. Indeed, there may be as broad a range in inositol requirements as there is the range of severity of diabetes. Recently, there have been reports in the medical literature that have suggested that the secondary complications of diabetes, that is, renal disease, could be ameliorated by dietary inositol supplementation. Some investigators have shown a reversal of the diabetes-induced increased glomerular filtration rate with a 7–10-fold increase in dietary levels of myoinositol. At any rate, it would appear that diabetics have a larger than normal need for dietary inositol because (1) they excrete more than do normal people; (2) when hyperglycemic, they synthesize less from glucose because less glucose is available inside the cell and because the first two steps in glucose metabolism are insulin dependent; (3) they absorb less from the diet and (4) when hyperglycemic, they have greater sorbitol production, which, in turn, inhibits the pathway for inositol synthesis.

Deficiency

In normal humans, inositol needs are presumed to be met by endogenous synthesis, so detailed studies have not been performed using healthy volunteers. Indirect evidence of need has been reported sparsely in the medical literature, but detailed controlled feeding studies have not been conducted. Such studies have been performed in laboratory rats and mice. In these animals, the most striking feature of the deficient state was the development of a fatty liver. This was reversed with dietary inositol supplements. Hair loss and poor growth were also reported for deficient animals. At the time these animal studies were conducted (1979–1980), the PIP cycle was not known. Researchers knew about the presence of PI in the cell membrane, but they did not recognize its importance in the lipid signal transduction process. Studies on the PIP cycle in rats made inositol deficient have yet to be conducted.

Is inositol essential in the human diet? In normal people, it probably is not, but in the diabetic, inositol may be an essential nutrient. As mentioned, the healthy human adult probably meets his or her daily need easily because of the ubiquitous presence of inositol in much of the food humans consume. Even in the event of inadequate intake, healthy humans can probably synthesize more than they need to maintain optimal health. However, just as there may be special circumstances that dictate an increased intake of other nutrients, so too can this occur with respect to inositol. This research arena is particularly active these days as we learn more about the PIP cycle and the nutritional implications of this signal system.

Needs

Many nutrition scientists argue that inositol is not an essential nutrient because the body can synthesize it from glucose. However, as we become more aware of the genetic diversity of humans (as well as other species), we have come to realize that some individuals vary in their needs for the required nutrients. This is particularly true for those nutrient needs that are partially satisfied through endogenous synthesis. In this category are niacin, arginine, histidine, choline, and inositol. Individuals who cannot synthesize these nutrients in the quantities they need must have a dietary supply. In addition, some individuals may excrete larger than normal amounts of the nutrient or catabolize it faster than usual. In all of these instances, the individual will require a far greater dietary supply of a given nutrient than other individuals of the same species. People with diabetes mellitus may have a need for inositol at a dose that exceeds the synthesizing capacity of their bodies. Research is needed to determine whether a nutrient recommendation should be developed for this group of people.

OTHER COMPOUNDS THAT MAY OR MAY NOT BE VITAMINS

The bulk of the work identifying and describing compounds we now know as vitamins occurred in the first part of the twentieth century. Recent work has suggested other compounds that may also be essential to the maintenance of normal metabolism. In this list are pyrroloquinoline quinone, ubiquinone, orotic acid, PABA, lipoic acid, and the bioflavonoids. Brief descriptions of these substances follow.

Pyrroloquinoline Quinone

Pyrroloquinoline quinone, sometimes called methoxatin, serves as a cofactor in the reaction catalyzed by lysyl oxidase. Lysyl oxidase catalyzes the cross-linking of collagen and elastin. It also requires copper as a cofactor.

Pyrroloquinoline quinone is a tricarboxylic acid with a fused heterocylic (*o*-quinone) ring system. Its C-5 carbonyl group is very reactive toward nucleophiles, and it is this action that allows this substance to function in collagen and elastin cross-linking. At present, information is scarce with respect to its food sources and essentiality. Likely, it can be endogenously synthesized, but whether or not this compound meets the definition of a vitamin has yet to be established.

Ubiquinone

Ubiquinone is another substance whose vitamin status is unclear. It is an essential component of the mitochondrial respiratory chain, and it has been assumed to be synthesized endogenously. Actually, ubiquinone is a group of related substances. They are a group of tetrasubstituted 1,4-benzoquinone derivatives with isoprenoid side chains of various lengths. The biochemists have termed these substances as coenzyme Q. They function as reversible donors/acceptors of reducing equivalents from NAD, passing electrons from flavoproteins to the cytochromes via cytochrome b_5. Because the ubiquinones can be synthesized endogenously in large amounts even when diets lacking the ubiquinones are offered, these substances fail to meet the definition of the word vitamin. However, synthesis may be reduced in persons consuming the statins that inhibit cholesterol synthesis at the HMG CoA reductase step. In so inhibiting this step, the synthesis of ubiquinone is inhibited. With more research, it may be that under these conditions a ubiquinone supplement may be needed.

Orotic Acid

Orotic acid is an important metabolic intermediate in the synthesis of pyrimidines. It is synthesized endogenously from *N*-carbamyl phosphate by dehydration and oxidation. It is another of those substances that fail to meet the definition of the word vitamin. However, when used as a dietary supplement (0.1% of diet), it has resulted in a fatty, enlarged liver and increased the levels of hepatic uracil presumably due to an influence on pyrimidine synthesis. Orotic acid–induced fatty liver is accompanied by falling plasma cholesterol levels and falling activity of HMG CoA reductase. This hepatic enzyme is greatly influenced by its product (cholesterol), and so if the liver does not export it, it feeds back to inhibit its synthesis.

Para-Aminobenzoic Acid

p-Amino benzoic acid is an essential growth factor for a number of bacteria that use it as a precursor of folacin. Animals, however, cannot synthesize folacin so *p*-amino benzoic acid does not meet the definition of the word vitamin. Its involvement in folacin use is discussed in the section on folacin.

Lipoic Acid

Lipoic acid is essential to oxidative decarboxylation of α-keto acids. It participates in pyruvate dehydrogenase complex. This is a multienzyme complex where lipoic acid is linked to the ε-amino group of a lysine residue from the enzyme dihydrolipoyl transacetylase. As lipoamide undergoes reversible acylation/deacylation, it transfers acyl groups to CoA and results in reversible ring opening/closing in the oxidation of the α-keto acid. Lipoic acid can be synthesized endogenously in amounts sufficient to meet the need. Therefore, it does not meet the definition of *vitamin*.

Bioflavonoids

Bioflavonoids are a group of compounds that augment the action of ascorbic acid in the prevention of scurvy. They are mixtures of phenolic derivatives of 2-phenyl-1,4-benzopyrone. The bioflavonoids are present in a large variety of foods and were first isolated by Szent-Gyorgy from lemon juice and red peppers. More than 800 different flavonoids have been found. They occur naturally as glycosides that are hydrolyzed by the gut flora prior to absorption. No single unique deficiency syndrome has been found or reported in animals fed a bioflavonoid-free diet. Furthermore, there has not been a unique response to the addition of bioflavonoids to the diet. On this basis, despite its activity as a potentiator of ascorbic acid, the bioflavonoids cannot be considered vitamins.

Pseudovitamins

The term vitamin was coined many years ago to designate those organic compounds that are needed to sustain normal growth and metabolism and that are needed in small amounts. This term developed by nutritional biochemists and physiologists has been used commercially as well as scientifically. Unfortunately, there have been (and continue to be) commercial uses of the term that are inappropriate. Hence, we have compounds such as laetrile (an extract from fruit pits), pangamic acid or vitamin B_{15}, and methylsulfonium salts of methionine called vitamin U and gerovital, also called vitamin H_3. Gerovital is advertized as an antiaging substance, but claims of its effects have not been substantiated. The advertised use of methylsulfonic salts of methionine to prevent peptic ulcers likewise has not been substantiated. Pangamic acid, another of these pseudovitamins, is not a chemically defined substance. Rather, it is a mixture of compounds. Of the materials labeled, pangamic acid is *N,N*-diisopropylamine dichloroacetate. This is a drug and when administered to normal rats caused death preceded by respiratory failure, extreme hypotension, and hypothermia. There is no evidence of essentiality for pangamic acid.

Lastly, laetrile is included in this list of pseudovitamins. This compound has been the focus of a number of litigations due to the claim by its suppliers that it can serve as an anticancer drug. This claim was investigated and found wanting by the U.S. Food and Drug Administration (FDA). The term laetrile has several synonyms: amygdalin and vitamin B_{17}. Amygdalin is a β-cyanogenic glucoside and is a major constituent in preparations named laetrile. Amygdalin is a substance found in peach pits, apricot pits, and the kernels and seeds of many fruits. Neither the U.S. FDA nor the Canadian equivalent of this regulatory agency recognizes laetrile as a vitamin.

SUMMARY

1. The water-soluble vitamins include ascorbic acid and the group of compounds that are called the B vitamins: thiamin, riboflavin, niacin, B_6, B_{12}, folacin, pantothenic acid, and biotin.
2. All are required in very small amounts.
3. Many are coenzymes in intermediary metabolism.
4. Skin lesions and anemia are symptoms of an inadequate intake.
5. Each of these vitamins has been isolated and their chemical and physical properties established.
6. Assays have been developed to quantify their presence in food.
7. The function of each of the vitamins has been established.
8. Carnitine, inositol, and choline are conditional vitamins. This means that they are required under certain conditions such as prematurity or trauma.
9. Other compounds are being studied to determine their essentiality but at present are not considered essential. These include pyrroloquinoline quinine, ubiquinone, PABA, lipoic acid, and the bioflavonoids.
10. A number of other compounds are considered to be pseudovitamins. These include pangamic acid, laetrile, methylsulfonium salts of methionine, and gerovital.

LEARNING OPPORTUNITIES

CASE STUDY 12.1 Uncle John Is an Alcoholic

Uncle John is 43 years old. He has always been rather lean but lately he has lost weight. He looks downright skinny. Uncle James is fun to visit. He tells lots of funny stories and is very convivial. He seldom is without a bottle of beer in his hand. He really loves his beer and the guys at work drink about the same amount. He does not think he is an alcoholic! In a given day, he might consume six packs of 12 oz bottles of beer, and he feels that his friends do likewise. Sometimes, he will snack on pretzels or potato chips to go along with the beer, and occasionally, he will have a hamburger with some fries. He says his appetite is poor. He seldom wants anything to eat preferring to drink his beer.

Lately, Uncle John has noticed some scaliness on his arms and also some other skin changes. He seems more tired than usual and his face seems paler than it used to be. He was always an outside guy. He loved to watch sports and cheer for his favorite team. Now, he is somewhat apathetic and listless. Analyze this situation and make some suggestions as to John's prognosis as well as the management of this situation.

CASE STUDY 12.2 Little Lizzie Has Scurvy

Lizzie is 2 years old. She has begun to walk but has a funny skeleton. Her mother has noticed that the ends of her ribs have little knobs on them. Lizzie has her baby teeth but her gums seem to bleed a lot and she is far more fussy than she used to be. When placed on her back in her bed, she spreads her legs with her little knees out. Her mom was concerned so she brought Lizzie to the well baby clinic at her local hospital. The doctors were dismayed because they realized that Lizzie's problem was scurvy. They promptly treated her with vitamin C and instructed Lizzie's mom to give her little girl fresh orange juice every morning. Thinking that the problem was fixed (the gums were healing and Lizzie's fussiness went away), they discharged Lizzie. Her mom took her home but a couple of weeks later, she was back at the hospital with the same symptoms. The doctors were so frustrated. They asked Lizzie's mom if she had followed their instructions about giving Lizzie orange juice every day. "Oh yes," Lizzie's mom said, "I ran down to the corner store every morning and got Lizzie a fresh bottle of orange pop!" What is the problem here? What would you do if this case was yours to manage?

MULTIPLE-CHOICE QUESTIONS

1. Anemia is one of the chief signs of malnutrition. In the context of this chapter, what nutrients are involved in anemia?
   a. Pyridoxine
   b. Folacin
   c. Vitamin V12
   d. All of the above
2. In people consuming a corn-based diet that is marginally adequate, what problem would develop?
   a. Pellagra
   b. Beriberi
   c. Scurvy
   d. Osteoporosis

3. What amino acid has a positive effect on niacin adequacy?
   a. Tyrosine
   b. Phenylalanine
   c. Tryptophan
   d. Valine
4. During World War 2, prisoners held in Asian camps were poorly fed. Their rations consisted mainly of white rice plus tiny amounts of vegetables and rarely a morsel of meat. The prisoners requested that they be given a lower-quality brown rice instead of the white polished rice. Their captors agreed because it was a cheaper foodstuff. What made the difference to these prisoners?
   a. They had a better intake of protein.
   b. They had more energy from the brown rice.
   c. The rations had a better flavor.
   d. The brown rice contained more B vitamins than the white rice.
5. Intermediary metabolism is dependent on
   a. NAD and NADH
   b. FAD and FADH
   c. Magnesium
   d. All of the above

REFERENCES

1. King, C.G. (1979) The isolation of vitamin C from lemon juice. *Fed. Proc.* 38: 2682–2682.
2. De Luca, L.M., Norum, K.R. (2011) Scurvy and cloudberries: A chapter in the history of nutritional sciences. *J. Nutr.* 141: 2101–2105.
3. Stevenson, N.R., Brush, M.K. (1969) Existence and characteristics of Na-dependent active transport of ascorbic acid in guinea pig. *Am. J. Clin. Nutr.* 22: 318–326.
4. Bowers-Komro, D.M., McCormick, D.B. (1991) Characterization of ascorbic acid uptake by isolated rat kidney cells. *J. Nutr.* 121: 57–64.
5. Hodges, R.E., Baker, E.M., Hood, J., Sauberlich, H.E, (1969) Experimental scurvy in man. *Am. J. Clin. Nutr.* 22: 535.
6. Kallner, A., Hartmann, D., Hornig, D. 1979. Steady state turnover and body pool of ascorbic acid in man. *Am. J. Clin. Nutr.* 32: 530.
7. Kallner, A.B., Hartmann, D., Hornig, D.H. (1981) On the requirements of ascorbic acid in man: Steady state turnover and body pool in smokers. *Am. J. Clin. Nutr.* 34: 1347.
8. Barja, G., Lopez-Torres, M., Perez-Campo, R., Rojas, C., Cadenas, S., Prat, J., Pamplona, R. (1994) Dietary vitamin C decreases endogenous protein oxidative damage, malonaldehyde, and lipid peroxidation and maintains fatty acid unsaturation in guinea pig liver. *Free Rad. Biol. Med.* 17: 105–115.
9. Padh, H. (1991) Vitamin C: Newer insights into its biochemical functions. *Nutr. Rev.* 49: 65–70.
10. Carr, A., Frei, B. (1999) Does vitamin C act as a pro-oxidant under physiological conditions? *FASEB J.* 13: 1007–1024.
11. Creagen, E.T., Moertel, C.G., O'Fallon, J.R., Schutt, A.J., O'Connell, M.J., Rubin, J., Frytak, S. (1979) Failure of high dose vitamin C therapy to benefit patients with advanced cancer. *N. Eng. J. Med.* 301: 687.
12. Michels, A.J., Hagen, T.M., Frei, B. (2010) A new twist on an old vitamin: Human polymorphisms in the gene encoding the sodium-dependent vitamin C transporter 1. *Am. J. Clin. Nutr.* 92: 271–272.
13. Herbert, V., Jacob, E. (1974) Destruction of vitamin B_{12} by ascorbic acid. *J. Am. Med. Assoc.* 230: 241.
14. Bieri, J.G. (1973) Effects of excessive vitamins C and E on vitamin A status. *Am. J. Clin. Nutr.* 26: 382.
15. Mayfield, H.L., Roehm, R.R. (1956) The influence of ascorbic acid and the source of B vitamins on the utilization of carotene. *J. Nutr.* 58: 203.
16. Harris, A.B., Hartley, J., Moor, R. (1973) Reduced ascorbic acid excretion and oral contraceptives. *Lancet* 2: 201.
17. McLeroy, V.J., Schendel, H.E. (1973) Influence of oral contraceptives on ascorbic acid concentrations in healthy, sexually mature women. *Am. J. Clin. Nutr.* 26: 191.

18. Rivers, J., Devine, M.M. (1970) Plasma ascorbic acid concentrations and oral contraceptives. *Fed. Proc.* 29: 295.
19. Will, J.C., Byers, T. (1996) Does diabetes mellitus increase the requirement for vitamin C? *Nutr. Rev.* 54: 193–202.
20. Snell, E.E. (1979) Lactic acid bacteria and identification of B-vitamins: Some historical notes, 1937–1940. *Fed. Proc.* 38: 2690–2693.
21. McCormick, D.B. (1989) Two interconnected B vitamins. *Physiol. Rev.* 69: 1170–1198.
22. McCormick, D.B. (1991) Coenzymes, biochemistry. In: *Encyclopedia of Human Biology* (R. Dulbecco, ed.), vol. 2. Academic Press, San Diego, CA, pp. 1009–1028.
23. Sklan, D., Trostler, N. (1977) Site and extent of thiamin absorption in the rat. *J. Nutr.* 107: 353–356.
24. McCormick, D.B. (1991) Coenzymes, biochemistry. In: *Encyclopedia of Human Biology* (R. Dulbecco, ed.), vol. 2. Academic Press, San Diego, CA, pp. 1029–1038.
25. Massey, V. (1994) Activation of molecular oxygen by flavins and flavoproteins. *J. Biol. Chem.* 269: 22459–22462.
26. Brin, M. (1980) Red cell transketolase as an indicator of nutritional deficiency. *Am. J. Clin. Nutr.* 33: 169–171.
27. Zhang, G., Ding, H., Chen, H., Ye, X., Li, H., Lin, X., Ke, Z. (2013) Thiamin nutritional status and depressive symptoms are inversely associated among older Chinese adults. *J. Nutr.* 143: 53–58.
28. Lonsdale, D., Shamberger, R.J. (1980) Red cell transketolase as an indicator of nutritional deficiency. *Am. J. Clin. Nutr.* 33: 205–211.
29. Molina, P.E., Yousef, K.A., Smith, R.M., Tepper, P.G., Lang, C.H., Abumrad, N.N. (1994) Thiamin deficiency impairs endotoxin-induced increases in hepatic glucose output. *Am. J. Clin. Nutr.* 59: 1045–1049.
30. Joseph, T., McCormick, D.B. (1995) Uptake and metabolism of riboflavin 5 α D glucoside by rat and isolated liver cells. *J. Nutr.* 125: 2194–2198.
31. Casirola, D., Gastaldi, G., Ferrari, G., Kasai, S., Rindi, G. (1993) Riboflavin uptake by rat small intestinal brush border membrane vesicles: A dual mechanism involving specific membrane binding. *J. Membr. Biol.* 135: 217–223.
32. Hoppel, C., DiMarco, J.P., Tandler, B. (1979) Riboflavin and rat hepatic cell structure and function. *J. Biol. Chem.* 254: 4164–4170.
33. McCormick, D.B., Zhang, Z. (1993) Cellular assimilation of water soluble vitamins in the mammal: Riboflavin B_6, biotin and C. *Proc. Soc. Exp. Biol. Med.* 202: 265–270.
34. Yao, Y., Yonezawa, A., Yoshimatsu, H., Masuda, S., Katsura, T., Inui, K.-I., (2010) Identification and comparative functional characterization of a new human riboflavin transporter hRFT3 expressed in the brain. *J. Nutr.* 140: 1220–1226.
35. Fujimura, M., Yamamoto, S., Murata, T., Yasujima, T., Inoue, K., Ohta, K.-Y., Yuasa, H. (2010) Functional characteristics of the human ortholog of riboflavin transporter 2 and riboflavin-responsive expression of its rat ortholog in the small intestine indicate its involvement in riboflavin absorption. *J. Nutr.* 140: 1722–1727.
36. Aw, T.Y., Jones, D.P., McCormick, D.B. (1983) Uptake of riboflavin by isolated liver cells. *J. Nutr.* 113: 1249–1254.
37. Addison, R., McCormick, D.B. (1978) Biogenesis of flavoprotein and cytochrome components in hepatic mitochondria from riboflavin deficient rats. *Biochem. Biophys. Res. Commun.* 81: 133–138.
38. Ross, N.S., Hansen, T.P.B. (1992) Riboflavin deficiency is associated with selective preservation of critical flavoenzyme-dependent metabolic pathways. *Biofactors* 3: 185–190.
39. Zaman, Z., Verwilghen, R.L. (1975) Effects of riboflavin deficiency on oxidative phosphorylation, flavin enzymes and coenzymes in rat liver. *Biochem. Biophys. Res. Commun.* 67: 1192–1198.
40. Muller, E.M., Bates, C.J. (1977) Effect of riboflavin deficiency on white cell glutathione reductase in rats. *Internat. J. Vit. Nutr. Res.* 47: 46–51.
41. Sebrell, W.H. (1979) Identification of riboflavin deficiency in human subjects. *Fed. Proc.* 38: 2694–2695.
42. Van Eys, J. (1991) Nicotinic acid. In: *Handbook of Vitamins* (L.J. Machlin, ed.), Marcel Dekker, New York, pp. 311–340.
43. Powers, H.J., Hill, M., Mushtaq, S., Dainty, J.R., Majsak-Newman, G., Williams, E.A. (2011) Correcting a marginal riboflavin deficiency improves hematologic status in young women in the United Kingdom (RIBOFEM). *Am. J. Clin. Nutr.* 93: 1274–1279.
44. Rose, R.C. (1990) Water soluble vitamin absorption in intestine. *Ann. Rev. Physiol.* 42: 157–171.
45. Horwitt, M.K., Harper, A.E., Henderson, L.M. (1981) Niacin-tryptophan relationships for evaluating niacin equivalents. *Am. J. Clin. Nutr.* 34: 423–427.

46. Zhang, J.Z., Henning, S.M., Swenseid, M.E. (1993) Poly (ADP-ribose) polymerase activity and DNA strand breaks are affected in tissues of niacin-deficient rats. *J. Nutr.* 123: 1349–1355.
47. Kirkland, J.B. (2010) Poly ADP-ribose polymerase-1 and health. *Exp. Biol. Med.* 235: 561–568.
48. Melax, H., Singh, D.N.P., Cookson, F.B., Jeria, M.J. (1981) Degeneration of the myocardium in rats fed nicotinic acid diet. *IRCS Med. Sci.* 9: 293–294.
49. Kamana, V.S., Ganji, S.H., Kashyap, M.L. (2009) Niacin: An old drug rejuvenated. *Curr. Atheroscler. Rep.* 11: 45–51.
50. Kamanna, V.S., Kashyap, M.L. (2008) Mechanism of action of niacin. *Am. J. Cardiol.* 101: 20B–26B.
51. Kamanna, V.S., Kashyap, M.L. (2008) Nicotinic acid: Recent developments. *Curr. Opin. Cardiol.* 23: 393–398.
52. Aktories, K., Jakobs, K.H., Shultz, G. (1980) Nicotinic acid inhibits adipocyte adenylate cyclase in a hormone like manner. *FEBS Lett.* 115: 11–14.
53. Jacob, R.A., Sweinseid, M.E., McKee, R.W., Fu, C.S., Clemens, R.A. (1989) Biochemical markers for assessment of niacin status in young men: urinary and blood levels of niacin metabolites. *J. Nutr.* 119: 591–598.
54. Leklem, J.E. (1991) Vitamin B_6. In: *Handbook of Vitamins* (L. Machlin, ed.), Marcel Dekker, New York, pp. 341–392.
55. Lepkovsky, S. (1979) The isolation of pyridoxine. *Fed. Proc.* 38: 2699–2700.
56. Schaumburg, H., Kaplan, J., Windebank, A., Vick, N., Rasmus, S., Pleasure, D., Brown, M.J. (1983) Sensory neuropathy from pyridoxine abuse. *N. Eng. J. Med.* 309: 445–448.
57. Allgood, V.E., Powell-Oliver, F.E., Cidlowski, J.A. (1990) Vitamin B_6 influences glucocorticoid receptor-dependent gene expression. *J. Biol. Chem.* 265: 12424–12433.
58. Tully, D.B., Allgood, V.E., Cidlowski, J.A. (1993) Vitamin B_6 modulation of steroid-induced gene expression. In: *Nutrition and Gene Expression* (C.D. Berdanier, J.L. Hargrove, eds.), CRC Press, Boca Raton, FL, pp. 547–567.
59. Thanassi, J.W., Nutter, L.M., Meisler, N.T., Commers, P., Chiu, J.-F. (1980) Vitamin B_6 metabolism in Morris hepatomas. *J. Biol. Chem.* 256: 3370–3375.
60. Zhang, Z., Gregory, J.F., McCormick, D.B. (1993) Pyridoxine-5′-α-D glucoside competitively inhibits uptake of vitamin B_6 into isolated liver cells. *J. Nutr.* 123: 85–89.
61. Ribaya-Mercado, J.D., Russell, R.M., Sahyoun, N., Morrow, F.D., Gershoff, S.N. (1991) Vitamin B_6 requirements of elderly men and women. *J. Nutr.* 121: 1062–1074.
62. Rogers, K.S., Mohan, C. (1994) Vitamin B_6 metabolism and diabetes. *Biochem. Med. Metab. Biol.* 52: 10–17.
63. Fox, H.M. (1991) Pantothenic acid. In: *Handbook of Vitamins* (L.J. Machlin, ed.), Marcel Dekker, New York, pp. 429–451.
64. Midtturn, O., Ulvik, A., Pedersen, E.V., Ebbing, M., Blieie, O., Schartum-Hansen, H., Nilsen, R.M., Nygard, O., Ueland, P.M. (2011) Low plasma vitamin B-6 status affects metabolism through the kynurenine pathway in cardiovascular patients with systemic inflammation. *J. Nutr.* 141: 611–616.
65. Morris, M.S., Sakakeeny, L., Jacques, P.F., Picciano, M.F., Selhub, J. (2009) Vitamin B-6 intake is inversely related to and the requirement is affected by, inflammation status. *J. Nutr.* 140: 103–110.
66. Shen, J., Lai, C.-Q., Mattei, J., Ordovas, J.M., Tucker, K.I. (2010) Association of vitamin B-6 status with inflammation, oxidative stress, and chronic inflammatory conditions: The Boston Puerto Rican Health Study. *Am. J. Clin. Nutr.* 91: 337–342.
67. Lamers, Y., O'Rourke, B., Gilbert, L.R., Keeling, C., Matthews, D.E., Stacpoole, P.W., Gregory, J.F. (2009) Vitamin B-6 restriction tends to reduce the red blood cell glutathione synthesis rate without affecting red blood cell or plasma glutathione concentrations in healthy men and women. *Am. J. Clin. Nutr.* 90: 336–343.
68. Zhao, M., Lamers, Y., Ralat, M.A., Coats, B.S., Chi, Y.-Y., Muller, K.E., Bain, J.R., Shankar, M.N., Newgard, C.B., Stacpoole, P.W., Gregory, J. (2012) Marginal vitamin B-6 deficiency decreases plasma (n-3) and (N-6) PUFA concentrations in healthy men and women. *J. Nutr.* 142: 1791–1797.
69. Fenstermacher, D.K., Rose, R.C. (1986) Absorption of pantothenic acid in rat and chick intestine. *Am. J. Physiol.* 250: G155–G160.
70. Eissenstat, B.R., Wyse, B.W., Hansen, R.G. (1986) Pantothenic acid status of adolescents. *Am. J. Clin. Nutr.* 44: 931–937.
71. Sugarman, B., Munro, H.N. (1980) ^{14}C pantothenate accumulation by isolated adipocytes from adult rats of different ages. *J. Nutr.* 110: 2297–2301.
72. Mock, D.M., Mock, N.I., Dankle, J.A. (1992) Secretory patterns of biotin in human milk. *J. Nutr.* 122: 546–552.
73. Mock, D.M., Mock, N.I., Langbehn, S.E. (1992) Biotin in human milk: Methods, location, and chemical form. *J. Nutr.* 122: 535–545.

74. Cole, H., Reynolds, T.R., Lockyer, J.M., Bucks, G.A., Denson, T., Spence, J.E., Hymes, J., Wolf, B. (1994) Human serum biotinidase. cDNA cloning sequence and characterization. *J. Biol. Chem.* 269: 6566–6570.
75. Vesely, D.L., Kemp, S.F., Eldres, M.J. (1987) Isolation of a biotin receptor from hepatic plasma membranes. *Biochem. Biophys. Res. Commun.* 143: 913–916.
76. Weiner, D., Wolf, B. (1991) Biotin uptake, utilization and efflux in normal and biotin deficient rat hepatocytes. *Biochem. Med. Metab. Biol.* 46: 344–363.
77. Li, S.-J., Cronan, J.E. (1992) The gene encoding the biotin carboxylase subunit of *E. coli* acetyl CoA carboxylase. *J. Biol. Chem.* 267: 855–863.
78. Xia, W.-L, Zhang, J., Ahmad, F. (1994) Biotin holocarboxylase synthetase: Purification from rat liver cytosol and some properties. *Biochem. Mol. Biol. Internat.* 34: 225–232.
79. Watanabe, T. (1993) Dietary biotin deficiency affects reproductive function and prenatal development in hamsters. *J. Nutr.* 123: 2101–2108.
80. Mock, D.M., Johnson, S.B., Holman, R.T. (1988) Effects of biotin deficiency on serum fatty acid composition: Evidence for abnormalities in humans. *J. Nutr.* 118: 342–348.
81. Utter, M.F., Sheu, K.-F.R. (1980) Biochemical mechanisms of biotin and thiamin action and relationships to genetic diseases. *Birth Defects* 16: 289–304.
82. Stokstad, E.L.R. (1979) Early work with folic acid. *Fed. Proc.* 38: 2696–2698.
83. Shane, B. (1982) High performance liquid chromatography of folates: Identification of poly-γ-glutamate chain lengths of labeled and unlabeled folates. *Am. J. Clin. Nutr.* 35: 598–599.
84. Shoda, R., Mason, J.B., Selhub, J., Rosenberg, I.H. (1990) Folate binding in intestinal brush border membranes: Evidence for the presence of two binding activities. *J. Nutr. Biochem.* 1: 257–261.
85. Rose, R.C., Koch, M.J., Nahrwold, D.L. (1978) Folic acid transport by mammalian small intestine. *Am. J. Physiol.* 235: E678–E685.
86. Halsted, C.H. (1979) Intestinal absorption of folates. *Am. J. Clin. Nutr.* 32: 846–855.
87. Antony, A. (1996) Folate receptors. In: *Annual Review of Nutrition* (D. McCormick, D. Bier, A. Goodridge, eds.), Annual Reviews, Palo Alto, CA, pp. 501–521.
88. Branda, R.F., Nelson, N.L. (1981) Inhibition of 5-methyltetrahydrofolic acid transport by amphipathic drugs. *Drug Nutr. Internat.* 1: 45–53.
89. Sadasivan, E., Rothenberg, S.P. (1988) Molecular cloning of the complimentary DNA for a human folate binding protein. *Proc. Soc. Exp. Biol. Med.* 189: 240–244.
90. Appling, D.R. (1991) Compartmentation of folate mediated one carbon metabolism in eukaryotes. *FASEB J.* 5: 2645–2651.
91. Balaghi, M., Horne, D.W., Wagner, C. 1993. Hepatic one carbon metabolism in early folate deficiency in rats. *Biochem. J.* 291: 145–149.
92. Schweitzer, B.I., Dicker, A.P., Bertino, J.R. (1990) Dihydrofolate reductase as a therapeutic target. *FASEB J.* 4: 2441–2452.
93. Chu, E., Takimoto, C.H., Voeller, D., Grem, J.L., Allegra, C.J. (1993) Specific binding of human dihydrofolate reductase protein to dihydrofolate reductase messenger RNA in vitro. *Biochemistry* 32: 4756–4760.
94. Iwakura, M., Tanaka, T. (1992) Dihydrofolate reductase gene as a versatile expression marker. *J. Biochem.* 111: 31–36.
95. Kim, Y.-L., Pogribny, I.P., Basnakian, A.G., Miller, J.W., Selhub, J., James, J., Mason, J.B. (1997) folate deficiency in rats induces DNA strand breaks and hypomethylation within the p53 tumor-suppressor gene. *Am. J. Clin. Nutr.* 65: 46–52.
96. Pitkin, R.M. (2007) Folate and neural tube defects. *Am. J. Clin. Nutr.* 85: 285S–288S.
97. Mason, J.B. (1994) Folate and colonic carcinogenesis: Searching for a mechanistic understanding. *J. Nutr. Biochem.* 5: 170–175.
98. Sirotnak, F.M., Burchall, J.J., Ensminger, W.B., Montgomery, J.A. (1988) *Folate Antagonists as Therapeutic Agents.* Academic Press, Orlando, FL, 460pp.
99. Green, J.M., Ballou, D.P., Matthews, R.G. (1988) Examination of the role of methylenetetrahydrofolate reductase in incorporation of methyltetrahydrofolate into cellular metabolism. *FASEB J.* 2: 42–47.
100. Purohit, P., Abdelmalek, M.F., Barve, S., Benevenga, N.J., Halsted, C.H., Kaplowitz, N., Kharbanda, K.K. et al. (2007) Role of S-adenosylmethionine, folate and betaine in the treatment of alcoholic liver disease: Summary of a symposium. *Am. J. Clin. Nutr.* 86: 14–24.
101. Chou, Y.-F., Yu, C.-C., Huang, R.-F.S. (2007) Changes in mitochondrial DNA deletion, content, and biogenesis in folate-deficient tissues of young rats depend on mitochondrial folate and oxidative DNA injuries. *J. Nutr.* 137: 2036–2042.

102. Kiefte-de Jong, J., Timmerman, S., Jaddoe, V.W.V., Hofman, A., Tiemeir, H., Steegers, E.A., de Jongste, J.C., Moll, H.A. (2012) High circulating folate and vitamin B12 concentrations in women during pregnancy are associated with increased prevalence of atopic dermatitis in their offspring. *J. Nutr.* 142: 731–738.
103. Wernimont, S.M., Raiszadeh, F., Stover, P.J., Rimm, E.B., Hunter, D.J., Tang, W., Cassano, P.A. (2011) Polymorphisms in serine hydroxymethyltransferase 1 and methylenetetrahydrofolate reductase interact to increase cardiovascular disease risk in humans. *J. Nutr.* 141: 255–262.
104. Choi, F.S. (2005) Gene nutrient interactions in one carbon metabolism. *Curr. Drug Metab.* 6: 37–46.
105. Caudill, M.A., Dellschaft, N., Solis, C., Hinkis, S., Ivanov, A.A., Naash-Barboza, S., Randall, K.E., Jackson, B., Solomitz, G.N., Vermeyleu, F. (2009) Choline intake, plasma riboflavin, and the phosphatidylethanolamine *N*-methyltransferase G5465A genotype predict plasma homocysteine in folate-deplete Mexican-American men with the methylenetetrahydrofolate reductase 677TT genotype. *J. Nutr.* 139: 727–733.
106. Wilson, C.P., Ward, M., McNulty, H., Strain, J.J., Trouton, T.G., Horigan, G., Purvis, J., Scott, J.M. (2012) Riboflavin offers a targeted strategy for managing hypertension in patients with the MTHFR677TT genotype: A 4 year followup. *Am. J. Clin. Nutr.* 95: 766–772.
107. Kim, J., Cho, Y.A., Kim, H.-J., Matsuo, K., Tajima, K., Ahn, Y.-O. (2012) Dietary intake of folate and alcohol, MTHFR C677T polymorphism and colorectal cancer risk in Korea. *Am. J. Clin. Nutr.* 95: 405–412.
108. Yang, Q, Bailey, L., Clarke, R., Flanders, W.D., Liu, T., Yesupriya, A., Khoury, M.J., Friedman, J.M. (2012) Prospective study of methylenetetrahydrofolate reductase (MTHFR) variant C677T and the risk of all-cause and cardiovascular disease mortality among 6000 US adults. *Am. J. Clin. Nutr.* 95: 1245–1253.
109. van Meurs, J.B.J. and 57 co authors. (2013) Common genetic loci influencing plasma homocysteine concentrations and their effect on risk of coronary artery disease. *Am. J. Clin. Nutr.* 98: 668–676.
110. Lai, C.-Q., Parnell, L.D., Troen, A.M., Shen, A.M., Shen, J., Caouette, H., Warodomwichit, D., Lee, Y.-C., Crott, J.W., Qiu, W.Q., Rosenberg, I.W., Tucker, K.L., Ordovas, J.M. (2010) MAT1A variants are associated with hypertension, stroke, and markers of DNA damage and are modulated by plasma vitamin B-6 and folate. *Am. J. Clin. Nutr.* 91: 1377–1386.
111. Strand, T.A., Taneja, S., Ueland, P.M., Refsum, H., Bahl, R., Schneede, J., Sommerfelt, H., Bhamndari, N. (2013) Cobalamin and folate status predicts mental development scores in North Indian children 12–18 mo of age. *Am. J. Clin. Nutr.* 97: 310–317.
112. Nguyen, C.T., Gracely, E.J., Lee, B.K. (2013) Serum folate but not vitamin B-12 concentrations are positively associated with cognitive test scores in children aged 6–16 years. *J. Nutr.* 143: 500–504.
113. Walker, J.G., Battercham, P.J., Mackinnon, A.J., Jorm, A.F., Hickle, I., Fenech, M., Kijakovic, M., Crisp, D., Christensen, H. (2011) Oral folic acid and vitamin B-12 supplementation to prevent cognitive decline in community-dwelling older adults with depressive symptoms: The beyond ageing project: A randomized controlled trial. *Am. J. Clin. Nutr.* 95: 194–203.
114. Ng, T.-P., Aung, K.C.Y., Feng, L., Scherer, S., Yap, K.B. (2012) Homocysteine, folate, vitamin B-12 and physical function in older adults: Cross sectional findings from Singapore Longitudinal Ageing Study. *Am. J. Clin. Nutr.* 96: 1362–1368.
115. Allen, R.H., Stabler, S.P., Savage, D.G., Lindenbaum, J. (1993) Metabolic abnormalities in cobalamin (vitamin B_{12}) and folate deficiency. *FASEB J.* 7: 1344–1353.
116. Smith, A.D. (2007) Folic acid fortification: The good, the bad, and the puzzle of vitamin B-12. *Am. J. Clin. Nutr.* 85: 3–5.
117. Ashokkumar, B., Mohammed, Z.M., Vaziri, N.D., Said, H.M. (2007) Effect of folate over supplementation on folate uptake by human intestinal and renal epithelial cells. *Am. J. Clin. Nutr.* 86: 159–166.
118. Ellenbogen, L. (1991) Vitamin B_{12}. In: *Handbook of Vitamins* (L.J. Machlin, ed.), Marcel Dekker, New York, pp. 491–536.
119. Sennett, C., Rosenberg, L.E. (1981) Transmembrane transport of cobalamin in prokaryotic and eukaryotic cells. *Ann. Rev. Biochem.* 50: 1053–1086.
120. Marcoullis, G., Rothenberg, S.P., Labombardi, V.J. (1980) Preparation and characterization of proteins in the alimentary tract of the dog which bind cobalamin and intrinsic factor. *J. Biol. Chem.* 255: 1824–1829.
121. Merzbach, D., Grossowicz, N. (1987) Absorption of vitamin B_{12} from the large intestine of rats. *J. Nutr.* 87: 41–51.
122. O'Sullivan, D. (1991) New studies pinpoint pathway of B_{12} biosynthesis. *C & E News* Feb. 4: 30–31.
123. Peifer, J.J., Lewis, R.D. (1981) Odd numbered fatty acids in phosphatidyl choline versus phosphatidyl ethanolamine of vitamin B_{12}-deprived rats. *Proc. Soc. Exp. Biol. Med.* 167: 212–217.
124. Watanabe, F., Saido, H., Toyoshima, S., Tamura, Y., Nekano, Y. (1994) Feeding vitamin B_{12} rapidly increases the specific activity of hepatic methylmalonyl CoA mutase in vitamin B_{12} deficient rats. *Biosci. Biotech. Biochem.* 58: 556–557.

125. Banerjee, R.V., Matthews, R.G. (1990) Cobalamin-dependent methionine synthase. *FASEB J.* 4: 1450–1459.
126. Scalabrino, G., Nicolini, G., Buccellato, F.R., Peracchi, M., Tredici, G., Manfridi, A., Pravettoni, G. (1999) Epidermal growth factor as a local mediator of the neurotropic action of vitamin B_{12} (cobalamin) in the rat central nervous system. *FASEB J.* 13: 2083–2090.
127. Brass, E.P., Ruff, L.J. (1989) Effect of carnitine on proprionate metabolism in the vitamin B_{12} deficient rat. *J. Nutr.* 119: 1196–1201.
128. Cullen, R.W., Oace, S.M. (1989) Fermentable dietary fibers elevate urinary methylmalonate and decrease propionate oxidation in rats deprived of vitamin B_{12}. *J. Nutr.* 119: 1115–1120.
129. Carmel, R. (2011) Biomarkers of cobalamin (vitamin B-12) status in the epidemiologic setting: A critical overview on context, applications, and performance characteristics of cobalamin, methylmalonic acid, and holotranscobalamin. *Am. J. Clin. Nutr.* 94: 348S–358S.
130. Nexo, E., Hoffmann-Lucke, E. (2011) Holotranscobalamin, a marker of vitamin B-12 status: Analytical aspects and clinical utility. *Am. J. Clin. Nutr.* 94: 359S–365S.
131. Yetley, E.A., Coats, P.M., Johnson, C.L. (2011) Overview of a roundtable on NHANES monitoring of biomarkers of folate and vitamin B-12 status: Measurement procedure issues. *Am. J. Clin. Nutr.* 94: 297S–302S.
132. Yetley, E.A. and 32 co authors. (2011) Biomarkers of vitamin B-12 status in NHANES: A roundtable summary. *Am. J. Clin. Nutr.* 94: 313S–321S.
133. Bock, J.L., Eckfeldt, J.H. (2011) Advances in standardization of laboratory measurement procedures: Implications for measuring biomarkers of folate and vitamin B-12 status in NHANES. *Am. J. Clin. Nutr.* 94: 332S–336S.
134. Bailey, R.L., Carmel, R., Green, R., Pfeiffer, C.M., Cogswell, M.E., Osterloh, J.D., Sempos, C.T., Yetley, E.A. (2011) Monitoring of vitamin B-12 nutritional status in the United States by using plasma methylmalonic acid and serum vitamin B-12. *Am. J. Clin. Nutr.* 94: 552–560.
135. Miller, J.W., Garrod, M.G., Allen, L.H., Haan, M.N., Green, R. (2009) Metabolic evidence of vitamin B-12 deficiency, including high homocysteine and methylmalonic acid and low holotranscobalamin in more pronounced in older adults with elevated plasma folate. *Am. J. Clin. Nutr.* 90: 1586–1592.
136. Peifer, J.J., Cleland, G. (1987) Metabolic demands for coenzyme B_{12}-dependent mutase increased by thiamin deficiency. *Nutr. Res.* 7: 1197–1201.
137. Borum, P. (1991) Carnitine. In: *Handbook of Vitamins* (L.J. Machlin, ed.), Marcel Dekker Inc., New York, pp. 557–563.
138. Xi, L, Brown, K., Woodworth, J., Shim, K., Johnson, B., Odle, J. (2008) Maternal dietary L-carnitine supplementation influences fetal carnitine status and stimulates carnitine palmitoyltransferase and pyruvate dehydrogenase complex activities in swine. *J. Nutr.* 138: 2356–2362.
139. Noland, R.C., Koves, T.R., Seiler, S.E., Lum, H., Lust, R.M., Ilkaeva, O., Hegardt, F.G., Muoio, D.M. (2009) Carnitine insufficiency caused by aging and over nutrition compromises mitochondrial functioning. *J. Biol. Chem.* 284: 22840–22852.
140. Murphy, M.M., Molloy, A.M., Ueland, P.M., Fernandez-Ballart, J.D., Schneede, J., Arija, V., Scott, J.M. (2007) Longitudinal study of the effect of pregnancy on maternal and fetal cobalamin status in healthy women and their offspring. *J. Nutr.* 137: 1863–1867.
141. Rebouche, C.J. (1992) Carnitine function and requirements during the life cycle. *FASEB J.* 6: 3379–3386.
142. Chan, M.M. (1991) Choline. In: *Handbook of Vitamins*. (L.J. Machlin, ed.), Marcel Dekker Inc., New York. pp. 537–556.
143. Zeisel, S.H. (1990) Choline deficiency. *J. Nutr. Biochem.* 1: 332–349.
144. Cermak, J.M., Holler, T., Jackson, D.A., Blusztajn, J.K. (1998) Prenatal availability of choline modifies development of the hippocampal cholinergic system. *FASEB J.* 12: 349–357.
145. Holler, T., Cermak, J.M., Blusztajan, J.K. (1996) Dietary choline supplementation in pregnant rats increases hippocampal phospholipase D activity of the offspring. *FASEB J.* 10: 1653–1659.
146. Albright, C.D., Liu, R., Bethea, T.C., DaCosta, K., Salganik, R.I., Zeisel, S.H. (1996) Choline deficiency induces apoptosis in SV40-immortalized CWSV-1 rat hepatocytes in culture. *FASEB J.* 10: 510–516.
147. Guerrerio, A.L., Colvin, R.M., Schwartz, A.K., Molleston, J.P., Murray, K.F., Diehl, A.M., Mohan, P. et al. (2012) Choline intake in a large cohort of patients with nonalcoholic fatty liver disease. *Am. J. Clin. Nutr.* 95: 892–900.
148. Pacelli, C., Coluccia, A., Grattagliano, I., Cocco, T., Petrosillo, G., Paradies, G., Der Nitto, A., Persichella, M., Borracci, P., Portincasa, P., Carratu, M.R. (2010) Dietary choline deprivation impairs rat brain mitochondrial function and behavioral phenotype. *J. Nutr.* 140: 1072–1079.
149. Craciunescu, C.N., Johnson, A.R., Zeisel, S.H. (2010) Dietary choline reverses some, but not all, effects of folate deficiency on neurogenesis and apoptosis in fetal mouse brain. *J. Nutr.* 140: 1162–1166.

150. Zeisel, S.H. (2011) Nutritional genomics: Defining the dietary requirement and effect of choline. *J. Nutr.* 141: 531–540.
151. Fischer, L.M., da Costa, K.-A., Kwock, L., Galanko, J., Zeisel, S.H. (2010) Dietary choline requirements of women: Effects of estrogen and genetic variation. *Am. J. Clin. Nutr.* 92: 1113–1119.
152. Mehlman, M.A., Therriault, D.G., Tobin, R.B. (1971) Carnitine-^{14}C metabolism in choline-deficient, alloxan diabetic choline deficient and insulin treated rats. *Metabolism* 20: 100–107.
153. Holub, B.J. (1986) Metabolism and function of myoinositol and inositol phospholipids. *Ann. Rev. Nutr.* 6: 563–597.
154. Best, L., Malaise, W.J. (1983) Phospholipids and islet function. *Diabetologia* 25: 299–305.
155. Farese, R.V. (1990) Lipid derived mediators in insulin action. *Proc. Soc. Exp. Biol. Med.* 312: 324.
156. Martin, T.F.J. (1991) Receptor regulation of phosphoinositidase C. *Pharmac. Ther.* 49: 329–345.
157. Saltiel, A.R. (1990) Signal transduction in insulin action. *J. Nutr. Biochem.* 1: 180–188.
158. Han, O., Failla, M., Hill, A.D., Morris, E.R., Smith, J.C. (1994) Inositol phosphates inhibit uptake and transport of iron and zinc by a human intestinal cell line. *J. Nutr.* 124: 580–587.
159. Flier, J.S., Underhill, L.H. (1990) Sorbitol, phosphoinositides, and sodium-potassium-ATPase in the pathogenesis of diabetic complications. *N. Eng. J. Med.* 316: 599–606.
160. Olgemoller, B., Schwaabe, S., Schleicher, E.D., Gerbitz, K.D. (1993) Upregulation of myoinositol transport compensates for competitive inhibition by glucose. *Diabetes* 42: 1119–1125.

13 Macrominerals

The term *macrominerals* refers to those elements needed by the body in milligram quantities on a daily basis. The category includes sodium, potassium, chloride, calcium, phosphorus, and magnesium. While the body content of the first three is relatively small because of high turnover, the body content of calcium and phosphorous, by comparison, is relatively large. All of the macrominerals serve as electrolytes, and their critical use relates to this function. While most minerals are found in the bones and teeth and thus have a structural function, they also serve as metabolic regulators.

SODIUM

Sodium is the major extracellular electrolyte. It circulates as a fully dissociated ion due to its +1 charge and is fully water soluble. It has been estimated that the adult body contains 52–60 mEq/kg (male) and 48–55 mEq/kg (female). One mEq/L equals one mmol/L. Thus, the average adult male would have about 83–97 g of sodium in his 70 kg body. Between 2/3 and 3/4 of this sodium is *fixed* in the mineral apatite of the bone. The remaining is part of a pool that undergoes considerable turnover as it participates in sodium–potassium exchange. The exchangeable sodium in the adult human body can be predicted using the following equation:

$$\text{Na}_e(\text{mEq}) = 163.2(\text{total body water}) - 69\text{-Ke}(\text{mEq})$$

where Ke is the exchangeable potassium.

Exchangeable potassium can be predicted as follows:

$$\text{Ke}(\text{mEq}) = 150(\text{intracellular body water}_L) + 4(\text{total body water} - \text{intracellular body water})$$

The body water (total and intracellular) can be determined using tracer techniques. Sodium is primarily an extracellular ion and as such the serum will contain 136–145 mEq/L. Normal sodium intake varies from less than 2 to 10 g/day. Most of this sodium comes from table salt, NaCl. Foods rich in added salt are usually snack foods such as potato chips, salted nuts, pretzels, and so forth (see www.nal.usda.gov/foodcomposition for food sodium content). Processed foods have more added salt than nonprocessed foods because salt not only improves the taste of the finished product but also serves as a preservative. Luncheon meats, cheese spreads, pickles, relishes, catsup, canned and frozen vegetables, crackers, breads, and frozen desserts are but a few of the foods that contain more sodium than their raw or nonprocessed components. Every living thing contains sodium and, except for pure fats and carbohydrates, no major food source lacks this element. Some people are especially sensitive to salt intake, and these people are at risk for developing hypertension when they consume excess amounts of sodium. There is a suggested acceptable intake (AI) figure for sodium (Table 13.1). These estimates presume that the individual has a moderately active lifestyle and lives in a temperate environment. Heavy work in a hot, dry environment and a variety of medical conditions will affect the need for sodium as well as for other electrolytes that are lost through the skin. While sodium intake can be highly variable, serum sodium is not. As described earlier, the normal range of serum sodium is quite small. Values in excess of 150 mEq/L (hypernatremia) are considered abnormal. Values below 135 mEq/L (hyponatremia) are also considered abnormal and are of clinical concern.

TABLE 13.1
Daily Dietary Reference Intakes and Acceptable Intakes of Various Age/Gender Groups

Group	Sodium (g)	Potassium (g)	Chloride (g)	Calcium (mg)	Hosphorus (mg)	Magnesium (mg)
Infants						
0–6 months	0.12*	0.4*	0.18*	210*	100*	30*
7–12 months	0.37*	0.7*	0.57*	270*	275*	75*
Children						
1–3 years	1.0*	3.0*	1.5*	500*	**469**	**80**
4–8 years	1.2*	3.8*	1.9*	800*	**500**	**130**
Males						
9–13 years	1.5*	4.5*	2.3*	1300*	**1250**	**240**
14–18 years	1.5*	4.7*	2.3*	1300*	**1250**	**410**
19–30 years	1.5*	4.7*	2.3*	1000*	**700**	**400**
31–50 years	1.5*	4.7*	2.3*	1000*	**700**	**420**
51–70 years	1.3*	4.7*	2.0*	1200*	**700**	**420**
70+	1.2*	4.7*	1.8*	1200*	**700**	**420**
Females						
9–13 years	1.5*	4.5*	2.3*	1300*	**1250**	**240**
14–18 years	1.5*	4.7*	2.3*	1300*	**1250**	**360**
19–30 years	1.5*	4.7*	2.3*	1000*	**700**	**310**
31–50 years	1.5*	4.7*	2.3*	1000*	**700**	**320**
51–70 years	1.5*	4.7*	2.0*	1200*	**700**	**320**
70+ years	1.5*	4.7*	1.8*	1200*	**700**	**320**
Pregnancy						
14–18 years	1.5*	4.7*	2.3*	1300*	**1250**	**400**
19–30 years	1.5*	4.7*	2.3*	1000*	**700**	**350**
31–50 years	1.5*	4.7*	2.3*	1000*	**700**	**360**
Lactation						
14–18 years	1.5*	5.1*	2.3*	1300*	**1250**	**360**
19–30 years	1.5*	5.1*	2.3*	1000*	**700**	**310**
31–50 years	1.5*	5.1*	2.3*	1000*	**700**	**320**

Source: www.nap.edu

Notes: Daily dietary reference intakes are indicated in bold and acceptable intakes (AI) are indicated with *.

There are several reasons why hypernatremia or hyponatremia can develop. These are summarized in Table 13.2. In normal individuals, the level of sodium in the serum is tightly controlled and this control is intertwined with the control of potassium concentration, chloride concentration, and water balance.

Regulation of Serum Sodium

The system that regulates sodium levels in the blood also is involved in the regulation of water balance, pH, and osmotic pressure. Both hormones and physical/chemical factors are involved. Table 13.3 lists the hormones and their role in sodium balance as well as in water balance. The hormones listed are all involved indirectly or directly because of the need to regulate the osmotic pressure within and around the cells. Osmolality, that is, the concentration of solutes on each side of a semipermeable membrane, is maintained by the passage of water through that membrane. This osmolality is maintained at roughly 270–290 mOsm. The proteins, many of which cannot

TABLE 13.2
Causes of Hypernatremia and Hyponatremia

Hypernatremia (Serum Na > 150 mEq/L)	Hyponatremia (Serum Na <135 mEq/L)
Dehydration—excess sweating, deficient water intake	Cachexia (any wasting disease, i.e., cancer)
Excess solute loading	Anorexia nervosa
Diabetes insipidus (too little ADH)	Ulcerative colitis
Brain stem injury	Liver disease
	Congestive heart failure
	Ascites, edema
	Major trauma
	Severe infection
	Excess water intake
	Inappropriate ADH release
	Diarrhea
	Certain drugs (chlorothiazide, mercurial diuretics, etc.)
	Adrenalectomy

TABLE 13.3
Hormones Involved in the Regulation of Serum Sodium

Hormone	Function
Vasopressin (ADH)	Serves to stimulate the reabsorption of water by the renal glomerulus and renal convoluted tubule.
Atrial natriuretic hormone	Counteracts vasopressin and thus induces water loss, sodium and potassium loss. It also decreases blood pressure and increases glomerular filtration rate. Suppresses renin release and aldosterone release. Antagonizes angiotensin II and norepinephrine.
Renin	Catalyzes the conversion of inactive angiotensin I to active angiotensin II.
Angiotensin II	At low serum sodium levels, it conserves sodium by stimulating its reabsorption. At high serum sodium levels, it has the reverse effect. Stimulates vasoconstriction which increases blood pressure. Reduces water loss and decreases glomerular filtration rate. Stimulates aldosterone release.
Aldosterone	Conserves sodium by increasing sodium resorption by the kidney.

pass through the plasma membrane, are part of this solute load. In the well-nourished, healthy individual, the intracellular and extracellular proteins are maintained at fairly constant levels. This leaves the small fully ionized solutes (Na^+, K^+, Cl^-) as major determinants of the osmotic pressure of the system. Osmotic pressure is the physical force required to keep the osmolality on both sides of the membrane approximately equal. If the solute load on one side exceeds that of the other, water and the small solutes (Na^+, K^+, Cl^-) will pass through the membrane to equalize the concentration of solutes.

Since the number of particles determines osmotic pressure, substances that ionize affect osmotic pressure according to the degree of dissociation. Thus, the fully dissociated NaCl produces the ions, Na^+ and Cl^- in such a fashion that at 0.154 M there are 1.85 particles of each ion that in turn exert a pressure of 286 mOsm.

There are several ways to measure osmolality in the laboratory using rather simple instruments called osmometers. For example, the osmolality of a solution can be determined using the effect of a solute on freezing point. The addition of 1 Osm to 1 L of water will depress the freezing point by 1.86°C.

Several of the hormones listed in Table 13.3 are released in response to changes in sodium concentration or to signals generated by osmoreceptors located in the anterolateral hypothalamus. The sodium ion, of all of the circulating ions, is the most potent of the solutes that activate the osmoreceptors. These in turn signal the release of hormones that regulate osmolality. Vasopressin (also called antidiuretic hormone [ADH]) is one of these; aldosterone is another. When the osmoreceptors sense a change (increase) in the solute load, ADH release is stimulated. This results in an increase in renal water resorption and thus dilution of the solute load.

The disorder *diabetes insipidus* develops in the relative absence of ADH. The disease is characterized by extreme urinary water loss (up to 30 L/day) and extreme thirst. In this disorder, the posterior pituitary may be diseased or may have a tumor that interferes with the production of ADH. In this disease, the resorption of water by the renal tubules is not stimulated and the patient excretes a large volume of very dilute urine. Patients with diabetes insipidus can be successfully treated. Interestingly, their treatment consists of providing the hormone in an aerosol that allows the patient to inhale the hormone through the nose. An even rarer disease of water balance is a form of diabetes insipidus that does not involve the production and release of ADH by the posterior pituitary but is primarily of renal origin. In this disorder, the kidney is unresponsive to the hormone. The reasons for this unresponsiveness are not known nor has a suitable treatment been devised.

Aldosterone release is stimulated by low serum sodium–high potassium levels in the blood. Aldosterone, released by the adrenal cortex, functions in sodium conservation by increasing the renal reabsorption of this ion. Of interest is the action of these ions at the level of the expression of the aldosterone synthetase gene. At low sodium–high potassium levels, the transcription of the aldosterone synthetase gene is stimulated. More messenger RNA is produced and more enzyme is synthesized.[1]

The pathway for the synthesis of aldosterone, as part of the steroid hormone synthetic network, is shown in Figure 13.1. Aldosterone synthesis from corticosterone via the enzyme 11β hydroxylase (an enzyme that catalyzes 11-deoxycorticosterone conversion to corticosterone) is enhanced by angiotensin II. Angiotensin II release is stimulated by low sodium levels. Figure 13.2 illustrates the roles of sodium and potassium in sodium conservation. Angiotensin II action requires the calcium ion and high potassium levels to facilitate calcium ion movement from outside the cell to the inside of the cell. As aldosterone levels increase, the calcium ion

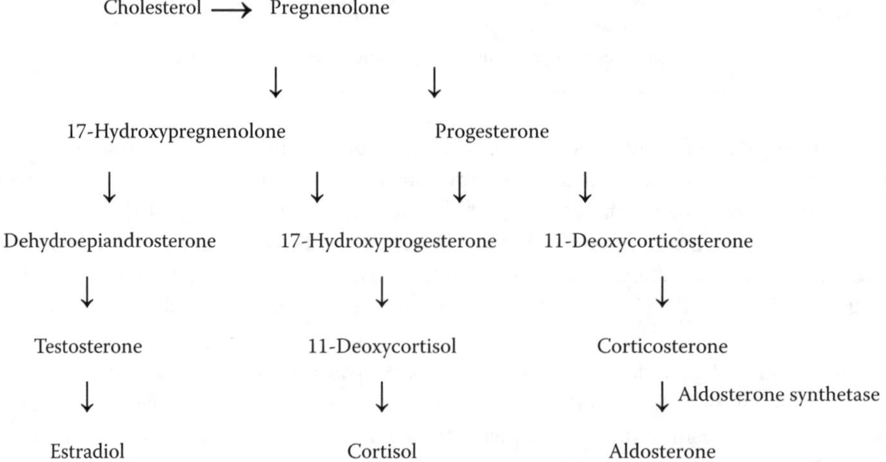

FIGURE 13.1 The steroid hormone synthetic pathway showing the synthesis of aldosterone as well as the other steroid hormones.

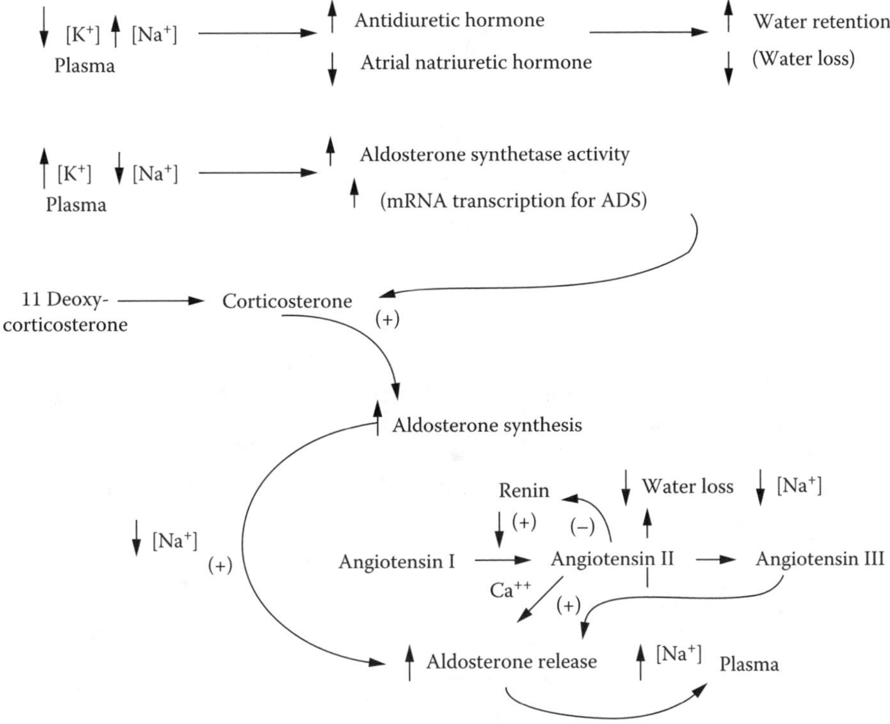

FIGURE 13.2 Schematic representation of how low-potassium, high sodium levels affect sodium conservation. Two systems are used: one involves the posterior pituitary, which releases antidiuretic hormone (ADH, also called vasopressin). ADH stimulates water and sodium retention. The other system involves the adrenal cortex, which is stimulated to release aldosterone, the mineral corticoid hormone responsible for sodium conservation.

facilitates its release by the cortex cell. Aldosterone then moves to the kidney where it stimulates electrolyte conservation. Thus, the circle is completed. Sodium is regulated by several hormones and in turn regulates the synthesis of these hormones through effects on gene transcription.[1] Sodium also stimulates the transcription of the genes for cholesterol SCC, a P450 enzyme, the gene for adrenodoxin, and, in hypertensive animals, has been found to stimulate the transcription of the gene for endothelin 1.[2] Endothelin 1 is an important vasoactive peptide that acts as a diuretic and as a natriuretic. It stimulates vasoconstriction and in genetic hypertension it seems to reduce sodium loss. Sodium conservation is a part of the regulation of water balance. This regulation is shown in Figure 13.3.

A major health consideration with respect to sodium is the role of this electrolyte in the development of hypertension (elevated blood pressure). Hypertension is defined as an elevation in the systolic/diastolic pressures and is due to an increase in the peripheral resistance of the vascular system. Hypotension is the reverse of hypertension; it is a depressed systolic/diastolic pressure. Normotension is <120/80 mm mercury. When the resistance against which the heart must pump is elevated for long periods, the heart muscle hypertrophies (enlarges). When this is coupled with the development of coronary vessel disease (constriction of the coronary vessels due to the development of atheromas and loss of vascular elasticity), the risk of developing a myocardial infarction or having a stroke increases. Thus, there is a close association between hypertension and vascular disease. There is also an association of cardiovascular disease and renal disease that is related to the regulation of blood pressure (see Chapter 8).

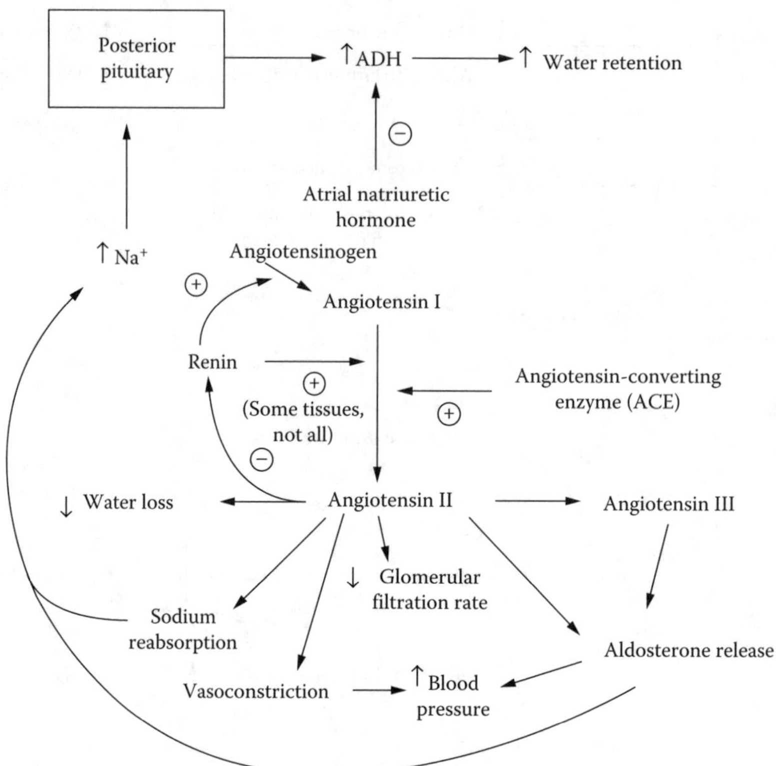

FIGURE 13.3 Water balance is controlled by a cascade of hormones. These hormones also have a role in the control of blood pressure. One of the drugs used for the control of blood pressure inhibits ACE. Another drug inhibits the activity of the ACE receptor. ACE inhibition lowers blood pressure. Diuretics also stimulate renal water loss and this lowers blood pressure.

Blood pressure increases with age and more than 50% of aging adults are hypertensive. As the ventricles pump out the blood from the heart, there is an expansion of the vascular tree shown by a rise in blood pressure. This is the systolic blood pressure. As the heart relaxes after pumping, the blood pressure falls. This is the diastolic pressure. Both systolic and diastolic pressures can rise with age. However, the rise in diastolic pressure is much less than that of systolic pressure. Diastolic pressure can fall as aging continues. The changes in pressure relate to changes in elasticity of the vascular tree. If the vascular system is stiff due to an accumulation of plaques and calcium deposits, it is not as flexible and responsive to the pumping action of the heart. This is shown by the increase in systolic pressure.

Population studies have shown that as sodium intake increases so too does blood pressure. In general, high sodium intakes are associated with an increased risk for developing hypertension as people age. Restricting sodium intake can have beneficial effects on blood pressure in some individuals. Salt restriction interacts with components of the rennin–angiotensin system.[3] The gene for the β_2-adrenergic receptor is one of the susceptibility loci for hypertension and polymorphisms at this site are related to salt sensitivity and low plasma renin activity.

One of the ways to reduce salt intake is through the use of the DASH (dietary approach to stop hypertension) diet. Its success depends on the polymorphism of the subject for the gene for the β_2 adrenergic receptor. Subjects with the β_2-AR G46A were more responsive to the DASH diet with respect to lowering blood pressure and aldosterone levels than subjects with the β_2-AR C46A polymorphism. Choosing a reduced sodium diet by people with this polymorphism could have some potential benefit with respect to a delay in the development of hypertension.[4]

Function

Indirectly, the function of the sodium ion as a participant in the regulation of osmotic pressure has already been discussed as the regulation of serum sodium levels was discussed. In addition to its function in this system, it also functions in nerve conduction, active transport both by the enterocyte and by other cell types, and plays a role in the formation of the mineral apatite of the bone. The common thread to its role in nerve conduction, active transport, and water balance is its function in the sodium–potassium ATPase. This enzyme, embedded in the plasma membrane of most cells, is perhaps the most thoroughly studied enzyme of the active transport systems. The ATPase transmembrane protein was first isolated in 1957 and consists of two subunits: a 110 kDa nonglycosylated α subunit that contains the enzyme's catalytic activity and ion-binding site and a 55 kDa glycoprotein β subunit. The enzyme has two of each of these subunits. Figure 13.4 illustrates the structure of this enzyme. The glycoprotein probably plays a role in recognition of appropriate substrates, but this probable role is speculative. The ATPase is frequently called the Na^+K^+ pump because it pumps sodium out as potassium returns to the cell, when this exchange takes place, there is a concomitant hydrolysis of ATP. The equation that describes this process is as follows:

$$3Na^+(in) + 2K^+(out) + ATP \leftrightarrow 3Na^+(out) + 2K^+(in) + ATP + Pi$$

The pump is an electrogenic system, illustrated in Figure 13.5, with the extrusion of three positively charged particles (the Na^+) in return for two negatively charged ones (the K^+). As an electrogenic system, the Na^+K^+ ATPase generates an electrochemical potential gradient that is responsible for nerve action. Signal transmission along a nerve path occurs via a depolarization/repolarization scheme whereby potassium leaves the neuron and sodium enters (depolarization) and through ATPase activity the reverse occurs (repolarization). Much of the ATP that cells produce by the mitochondria is used by this ATPase. In fact, in nerve cells, up to 70% of their ATP production is consumed by the sodium pump as it functions in signal transmission. Other tissues as well use the ATPase to sustain the resting electric potential of the cells within them.[5] Other cell types use the pump for other purposes. As mentioned, the active transport of needed nutrients into the enterocyte uses the pump. Should the pump malfunction, these nutrients will not be absorbed and create an osmotic pull of water into the colon. In turn this will stimulate evacuation of the colon contents (diarrhea). This mechanism can explain the diarrhea associated with malabsorption syndromes such as those described in earlier chapters. However, it can also explain the symptoms of food-borne illness. In these instances, the ATPase is temporarily compromised with the result of an accumulation of unabsorbed nutrients that, as explained earlier, draw water into the colon and then diarrhea.

Various organisms such as those from the Salmonella family or the *Vibrio cholerae* can cause massive diarrhea and fluid loss. In the case of the latter, the cholera causing organism produces a toxin that binds to specific receptors on the intestinal cell wall. The toxin activates adenylyl

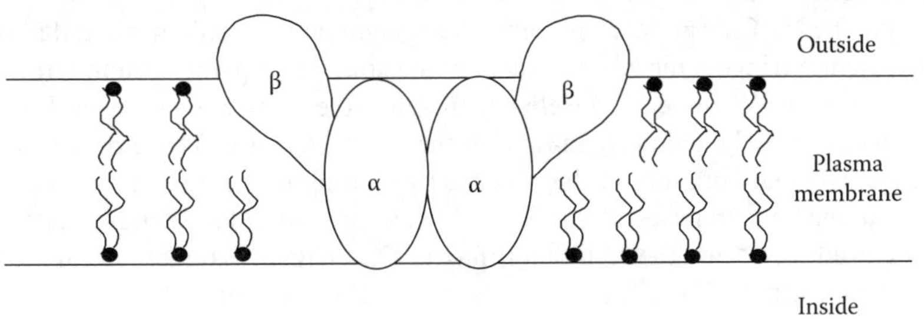

FIGURE 13.4 Structure of the membrane-bound Na^+K^+ ATPase.

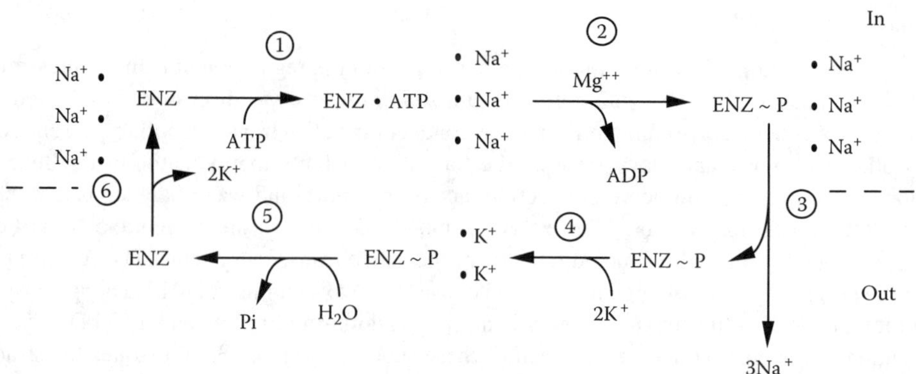

FIGURE 13.5 Mechanism of action of the Na^+K^+ ATPase. The ion exchange occurs via a series of reactions utilizing the α subunits of the enzyme, which has an inward-facing high-affinity Na+-binding site that reacts with ATP to form the activated ENZ~P only when Na^+ is bound to it. On the exterior aspect of the α subunits is a high-affinity K^+-binding site that will hydrolyze releasing inorganic phosphate only when K^+ is bound to it. The obligatory sequence begins with the sodium ATP binding and ends with the K^+ import into the cell. The sequence of these steps is numbered in this illustration.

cyclase by causing ADP-ribosylation of the GαS protein involved in regulating the cyclase. This results in an elevation in cAMP levels, which turns on electrolyte secretion and thereby inhibits the active transport processes necessary for the absorption of nutrients (and water) from the gut. While the water can pass freely from the intestine, other materials cannot and, as such, create an osmotic pull on the water. In turn, the water and unabsorbed nutrients fill the intestine stimulating peristalsis and evacuation of the colon. If the massive fluid and electrolyte losses are not replaced, the cholera victim does not survive and recover. Cholera victims can be given an oral solution rich in glucose (~110 mM), sodium (99 mM), chloride (74 mM), bicarbonate (39 mM), and potassium (4 mM). The World Health Organization (WHO) recommends a solution containing 20 g glucose, 3.5 g NaCl, 2.5 g $NaHCO_3$, and 1.5 g KCl/L of clean drinking water. This solution takes advantage of the fact that the cholera toxin does not *poison* the sodium-dependent ATP-dependent glucose uptake system. By giving excess glucose, sodium is *pushed in* to the cell and electrolyte balance is restored. If the victim cannot swallow, an intravenous replenishment must be followed. If untreated, the victim becomes severely dehydrated and death ensues. In countries where fresh human excreta is used as fertilizer for the fields, epidemics of cholera occur frequently. Epidemics are particularly evident in very warm climates since the cholera organisms multiply very rapidly under these conditions. Food contamination by organisms other than *V. cholerae* is also common in areas where both animal and human excreta are used in the untreated state. If the excreta is allowed to ferment, the heat generated by the fermentation process will kill most of the organisms likely to cause food-borne illness.

Muscle contraction/relaxation also uses an Na^+K^+ ATPase or pump. In the muscle, there is an additional pump, the Na^+Ca^{++} antiport system. This system pumps sodium out and allows calcium into the cell. Calcium triggers muscle contraction and so the two pump systems work together to regulate muscle action. When heart muscle degenerates, the clinician has several drugs that can be used to stimulate muscle action by inhibiting the Na^+K^+ ATPase. These drugs, called cardiac glycosides (digitalis, ouabain), inhibit the ATPase by binding to the α subunits (see Figure 13.4). This results in an increase in intracellular Na^+, which in turn stimulates the Na^+Ca^{++} antiport system. The cell extrudes Na^+ and the resultant influx of Ca^{++} triggers an increase in the force of the cardiac muscle contraction. The drug dose must be carefully monitored because too much Ca^{++} influx could be lethal unless counteracted. The regulation of intracellular calcium levels together with its role in metabolic regulation is the topic of intense interest by nutritionists, biochemists, and physiologists.

POTASSIUM

Potassium is the major intracellular electrolyte.[6] The healthy young adult male has between 42 and 48 mEq K^+/kg body weight or 2940–3360 mEq in the 70 kg man. Persons with above average muscle mass, that is, athletes, will have more body potassium than persons of average muscle mass. Virtually all the body potassium is exchangeable with the exception of small amounts that are irretrievably bound up in the bone mineral. Since potassium is primarily an intracellular ion, the number of cells in the body can be estimated using an infusion of heavy isotope K^{40}. The infused and exchangeable potassium equilibrates and by determining the dilution of the isotope one can determine cell number and mass while correcting for fat mass. The Na^+K^+ ATPase actively works to ensure that K^+ stays within the cell and that very little (3.5–5.0 mEq/L) is present in extracellular fluids.[7,8]

Just as all living things serve as sources of sodium, so too are they sources of potassium. The content of potassium in a wide variety of foods can be found at the USDA website, www.nal.usda.gov/foodcomposition. Only highly refined food ingredients, that is, pure sugars, fats, and oils, lack this essential nutrient. Especially good sources are milk and milk products, orange juice, avocados, fish, and bananas.[9] Potassium passes freely from the gastrointestinal system into the enterocyte and thence into the body. Potassium is distributed in response to energy-dependent Na^+ redistribution. Almost all of the consumed potassium is excreted in the urine with a very small amount found in the feces in healthy, normal adults. In persons experiencing diarrhea, however, the loss of potassium can be quite large and debilitating. If the diarrhea is of short duration (less than 12 h), the body will compensate and the person will survive. However, should this condition persist, potassium supplementation will be needed. Such is the case with the food-borne illness and for a number of the malabsorption syndromes. The plasma or serum level of potassium is not a reliable index of whole-body potassium status simply because potassium within the cell (not the serum) is what is needed. Causes for concern with too little potassium (hypokalemia) or too much (hyperkalemia) have to do with muscle contractility. If hypokalemia persists, the person could die of cardiac arrest. This occurs because too much K^+ has left the contractile unit and the heart muscle loses its ability to contract. Common causes of hypo- and hyperkalemia are listed in Table 13.4. The regulation of potassium balance follows that of sodium balance, and its participation in the sodium potassium pump has already been discussed.

CHLORIDE

Chloride is the third leg upon which osmotic pressure and acid–base balance rests.[10] Normal chloride levels in plasma are 100–106 mEq/L and vary very little. The glomerular filtrate contains 108 mEq/L and urine contains 138 mEq/L. Sweat can contain as much as 40 mEq/L but usually contains only trace amounts. The intracellular fluid contains very little Cl^- (~4 mEq/L) whereas intestinal juice contains 69–127 mEq/L. In instances of secretory diarrhea, the chloride content of the excrement

TABLE 13.4
Causes of Hypokalemia and Hyperkalemia

Hypokalemia (Plasma Levels <3.5 mEq/L)	Hyperkalemia (Plasma Levels >7 mEq/L)
Vomiting in excess (loss of chloride)	Chronic renal failure
Diuretics that enhance K^+ loss	Addison's disease (no aldosterone)
Cushing's disease (excess steroids)	Major trauma, infection
Rehydration therapy without K^+	Metabolic acidosis
Chronic renal disease	
Metabolic alkalosis	
Diarrhea	

TABLE 13.5
Causes of Hypochloremia and Hyperchloremia

Hypochloremia	Hyperchloremia
Increased extracellular water volume due to trauma and/or cachexia	Dehydration
Vomiting with large loss of gastric HCL	Diabetes insipidus
Overuse of diuretics	Brain stem injury
Overuse of adrenal steroids with retention of Na^+	Ureterointestinal anastomoses due to reabsorption of Cl^-
Chronic respiratory acidosis (high CO_2, low pH)	
Chronic renal disease, renal failure	

can be as high as 45 mEq/L. Most of the chloride in the intestinal tract does not appear in the feces of normal individuals. Rather, this ion recirculates as sodium and potassium are carried into the body. The main excretory pathway is urine. This ion, a member of the halogen family of elements that includes fluoride, iodide, and bromide in addition to chloride, although very reactive, is passively distributed throughout the body. As mentioned, it moves to replace anions lost to cells via other processes. It is the other half of table salt, NaCl, and as such is found in abundance in most foods. Dietary intake is in excess of that of sodium, yet the usual plasma Na^+:Cl^- ratio is about 3:2. This imbalance is due to the passive nature of chloride transfer between water compartments and to the active system that serves to retain Na^+.[11] Instances of below and above normal plasma levels of Cl^- are not diet related but are due to metabolic reasons usually related to Na^+ and K^+ homeostasis. Cystic fibrosis, for example, is a disease where chloride transport is abnormal.[12–14] In these patients, there are abnormalities in chloride transport in the epithelia of the respiratory tract, sweat glands, and intestinal tract. The disease is characterized by defective chloride channels.[15] Actually, cystic fibrosis is just one of several diseases in the group of diseases called channelopathies.[16] Not only can chloride channels be abnormal, so too can potassium channels. Altogether, problems in ion exchange can have marked effects on normal cell function. Listed in Table 13.5 are reasons why hypochloremia and hyperchloremia develop. Note the similarities between these causes and those listed for sodium in Table 13.2 and those for potassium in Table 13.4.

FUNCTION

As an electronegative element, Cl^- is a good oxidizing agent. In typical reactions, it is reduced to its electronegative form. One of its main functions is as an essential ingredient of the gastric acid, hydrochloric acid. This is completely dissociated into a strong electron donor (H^+) and a strong electron acceptor (Cl^-). Gastric juice contains 120–160 mEq/L. The function of chloride aside from its passive participation in electrolyte balance has to do with hemoglobin and its function as a carrier for oxygen and carbon dioxide. The process is called the chloride shift. The Cl^- is bound more tightly to deoxyhemoglobin than to oxyhemoglobin. Hence, the affinity of hemoglobin is directly proportional to the concentration of Cl^-. The carbonate ion, HCO_3^-, freely permeates the erythrocyte membrane so that once formed it equilibrates with the plasma. The need for charge neutrality on both sides of the red cell membrane requires that Cl^- replace HCO_3^- as it leaves the erythrocyte. Consequently, because cations do not shift, the Cl^- ion in the venous blood erythrocyte is higher than that in the arterial blood erythrocyte. Thus, the Cl^- modulates hemoglobin oxygen affinity.

CALCIUM

Calcium is the fifth most abundant element in the body exceeded only by carbon, hydrogen, oxygen, and nitrogen. It is the primary mineral in bones and teeth where it is present as hydroxyapatite ($3Ca_3(PO_4)_2 \cdot Ca(OH)_2$). On a dry weight basis, bone contains about 150 mg calcium/gram bone.

By comparison, soft tissues such as liver, muscle, or brain contain less than 35 μg calcium/g tissue. A normal 70 kg man will have about 22 g calcium/g fat-free tissue or a total of 1.54 kg calcium. While the calcium in the teeth is seldom mobilized, that which is in the skeletal muscle is mobilized and replaced at about 0.5 g/day. This daily turnover of calcium is essential to the maintenance of metabolic homeostasis because not only does calcium serve as a structural element, it also serves, in its ionized form, as an essential element in cell signaling systems. Of the total body calcium, 1% serves as an intracellular/intercellular messenger/regulator. Calcium mobilization and deposition changes with age, diet, hormonal status, and physiological state. Bone calcium homeostasis is related to bone strength, and if mobilization exceeds deposition, the bones will become porous (osteoporosis) and break easily.

Sources

The average daily calcium intake for adults in the United States ranges from 500 to 1200 mg. The range is quite broad because it depends on the percentage of the diet that comes from dairy products. Milk, cheese, ice cream, yogurt, sour cream, buttermilk, and other fermented and nonfermented milk products can provide as much as 72% of the daily calcium intake. Nuts and whole grain products are also good sources of calcium while other foods are relatively poor sources of this mineral. Shown in Table 13.6 are a number of foods and their calcium content. An extensive list of foods and their calcium content can be found on the USDA website: www.nal.usda.gov/foodcomposition. Some foods contain calcium-binding agents that reduce the availability of the calcium to the enterocyte. For example, some plant foods contain calcium in measurable quantities, but these same foods also contain phytate, a six-carbon anomer of glucose having six phosphate groups. Phytate will bind calcium reducing its availability for absorption. Once the phytate is degraded by the enzyme phytase, the bound calcium is then released and is once again available for absorption. Unfortunately, this release occurs in the lower third of the intestine and in the large intestine, areas that are less active in terms of calcium absorption. Phytate binds other divalent ions (Zn, Fe, Mg) as well and has a similar effect on their absorption. In addition, oxalate and some tannins can have this effect.

TABLE 13.6
Food Sources of Calcium in 100 g Portions

Source	mg	Weight of Average Serving (g)
Skim milk	123	245
Whole milk	119	244
Ice cream	129	66
Yogurt	120	227
Oysters	45	84
Cheddar cheese	728	28
Spinach	135	90
Mustard greens	74	70
Broccoli	48	44
White bread	125	24
Whole wheat bread	72	25
Carrots	26	72
Potatoes	10	202
Winter squash	14	102
Egg	50	50
Hamburger	10	100
Hot dog	19	57

Source: www.nal.usda.gov/foodcomposition.

Food Mixtures

Milk and milk products are excellent sources of calcium, as mentioned earlier. The reason why milk calcium absorption is so good is because of the type of protein found in these foods.

Casein, the main protein in milk, is a relatively small protein (molecular weight 23,000) having numerous phosphorylated serine residues. These residues have a negative charge to them, which enables the protein to bind the positively charged calcium ions. Lactalbumin, another milk protein, is also a calcium-binding protein. In addition to calcium, it will also bind zinc. This is true for a number of proteins; those that bind one divalent ion will also bind other divalent ions. Hence, there could be a competition for binding that would affect the availability of the minerals involved. As the food proteins are degraded by the digestive enzymes, these protein-bound minerals become available for uptake by the enterocyte. In mixtures of foods, this availability can be enhanced or compromised depending on the food mixture. As mentioned, cereal foods and green leafy vegetables contain oxalates or phytate that bind calcium. When these foods are mixed with dairy foods, one could anticipate a reduction in the availability of the calcium in the dairy food. In contrast, foods that are rich in vitamin C enhance calcium availability probably due to the redox nature of ascorbic acid. This vitamin readily changes from an oxidized to a reduced form and assists not only calcium absorption but also assists the absorption of those minerals that have more than one charged state (Fe^{++}, Fe^{+++}, Cu^{++}, Cu^{+++}, etc.).

Foods and food mixtures that provide calcium and phosphorus together in a ratio of 2:1–1:2 optimize calcium absorption. Both minerals are actively transported and yet do not share a single transport mechanism (see absorption, in a later section). When food mixtures are unbalanced with respect to this ratio, then calcium uptake will be impaired. Table 13.7 summarizes the influence of food components on calcium availability.

Bioavailability

In contrast to the macronutrients, the vitamins and sodium, potassium and chloride, not all of the calcium that is consumed is absorbed. The fraction that is absorbed can vary depending on the food source, the mixture of foods consumed, and the physiological status of the individual. That which is actually involved in biological processes is the bioavailable fraction.[17] The determination of calcium

TABLE 13.7
Food Components That Affect Calcium Absorption

Component	Effect
Alcohol	Decrease
Ascorbic acid	Decrease followed by an increase
Cellulose	Decrease
Fat[a]	Decrease followed by an increase
Fiber	Decrease
Lactose	Increase
Medium chain triglycerides	Increase
Oxalates	Decrease
Pectin	Decrease followed by an increase
Phytate	Decrease
Protein[b]	Decrease followed by an increase
Sodium alginate	Decrease
Uronic acid	Decrease

[a] In cases of steatorrhea, calcium absorption is reduced.
[b] Certain proteins, that is, those in milk, enhance calcium availability while others, that is, those in plants, reduce it.

bioavailability and absorption efficiency is a complicated process that involves careful food analysis to determine calcium content, careful measurements of the food consumed followed by feces and urine analysis of calcium excretion, corrected for calcium recycling. While the amount of calcium in the urine reflects the calcium that is absorbed, it does not indicate the amount of calcium that has been recycled. Likewise, the calcium in the feces reflects not only the calcium that was not absorbed from the food but also the calcium that was secreted into the intestine and not reabsorbed. The use of the calcium balance technique likewise does not measure the amount of calcium deposited in the bones and teeth, nor does it provide an estimate of the amount of calcium that is mobilized from these depots. However, the balance technique can be combined with tracer techniques and this provides a reasonably good estimate of absorption and bioavailability. Bioavailability estimates can be obtained using isotopes of calcium as tracers.[18,19] The heavy isotope Ca (^{46}Ca, ^{48}Ca) or the radioisotope calcium (^{45}Ca, ^{47}Ca) can be incorporated into a food and its presence in blood, urine, and feces monitored over time. If a plant food, the plant can be grown in an isotope-enriched growth medium and the edible portions provided to the subject or animal. If an animal food, the animal either consumes an isotopically labeled feed or is infused with a solution of labeled $CaCl_2$. Knowing the total food calcium and the percent that was isotopically labeled will then allow for calculations of intestinal uptake, recycling, excretion, storage, and use. The double isotope technique involves the consumption of a ^{45}Ca-enriched food followed by an infusion of $^{47}CaCl$ in the vein. ^{47}Ca has a short half-life (~4.7 days) while ^{45}Ca has a much longer one (~163.5 days). The stable isotopes (^{48}Ca, ^{49}Ca) can be substituted for the radioisotopes. The infused ^{47}Ca will be diluted in the blood by the calcium mobilized from the depots as well as by the absorbed calcium that also dilutes the food ^{45}Ca. The fraction that is absorbed is calculated as follows:

$$J_{ms} = \frac{J_{max}\left[Ca_L^{++}\right] + A\left[Ca_L^{++}\right]}{K_T + \left[Ca_L^{++}\right]}$$

where

J_{ms} is the total calcium flux from lumen
J_{max} is the maximum saturable flux
Ca^{++} is the lumen, $J_{max}/2$ is observed
A is the diffusion constant

In practice, absorption = fraction of oral ^{45}Ca in urine/fraction of ^{47}Ca in urine. The use of ^{47}Ca assumes that the infused calcium will behave as though it had been absorbed. In each instance, the measurement is a single time point. Urine is collected for 24 h after isotope administration. To obtain an estimate of recycling, the investigator will collect blood, urine, and feces at intervals over a 2- to 4-day period, monitor the dilution of the consumed and infused labels, and using this information, calculate rate constants for each calcium pool. Absorption can also be calculated from the feces using the loss of the consumed label to estimate the absorption. However, since there is considerable individual variation in gut passage time that can influence calcium absorption, feces must be collected for periods of up to 12 days. Given the shorter half-life of ^{47}Ca that is infused to provide the estimate of recycling, this method for determining apparent absorption is not as popular.

Combining the use of both radioactive and stable isotopes also has some problems. The stable isotope ^{48}Ca degrades to ^{49}Ca with the emission of a γ ray. ^{49}Ca has a half-life of 8.8 min. ^{46}Ca converts to ^{47}Ca, which has radioactivity. The use of heavy isotopes requires the use of mass spectrometry to detect their presence while liquid scintillation or gamma counters are needed for detecting the radioisotopes. Small animals such as the rat, mouse, and chicken with their smaller body sizes, faster rates of growth, and faster metabolic rates reduce the expense and increase the number of measurements, as well as the validity of these measurements due to their genetic homogeneity.

Apparent Absorption

Apparent absorption is the fraction of the consumed calcium that disappears from the gastrointestinal tract. Thus, it is the net movement of calcium from the lumen into the animal. This movement can be tracked in vitro using an intestinal segment and a calcium isotope. The apparent absorption is calculated:

$$\text{Apparent absorption} = \frac{V\left[{}^{40}\text{Ca}_i - \left({}^{40}\text{Ca}_f\right)(\text{PRR})\right]}{\text{L or W}}$$

The subscripts i and f refer to initial and final concentrations of calcium in μmol/mL. PRR is the ratio of phenol red in the initial and final samples. L is the length, W is the weight of the intestinal segment, and V is the volume perfused in milliliters. The lumen to plasma flux is unidirectional and can be calculated as follows:

$$\text{Flux} = \frac{V\left[{}^{45}\text{Ca}_i - \left({}^{45}\text{Ca}_f\right)(\text{PRR})\right]}{\left[\left(\text{SA}_i + \text{SA}_f\right)/2\right]W}$$

In this calculation, SA refers to the specific activity of the calcium isotope and W is the dry weight of the intestinal segment. All the other definitions are the same as in calculation of apparent absorption. These equations have been successfully used to calculate calcium absorption in normal rats as shown in Table 13.8.

Physiological Status

Absorption efficiency is greater in the young growing individual than in the mature adult, which in turn is greater than in the aged individual.[20] As well, there are gender differences due in part to hormonal status. Postmenopausal females have a less efficient calcium absorption than premenopausal females.[21,22] Men, both young and mature, have a greater calcium absorption efficiency than females of the same age.[17,22] Testosterone has been shown to enhance calcium absorption.[22] Calcium absorption is impaired in vitamin D–deficient individuals,[23,24] as well as in persons with insulin-dependent diabetes mellitus.[25] Clearly the endocrine status of the individual has effects on calcium uptake and this in turn can influence calcium status in terms of bone structure and calcium content.

TABLE 13.8
Apparent Absorption of Calcium In Vitro by Duodenal Loops in Normal Rats

Volume perfused	240 mL
Duration of perfusion	2 h
Conc. Ca	0.8 mM
Conc. ^{45}Ca (sp act., 2000 μCi/mg)	12 μCi/L
Length of intestine	87 cm
Weight of intestine	5.4 g
Mucosal dry weight	7.2 mg/cm
Net absorption, μmol/h	
Per cm segment length	0.140
Per g dry weight mucosa	20.1
Lumen to plasma flux	
Per cm segment length	0.196
Per g dry weight mucosa	27.6

Mechanisms of Absorption

Only 20%–50% of ingested calcium is absorbed yet this mineral is so important to metabolism that two mechanisms exist for its uptake.[26,27] One of these is vitamin D dependent while the other is not. The latter is one that uses passive diffusion. The former is an energy-dependent active transport system and is illustrated in Figure 13.6. This is a saturable system that operates actively when calcium is in short supply in the diet. Thus, when the diet is calcium poor, this system is more active than when a calcium-rich diet is consumed. A wide range of apparent calcium absorption exists. In the active system, calcium diffuses across the brush border down its thermodynamic gradient into the cell as free unbound Ca^{++}. This calcium is then bound by an intracellular protein called calbindin D_{9k}, which serves to maintain the level of calcium in the cell at a low, nontoxic level.[25,27] Calcium released from calbindin enters and leaves the subcell compartments such as the mitochondria[28,29] and endoplasmic reticulum.[30] This occurs in an orderly oscillatory manner.[31] The calcium ion leaves the enterocyte either in exchange for sodium or is extruded from the cell by a calcium-activated ATPase. This ATPase has been found in both the brush border and at the basal-lateral membrane. As calcium is extruded, ATP is cleaved to ADP and Pi. Hence, the energy dependence of this system. Because the sodium that is exchanged for calcium must be actively removed from the intracellular compartment by the Na^+K^+ ATPase, this process is also part of this energy-dependent system.

Absorption of calcium by the enterocyte is but one of the roles of vitamin D (see Chapter 11). Other roles include renal calcium conservation, intracellular calcium movement, bone calcium deposition, as well as bone calcium mobilization. Vitamin D or 1,25 dihydroxycholecalciferol has these effects on calcium homeostasis due to its effects on the synthesis of calcium-binding proteins (Table 13.9). In the intestine, the protein of interest is calbindin D_{9k}. Vitamin D binds to its cognate receptor in the enterocyte and this steroid–receptor complex migrates to the nucleus where it binds to a specific DNA sequence, which encodes the protein, calbindin D_{9k}. Studies of vitamin D–deficient animals have shown a rapid induction of calbindin mRNA transcription when the missing vitamin was provided. This was followed by a restoration of normal calcium absorption in these

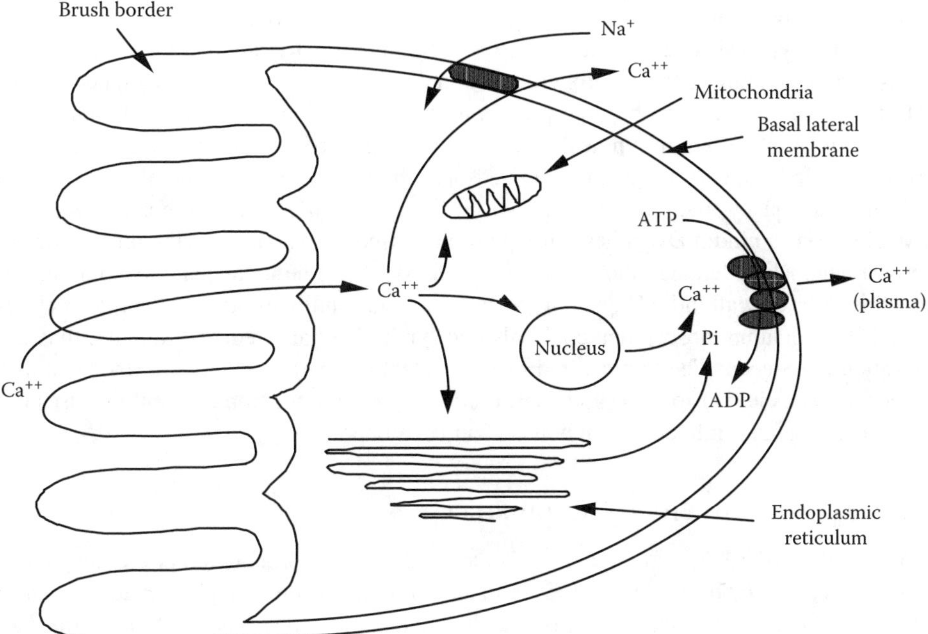

FIGURE 13.6 Calcium absorption by the enterocyte. Both the $Ca^{2+}Na^+$ exchange and the energy-dependent systems are shown.

TABLE 13.9
Calcium-Binding Proteins

Protein	Function
α Lactalbumin	Carries calcium in milk
Casein	Carries calcium in milk
Calmodulin	Serves as major intracellular calcium receptor; activates cyclic nucleotide phosphodiesterase
Calbindin—D_{9k} and D_{28k}	Facilitates intracellular Ca^{++} translocation
Osteocalcin	Essential for calcium deposition in bone
$Ca^{++}Mg^{++}$ ATPase	Essential to movement of calcium across membranes
Prothrombin	Essential to blood clot formation
Calcitonin	Inhibits osteoclast-mediated bone resorption; regulates blood calcium levels by preventing hypercalcemia
Parathyroid hormone	Stimulates calcitonin synthesis, bone Ca resorption, renal Ca conservation
Albumin	Carries calcium in the blood
Globulin	Carries calcium in the blood
Osteopontin	Essential for calcium mobilization from bone
Troponin C	Muscle contraction
Alkaline phosphatase	Mineralization of bone
Sialoprotein	Embryonic bone growth
GLA-rich clotting proteins	Binds calcium in the coagulation cascade (see vitamin K)
Villin, gelsolin	Cytoskeleton stabilization

repleted animals. In addition to the rapid increase in transcription was an effect of the vitamin on calbindin mRNA half-life. There was an increase in this half-life, which indicates a vitamin effect on mRNA stability. Thus, the vitamin both stimulates transcription and has a posttranscriptional effect on calbindin synthesis.

Vitamin D is not the only hormone involved in calbindin synthesis. Testosterone, retinoic acid, growth hormone, progesterone, insulin-like growth factor 1, and estrogen augment while glucocorticoids inhibit the synthesis of calbindin D_{9k}.[21,22,32,33,34] Calbindin D_{28k}, another vitamin D–dependent calcium-binding protein in the enterocyte and renal cell, has its synthesis regulated by retinoic acid. In the brain, this calcium-binding protein is not regulated by vitamin D. The multiplicity of hormonal controls of calbindin synthesis explains in part the gender and age differences in calcium absorption and indeed helps to elucidate the reasons why postmenopausal females are more at risk for calcium inadequacy than are young growing males and females. Those hormones that have a positive effect on calbindin D synthesis are the same hormones that are missing (or in short supply) in the postmenopausal female. Should calbindin D_{9k} synthesis be inadequate, calcium absorption will decline. As well, calbindin D_{28k}, an important calcium-binding protein in the renal cell responsible for renal calcium reabsorption, could also be synthesized at a reduced rate and thus calcium conservation is reduced. The two calbindins are subject to nearly the same hormonal influences. With decreased calcium absorption and conservation, bone calcium mobilization increases with the result of an age-/gender-related loss in bone calcium, osteoporosis.

Calcium Transport and Blood Calcium Regulation

The concentration of calcium in the plasma is the result of three processes that are integrated so as to maintain a constancy of calcium in the circulation. Blood calcium is regulated at 100 mg/L (2.50 mmol/L) across the lifespan although in late adulthood there may be a small (10%) decline due to an age-related decline in the total calcium-binding capacity of the serum proteins. Most (80%) of the blood calcium bound to protein is carried by albumin with the remainder bound to a variety of globulins. Sixty percent of blood calcium circulates as the free ion or as an ion complex. Calcium levels in the

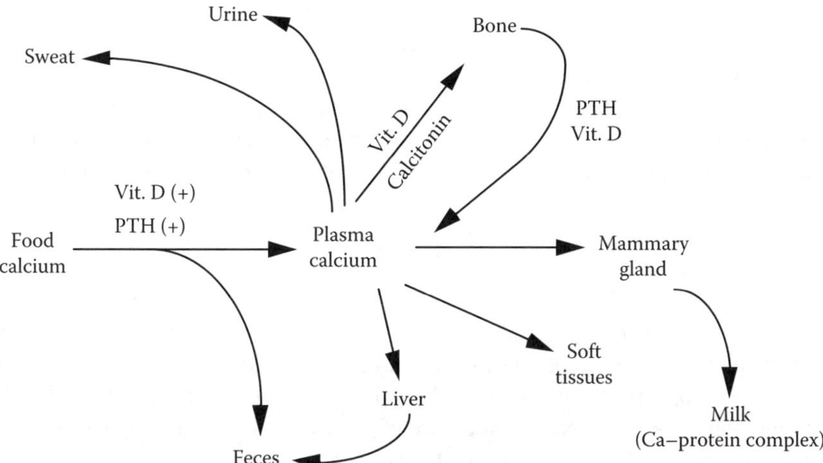

FIGURE 13.7 Pathways of calcium use.

blood are regulated mainly by three hormones: active vitamin D (1,25 dihydroxycholecalciferol), calcitonin, and parathyroid hormone (PTH), a hormone released by the parathyroid glands. These glands are embedded in the thyroid gland and are stimulated by falling calcium levels to release PTH. PTH acts on the bone and the kidneys. In the kidneys, PTH reduces calcium loss by stimulating its reabsorption. In the bone, PTH stimulates calcium release. It also inhibits collagen synthesis by osteoblasts. Osteoblasts, through the synthesis of collagen, provide the organic matrix on which the minerals of the bone are deposited. Osteoclasts, in contrast, are those bone cells responsible for bone resorption. PTH stimulates osteoclast activity indirectly because PTH stimulates renal inorganic phosphate loss. Since phosphate is the counter ion of Ca^{++} in the bone, phosphate loss causes $Ca_5(PO_4)_3OH$ to leach out of the bone and thus raise serum calcium levels. Finally, PTH has one other effect. It stimulates the synthesis of 1,25 dihydroxycholecalciferol, which in turn stimulates intestinal calcium uptake.

Counteracting PTH is calcitonin.[35] Calcitonin, synthesized by C cells in the thyroid gland, inhibits osteoclast-mediated bone resorption. Calcitonin also inhibits the activation of vitamin D and inhibits renal calcium conservation. Altogether PTH, active vitamin D, and calcitonin regulate blood calcium levels such that there is little variation in normal individuals.[35] Should blood levels fall below the 2.2–2.5 mmol/L level, calcium tetany will occur. In newly lactating females, this is called milk fever. It can quickly be reversed with an infusion of a calcium lactate or gluconate. Milk fever develops because of a great demand for calcium by the mammary gland. When the demand exceeds the elasticity of the blood calcium homeostatic system, hypocalcemia results. As mentioned, this is usually temporary and reversible.

Hypocalcemia due to underactive parathyroid glands or to chronic renal failure, vitamin D deficiency or hypomagnesemia, is more difficult to manage because the underlying causes are more difficult. Hormone replacement, renal transplant, or correction of blood magnesium levels are the usual strategies followed. With respect to the low blood magnesium, this is one of the consequences of alcoholism.[36] Excess ethanol intake can interfere with the intake and use of magnesium, which in turn results in a loss of responsiveness of osteoclasts to PTH. This interrupts or interferes with the homeostatic mechanisms needed to control blood calcium levels. The pathways of calcium use are illustrated in Figure 13.7.

Function

Bone Mineralization

Ninety-nine percent of the total body calcium is found in the bones and teeth. This calcium is part of a mineral complex that is deposited on an organic matrix comprised primarily of type I collagen.

This collagen has a unique amino acid composition consisting of large amounts of glycine, proline, and hydroxyproline.[37] A single molecule of type I collagen has a molecular mass of ~285 kDa, a width of ~14 Å, and a length of ~300 Å. There are at least 17 different polypeptides found in collagen. The polypeptides used vary throughout the body and each collagen uses at least three of them. Collagen is about 30%–33% glycine with another 15%–30% of the amino acid residues as proline and 3, 4, or 5 hydroxyproline. Collagen is a left-handed triple helix stabilized by hydrogen bonding. These bonds may involve bridging water molecules between the hydroxyprolines. The collagen fibrils are also held together by covalent cross-linking. These cross-links are between the side chains of lysine and histidine and the linkage is catalyzed by the copper-dependent enzyme, lysyl oxidase. Up to four side chains can be covalently bonded to each other. All in all, this collagen provides a network of fibers upon which the crystals of hydroxy apatite ($Ca_3(PO_4)_3OH$) are deposited. The hydroxy apatite is by no means pure calcium phosphate. Some ions (magnesium, iron, sodium, and chloride) are adsorbed on to the surface of the hydroxyapatite crystallites while other ions (strontium, fluoride, and carbonate) are incorporated into the mineral lattice. The presence of these other ions affects the chemical and physical properties of the calcified tissue. Solubility, for example, is decreased when strontium and fluoride ions are present. Hardness is enhanced by the presence of fluoride.

Bone formation begins in the embryo and continues throughout life. The nature of the process and the cells involved change as the individual ages. Osteoprogenitor cells in early development synthesize the extracellular matrix described earlier and also regulate the flux of minerals into that matrix. As the calcified tissue begins to form, osteoclasts appear on the surface of this tissue and osteoblasts, connected to one another by long processes are totally surrounded by mineralizing matrix. Each type of mineralized tissue has some unique properties but all share several histological features in the early mineralization process. Hunziker et al.[37] have described this process in the epiphysial growth plate during the ossification of the endochondral cartilage as it becomes bone. Initial mineral deposition occurs at discrete sites on membrane-bound bodies (matrix vesicles) in the extracellular matrix. These initial deposits are diffuse and lack orientation. The mineral crystals proliferate and mineralization proceeds filling the longitudinal but not the transverse septa. Changes in the activities of enzymes that catalyze the hydrolysis of phosphate esters and those that catalyze certain proteolytic reactions follow or accompany this mineralization. These reactions are prerequisite to vascular invasion. Following vascular invasion, lamellar bone is formed by osteoblasts directly on the surface of the pre-existing mineralized cartilage. These osteoblasts secrete type I collagen with very little proteoglycan and few extracellular matrix vesicles. This process is repeated over and over until the bone has finished growing. At this point, the growth plate closes and the mature length and shape of the bone is apparent. This bone, however, is not at all metabolically inert. It continues to lose and gain mineral matter; that is, it is continuously remodeled through the action of the osteoblasts that synthesize the collagen matrix and the osteoclasts that are stimulated by PTH to reabsorb calcium (and other minerals) in times of need. While the number of osteoblasts declines with age, the number of osteoclasts increases especially in postmenopausal females. This helps to explain some of the age-related loss in bone mineral that occurs in aging females. Osteoclasts act first during bone remodeling by producing cavities on either the cortical or cancellous (trabecullar) bone surfaces. When these cavities develop, osteoblasts are recruited for bone remineralization, thereby filling (or refilling) the cavities. The bone matrix reforms and remineralizes as described earlier with the result of new bone formation. The remodeling process is an ongoing one with rates of resorption equaling the rates of new bone formation as long as the hormones controlling each process are in balance and as long as the nutrients needed to support this ongoing process are provided. Figures 13.8 and 13.9 illustrate calcium turnover in bone and the influence of hormones on this process.

Bone mass can remain constant for many decades. However, once the hormone balance changes, this constancy changes. In females, bone mass declines by an estimated 1%–2% per year after menopause. In senile men, bone mass loss also occurs. In fact, both senile males and females experience about a 1% loss per year. Not only is there a loss in bone mass but there is a loss in structural integrity. The bones lose their mineral apatite and become porous (osteoporosis) as well lose their

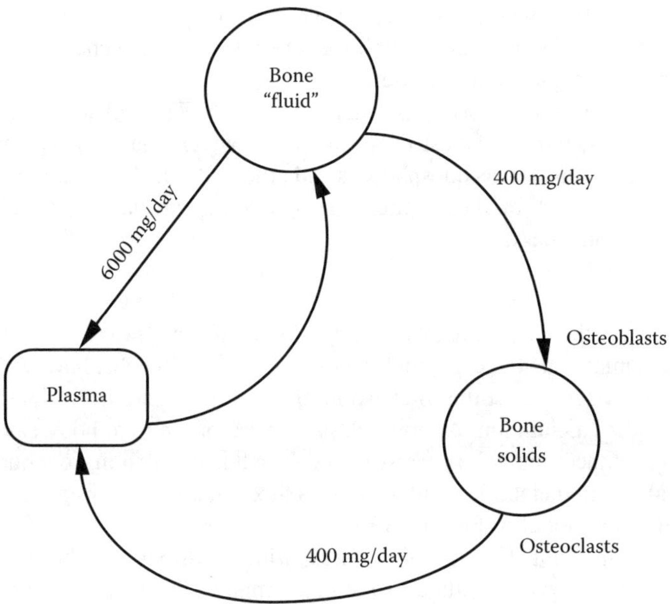

FIGURE 13.8 Calcium turnover in bone.

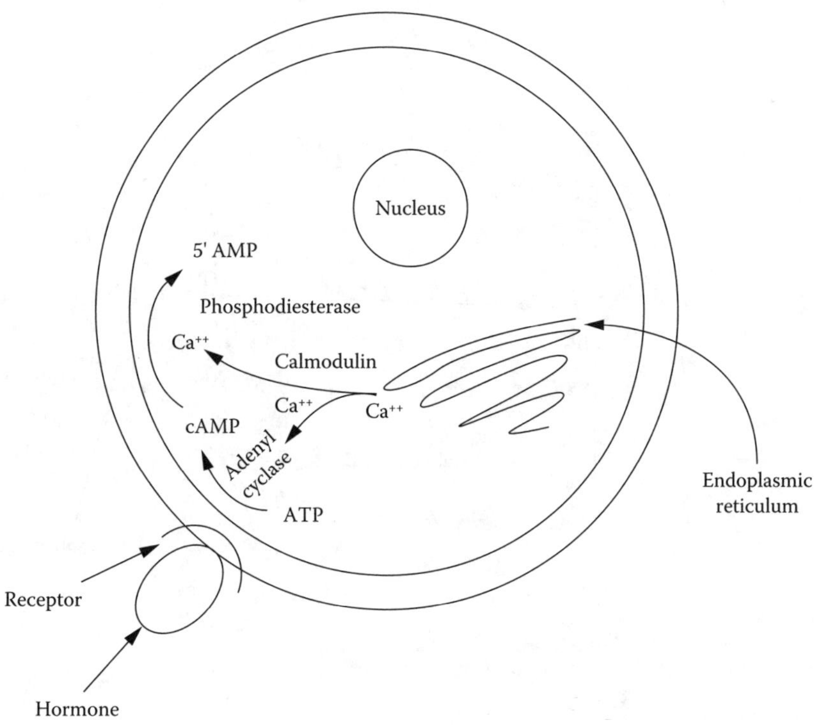

FIGURE 13.9 Calmodulin moves Ca^{++} from the endoplasmic reticulum to serve as a cofactor in reactions catalyzed by phosphodiesterase and adenyl cyclase in the cylic AMP second messenger system.

architecture upon which the mineral has rested.[38] The very compact cortical portions of the bone disappear, leaving a fragile, largely trabecular bone. The result of these changes is a fragile skeletal system subject to non-trauma-related fracture.

While the importance of appropriate hormone balance (PTH, calcitonin, active vitamin D, Insulin-like growth factor (IGF_1) and estrogen) cannot be overemphasized, it should also be recognized that dietary calcium (as well as phosphorous and other nutrients) plays an important role in the maintenance of bone mass.[39–42] Intakes at or exceeding 800 mg/day have been shown to counteract the age-related loss in bone mass.

Cell Signaling

Metabolic regulation and the integration of a variety of metabolic pathways and cell systems depends largely on the communications the cells, and the organelles within cells, have within and between each other. Signaling systems exist that orchestrate this communication. An integral part of these signaling systems is the calcium ion. Although less than 1% of the total body calcium store serves this function, its importance cannot be overestimated. The flux of calcium from one compartment to another plays a vital role in metabolic regulation. This flux is facilitated by an intracellular calcium-binding protein called calmodulin (Figure 13.10).

Calmodulin contains four Ca^{++}-binding sites with affinities in the micromolar range. It is ubiquitous in all eukaryotic cells and mediates many of calcium's effects. Among these

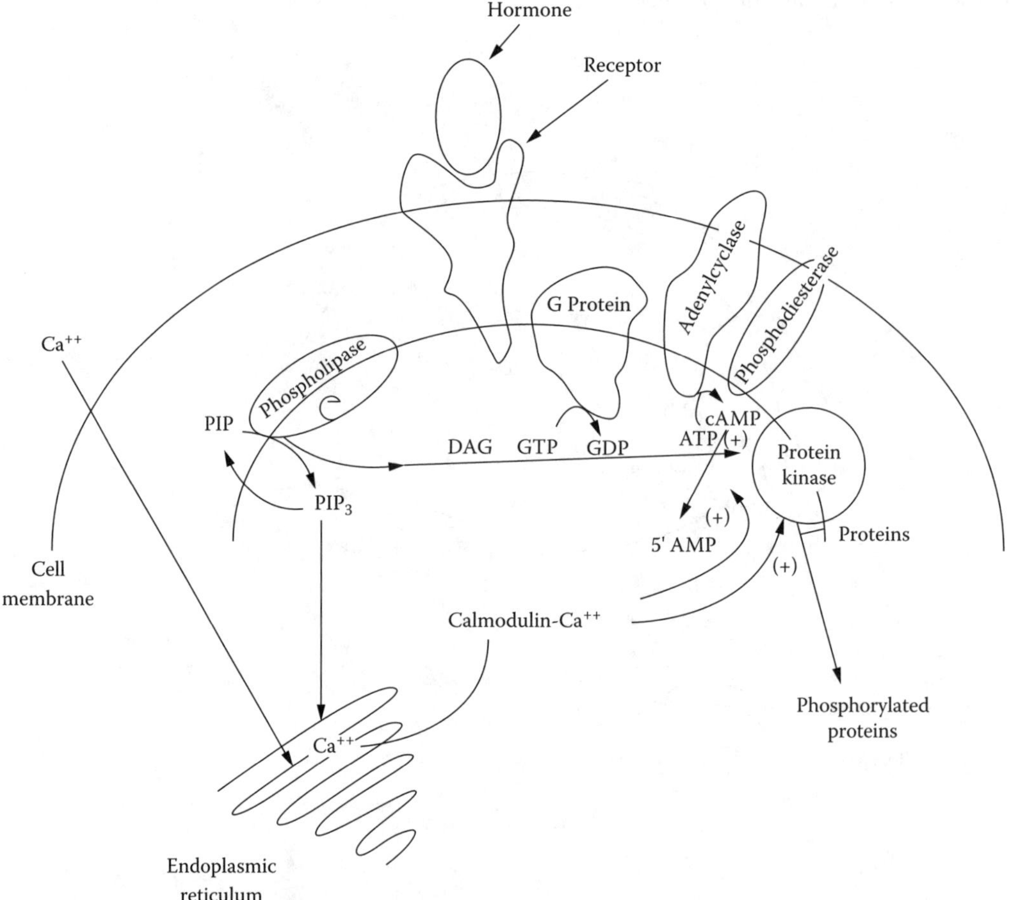

FIGURE 13.10 Integration of cAMP and PIP second messenger systems showing the role of calcium in both.

are the activation of phosphodiesterase, a component of the cAMP second messenger system. Phosphodiesterase catalyzes the conversion of cAMP to 5′ AMP and requires calcium as a cofactor. Calcium is translocated from its storage site on the endoplasmic reticulum by calmodulin to the interior aspect of the plasma membrane whereupon it is released to serve as a cofactor for phosphodiesterase. A similar mechanism exists for the action of calcium in another cell second messenger system, the phosphatidyl inositol system (see Chapter 12). In this instance, phospholipase C, a membrane-bound protein, is activated by the binding of an external compound to its cognate receptor. Phospholipase C catalyzes the release of inositol 1,4,5 phosphate from phosphatidylinositol, one of the plasma membrane's phospholipids. Diacylglycerol and inositol 1,4,5 phosphate then migrate forward into the cytoplasm. DAG binds to protein kinase C and activates it with the help of the calcium ion. Inositol 1,4,5 phosphate in the meantime migrates to the endoplasmic reticulum, stimulating the release of more calcium, which in turn further stimulates protein kinase C. Protein kinase C catalyzes the phosphorylation of a variety of proteins. Some of these are enzymes that must be phosphorylated to increase or decrease their metabolic activity whereas others are necessary for secretion processes, that is, gastric acid release or hormone release, or for substrate uptake, that is, glucose transport or for any of a number of energy-driven processes.

Calcium and the cAMP signaling system together with the phosphatidylinositol signaling system have been shown to explain the action of many hormones and cell regulators. Figure 13.11 illustrates these two systems. Angiotensin, cholecystokinin, acetylcholine, insulin-like growth factors, insulin, and glucagon are but a few hormones whose mode of action involve the calcium ion in one or the other of these signaling systems. There is considerable cross-talk between these systems as a result of their mutual need for Ca^{++}.[43,44]

In addition to its role in these second messenger systems, Ca^{++} flux between cytoplasm and mitochondria regulates mitochondrial activity. Ca^{++} uptake by mitochondria is energetically less demanding than its export.[28] Uptake followed by active export is an oscillatory process. Ca^{++} flows in until a 200 μM concentration is reached whereupon it is actively pumped out using the energy of ATP. This active system costs about 63% of the ATP hydrolysis energy. There are three separate Ca^{++} transport mechanisms at work (Figure 13.11). One is the calcium

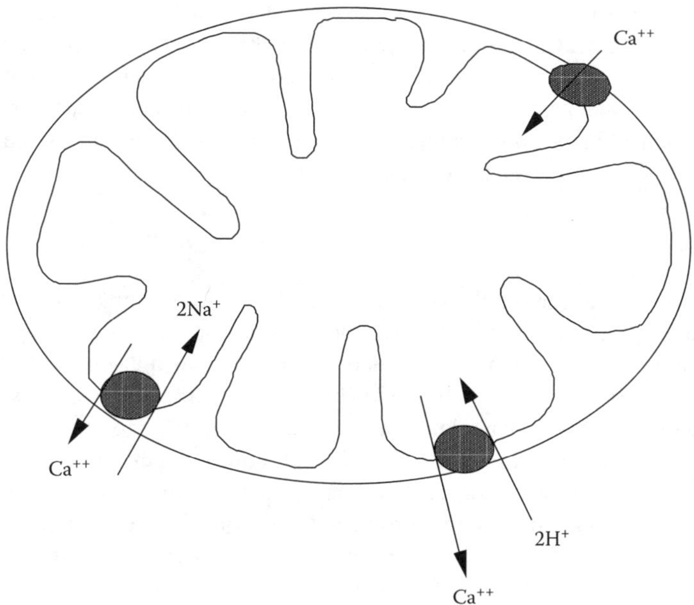

FIGURE 13.11 Ca^{++} flux in the mitochondrial compartment.

TABLE 13.10
Ca^{++} as a Metabolic Regulator: Reactions or Reaction Sequences Stimulated by Ca^{++}

Fatty acid oxidation
Amino acid transport into hepatocytes
Citric acid cycle (isocitrate dehydrogenase, α ketoglutarate dehydrogenase)
Pyruvate dehydrogenase
ATP-Mg/Pi carrier (mitochondrial carrier)
Glucose-stimulated insulin release
Phosphodiesterase
Stimulation of olfactory neurons
Trypsinogen conversion to trypsin
Pancreatic α amylase activation
Pancreatic phospholipase A_2
Hydrolysis of troponin in muscle to tropomyosin
Phospholipase C
Blood clotting (binding of calcium to GLA-rich proteins)

uniporter. The uniporter rapidly sequesters external Ca^{++} into the mitochondrial matrix and in a similar fashion also sequesters Fe^{++}, Sr^{++}, Mn^{++}, Ba^{++}, and Pb^{++}. Mg^{++} uptake is much slower than Ca^{++} and is probably not mediated by this uniporter system. The other two Ca^{++} transport mechanisms facilitate Ca^{++} efflux rather than influx. There is a sodium-independent and a sodium-dependent mechanism. The latter is more powerful of the two for facilitating Ca^{++} efflux. Its velocity is much higher than the sodium-independent mechanism. Altogether these three mechanisms function to control Ca^{++} flux and hence mitochondrial metabolism, particularly oxidative phosphorylation.

The mitochondrial Ca^{++} cycle is designed to regulate intramitochondrial Ca^{++} levels and to relay changes in cytosolic Ca^{++} to the mitochondrial matrix. Surges in cytosolic Ca^{++} via the cell signaling systems activate a variety of ATP requiring reactions. In turn, as ATP is used, its metabolic end product, ADP or AMP, is transported back into the mitochondria whereupon it is rephosphorylated and exported (along with the Ca^{++}) to the cytosol. This multifaceted system provides flexibility and responsivity to changing cellular environments and has considerable control strength with respect to the balance of catabolic and anabolic metabolic pathways. In this instance, Ca^{++} is more than a mere signal; it is a key element in metabolic control. Shown in Table 13.10 are some of the many reactions or reaction sequences that are activated or suppressed by Ca^{++}.

Calcium and Cell Death

Just as Ca^{++} is important to the regulation of cell metabolism, it has another role: it can mediate the death of a cell or a group of cells.[45] When the integrity of the cell's membrane is breached either through injury, sepsis, chemical insults or anoxia, the normal flux of Ca^{++} from storage depots to sites of use and return is interrupted. Just as the extracellular Ca^{++} is carefully regulated so as not to exceed that very narrow range of 2.2–2.5 mmol so too is the intracellular Ca^{++} concentration. As described earlier, Ca^{++} flows into the mitochondria but is actively exported. If the injury to the cell interrupts this active energy-driven export, the Ca^{++} will continue to flow into the mitochondria and raise the ionic concentration of the mitochondrial matrix. This has negative effects on oxidative phosphorylation and the stage is set for a downward spiral toward mitochondrial dysfunction. Ca^{++} influx into the cytosol as well as the nucleus also occurs because it is downward energetically under these conditions. When sufficient calcium accumulates, the cell dies. While the loss of one cell is not devastating, the loss of many cells can be and is. Of particular concern is the accumulation of Ca^{++} by interconnected muscle such as the heart. Muscle contraction is a Ca^{++}-mediated event. Ca^{++} flows into the myocyte mitochondria and is pumped out using ATP. If Ca^{++} accumulates in the myocyte and is not actively pumped out, the myocyte dies.

Counteracting this Ca^{++} movement in cells under duress is a class of pharmaceutical agents called calcium blockers. These drugs postpone cell death by interfering with Ca^{++} influx. Since their discovery, they have been very useful in the management of hypertension, the management of heart disease, and have been found useful in several other settings. Calcium ionophores, agents that facilitate Ca^{++} flux, have also been discovered. The most widely used one is A23187. Two molecules of this compound surround Ca^{++} and because the agent is lipophilic it is able to passively cross the plasma membrane and deliver the Ca^{++} to the cytosol.

Other functions of calcium, particularly those relating to clot formation and embryonic development, have been discussed in the sections on vitamin K and vitamin A, respectively. In these sections, the synthesis of specific proteins that bind calcium and that perform specific roles in the processes of interest is described.

Muscle Contraction

The muscle cell has a unique calcium storage site called the sarcoplasmic reticulum. This reticulum is similar to that found in other cell types but is highly specialized. It contains ribosomes, and many of the same enzymes found in the endoplasmic reticulum of other cell types but in addition also contains large quantities of calcium-activated ATPase. Approximately 75% of the sarcoplasmic reticulum is this ATPase. The ATPase also requires magnesium so its name is $Ca^{++}Mg^{++}$ ATPase. It serves as a calcium pump using the energy released by ATP to drive the calcium ion from the cytosol to the sarcoplasmic reticulum. There the calcium resides until needed for muscle contraction. Upon receipt of a signal to contract, a Ca^{++} channel is opened and Ca^{++} flows into the cytoplasm of the muscle cell whereupon it binds to troponin, a contractile protein of skeletal and cardiac muscle. This protein is a long rod-like structure that extends over the length of the muscle fiber. When Ca^{++} binds to it, it changes its shape becoming shorter. The muscle cell contains two other filaments, actin and myosin, which interact when troponin shortens due to Ca^{++} binding. When troponin is in the relaxed state, these two filaments are too far apart to interact.

Muscles are signaled to contract by a wave of depolarization–repolarization flowing down the muscle fiber from its point of contact at the neuromuscular junction. During depolarization of skeletal muscle, extracellular Na^+ flows into the cell and potentiates the Ca^{++} release from the sarcoplasmic reticulum. In the heart muscle, with its slightly different muscle fiber organization the signal for contraction is generated by the AV sinus node on the right side of the heart. This signal is regularly spaced and results in depolarization–repolarization just as happens in skeletal muscle. However, with depolarization Ca^{++} flows into the cytosol from the extracellular fluid as well as from the sarcoplasmic reticulum. This has the result of increasing the strength of the contraction because more calcium is present. During repolarization, Ca^{++} is then pumped, via the Ca^{++} Mg^{++} pump, back into the sarcoplasmic reticulum. In heart muscle, there are many more mitochondria providing ATP than are found in skeletal muscle, hence the need for Ca^{++} by the heart muscle is greater than that of skeletal muscle.

In contrast to the heart and skeletal muscle, smooth muscle does not contract and relax strongly. These muscles can sustain contraction for a longer period of time and are far less dependent on calcium for contractile strength. Rather, the chief role of calcium in this muscle type is that of serving in the various hormone-mediated cell signaling systems.

Calcium Deficiency

Considering the vital role of vitamin D and other micronutrients in determining calcium status, it is truly difficult to produce a *pure* calcium-deficient state.[39,44] Calcium deficiency does indeed occur, but it is usually due to other factors: lack of vitamin D activation, loss of estrogen production, adrenal dysfunction, parathyroid gland dysfunction, and so forth. If any of these conditions develop, then signs of calcium deficiency occur. These signs include inadequate bone calcification and growth in children (rickets) and weak porous bones in adults (osteoporosis).[46–50] Rickets characterized by malformed poorly calcified bones is more of a disease of inadequate vitamin intake than one of inadequate calcium intake. Should blood calcium levels fall acutely, calcium tetany will result and unless calcium is provided quickly by the intravenous route, death will ensue.

Need

Because calcium absorption is dependent on so many different factors, there has been vigorous discussion among experts as to what the recommended intake of calcium should be. Acceptable intakes have been devised (Table 13.1), and these figures should be used as guidance for intake targets. Racial differences in calcium need have been reported.[47] In addition, there are a number of dietary factors (excess protein, calcium:phosphorus ratio, calcium:magnesium ratio, oxalates, phytates) that increase calcium loss from the system and these are hard to quantitate such that an age-appropriate recommendation can be made. Several diseases stem from or affect calcium use and these must be considered. For example, hypertension has been linked to inadequate milk product calcium intake.[48,49] Critical experiments that would irrefutably support such a linkage have yet to be conducted; nonetheless, there are suggestions arising from population studies that those who consume calcium by way of dairy foods have less hypertension than those who avoid dairy foods. Follow-up studies in hypertensive rats have shown that increasing dietary calcium reduces the hypertensive state.

As mentioned earlier, vitamin D and estrogen status affect calcium use. Increasing the calcium intake can compensate for a reduction in absorption efficiency, and thus, the postmenopausal female could benefit from increasing the calcium intake. More recently, it has been noted that postmenopausal women given calcium and vitamin D supplements have a reduced risk of postmenopausal weight gain.[50] The relationship between obesity or weight gain and food intake control as affected by dietary calcium intake[51] as well as the relationship between calcium and insulin resistance[52] is an interesting consideration with respect to calcium need. Pittas et al.[53] reviewed the role of vitamin D and calcium in type 2 diabetes. They used a meta-analysis to systematically review a variety of studies of people with diabetes. They concluded that vitamin D and calcium insufficiency may have a negative impact on glucose homeostasis. Results of the CARDIA study[53] showed that dietary patterns characterized by increased dairy consumption (increased vitamin D and calcium with increased milk consumption) had a strong inverse association with insulin resistance in young adults who were overweight. This same dietary characteristic has also been reported to reduce obesity and to have a beneficial effect on weight loss by nondiabetic overweight and obese subjects[54–56] and genetically obese mice.[57] The mechanism of action of vitamin D and calcium in the problem of excess fat stores has yet to be elucidated; however, it is apparent that hypocaloric diets that include calcium–vitamin D–rich foods have positive effects on weight loss.

Note in Table 13.1 that older people have a larger DRI for calcium than young adults. In part, this may be an indirect indication that increased calcium intakes could ameliorate the age-related increase in fat accumulation and its effect on type 2 diabetes. It could also be a compensatory dietary recommendation for the older adult that often becomes more sedentary with age. Physical activity influences calcium turnover through increases in calcium retention. Bedridden individuals tend to lose calcium, whereas the person who maintains a moderately active lifestyle optimizes his/her calcium retention.

PHOSPHORUS

Calcium and phosphorus are essential minerals that are usually considered together because the formation of bone and the uptake of calcium for this purpose is closely tied to an optimal ratio of calcium:phosphorus of 1:2–2:1.[39] However, phosphorus has other functions in addition to bone formation. Since bone formation was discussed in the preceding section concerning calcium, this section will present information about other aspects of the need for phosphorus.

Phosphorus is a member of Group V in the fourth period of the periodic table. It has an atomic number of 15 and an atomic weight of 31. There are no heavy isotopes but there are some useful radioisotopes. ^{32}P is the radioisotope most frequently used in biological systems. It has a short half-life (14.3 days).

Little free phosphorus is found in the living body.[58,59] Most phosphorus is in the form of phosphate PO_4^-. The phosphate ion has a central atom of phosphorus surrounded by four atoms of oxygen. At pH 7, hydrogen is joined to the phosphorus and oxygen to form HPO_4^-. At low pH, it is phosphoric acid, H_3PO_4. Other phosphates include H_3PO_4, H_2PO_{4-}, and PO_4^-. Phosphate in the free form is called inorganic phosphate with the abbreviation Pi. Phosphates are widely distributed in nature and, thus, a deficiency due to inadequate intake is highly unlikely. Soft drinks, processed foods, and foods of animal origin are excellent sources of phosphate. The usual intake of humans consuming a mixed diet is about 1 g/day for females and 1.5 g/day for males. Even though a deficiency is unlikely, a daily DRI very close to that of calcium is available as shown in Table 13.1. Symptoms of deficiency have been observed in premature infants fed a low phosphorus milk.[59,60] These symptoms include anorexia, muscle weakness, rickets, impaired growth, and bone pain. Adults consuming large amounts of aluminum oxide anti acids and a low phosphate diet can also develop some of these same symptoms.[60] Rickets, of course, is only seen in the young. There is a genetic disease (Fanconi Syndrome) related to phosphate deficiency carried on the X chromosome that phenotypes as phosphate deficiency. These symptoms can be ameliorated by phosphate supplements, and it is clear from the biochemical studies made using tissues from these patients that many of their symptoms are due to phosphate-related deficits in intermediary metabolism. The bone pain and poor skeletal growth and mineralization is due to a lack of phosphate and hence hydroxyapatite for deposition in the bone matrix. Phosphates are readily absorbed with little loss except that which is tightly bound in indigestible portions of food. Phytic acid, a hexose containing 6 phosphate groups, a component of some plant foods, can form insoluble salts with calcium, magnesium, and iron rendering these minerals unavailable for absorption. However, there is a phytase lower in the intestinal tract that will dephosphorylate phytic acid and when this happens these minerals are released. Usually this happens too far away from their absorption sites to be of benefit.

Phosphorus as phosphate is readily absorbed via an active saturable sodium-dependent mechanism. Calcitriol (active vitamin D) facilitates the absorption as it facilitates calcium uptake. Of the total body pool of phosphorus (~750 g), ~600 g is found in the bones and teeth. One gram is found in the extracellular compartment while the remainder (~150 g) is found within the cells. Urinary excretion is the route for excretion although up to 25% of the food phosphorus can appear in the feces. Renal conservation of phosphorus is the main mechanism for phosphorus homeostasis. Vitamin D, glucocorticoids, and growth hormone enhance, while estrogen, thyroid hormones, parathyroid hormones, and elevated plasma Ca^{++} levels inhibit renal phosphate conservation.

Function

A principal use for phosphorus is as the anion in hydroxyapatite used in bone mineralization. However, more important is the role of phosphate in intermediary metabolism. It is a crucial part of the genetic material DNA and RNA. It is a key component of the phospholipids, the phosphoproteins, the adenine nucleotides (ATP, ADP, AMP), the guanine nucleotides (GTP, GDP, GMP), and second messenger systems. As such it plays a critical role in all anabolic and catabolic pathways.

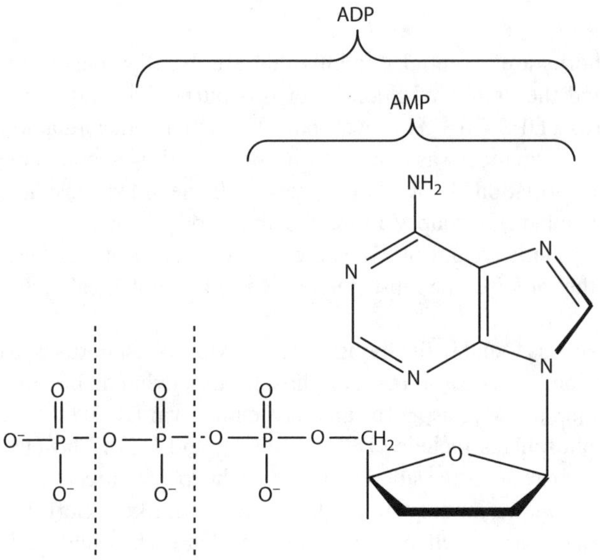

FIGURE 13.12 Structure of ATP. ADP has two phosphate groups while AMP has only one.

In the genetic material, the purine and pyrimidine bases are linked together by deoxyribose or ribose and phosphate groups (see Chapter 7 for structure). The phosphate groups serve as the links between the bases and because of the polarity of the phosphate group serve to stabilize the structure. The DNA polymer is very stable under nonenzymatic conditions. It owes its stability to the fact that the phosphate group can bind the bases yet still have sufficient polarity to retain a negative charge repelling other negatively charged molecules such as peroxides. Of course, the phosphate group is not the only negatively charged group in the DNA molecule. Hydrogen bonding leaves some atoms vulnerable to attack, but overall, the phosphate group is the important group when nonenzymatic degradation is considered.

The ATP molecule (Figure 13.12) is another important use of phosphate. The bonds that hold the phosphate groups to the ribose and thence to the adenine are called high-energy bonds represented by the symbol $\approx$. When broken, these bonds release about twice the energy of a normal bond. As such, ATP and its related high-energy compounds GTP and CTP are the keystones of energy transfer from one metabolite to another. A full discussion of ATP synthesis and degradation can be found in the section on energy in Chapter 1. The phosphorylation of intermediates in both catabolic and anabolic pathways is the important use of phosphate. Again because of its unique structure, it provides a necessary electronegative charge that in turn creates a vulnerable position in the molecule to which it is attached. For example, glucose could not be metabolized to pyruvate unless it was phosphorylated. The glucokinase (or hexokinase) using the high-energy phosphate group from ATP phosphorylates glucose at carbon #6. In so doing the molecule becomes somewhat unstable such that in the next few steps it can be rearranged to form fructose (a five-member ring) 6-phosphate. This structure now has a vulnerable carbon at position one and the next step is to attach another phosphate group at position 6. With two strong electronegative centers, one at each end of the molecule, this six-carbon structure can be split in half to two phosphorylated 3 carbon structures and on it goes. The phosphate group is reused over and over and in each use it provides a means for subsequent reactions in metabolism only to be discarded by the resultant metabolic product.

Use and reuse also applies to the role of phosphate in the structure and function of the membrane phospholipids. Phospholipids have both a lipophilic and a lipophobic portion in their structure. The lipophilic portion (see Figure 13.13) is the fatty acid portion while the phosphatidylated compounds provide the lipophobic portion. This structure is absolutely required for the functional attributes

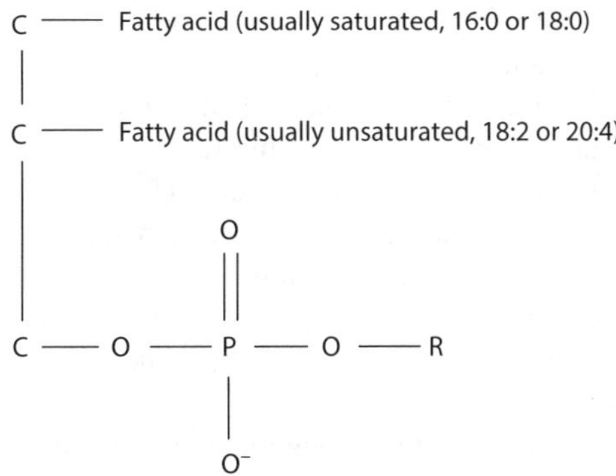

FIGURE 13.13 Structure of a phospholipid.

of the membranes. The membranes serve as geographical barriers around the cells and organelles. As such some materials are refused entry into the cell or organelle while other materials are either embedded in these phospholipids and held there or are allowed to pass into or out of the cell or organelle. Lipid-soluble materials can diffuse through the lipophilic portion of the phospholipid while lipophobic materials are excluded unless carried through by one of the embedded proteins. The charge contributed by the phosphate group in the phospholipid is what holds the proteins in place and that in turn functions to permit entry or exit of lipophobic metabolites and substrates. It should be noted, however, that highly charged metabolites such as the phosphorylated intermediates do not cross membranes. They are repelled by the phosphate group of the phospholipids.

From the aforementioned discussion of the function of phosphorus in living systems, it is easy to understand why phosphorus is so widely distributed in the food supply. Every living thing must have phosphorus in its cells or it would not survive. It is as essential to life as oxygen, carbon, and nitrogen.

MAGNESIUM

Magnesium is an alkaline earth metal with an atomic number of 12 and an atomic weight of 24. It is in group II of the third period of the periodic table. Magnesium has two naturally occurring isotopes, ^{25}Mg and ^{26}Mg, and seven radioisotopes. ^{28}Mg is the most commonly used radioisotope with a half-life of 21 h.

Magnesium is the most abundant divalent cation in living systems. As such its distribution in the food supply is broad. Both vegetables and meats are good sources of magnesium while milk and milk products are relatively poor sources of this mineral. Magnesium stabilizes mammalian membranes and in plants this mineral is ionically bound in the center of the chlorophyll molecule. In addition, magnesium is a cofactor in almost all phosphorylation reactions involving ATP. Because of the universality of its presence in the food supply, deficiency states are unlikely to develop in persons consuming a variety of foods.

Absorption, Metabolism, Excretion

Magnesium is absorbed by both passive diffusion and active transport. While there are two systems for Mg^{++} uptake, neither is particularly efficient. Between 30% and 70% of that consumed in food is absorbed. When food is supplemented with Mg^{++}, the percent absorbed falls. Thus, a meal containing 40 mg in food will result in 28 mg actually entering the enterocyte and appearing in the blood whereas in an enriched Mg^{++} containing meal (40 mg + a 920 mg magnesium salt) only 11%–14% will be absorbed, or 105–134 mg. The usual ~300 mg Mg^{++} intake has an apparent absorption of about 100 mg, a 33% efficiency.

Magnesium is recirculated via biliary secretion into the intestinal contents. The recirculated mineral can be reabsorbed, and in times of need, this reabsorption can be very efficient. If not reabsorbed, this magnesium will be excreted via the feces. The usual excretory route for absorbed magnesium is via urine. In fact, the renal absorption mechanism is the main means for regulating magnesium status. About 100 mg of magnesium is lost via the urine per day by normal adults consuming about 300 mg/day in the food. In times of need, magnesium reabsorption by the renal tubules will occur and urinary magnesium levels will fall. In the deficient state, the level will fall to zero as the deficiency proceeds.

After magnesium is absorbed, it circulates throughout the body; about 30%–35% of the circulating magnesium is protein bound while the remaining circulates as magnesium salts (13% as citrate or phosphate complexes) or as free magnesium (~55%). Magnesium is principally an intracellular ion occupying a central role in intermediary metabolism as described in the next section.

Function

More than 300 metabolic reactions require magnesium as a cofactor. The role of magnesium is one of forming a labile association with a substrate allowing the enzyme to complex with it and then once a product is formed the product, the magnesium and the enzyme separate for further use. This is illustrated in Figure 13.14.

Mg^{++} reduces the high negative charge of the substrate (usually ATP) by chelate formation with two phosphate groups (the β and γ P). The adenine ring is not involved. Actually the aforementioned reaction sequence occurs concurrent with the transfer of the liberated phosphate group to another substrate such as glucose. This coupled reaction sequence is facilitated by the enzyme hexokinase or glucokinase. Any kinase, however, will use this same reaction sequence as will a number of other reactions involving a cleavage of high-energy bond and the use of that energy to activate via attachment of a reactive electronegative group to a formerly inactive metabolic substrate or intermediate. Thus, in the instance of the phosphorylation or glucose, the coupled reaction is represented in Figure 13.15.

Some coupled reactions use more than one Mg^{++}. Enolase, for example, uses 4 Mg^{++}. The Mg^{++} ion binds to enolase activating it by keeping it in its active conformation. Magnesium is probably binding to the sulfur group of sulfur-containing amino acids in the enzyme structure, thus favoring the reaction by polarizing the P–O bonds. Conformational change likely explains the Mg^{++} in many of the enzymes in which it is a required cofactor for activation. In contrast, Mg^{++} can be an inhibitor; it can bind with tyrosyl residues. If these residues are part of the active site of an enzyme, then the

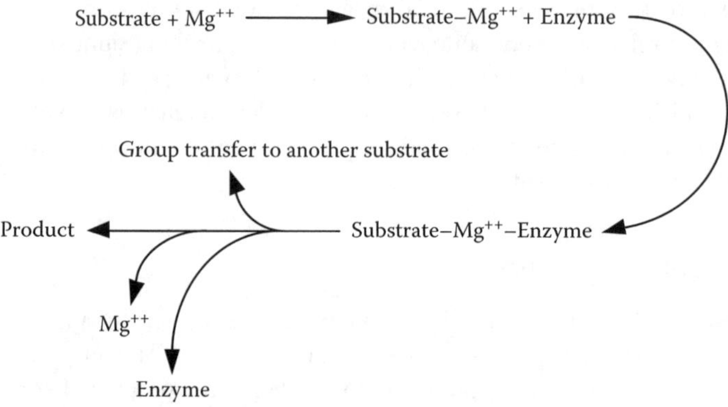

FIGURE 13.14 Use of magnesium as a cofactor in metabolic reactions.

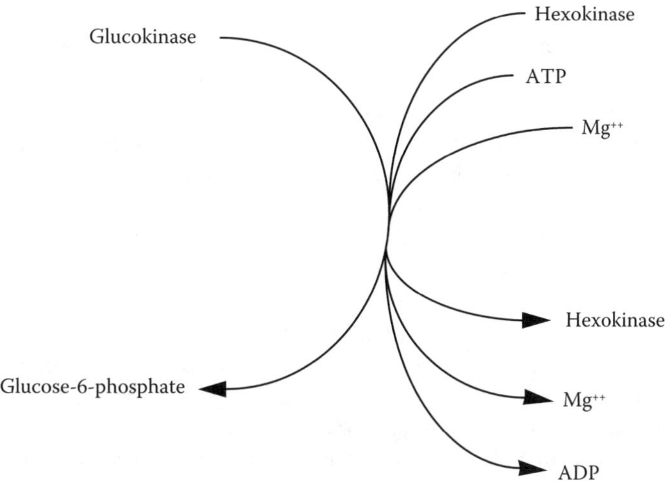

FIGURE 13.15 Example of the role of magnesium as a cofactor in the phosphorylation of glucose.

enzyme will be less active. Actually, the binding of Mg^{++} to the tyrosyl residue of albumin accounts for its transport in the blood. Much (32%) of the magnesium in the blood is carried by albumin.

Phospholipids form complexes with both Mg^{++} and Ca^{++}. These phospholipid complexes are integral parts of the various membranes in the cell (plasma membrane, endoplasmic reticulum, mitochondrial membrane, nuclear membrane). The degree to which these minerals are held by the membrane depends on the type of phospholipid in that membrane. The phospholipids are not uniformly distributed. The plasma membrane, for example, has very little cardiolipin while the mitochondrial membrane has very little phosphatidyl serine (see Chapter 10). Highly negative phospholipids will attract and bind more Ca^{++} and Mg^{++} than phospholipids having a lesser charge. In addition, Ca^{++}, due to its stronger 2^{++} charge, will be more attracted than will Mg^{++}. Nonetheless, the attraction of these minerals lends a stabilizing effect to an otherwise labile and mobile membrane constituent.

Bone accounts for 60%–65% of the total magnesium in the body. It is deposited in the bone matrix along with calcium phosphate as part of the mineral apatite. Hormones that affect calcium deposition and mobilization also affect magnesium deposition and mobilization.

Deficiency

Deficiency states have been produced in animals under stringent magnesium exclusion conditions. As early as 1926, mice were shown to develop magnesium deficiency using a magnesium-deficient diet. Cattle, and later rats, were also made deficient. The first clinical evidence in man appeared in 1934, and subsequent studies have shown that persons experiencing prolonged malabsorption, renal dysfunction or failure, alcoholism, and a number of endocrine disorders can become magnesium deficient.[36,61–65] Magnesium deficiency is characterized by very low blood levels of magnesium and neuromuscular symptoms such as muscle spasms, twitching, muscle fasciculations, tremor, personality changes, anorexia, nausea, and vomiting. Acutely deficient individuals may have convulsions and lapse into coma. In almost every instance of clinically evident magnesium deficiency, there has been a clinically important predisposing condition as cited earlier. Marginally deficient states have also been suggested in patients with normal serum or blood levels but depleted tissue levels of magnesium. In these patients, the symptoms are varied and may be difficult to assign magnesium deficiency as their cause unless tissue samples (muscle) are obtained and assayed. A positive magnesium balance of 1 mEq/kg can be demonstrated in such individuals. Persons at risk are those with diabetes, renal disease, or malabsorption syndrome, which in turn reduces magnesium conservation in the former and decreases magnesium absorption in the latter. Chronic ulcerative colitis and chronic granulomatous enteritis are the most common causes of the diarrhea of malabsorption syndrome. Other causes are gluten-induced enteropathy, celiac disease, and unrecognized lactose intolerance. Frequently, magnesium deficiency is accompanied by hypocalcemia. This appears to be due to a failure of bone to exchange calcium for magnesium. The osteoclast receptor for PTH loses its responsiveness to this hormone with the resultant loss in active bone resorption. This means that there is a failure in the system used to maintain blood calcium levels and also that magnesium is a key feature in the PTH-calcium regulatory pathway. Once magnesium is restored, the sensitivity of the osteoclast receptor to PTH is restored and the serum calcium returns to normal levels.

Magnesium deficiency also has effects on the vitamin D–calcium relationship. Vitamin D (1,25 dihydroxycholecalciferol) is not as active in promoting intestinal calcium uptake in the absence of magnesium. Even though neither ion is absorbed very efficiently, this efficiency is further reduced when one or the other is absent or in short supply. Both are poorly absorbed in vitamin D–deficient states because vitamin D mediates the uptake of both.

The use of mercurial or thiazide diuretics in the management of hypertension can result in excess magnesium loss. These diuretics interfere with renal magnesium conservation. They also enhance potassium loss as do some other drugs, that is, furosemide, ethacrynic acid, goutamicin, cabenicillin, cisplatin, and amphotericin B. Many of these drugs are cytotoxic drugs used in cancer chemotherapy and, as such, are used over a short time span. While minerals are lost through the use of these drugs, they can be replaced from the body store or through supplementation. Many physicians using these therapies may elect to supplement the patient's diet after the chemotherapeutic regimen is complete, anticipating that the cancer cell also needs magnesium. Chemotherapy consists of using highly toxic materials anticipating that the fast growing cancer cell will be more likely to take up the drug and die than will the normal cell. Part of the drug action is to interfere with cell replication, which, in turn, requires magnesium. If the cancer cell becomes magnesium deficient, then the drug will be a more effective chemotoxic agent.

Magnesium deficiency in rats has been shown to result in elevated blood lipids as well as proliferation of smooth muscle cells.[61–65] These responses are key elements in the atherogenic process, and it has been proposed that a relative magnesium deficiency in humans could pave the way for atherosclerosis or other degenerative diseases. However, other studies of alcoholism, renal disease, and various endocrinopathies have shown that these conditions must be in place prior to the development of magnesium deficiency. Thus, atherosclerosis could occur as a secondary complication of alcoholism or renal disease or diabetes, etc., and this secondary complication might develop as a result of an induced magnesium deficiency.

Need

As mentioned, magnesium is widely distributed in the food supply and thus a deficiency in an individual having access to a variety of foods is unlikely. Nonetheless, the Food and Nutrition Board of the National Academy of Sciences (www.nap.edu) has recommended intakes based on age and gender of 40–400 mg/day as detailed in Table 13.1.

SUMMARY

1. Minerals are divided into two groups based on the amounts needed on a daily basis. Included in the macromineral group are sodium, potassium, chloride, calcium, phosphorus, and magnesium.
2. All of the macrominerals can be found in the bones and teeth. Yet each has some very specific functions in the body aside from their incorporation in the skeleton.
3. Sodium is the chief extracellular ion; potassium is the chief intracellular ion.

4. Sodium intake is of concern in the development of hypertension; high sodium intakes are associated with increases in systolic pressure.
5. Sodium and potassium are important in the function of the sodium-potassium ATPase.
6. Calcium is a major player in cell signaling system and in the intracellular metabolic control.
7. Calcium homeostasis is controlled by vitamin D.
8. Phosphorus is a critical component of high-energy compounds such as ATP. It is also critical to the formation of membrane phospholipids and phorylated intermediates.
9. Magnesium is an important cofactor in phosphorylation reactions.

LEARNING OPPORTUNITIES

CASE STUDY 10.1 Aunt Tillie Is Getting Shorter

Aunt Tillie is 94 years old. She is mentally alert and emotionally stable. She has a problem however. As the years have passed, she has become shorter. Her niece, Nancy, noticed that whereas she used to be able to look Aunt Tillie in the eye, now she has to look down in order to meet Aunt Tillie's gaze. Aunt Tillie seems to have gotten frail as well. Concerned, Nancy took Aunt Tillie for a checkup. A DEXA scan showed that for her age, Aunt Tillie's bones were reasonably dense. No real evidence for osteoporosis. Analyze this situation. What can you conclude about Aunt Tillie's health and her bone structure? Why is her skeleton shrinking?

CASE STUDY 10.2 Mike Writhes on the Floor

Mike is a vigorous man, age 40, who enjoys the outdoors. He has a small horse farm and regularly works his horses. He is also a part-time builder performing small renovation jobs for his friends and neighbors. One day as he was drinking coffee with his neighbor, he suddenly bends over and cries out in pain. The pain is so intense he is soon on the floor writhing in agony. His neighbor calls 911, and Mike is rushed to the hospital. Pain relief is accomplished with some very heavy doses of medication and the doctors set about trying to find out the source of his pain.

Initially, Mike's pain began with a dull intermittent discomfort in his flank and in the lumbar region of his back. Then, it intensified across his abdomen as he was drinking coffee with his friend. It ran down the middle of his abdomen to his genitalia and to the inner aspect of his thigh. He began to sweat profusely, felt nauseous, and was faint. He teetered on the edge of shock. He felt the urge to urinate but very little urine was passed. By this time he was in the hospital and, with medication, the pain receded. A sample of urine was obtained. It was tinged with blood and there was evidence of albuminuria. An x-ray of his pelvic region was done but the shadows were inconclusive. Analyze this situation. What do you think is happening? If you were the clinical detective, how would you proceed?

CASE STUDY 10.3 Bertha Takes a Fall

Bertha is 75 years old. One day as she was walking to her kitchen she fell. She was able to summon help and was transported to the hospital. X-rays of her hip revealed a fracture. She had not tripped or slipped and was puzzled as to the reason for her fall. Bertha was not overweight and she had been fairly active for a woman of her age. Why did Bertha fall? What happened? Where does her physician go next?

MULTIPLE-CHOICE QUESTIONS

1. There are a number of ATPases in the body.
   a. They provide the energy for the transport of electrolytes across membranes
   b. ATP is an essential component of these complexes
   c. They facilitate the exchange of metabolites as well as electrolyte exchange
   d. All of the above
2. Aldosterone and ADH are
   a. Essential to the regulation of sodium balance
   b. Essential to the regulation of water balance
   c. Hormones
   d. All of the above
3. Hyponatraemia is
   a. Low levels of sodium in the blood
   b. High levels of sodium in the blood
   c. High levels of potassium in the blood
   d. Low levels of potassium in the blood
4. The DASH diet is useful in
   a. Reducing the energy intake
   b. Reducing the protein intake
   c. Reducing the sodium intake
   d. Increasing the sodium intake
5. Magnesium functions in
   a. ATP-related reactions
   b. Bone formation
   c. Nerve conduction
   d. Muscle strength

REFERENCES

1. Holland, O.B., Carr, B. (1993) Modulation of aldosterone synthase mRNA levels by dietary sodium and potassium and by adrenocorticotropin. *Endocrinology* 132: 2666–2673.
2. Feron, O., Salomone, S., Godfraind, T. (1995) Influence of salt loading on the cardiac and renal prepro-endothelin-1 mRNA expression in stroke-prone spontaneously hypertensive rats. *Biochem. Biophys. Res. Commun.* 209: 161–166.
3. Sun, B., Williams, J.S., Svetkey, L.P., Kolatkar, N.S., Conin, P.R. (2010) β_2-Adrenergic genotype affects the rennin-angiotensin-aldosterone system response to the dietary approaches to stop hypertension (DASH) dietary pattern. *Am. J. Clin. Nutr.* 92: 444–449.
4. Guenther, P.M., Lyon, J.M.G., Appel, L.J. (2013) Modeling dietary patterns to asses sodium recommendations for nutrient adequacy. *Am. J. Clin. Nutr.* 97: 842–847.
5. Veech, R.L. Kashiwaya, Y., Gates, D.N., King, M.T., Clarke, K. (2002) The energetics of ion distribution: The origin of the resting potential of cells. *IUBMB Life* 54: 241–252.
6. Bieri, J.G. (1977) Potassium requirement of the growing rat. *J. Nutr.* 107: 1394–1398.
7. Dow, S.W., Fettman, M.J., Smith, K.R., Hamar, D.W., Nagode, L.A., Refsal, K.R., Wilke, W.L. (1990) The effects of dietary acidification and potassium depletion on acid-base balance, mineral metabolism and renal function in adult cats. *J. Nutr.* 120: 569–578.
8. Mann, M.D., Bowie, M.D., Hansen, J.D.L. (1975) Total body potassium, acid-base status and serum electrolytes in acute diarrhoeal disease. *S. Afr. Med. J.* 49: 709–711.
9. McGill, C.R., Fulgoni, V.L., DiRenzo, D., Huth, P.J., Kurilich, A.C., Miller, G.D. (2008) Contribution of dairy products to dietary potassium intake in the United States population. *J. Am. Coll. Nutr.* 27: 44–50.
10. Simopoulos, A.P., Bartter, F.C. (1980) The metabolic consequences of chloride deficiency. *Nutr. Rev.* 38: 201–205.
11. Kays, S.M., Greger, J.L., Marcus, M.S.K., Lewis, N.M. (1991) Blood pressure, fluid compartments and utilization of chloride in rats fed various chloride diets. *J. Nutr.* 121: 330–337.

12. Berschneider, H.M., Knowles, M.R., Azizkhan, R.G., Boucher, R.C., Tobey, N.A., Orlando, R.C., Powell, D.W. (1988) Altered intestinal chloride transport in cystic fibrosis. *FASEB J.* 2: 2625–2629.
13. Liedtke, C.M. (1992) Electrolyte transport in the epithelium of pulmonary segments of normal and cystic fibrosis lung. *FASEB J.* 6: 3076–3084.
14. Quinton, P.M. (1990) Cystic fibrosis: A disease in electrolyte transport. *FASEB J.* 4: 2709–2717.
15. Valverde, M., Hardy, S.P., Sepulveda, F.V. (1995) Chloride channels: A state of flux. *FASEB J.* 9: 509–515.
16. Abraham, M.R., Jahangir, A., Alekseev, A.E., Terzic, A. (1999) Channelopathies of inwardly rectifying potassium channels. *FASEB J.* 13: 1901–1910.
17. Allen, L.H. (1982) Calcium bioavailability and absorption: A review. *Am. J. Clin. Nutr.* 35: 783–808.
18. DeGrazia, J.A., Ivanovich, P., Fellows, H., Rich, C. (1965) A double isotope method for measurement of intestinal absorption of calcium in man. *J. Lab. Clin. Med.* 66: 822–829.
19. Koo, J.O., Weaver, C.M., Neylan, M.J., Miller, G.D. (1993) Isotopic tracer techniques for assessing calcium absorption in rats. *J. Nutr. Biochem.* 4: 72–76.
20. Weaver, C.M. (1994) Age related calcium requirements due to changes in absorption and utilization. *J. Nutr.* 124: 1418S–1425S.
21. Hope, W.G., Bruns, M.E.H., Thomas, M.L. (1992) Regulation of duodenal insulin-like growth factor 1 and active calcium transport by ovariectomy in female rats. *Proc. Soc. Exp. Biol. Med.* 200: 528–535.
22. Hope, W.G., Ibarra, M.J., Thomas, M.L. (1992) Testosterone alters duodenal calcium transport and longitudinal bone growth rate in parallel in the male rat. *Proc. Soc. Exp. Biol. Med.* 200: 536–541.
23. DeLuca, H.F. (1988) The vitamin D story: A collaborative effort of basic science and clinical medicine. *FASEB J.* 2: 224–229.
24. Henry, H.L., Norman, A.W. (1984) Vitamin D: Metabolism and biological action. *Ann. Rev. Nutr.* 4: 493–520.
25. Walker, B.E., Schedl, H.P. (1979) Small intestinal calcium absorption in the rat with experimental diabetes. *Proc. Soc. Exp. Biol. Med.* 161: 149–152.
26. Bronner, F. (1984) Role of intestinal calcium absorption in plasma calcium regulation of the rat. *Am. J. Physiol.* 246: R680–R683.
27. Bronner, F., Peterlik, M. (Eds.) (1995) Proceedings of an international conference on progress in bone and mineral research. *J. Nutr.* 125 (Supplement): 1963S–2037S.
28. Garlid, K.D. (1994) Mitochondrial cation transport: A progress report. *J. Bioenerg. Biomembr.* 26: 537–542.
29. Gunter, K.K., Gunter, T.E. (1994) Transport of calcium by mitochondria. *Am. J. Physiol.* 267: C313–C339.
30. Foletti, D., Guerini, D., Carafoli, E. (1995) Subcellular targeting of the endoplasmic reticulum and plasma membrane. Ca^{++} pumps: A study using recombinant chimeras. *FASEB J.* 9: 670–680.
31. Sneyd, J., Keizer, J., Sanderson, M.J. (1995) Mechanisms of calcium oscillations and waves: A quantitative analysis. *FASEB J.* 9: 1463–1472.
32. Duflos, C., Bellaton, C., Baghdassarian, N., Gadoux, M., Pansu, D., Bronner, F. (1996) 1,25 dihydroxycholecalciferol regulates rat intestinal calbindin. D_{9k} posttranscriptionally. *J. Nutr.* 126: 834–841.33.
33. Wang, Y.-Z., Christakos, S. (1995) Retinoic acid regulates the expression of the calcium binding protein, calbindin D_{28k}. *Mol. Endocrinology* 9: 1510–1521.
34. Broess, M., Riva, A., Gerstenfeld, L.C. (1995) Inhibitory effects of $1{,}25(OH)_2$ vitamin D_3 on collagen type 1, osteopontin, and osteocalcin gene expression in chicken osteoblasts. *J. Cellular Biochem.* 57: 440–451.
35. Jaros, G.G., Belonje, P.C., van Hoorn-Hickman, R., Newman, E. (1984) Transient response of the calcium homeostatic system: Effect of calcitonin. *Am. J. Physiol.* 246: R693–R697.
36. Rivlin, R.S. (1994) Magnesium deficiency and alcohol intake: Mechanisms, clinical significance and possible relation to cancer development. *J. Am. Coll. Nutr.* 13: 416–423.
37. Hunziker, E.B., Herrmann, K.W., Schenk, R.K., Mueller, M., Moor, H. (1984) Cartilage ultrastructure after high pressure freezing, freeze substitution and low temperature embedding. 1. Chondrocyte ultrastructure-implications for the theories of mineralization and vascular invasion. *J. Cell. Biol.* 98: 267–276.
38. Bronner, F. (1994) Calcium and osteoporosis. *Am. J. Clin. Nutr.* 60: 831–836.
39. Anderson, J.B. (1991) Nutritional biochemistry of calcium and phosphorus. *J. Nutr. Biochem.* 2: 300–307.
40. Kasukawa,Y., Baylink, D.J., Wergedal, J.E., Amaar, Y., Srivastava, A.K., Guo, R., Mohan, S. (2003) Lack of insulin-like growth factor I exaggerates the effect of calcium deficiency on bone accretion in mice. *Endocrinology* 144: 4682–4689.

41. Mohan, S., Baylink, D.J. (2005) Impaired skeletal growth in mice with haploinsufficiency of IGF-I: genetic evidence that differences in IGF-I expression could contribute to peak bone mineral density differences. *J. Endocrinol.* 185: 415–420.
42. Biand, T., Glatz, Y., Bouillon, R., Froesch, E.R., Schmid, C. (1998) Effects of short term insulin-like growth factor-I (IGF-I) or growth hormone (GH) treatment on bone metabolism and on production of 1,25-dihydroxycholecalciferol in GH-deficient adults. *J. Clin. Endocrinol. Metab.* 83: 81–87.
43. Bygrave, F.L., Benedetti, A. (1993) Calcium: Its modulation in liver by cross-talk between the actions of glucagon and calcium mobilizing agonists. *Biochem. J.* 296: 1–14.
44. Bygrave, F.L., Roberts, H.R. (1995) Regulation of cellular calcium through signaling cross-talk in intricate interplay between the actions of receptors g-proteins and second messengers. *FASEB J.* 9: 1297–1303.
45. Farber, J.L. (1981) The role of calcium in cell death. *Life Sci.* 29: 1289–1295.
46. Fujita, T. (1992) Vitamin D in the treatment of osteoporosis. *Proc. Soc. Exp. Biol. Med.* 199: 394–399.
47. Walker, M.D., Novotny, R., Bilezikian, J.P., Weaver, C.M. (2008) Race and diet interactions in the acquisition, maintenance and loss of bone. *J. Nutr.* 138: 1256S–1260S.
48. Ayachi, S. (1979) Increased dietary calcium lowers blood pressure in the spontaneously hypertensive rat. *Metabolism* 28: 1234–1238.
49. Hamet, P. (1995) Evaluation of the scientific evidence for a relationship between calcium and hypertension. *J. Nutr.* 125 (Supplement): 311S–400S.
50. Caan, B., Newhouser, M., Aragaki, A., Lewis, C.B., Jackson, R., LeBoff, M.S., Margolis, K.L. et al. (2007) Calcium plus vitamin D supplementation and the risk of postmenopausal weight gain. *Arch Med.* 167: 893–902.
51. Lorenzen, J.K., Nielsen, S., Holst, J.J., Tetens, I., Rehfeld, J.F., Astrup, A. (2007) Effect of dairy calcium or supplementary calcium intake on postprandial fat metabolism, appetite, and subsequent energy intake. *Am. J. Clin. Nutr.* 85: 678–687.
52. Pereira, M.A., Jacobs, D.R., Van Horn, L., Slattery, M.L., Kartashov, A.I., Ludwig, D.S. (2002) Dairy consumption, obesity, and the insulin resistance syndrome in young adults. The CARDIA study. *JAMA* 287: 2081–2089.
53. Pittas, A.G., Lau, J., Hu, F.B., Dawson-Hughes, B. (2007) Review: The role of vitamin D and calcium in type 2 diabetes. A systematic review and meta-analysis. *J. Clin. Endocrinol. Metab.* 92: 2017–2029.
54. Zemel, M.B., Thompson, W., Milstead, A., Morris, K., Campbell, P. (2004) Calcium and dairy acceleration of weight and fat loss during energy restriction in obese adults. *Obes. Res.* 12: 582–590.
55. Zemel, M.B. (2003) Mechanisms of dairy modulation of adiposity. *J. Nutr.* 133: 252S–256S.
56. Zemel, M.B., Richards, J., Milsted, A., Campbell, P. (2005) Effects of calcium and dairy on body composition and weight loss in African-American adults. *Obes. Res.* 13: 1218–1225.
57. Sun, X., Zemel, M.B. (2004) Calcium and dairy products inhibit weight and fat regain during ad libitum consumption following energy restriction in AP2-agouti transgenic mice. *J. Nutr.* 134: 3054–3060.
58. Westheimer, F.H. (1987) Why nature chose phosphates. *Science* 235: 1173–1178.
59. Knochel, J.P. (1977) Pathophysiology and clinical characteristics of severe hypophosphatemia. *Arch. Intern. Med.* 137: 203–220.
60. Berner, Y.N., Shike, M. (1988) Consequences of phosphate imbalance. *Ann. Rev. Nutr.* 8: 121–148.
61. Bussiere, L., Mazur, A., Gueux, E., Rayssigiuer, Y. (1994) Hypertriglyceridemic serum from magnesium deficient rats induces proliferation and lipid accumulation in cultural vascular smooth muscle cells. *J. Nutr. Biochem.* 5: 585–590.
62. Corica, F., Ientile, R., Allegra, A., Romano, G., Cangemi, F., DiBenedetto, A., Buemi, M., Cucinotta, D., Ceruso, D. (1996) Magnesium levels in plasma, erythrocyte, and platelets in hypertensive and normotensive patients with type II diabetes mellitus. *Biol. Trace Element Res.* 51: 13–21.
63. Flink, E.B. (1981) Magnesium deficiency. Etiology and clinical spectrum. *Acta Med. Scand. Suppl.* 647: 125–137.
64. Rayssiguier, Y. (1981) Magnesium and lipid interrelationships in the pathogenesis of vascular diseases. *Magnesium Bull.* 12: 165–177.
65. Robeson, B.L., Martin, W.G., Freedman, M.H. (1980) A biochemical and ultrastructural study of skeletal muscle from rats fed a magnesium deficient diet. *J. Nutr.* 110: 2078–2084.

14 Trace Minerals

In addition to the minerals already described as members of the macromineral class of nutrients, there are two groups of minerals needed in far smaller amounts.[1,2] These groups fall into the general class of microminerals. One of these is the trace mineral group that includes iron, copper, and zinc, while the other group, the ultra trace minerals, includes chromium, manganese, fluoride, iodide, cobalt, selenium, silicon, arsenic, boron, vanadium, nickel, cadmium, lithium, lead, and molybdenum. Dietary reference intakes (DRIs) or suggested adequate intakes (AIs) have been made for iron, zinc, iodide, chromium, fluoride, selenium, manganese, and molybdenum (www.nap.edu). With some of these minerals, there are recommendations for intakes for some of the population groups but not for all. There are insufficient data for intake recommendations for silicone, sulfate, vanadium, potassium, arsenic, and chromium. Table 14.1 gives the recommended intakes (in bold type) and suggested AIs (indicated by an asterisk). For some of the minerals, an excess intake could be toxic. For these minerals, an upper intake limit has been set that defines the upper intake at which no adverse effects would be expected. Thus, the National Academy of Sciences, Food and Nutrition Board has developed a table of tolerable upper limits (TUL or UL). These are shown in Table 14.2. Tolerable upper limits also exist for nonmineral nutrients as discussed in earlier chapters.

Figures in bold type are the DRIs while figures followed by an asterisk are those of AIs. The latter are extrapolated figures and are based on observed or experimentally determined approximations or estimates of nutrient intake by a group (or groups) of apparently healthy people that are assumed to be adequate. These figures are used when the DRIs cannot be determined directly. For further information, see http://www.nap.edu.

ESSENTIAL MICROMINERALS

The definition of essentiality for the trace and ultra trace minerals is different from that used for amino acids, vitamins, and essential fatty acids. That difference is due to the problem of not having clear, incontrovertible evidence of the essentiality of each of these minerals compared with that published for the other nutrients.[2] A mineral is thought to be essential if its lack adversely affects an essential biological function that can be reversed by the replacement of that mineral in the diet. A mineral is also considered essential if its lack interrupts an essential phase of the life cycle, for example, the completion of a normal pregnancy. The latter definition has been disputed, however, because not all trace minerals with a defined biochemical function interfere with the completion of a normal pregnancy. Lastly, some of the trace minerals become essential only when there is some other disturbance in the normal physiology of the individual. In these instances, there might be genetic diseases that interfere with the absorption or transport of a given mineral or there might be some disease that interferes with the use of that mineral. An example of the latter is seen in pernicious anemia. In this disease, the individual lacks the intrinsic factor needed for the absorption of vitamin B_{12}. Cobalt is an essential component of this vitamin and constitutes 4% of its molecular weight. If the vitamin is not absorbed, then cobalt is not absorbed.

In addition, there may be temporary changes in micronutrient status as part of a systemic inflammatory response. When the inflammatory response is suppressed, micronutrient status is normalized.[3] Plasma zinc, copper, and selenium levels have been determined in subjects with an acute

TABLE 14.1
Daily DRIs for Iron, Zinc, Iodide, Selenium, Chromium, Copper, Fluoride, Manganese, and Molybdenum

		DRI								
Group	**Age**	**Iron (mg)**	**Zinc (mg)**	**Iodide (μg)**	**Selenium (μg)**	**Chromium (μg)**	**Copper (μg)**	**Fluoride (mg)**	**Manganese (mg)**	**Molybdenum (μg)**
Infants	0–6 months	0.27*	2*	110*	15*	0.2*	200*	0.01*	0.003*	2*
	7–12 months	**11**	**3**	130*	20*	5.5*	220*	0.5*	0.6*	3*
Children	1–3 years	**7**	**3**	**90**	**20**	11*	**340**	0.7*	1.2*	**17**
	4–8 years	**10**	**5**	**90**	**30**	15*	**440**	1.0*	1.5*	**22**
Males	9–13 years	**8**	**8**	**120**	**40**	25*	**700**	2.0*	1.9*	**34**
	14–18 years	**11**	**11**	**150**	**55**	35*	**890**	3.0*	2.2*	**43**
	19–30 years	**8**	**11**	**150**	**55**	35*	**900**	4.0*	2.3*	**45**
	31–50 years	**8**	**11**	**150**	**55**	30*	**900**	4.0*	2.3*	**45**
	50–70 years	**8**	**11**	**150**	**55**	30*	**900**	4.0*	2.3*	**45**
	70 + years	**8**	**11**	**150**	**55**	30*	**900**	4.0*	2.3*	**45**
Females	9–13 years	**8**	**8**	**120**	**40**	21*	**700**	2.0*	1.6*	**34**
	14–18 years	**15**	**9**	**150**	**55**	24*	**890**	3.0*	1.6*	**43**
	19–30 years	**18**	**8**	**150**	**55**	25*	**900**	3.0*	1.8*	**45**
	31–50 years	**18**	**8**	**150**	**55**	20*	**900**	3.0*	1.8*	**45**
	51–70 years	**8**	**8**	**150**	**55**	20*	**900**	3.0*	1.8*	**45**
	70 + years	**8**	**8**	**150**	**55**	29*	**1000**	3.0*	2.0*	**50**
Pregnancy	14–18 years	**27**	**12**	**220**	**60**	30*	**1000**	3.0*	2.0*	**50**
	19–30 years	**27**	**11**	**220**	**60**	30*	**1000**	3.0*	2.0*	**50**
	31–50 years	**27**	**11**	**220**	**60**	44*	**1300**	3.0*	2.6*	**50**
Lactation	14–18 years	**10**	**13**	**290**	**70**	45*	**1300**	3.0*	2.6*	**50**
	19–30 years	**9**	**12**	**290**	**70**	45*	**1300**	3.0*	2.6*	**50**
	31–50 years	**9**	**12**	**290**	**70**					

TABLE 14.2
Daily Tolerable Upper Limits of Copper, Fluoride, Iodide, Iron, and Magnesium

Group	Copper (μg)	Fluoride (mg)	Iodide (μg)	Iron (mg)	Magnesium (mg)
Infants					
0–6 months	ND	0.7	ND	40	ND
7–12 months	ND	0.9	ND	40	ND
Children					
1–3 years	1,000	1.3	200	40	65
4–8 years	3,000	2.2	300	40	110
Males and females					
9–13 years	5,000	10	600	40	350
14–18 years	8,000	10	900	45	350
19–70 years	10,000	10	1100	45	350
70 + years	10,000	10	1100	45	350
Pregnancy					
14–18 years	8,000	10	900	45	350
19–50 years	10,000	10	1100	45	350
Lactation					
14–18 years	8,000	10	900	45	350
19–50 years	10,000	10	1100	45	350

Source: www.nap.edu.

inflammatory response. Levels of vitamins A and E, pyridoxine, ascorbic acid, and vitamin D were also examined. Except for copper and vitamin E, the plasma levels of these micronutrients declined with increasing severity of the inflammatory response and these levels were reversed once the response was reversed.

Almost all of the trace and ultra trace minerals can be found in the bones and teeth. These minerals are deposited in the organic matrix of these structures along with calcium phosphate. Bone mineralization (the formation of the bone apatite) involves many of the trace and ultra trace minerals known to be consumed by man and other animals. These minerals can be mobilized from the bones, but the extent of this mobilization is variable. To a large degree, the mobilization of the trace elements is very slow. This results in a long residence time in the bones and teeth and a long half-life. When coupled with a low absorption efficiency,[4] this long residence time is part of a system designed to protect the body from excess mineral exposure: mineral toxicity. For many of the trace elements, their discovery as essential nutrients was preceded by their recognition as toxic elements. A summary of the functions of the trace and ultra trace minerals is provided in Table 14.3.

TRACE MINERAL TOXICITY

Excess exposure to many of the essential minerals, whether it be via inhalation, absorption through the skin, or ingestion with food or drink, can elicit a toxic response. Some of the essential minerals can be toxic if subjects are exposed to high quantities. As indicated in Table 14.2, there are tolerable upper limits to these minerals that if exceeded, might elicit an undesirable set of symptoms. There are other minerals whose essentiality for man has yet to be proven. Some of these have been shown to be needed by other species. As with the essential minerals, excess exposure can elicit an adverse (toxic) response. Minerals in this category include arsenic, vanadium, nickel, silicone, tin,

TABLE 14.3
Trace Elements and Key Features of Their Use

Micromineral	Function	Remarks
Trace minerals		
Copper	Essential cofactor for a variety of enzymes involved in iron use, collagen synthesis, and antioxidants.	Wilson's disease results from excess intake.
Iron	Essential for hemoglobin synthesis, cytochrome activity, urea cycle activity, lipogenesis, and cholesterogenesis.	Hemochromatosis results from excess intake. Anemia is the major sign of inadequate intake.
Zinc	Essential to the function of over 70 enzymes; important to activity of DNA and RNA polymerase; essential to zinc finger proteins need for gene expression.	Poor growth in children with renal disease due to excess zinc loss during dialysis. Deficiency may occur with the use of diuretics. Zinc loss is increased in traumatized patients.
Ultra trace minerals		
Arsenic	Needed for growth and optimal iron use.	Toxic; well-known metabolic poison.
Chromium	Needed for optimal action of insulin at target tissue.	Widely dispersed in a variety of foods. Brewer's yeast and beer are good sources. Deficiency is unlikely.
Cobalt	Important component of vitamin B_{12}; deficiency symptoms are those of B_{12} deficiency.	Large excess intake can block iron absorption.
Fluorine	Increases the hardness of bones and teeth, activates adenylate cyclase.	Fluorosis (mottling of teeth) results from excess intake.
Iodine	Needed for thyroid hormone synthesis.	Goiter and cretinism result from inadequate intake.
Manganese	Cofactor in a wide variety of enzymes; essential to reactions using ATP or UTP.	Widely distributed throughout the body. Deficiency is unlikely.
Molybdenum	Activates adenylate cyclase; cofactor in sulfite oxidase and xanthine oxidase.	Widely distributed in the food supply. Deficiency is unlikely.
Nickel	The need for this element has not been shown for humans.	Widely distributed in the food supply. Deficiency is unlikely.
Selenium	Essential to glutathione peroxidase and thyroxine deiodinase.	Toxicity and need are influenced by environmental factors.
Silicon	The need for this element has not been shown for humans but has been shown for animals.	Widely distributed in the food supply. Deficiency is unlikely.
Vanadium	The need for this element has not been shown for humans but has been shown for animals.	Widely distributed in the food supply. Deficiency is unlikely.

aluminum, boron, cadmium, lead, germanium, lithium, asbestos, mercury, and rubidium. Mercury, used in the silver amalgam of tooth fillings, has been identified as a toxic element.[5] It has been found in fish such as those at the top of the marine food chain, for example, tuna, swordfish, and shark. When consumed or released from tooth amalgam fillings, it is sequestered in the bone, brain, and kidney. If the individual is pregnant, the mercury crosses the placental barrier and can be found in the fetal liver and kidney. Mercury is usually excreted through the kidneys and urinary mercury can be used as an index of exposure.

With most minerals, the first line of defense against food-borne mineral toxicity is that offered by the gastrointestinal system: vomiting and diarrhea. Through vomiting, contaminated food is expelled. Through diarrhea, malabsorption as well as excretion of recirculated (via bile) mineral is facilitated, reducing the intestinal exposure and subsequent uptake of the mineral. Failing to ablate the toxic state, the kidney tubules will attempt to reduce the body load and some minerals are excreted in the urine. However, some minerals, that is, copper, iron, zinc, and lead, are not as subject to renal filtration as are other minerals, that is, selenium, magnesium, calcium, molybdenum, and mercury.[5–15] Reduction of the body load that is in circulation then is accomplished by depositing the excess mineral in the bones. Bone mineral content has been used to document cases of suspected toxicity. Accidental or intentional poisoning can sometimes be masked by other nonspecific symptoms, but bone analysis can provide the documentation needed to support or deny a supposition of toxicity.

To a lesser extent, hair analysis together with blood analysis can reveal the mineral status of an individual. The difficulty in using these analyses is that the mineral content can be transient.[16] That is, blood levels of trace minerals represent the immediate mineral intake rather than long-term exposure, whereas hair mineral content can represent not only food or drink mineral but also airborne mineral. Hair mineral can be contaminated by shampoos and other hair treatments.

The adverse effects of trace minerals are as diverse as the minerals themselves. Each mineral has its preferred target in the body. For some, the target is DNA.[9,17–19] Certain minerals (copper, arsenic, nickel, chromium) bind to DNA. The binding is a covalent one and produces either a nonfunctional DNA or a DNA that cannot repair itself. Evidence of this cross-linking has been demonstrated in vitro using a variety of cell types. Chinese hamster cells have been used to show copper-, chromium-,[20] arsenic-, and nickel-induced DNA cross-linking in human fibroblasts and epithelial cells.[17,21]

The concept of chemically induced cross-linkage of DNA as a factor in carcinogenesis has been proposed to explain the role of asbestos and the development of mesothelioma. Mesothelioma is a malignant growth within the pleural and peritoneal cavities. These tumors are stimulated to grow by the presence of asbestos fibers that act as artificial linkers of DNA, resulting in mutations within the pleural and peritoneal cells. Changes in the CDKN2 (p16) gene seem to be involved. This gene is either lost or mutated. Its gene product is a regulator of the phosphorylation of protein 105, a tumor suppresser. Unphosphorylated p105 can inhibit passage from G1 to S phase of the cell cycle, whereas phosphorylated 105 permits this passage. Passage inhibition is a common feature of cancer cell initiation. Thus, any substance that interferes with this passage could be regarded as a carcinogen. Minerals in excess can have this effect and excess intakes of some have been linked with certain forms of cancer. Iron, for example, has been linked to colon cancer.[8] The mechanism whereby excess iron has its effect is far from clear. It may induce DNA cross-linking as described earlier, but it may also act as an ion that stimulates free radical formation and attacks cells and their DNA, causing them to mutate. In either scenario, excess iron and colon cancer are associated.

ANTAGONISMS AND INTERACTIONS AMONG TRACE MINERALS

No general discussion of trace minerals would be complete without mention of mineral interactions. Numerous antagonisms and synergisms have been reported. This should be expected as one realizes that many of the trace minerals have more than one charged state and that living cells have preferences with respect to these states. For example, the uptake of iron is much greater when the iron is in the ferrous (+2) state than when in the ferric (+3) state. Minerals that keep iron in the ferric state will interfere with its absorption and use. Minerals that do the reverse will enhance iron uptake. Such is the beneficial action of copper on iron. The cuprous ion keeps the ferrous ion from losing electrons, becoming the ferric ion. In addition, there is an interaction among nickel, copper, and iron[22] and between nickel and copper[23] and between zinc and copper.[24] These interactions make it difficult to assess the relative need for each of these minerals. Nickel supplementation accentuates copper deficiency, and this effect is influenced by iron. In the ruminant, the potency of molybdenum as a copper antagonist depends on an adequate supply of sulfur.[19] Tin, copper, iron, zinc, and calcium also interact, affecting the needs for each.[22–26] Copper and zinc mutually antagonize each other with respect to their absorption.[26] Iron transporters are differentially regulated by dietary iron, and this in turn is associated with changes in manganese metabolism.[27] The interactions of essential minerals are best illustrated in Figure 14.1. To the nutrition scientist seeking to design a purified diet providing all the known nutrients in needed amounts, these mineral interactions can be quite a problem. Sometimes the so-called purified ingredients contain (or fail to contain) minerals unknown to the producer or user. This is especially a problem in the protein portion of the diet. Proteins can bind

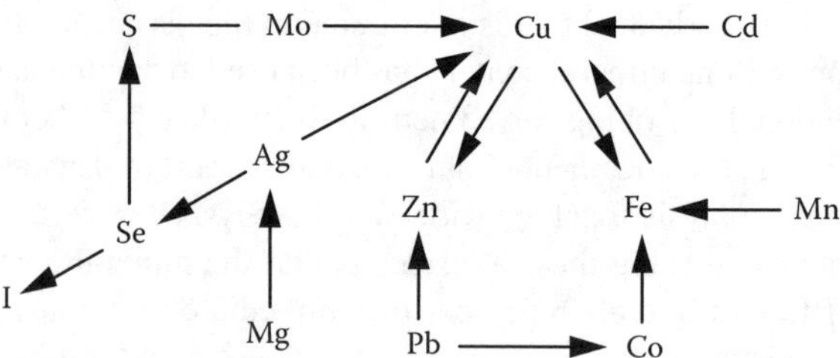

FIGURE 14.1 Trace mineral interactions.

minerals (as described in each of the sections on each of the minerals), and these minerals are found in the proteins. Soybean protein can contain phytate-bound phosphorus and magnesium; casein and lactalbumin, depending on origin, contain variable amounts of calcium, magnesium, and selenium. Unless the investigator determines the mineral content of the diet ingredients before using them, there is the possibility that an unexpected mineral imbalance could occur and this imbalance could affect the outcome of the experiment. The specifics of these imbalances and interactions will be detailed as each of the trace and ultra trace minerals is discussed.

IRON

Iron, element 26 in the periodic table, is the fourth most prevalent mineral in the earth's crust. Neolithic man learned to mine iron and forge tools from it. The Romans used iron preparations as tonics, but the clinical recognition of iron as an essential nutrient was not accomplished until the seventeenth century.[28] Sydenham was the first to propose that chlorosis (a sickness in adolescent females characterized by a pale skin color) was due to iron deficiency anemia. He showed that iron salts were an effective treatment.

In 1713, Remmery and Jeffrey demonstrated the presence of iron in the mineral matter of blood, and in 1852, Funke showed that this mineral was contained by the red cell.[28] Thus, it was learned that iron and red cell number were related and that the red cell function of carrying oxygen depended on its hemoglobin content.

Iron is present in a variety of inorganic salts in the environment. It exists mainly in a trivalent form as ferric oxide or hydroxide or its polymers. Absorption of these salts is very limited unless they can be dissolved and ionized by the intestinal contents. Both ferric and ferrous salts are present in the diet, but only the ferrous salts are absorbed from the gastrointestinal tract. Ferric compounds must be reduced in order to be absorbed. This is accomplished in the stomach by the low pH of the gastric juice.

The availability of iron from food depends on its source.[29–32] Soybean protein, for example, contains an inhibitor of iron uptake. Diets such as those in Asia contain numerous soybean products, and iron absorption is adversely affected. Tannins, phytates, certain fibers (not cellulose), carbonates, phosphates, and low-protein diets also adversely affect the apparent absorption of iron. In contrast, ascorbic acid, fructose, citric acid, high-protein foods, lysine, histidine, cysteine, methionine, and natural chelates, that is, heme, all enhance the apparent absorption of iron. Zinc and manganese reduce iron uptake by about 30%–50% and 10%–40%, respectively. Excess iron reduces zinc uptakes by 13%–22%. Stearic acid, one of the main fatty acids in meat, enhances iron uptake.

In foods, as well as in animal tissues, iron is present in a variety of metalloproteins that include hemoglobin, myoglobin, the cytochromes, transferrin, ferritin, hepcidin, and a variety of other iron-binding proteins.[33] In the heme proteins, iron is coordinated within a tetraporphyrin moiety, which, in turn, is bound to a polypeptide chain. Hemoglobin is a tetramer with a molecular weight of 64,500 and contains two α-subunits and two β-subunits, which gives the protein allosteric properties in the uptake and release of oxygen. Each polypeptide subunit contains 1 atom of ferrous iron, which amounts to 0.34% of the protein by weight.

Absorption, Metabolism, Excretion

Iron uptake by the gut, iron use and reuse, and iron loss are components of an essentially closed system.[33,34] The gain through the gut is very inefficient, and there is virtually no mechanism aside from blood loss that rids the body of iron intake excess. This system is shown in Figure 14.2. The total iron content of the body averages 4.0 g in men and 2.6 g in women. As shown in Table 14.4, there are two groups of iron-containing compounds that are considered essential to life.

Hemoglobin is the most abundant and easily sampled of the heme proteins and accounts for greater than 65% of body iron. The second group of molecules are those involved in iron transport (transferrin) and storage (ferritin, hemosiderin).[34] In addition, there are a number of enzymes whose active sites have an iron–sulfur center.

Transferrin is the iron-transport protein that carries the ferric iron between the sites of its absorption, storage, and utilization. It is a β-glycoprotein, MW 76,000, which binds two atoms of ferric iron per mole. Iron is transferred from the intestinal mucosa to transferrin and is carried through the blood to peripheral tissues containing receptor sites for transferrin. Transferrin is synthesized in the liver, brain, and testes, as well as other tissues. The regulation of the gene for transferrin varies from

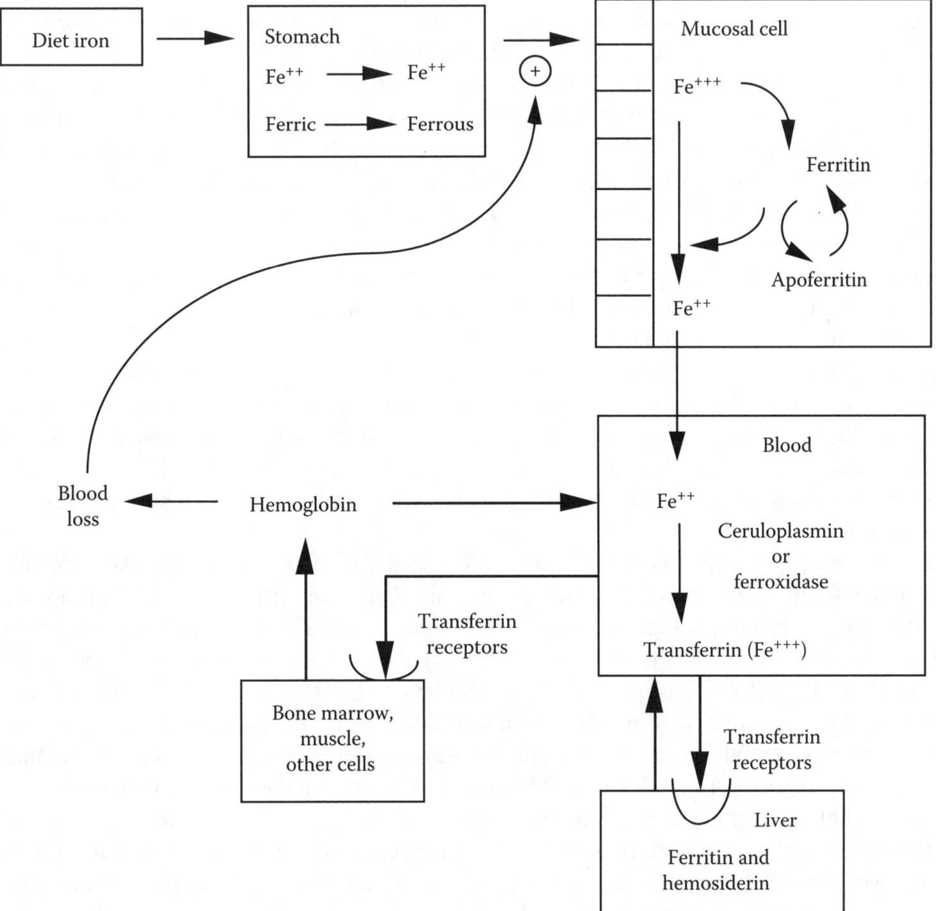

FIGURE 14.2 Overview of iron uptake and use. This is an apparently closed system with the recycling and conservation of iron absorbed from the gut.

TABLE 14.4
Body Content of Iron

Types of Iron	Male 70 kg	Female 60 kg
Essential iron	3.100 g	2.100 g
Hemoglobin	2.700	1.800
Myoglobin, cytochromes, and other enzymes	0.400	0.300
Storage and transport iron	0.900	0.500
Ferritin, hemosiderin	0.897	0.497
Transferrin	0.003	0.003
Total iron	4.000	2.600

cell type to cell type and each cell type has its own array of promoters and transcription factors that control the amount of transferrin synthesized. The amount of transferrin synthesized is inversely related to the iron supply. In times of low intake, more transferrin is produced so as to optimize iron uptake.[35,36]

Once iron enters the cell, it is chelated to a protein called ferritin. The enzyme that catalyzes this chelation is called ferrochelatase. This reaction then represents the ultimate destination for the majority of the iron that enters the cell. Chelation of iron to its storage protein occurs at the outer aspect of the mitochondrial membrane. Ferritin has a molecular weight of 450,000. It is composed of 24 subunits, which form an outer shell within which there is a storage cavity for polynuclear hydrous ferric oxide phosphate. Its synthesis is highly regulated at the level of translation by the ferric atom[37–39] and posttranscriptionally by a cytoplasmic protein called the iron regulatory protein.[40] When iron is present, the mRNA is available for translation. In the absence of iron, the mRNA folds up on itself such that the start site for translation is covered up. Over 30% of the weight of ferritin may be iron. It is present in the liver, gut, reticuloendothelial cells, and bone marrow. Hemosiderin is a form of denatured ferritin that contains about one-third of the iron stores. The posttranscriptional regulation of ferritin synthesis is regarded as a protective mechanism when excess iron is present. In this situation, the iron regulatory protein binds to the iron-responsive element in the ferritin mRNA decreasing ferritin synthesis. When the iron-responsive protein dissociates from the iron-responsive element, ferritin synthesis resumes. Aconitase, an enzyme that catalyzes the dehydrogenation of citrate to α-ketoglutarate, has been found to serve as an iron regulatory protein.[41] Ferritin also serves as a zinc detoxicant and a zinc ion donor.[42] This is important in instances where a zinc overload has occurred.

The hormone, hepcidin, has emerged as the key to the regulation of iron balance. When elevated, it serves to increase iron in macrophages and decrease gastrointestinal iron uptake.[43,44] The synthesis of hepcidin is induced by infection, inflammation, and elevated iron intake. Lower levels of hepcidin are associated with anemia, hypoxia, iron deficiency, and hereditary hemochromatosis. Hepcidin mRNA falls quickly after blood loss.[44] In response to inflammation, IL6 levels rise followed by rises in hepcidin.[43] Hepcidin inhibits iron release by the macrophages, and this inhibition results in a fall in serum iron. The export of iron from enterocytes and macrophages is mediated by ferroportin. Hepcidin acts by binding ferroportin on the plasma membranes, causing it to be internalized and degraded. This increases enterocyte iron that eventually passes this iron into the lumen of the gastrointestinal tract. Hepcidin deficiency seems to be the basis for hemochromatosis. Plasma hepcidin is a modest predictor of dietary iron bioavailability in humans, whereas oral iron loading, measured by stable-isotope appearance curves, increases plasma hepcidin.[45] While hepcidin predicts dietary iron availability, it also predicts the interindividual variability in iron absorption.[46–49]

Other Iron-Containing Compounds

The cytochromes are enzymes involved in the electron transport system that is located principally in the mitochondria. Cytochrome P-450, a specialized cytochrome, is used to oxidize organic compounds. This cytochrome is located in the endoplasmic reticulum. While the cytochrome P-450 enzymes are active in the detoxification of drugs and chemicals, these enzymes also activate carcinogens. The cytochrome P-450I has this function while P-450IIE has a propensity to form oxygen radicals that are both cytotoxic and carcinogenic.[50] Other cytochromes generate oxygen radicals by futile cycling. In some respects, the ability to generate peroxides has a protective effect in that peroxides will kill invading pathogens. Peroxide formation is in fact the first line of defense against such an invasion. Other enzymes in which iron is not bound to heme include iron sulfur proteins, metalloflavoproteins, and certain glycolytic enzymes.

The lifetime of a red cell is about 120 days in humans. The red cell contains the iron-containing hemoglobin. The flow of iron through the plasma space amounts to about 25–30 mg/day in the adult (about 0.5 mg/kg body weight).[48,51] This amount of iron corresponds to the degradation of about 1% of the circulating hemoglobin mass per day. Iron is conserved in the body in males and postmenopausal females to a greater degree than in growing children and menstruating women; only 10% of the iron in the body is lost per year in normal men.[48] This amounts to about 1 mg/day. This loss of 1 mg/day has to be made up by absorption of iron from the diet, which is only about 10% efficient, requiring about 10 mg of dietary iron/day. In menstruating females, the loss is increased to 2 mg/day, which means that the intake and absorption of iron must be increased or these females will develop iron deficiency.

In contrast to the turnover of hemoglobin in the red cell, tissue iron compounds, which include the cytochrome enzymes and a variety of other nonheme enzymes, are heterogeneous in respect to lifespan. Furthermore, these compounds are subject to degradation at exponential rates similar to the rate of turnover of the subcellular organelle with which they are associated. For example, in rats, mitochondrial cytochrome C has a half-life of about 6 days, whereas hemoglobin has a half-life of about 63 days.

The apparent absorption of iron, that is, the amount absorbed from food, can vary from less than 1% to more than 50%. The percentage that is absorbed depends on the nature of the diet, on the type of iron compound in the diet, and on regulatory mechanisms in the intestinal mucosa that reflect the body's physiological need for iron.

Two types of iron are present in the food: heme iron, which is found principally in animal products, and nonheme iron, which is inorganic iron bound to various proteins in plants. Most of the iron in the diet, usually greater than 85%, is present in the nonheme form. The absorption of nonheme iron is strongly influenced by its solubility in the upper part of the intestine. Absorption of nonheme iron depends on the composition of the meal and is subject to enhancers of absorption such as animal protein and by reducing agents such as vitamin C. On the other hand, heme iron is absorbed more efficiently. It is not subject to these enhancers. Although heme iron accounts for a smaller proportion of iron in the diet, it provides quantitatively more iron to the body than dietary nonheme iron.

The regulation of iron entry into the body takes place in the mucosal cells of the small intestine. Its iron gate is very sensitive to the iron stores, so if the iron stores are low, which is true for many women[47] and children, the intestinal mucosa takes up iron and increases the proportion absorbed from the diet. On the other hand, if the body is replete with iron, as is typical of healthy men[48] and postmenopausal women, then the percentage of iron absorbed is low. This mechanism offers some protection against iron overload. In infancy, lactoferrin, an iron-binding protein in human milk, promotes the absorption of iron through lactoferrin receptors on the surface of the intestinal mucosa of infants. This may explain why iron is well absorbed from human milk. Milk is not usually considered a good source of iron, but for the breastfed infant, this lactoferrin-iron mechanism prevents deficiency from developing. As the infant matures, however, this mechanism becomes inadequate.

On the average, only about 10% of dietary iron is absorbed. In order to be absorbed, the iron must be in the ferrous state. Upon entry into the enterocyte, it is incorporated (in part) into ferritin in which the iron is in the ferric state. When the iron is transported from the mucosal to the serosal side of the enterocyte, it is transported in the ferrous state, probably bound to cytoplasmic proteins. The iron transporters play an important role here. Hepcidin decreases iron transporter expression in several cell types, including intestinal cells.[49] Hepcidin is thought to control iron metabolism by interacting with the iron efflux transporter, ferroportin. In macrophages, hepcidin directly regulates ferroportin gene expression. Intestinal enterocytes have significantly less ferroportin when hepcidin levels are elevated.[49] This suggests that hepcidin regulates iron release from the enterocytes. When the iron is pumped out of the enterocyte, it must be oxidized to the ferric state in order to bind to transferrin. This is accomplished by ceruloplasmin (MW 160,000), which contains eight copper ions in the divalent state. Ceruloplasmin copper is reduced by the iron, resulting in the formation of cuprous ions in ceruloplasmin and ferric iron in transferrin. As mentioned earlier, transferrin is recognized in the periphery by cells that have transferrin receptors. The transferrin receptors vary, depending on the tissue and the condition. Tissues such as erythroid precursors, placenta and liver that have a large number of transferrin receptors, have a proportionately high uptake of iron. When these cells are in an iron-rich environment, the number of receptors decreases and conversely, when they are in an iron-poor environment, the number of receptors increases. The up- and down-regulation of transferrin receptors is accomplished at the level of transcription.[37,38] Measurements of messenger RNA for the transferrin receptors indicate that there can be as much as a 20-fold change in messenger RNA and, presumably, as much as a 20-fold difference in transcription of the transferrin receptor gene. The change in mRNA and its transcription is related to the concentration of iron. When the iron is delivered to an erythroid precursor cell in the bone marrow, the ferric iron has to be again reduced to the ferrous state in order to be incorporated into the heme prosthetic group. The reduction is accomplished by an NADH-dependent reductase, and the insertion of iron in the heme ring is accomplished by another enzyme known as chelatase. When the ferrous iron is inserted into heme associated with specific subunits in hemoglobin, the various subunits polymerize to form the tetramer of hemoglobin A.

The presence of oxygen, of course, tends to oxidize a certain small percent of the iron each day and the formation of ferric iron in the hemoglobin molecule results in its conversion to methemoglobin, which has no capacity to take up and release oxygen. In order to minimize this effect of the oxidation of ferrous iron in hemoglobin by cellular oxygen concentrations, methemoglobin reductase, which is also an NADH-dependent enzyme, reduces the ferric iron in methemoglobin back to the ferrous state that regenerates ordinary hemoglobin.

Iron Needs

As mentioned earlier, the normal red cell lasts for about 120 days in the circulation of man and is then taken up by the reticuloendothelial system and degraded into bile pigments and ferric ion. The ferric ion enters the transferrin pool and is recirculated to the extent of about 25 mg/day. Thus, the turnover of iron within the body is 10–20 times the amount absorbed. A similar small amount, ~1 mg/day, is lost by the sloughing of G.I. cells and by skin cells. Fecal losses of iron are about 0.6 mg/day. Urinary losses are essentially nil.

In menstruating women, or in individuals with hemorrhage, the iron losses can be considerable and anemia can occur as a result of menstrual losses or bleeding. This is the basis for the chlorosis (chronic hypochromic microcytic anemia) that was first observed in adolescent girls in the seventeenth century. Females, during the childbearing years, must replace the iron lost in menstrual blood, which over a month amounts to about 1.4 mg/day. During infancy and childhood, about 40 mg of iron are required for the production of essential iron compounds associated with the gain of 1 kg of new tissue. Obviously, the iron needs are great in the rapid growth phases of infancy and adolescence. The needs of pregnant women are also great because during pregnancy a total of about 1.0 g of iron is needed to cover the growth need of the fetus and that of the mother as she prepares for delivery and lactation. It is difficult to obtain this amount of iron from the usual diet. It is estimated that about 27 mg/day of elemental iron is needed in the diet to provide sufficient iron to the pregnant female. The elderly in good health have no apparent increase in their needs for iron[51]; however, their need might be increased should they develop chronic disease. Table 14.1 gives the DRIs for iron.

Iron Deficiency

Iron deficiency is probably the most common nutritional deficiency present in the world population. This is true because iron is poorly absorbed and because many diets, especially those consumed by Third World populations, are iron poor. Low- or no-meat diets rich in whole grain cereals and legumes contain only nonheme iron and this iron is poorly absorbed. Furthermore, menstruating women and growing children are more at risk for iron deficiency than are adult men.[47,48,51] Pregnant women also are at risk, especially if they are multiparous. Women who are deficient during pregnancy are likely to give birth to deficient infants. Assessment of deficiency includes the determination of levels of tissue ferritin, transferrin, transferrin receptor activity, heme iron, red cell number and hemoglobin levels.

The appearance of clinical iron deficiency anemia occurs in three stages: the first involves depletion of iron stores as measured by a decrease in serum ferritin. Serum ferritin reflects the magnitude of the iron store in the body, Low serum ferritin levels can be observed in a deficient individual without a loss of essential iron compounds and without any evidence of anemia. The second stage is characterized by biochemical changes that reflect the lack of iron sufficient for the normal production of hemoglobin and other iron compounds. This is indicated by a decrease in transferrin saturation levels and an increase in erythrocyte protophyrin. In the final stage, the appearance of iron deficiency anemia occurs with depressed hemoglobin production and a change in the mean corpuscular volume of the RBC to produce a microcytic hypochromic anemia. This is expressed clinically as pallor and weakness. There are also changes in the nails, which take on a spoon shape when the iron-deficient state is severe. In rats and chicks made iron deficient, several changes in intermediary metabolism have been reported.[52,53] These include an increase in peripheral tissue sensitivity to insulin, an increase in hepatic glucose production (gluconeogenesis), a decrease in the conversion of thyroxine to triiodothyronine, impaired fatty acid oxidation and ketogenesis, an increased need for carnitine, evidence of oxidative damage to the erythrocyte membrane, abnormal monoamine metabolism in the brain (increased dopamine synthesis and down regulation of dopamine receptors), increased serum triglycerides and cholesterol and slightly less pentose shunt activity. In addition to these metabolic changes, iron-deficient rats had an impaired immune response to a pathogen challenge. There was a decrease in antibody production and a decrease in the natural killer cell population. Iron deficiency in chicks results in a compromised development of the elastic fibers in the aorta and lungs.[52] Whether these same responses also exist in iron-deficient humans is not certain; however, it is likely that there are numerous similarities.

Pharmacological Treatment of Iron Deficiency

The treatment of iron-deficiency anemia is a pharmacological activity and involves giving doses of iron, usually equivalent to 60 mg of elemental iron or 300 mg of ferrous sulfate, once or twice a day. It is usually given between meals to minimize gastrointestinal side effects. Fortunately, the smaller the dose and the more severe the anemia, the greater will be the percentage of iron absorbed. This treatment is usually continued for 2–3 months to normalize hemoglobin levels and iron stores. These should be monitored until satisfactory values are obtained. Iron intake should then be assessed periodically to ensure that an excess intake is avoided.

Excess Iron Intake: Toxicology

Iron toxicity is a result of excess iron intake. This can occur acutely in children who ingest iron pills or iron–vitamin supplements. Severe iron poisoning is characterized by damage to the intestine with bloody diarrhea, vomiting, acidosis, and, sometimes, liver failure. Effective treatment includes induced emesis, food and electrolyte treatment to prevent shock, and the use of iron-chelating agents to bind the iron. These treatments have substantially decreased the mortality due to iron overdose from about 50% in 1950 to less than a few percent in recent years. Table 14.2 provides information on the upper tolerable limit for iron intake, and when these intakes are exceeded, toxicity results.

Chronic overload of iron can result either from chronic excess intake or from a genetic disorder, hemochromatosis. Hemochromatosis is intermittent in nature. The genetic disorder is carried on chromosome 6. Two descendants of the British King George III have been diagnosed with the disease, and it has been suggested that the intermittent psychiatric state of King George III during the American Revolution might have been due to hemochromatosis. Hemochromatosis is characterized by increased iron absorption with damage to the pancreas, liver, brain, and heart. This damage has been associated with diabetes, liver failure, and heart failure. There is also an associated psychiatric abnormality that is likewise intermittent in character. Persons with hemochromatosis may also develop hepatocellular carcinoma and colon cancer. Two lines of evidence have been put forth that support this suggestion. The first line concerns the production of free radicals.[8,17] Iron, in excess, can catalyze the production of free radicals, which in turn can damage cell membranes as well as act as mutagens through damaging DNA. The DNA can repair itself, but the free radical damage could be so great that the repair is inadequate. The second line concerns the fact that cancer cells, like normal cells, require iron as an essential ingredient of metabolism. Having a surplus of iron in the system could increase the survival and proliferation of the cancer cell. Several population studies have provided support for this line of thought. In these studies, a dose–response relationship, that is, a correlation of iron intake, ferritin levels, and the development of colon cancer, was found that was highly suggestive of a causal role for excess iron intake in colon cancer development.

Carcinogenesis can also be instigated by other minerals. Nickel subsulfide, for example, is a potent carcinogen having the renal tissue as a target.[21] In the presence of high-to-moderate iron levels, the activity of the nickel compound is increased. In copper excess due to a genetic disorder involving the protein that transports copper, hepatic cancer develops and this cancer is potentiated by high iron levels.[18,19] It would appear in these last examples that the role of iron is that of a cancer promoter rather than that of an initiator as described for colon cancer.

Although high iron intakes can be harmful, it should be noted that optimal iron intakes can protect against lead toxicity. Lead competes with iron for uptake by the enterocyte. If the transporter is fully saturated by its preferred mineral, iron, then the lead will be poorly absorbed and excreted in the feces. Well-nourished individuals with respect to iron nutriture are at less risk for lead toxicity than are those whose iron intake is marginal or deficient.

ZINC

Zinc is the last transition element in the series of the fourth period of the periodic table. It has an atomic number of 30 and an atomic weight of 65.4. There are 15 isotopes of which ^{65}Zn is the most useful. This radioisotope has a half-life of 244 days. Zinc is a good reducing agent and will form stable complexes with other ions as well as form a wide range of salts with members of the halogen family as well as with carbonates, phosphates, sulfates, oxalates, and phytate.

Absorption, Metabolism, Excretion

Like iron, zinc absorption is relatively poor.[53–55] Of the approximately 4–14 mg/day consumed, only 10%–40% is absorbed. Zinc supplements differ in their availability and absorption.[56]

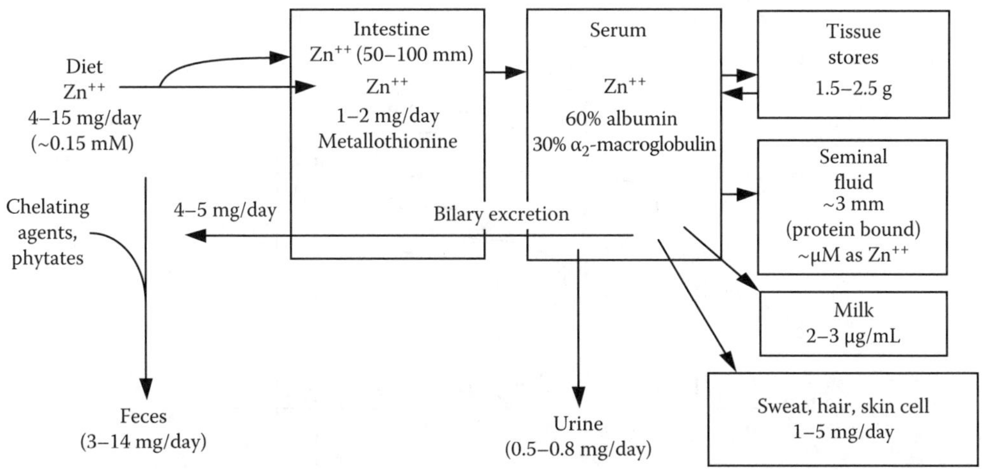

FIGURE 14.3 Zinc balance in normal adult humans.

Zinc gluconate, zinc citrate, acetate, or sulfate is absorbed more readily than zinc oxide. Absorption is decreased by the presence of binding agents or chelating agents that render the mineral unabsorbable. Zinc binds to ligands that contain sulfur, nitrogen, or oxygen. Zinc will form complexes with phosphate groups (PO_4^-), chloride (Cl^-), and carbonate groups (HCO_3^-), as well as with cysteine and histidine. Buffers such as *N*-(2-hydroxyethyl)-1-piperazine ethane sulfonic acid (HEPES) have little effect on zinc binding to these ligands. Clay, a mixed mineral soil component, for example, can render zinc unavailable. So too can fiber, phosphate, and phytate (inositol hexaphosphate). Zinc bound in this fashion is excreted via the feces. People who are geophagic (Pica) and/or who consume large amounts of phytate-containing foods (mainly cereal products) are at risk for developing zinc deficiency. Oberleas[54] has calculated that diets having a phytate to zinc ratio greater than 10 will induce zinc deficiency regardless of the total zinc content in these diets. Unlike iron, zinc exists in only one valence state: Zn^{++}. The normal 70 kg human absorbs 1–2 mg/day (Figure 14.3) using both a nonsaturable and a saturable process. The former is passive diffusion while the latter involves zinc-binding metallothionein protein. Studies on the mechanisms of zinc absorption by the enterocyte have shown that fast zinc uptake is attributable to extracellular binding of zinc followed by internalization of the zinc ligand mediated by an unknown molecular entity. After entry into the enterocyte, zinc is bound to a cysteine-rich intestinal protein (CRIP), which in turn transfers the zinc to either metallothionine or through the serosal side of the enterocyte to albumin that carries it to its site of use. Figure 14.4 shows this proposed uptake system. Vitamin D enhances zinc uptake probably due to an effect of the vitamin on the synthesis of metallothionine. From the enterocyte, it is transferred to the serum where ~60%–77% is loosely bound to albumin.[57] Approximately 20%–30% is tightly bound to an α_2-macroglobulin and 2%–8% (1–0.1 nm) is ultrafilterable.[57] This ultrafiltrate is excreted either in the urine (0.5–0.8 mg/day) or in the feces via biliary excretion. The liver appears to be a major site of Zn^{++} uptake after it has been absorbed. There is both rapid uptake ($t_{1/2}$ = 20 s) and a slower linear uptake.[55]

Function

Zinc has two important functions. One is that of serving as an essential cofactor for more than 70 enzymes. Table 14.5 provides a partial list of these enzymes. In this role, zinc binds to the histidine and cysteine residues of the enzyme proteins (Figure 14.5) and in so doing stabilizes and exposes the active sites of these enzymes such that catalysis of the reaction in question can take place. Even though these enzymes require zinc as a cofactor, these enzymes appear to function at

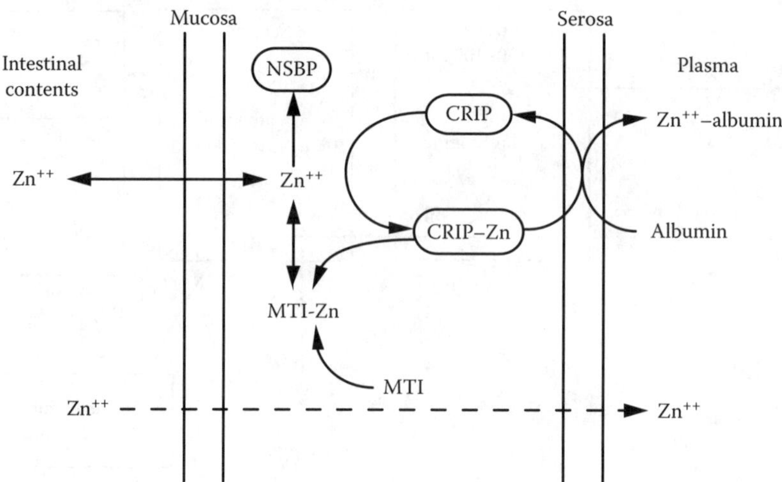

FIGURE 14.4 Intestinal zinc absorption. Passive diffusion is shown at the lower part of the diagram while mediated transport involving metallothionine (MTI), the cysteine-rich protein (CRIP), and the nonspecific binding protein (NSBP) are shown in the upper part of the diagram.

TABLE 14.5
Enzymes Requiring Zinc as a Cofactor

Alcohol dehydrogenase	δ-Amino levulinate dehydrase
Lactate dehydrogenase	Fructose-1,6 bisphosphatase
Alkaline phosphatase	Transcarboxylases
Angiotensin-converting enzyme	Reverse transcriptase
Carbonic anhydrase	Leukotriene hydrolase
Carboxypeptidase A, B, and DD	Phosphodiesterase
Cytoplasmic superoxide dismutase (also requires copper)	Elastase
DNA and RNA polymerases	Adenosine deaminase
Pyruvate dehydrogenase	5′ Nucleotidase
Proteases and peptidases	Glyoxalase
Aspartate transcarbamylase	Transcription factor Sp1
Thymidine kinase	Thymulin

near normal levels in deficient animals. In part, this occurs because these enzymes are intracellular enzymes and tenaciously retain their zinc so as to continue to function. There obviously is a hierarchy of zinc need by the living body. Tissue stores and dispensable zinc uses are raided well before the store of the intracellular zinc needed by these enzymes. Furthermore, deficient states are characterized by an increase in zinc absorption efficiency further protecting the system from self-destruction. The enzymes listed in Figure 14.5 are representative of the many requiring zinc for activity. Equally important is the binding of zinc to specific DNA-binding proteins found in the nucleus. These proteins are called zinc finger proteins or simply zinc fingers.[9] They have an important role in transcription. A number of nutrients, that is, vitamin A, vitamin D, and hormones, that is, steroids, insulin-like growth factor I, growth hormone and others, have their effects on the expression of specific genes because they can bind to very specific DNA-binding proteins that in turn bind to very specific DNA sequences. More than 500 zinc-binding proteins have been identified that have important roles in gene expression.[58–60] In this role, zinc again binds to histidine and cysteine residues of the linear portions of the binding proteins giving these proteins a sausage-like shape (Figure 14.6). If there is a mutation in the gene that encodes

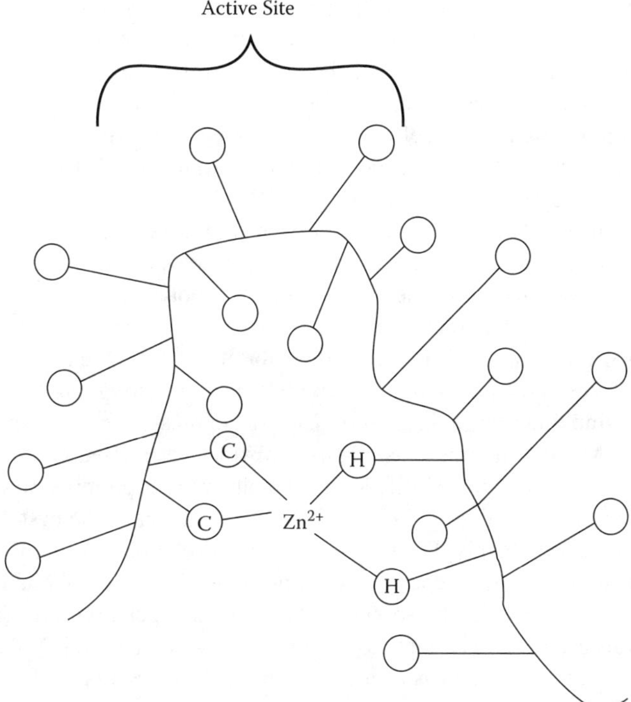

FIGURE 14.5 Zinc binds to cysteine (C) and histidine (H) residues of an enzyme protein stabilizing it so as to expose its active catalytic site. The rods and balls shown in this illustration are used to represent the various amino acid residues sticking out from the amino acid chain of the enzyme.

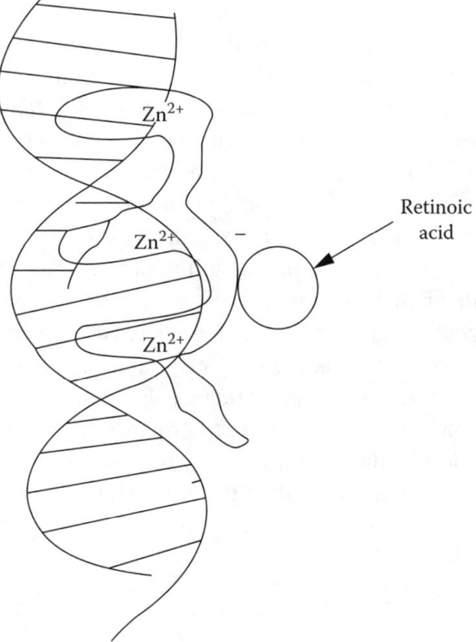

FIGURE 14.6 A zinc-DNA-binding protein in action. In this instance, retinoic acid is bound to its zinc-containing DNA-binding protein.

a specific DNA-binding protein such that the protein lacks one or more of the requisite residues of histidine and cysteine in the linear part of its structure, then the functional attribute of ligand, vitamin or hormone, at the genetic level will be ablated. Instances of such mutations have been published as well as instances where these zinc fingers have been purposefully modified as a therapeutic approach to disease control.[61] Zinc-containing transcription factor Zif268 has been modified with the result of a loss in sequence-specific recognition of DNA by viruses, thus ablating the viral invasion and takeover of their target cells. Although this modification was done in vitro and not tested in whole animals, this approach might have therapeutic application in the future as a means to avert the consequences of viral diseases such as AIDS.[61]

Zinc by itself may have effects on gene expression.[60,62–69] For example, the expression of the gene for the zinc transport protein, metallothionine, is influenced by zinc inake.[60,62–68] Total zinc intake can modify the glucose-raising effect of a zinc transporter variant. One of these variants is associated with type 2 diabetes and an increase in zinc intake lowers fasting glucose levels.[69]

Zinc as part of a zinc finger or by itself stimulates the expression of its own transporter protein, metallothionine.[62–68] Metallothionine exists as two distinct yet related compounds termed MT-1 and MT-2. These proteins are hydrophilic, low molecular weight proteins (6–7 kDa) containing a high percentage of cysteine residues (23–22 mol%). The function of the cysteine is to bind heavy metals via clusters of thiolate bonds. The synthesis of metallothionines is regulated by zinc through its action on the expression of the genes for these proteins. The level of MT-1 is a very sensitive indicator of zinc deficiency.[62–68] In the absence of dietary zinc, gene transcription is impaired and metallothionine levels are low.[68] The metallothionine gene was identified by Palmiter et al.[63–66] By combining the results of DNA sequence information with the results of deletion mapping studies, unique short sequences of DNA were found that mediated the role of zinc in metallothionine gene expression.[63–68] The metal response units were sites for trans-acting transcription factors that bind and enhance the basal rate of transcription of the genes for metallothionine. In addition, in zinc-deficient animals, numerous breaks in single-strand DNA have been observed.[70] This can be reversed when dietary zinc is restored. Incidentally, transgenic mice that overexpress metallothionine I are very resistant to zinc deficiency.[63] The overexpression of metallothionine increases the absorption efficiency of these mice, thus compensating for inefficient absorption. The cytokine, interleukin 1, has been shown to direct and regulate zinc metabolism in the traumatized or septic individual as well as in normal people.[62] Interleukin 1 increases the expression of the metallothionine gene, thereby increasing zinc uptake through the gut and its transport to and uptake by bone marrow and thymus with relatively less zinc taken up by other body components. Trauma and sepsis both require zinc for new protein synthesis for tissue repair and both conditions are characterized by a rise in interleukin 1 levels in the blood. In addition to its function in metallothionine transcription, as a component of numerous enzymes and in the zinc fingers, zinc also is important for the stabilization of membranes and provides structural strength to bone as part of the bone mineral apatite.[71] Zinc also plays a role in alleviating inflammation. It also functions as an anti-inflammatory agent and as an antioxidative agent. Zinc supplementation decreases c-reactive protein, lipid peroxidation, and the levels of inflammatory cytokines in elderly subjects.[72] In rats, zinc deficiency results in DNA damage, an increase in oxidative stress markers, a decrease in the activity of their antioxidant defense systems, and an inhibition of their DNA repair capability.[73] Healthy young men when zinc restricted had a measure of loss in their DNA integrity that was reversed once their zinc intake was normalized.[74] All of these observations speak to the multiplicity of functions of this important and essential trace mineral.

Storage

Zinc is found in all cell types and tissues; however, it is notably stored in the β cells of the islets of Langerhans in the pancreas.[75] There, zinc is incorporated into the hormone insulin. Insulin contains two to four atoms of zinc as part of its crystalline structure. Zinc may play a role in insulin release, but the details of this role have not been completely elucidated. Pharmaceutical preparations of insulin needed by diabetics for hormone replacement therapy contain zinc. It should be noted that not all species incorporate zinc in their insulin structure.

Zinc Interactions

Zinc can sometimes be displaced on the zinc fingers by other divalent metals. Iron, for example, has been used to displace zinc on the DNA-binding protein that binds estrogen. This protein binds to the estrogen response element of the DNA in the promoter regions encoding estrogen-responsive gene products. When this occurs in the presence of H_2O_2 and ascorbic acid, damage to the proximate DNA, the estrogen response element, occurs. It has been suggested that in this circumstance of an iron-substituted zinc finger, free radicals are more readily generated with the consequence of genomic damage.[9] This suggestion has been offered as an explanation of how excess iron (iron toxicity) could instigate the cellular changes that occur in carcinogenesis.

In excess, cadmium can also substitute for zinc in the zinc fingers. In this substitution, the resultant zinc fingers are nonfunctional. Because of the importance of these fingers in cell survival and renewal, a cadmium substitution is lethal. Cadmium toxicity is an acute illness with little lag time needed for the symptom of cell death to manifest itself. Cadmium is also bound by the metallothionine transport protein. The metallothionine proteins in addition to binding zinc and copper also bind other heavy metals such as mercury. This occurs when the individual is acutely exposed to toxic levels of these metals.

Excess zinc intake can adversely affect copper absorption and also affect iron absorption. Further, excess zinc can interfere with the function of iron as an antioxidant and can interfere with the action of cadmium and calcium as well. Ferritin, the iron storage protein, can also bind zinc. In zinc excess, zinc can replace iron on this protein. Other interactions include the copper–zinc interaction. Copper in excess can interfere with the uptake and binding of zinc by metallothionine in the enterocyte. In humans consuming copper-rich diets, the apparent absorption of zinc is markedly reduced. In part this is due to a copper–zinc competition for enterocyte transport and in part due to a copper effect on metallothionine gene expression. Metallothionine has a greater affinity for copper than for zinc, and thus, zinc is left behind while copper is transported to the serosal side of the enterocyte for export to the plasma whereupon the copper rather than the zinc is picked up by albumin and transported to the rest of the body. Fortunately, excess copper in the normal diet is not common. Zinc is usually present in far greater amounts, and so this interaction is of little import in the overall scheme of zinc metabolism.

Deficiency

Until the early 1960s, zinc as an essential nutrient for humans had not been demonstrated. Prasad in 1961[76] and Halsted[53] described conditions in humans later found to be due to inadequate zinc intake. Among the symptoms were growth failure, anemia, hypogonadism, enlarged liver and spleen, rough skin, and mental lethargy. These features can be attributed both to the loss of zinc as a cofactor in many enzymatic reactions *and* to the loss of zinc as an essential component of the DNA-binding zinc fingers. Detailed studies of populations having these symptoms among its members revealed the custom of clay eating as well as diets that were very low in animal protein and high in cereal products. Geophagia (clay eating or pica) can affect the bioavailability of not only zinc but also iron and other minerals needed for optimal growth and development. In Iran, Prasad and also Halsted found that the provision of iron and protein supplements corrected the anemia and enlarged spleen and liver associated with zinc deficiency. Pubic hair and the gonads also began to develop. It was difficult to explain all of the clinical features (and their reversal) solely on the basis of iron deficiency and/or protein deficiency since other investigators had not reported the features of hypogonadism as part of the iron- or protein-deficient state. However, studies in animals showed that this feature is characteristic of zinc deficiency. Later, Prasad in Egypt reported on growth retardation and testicular atrophy in young men. Geophagia was not a custom in this group nor were there signs of enlarged spleens and livers. The dietary patterns were similar to those found in Iran in that the diets were high in cereals and low in animal protein. Zinc concentrations in hair, plasma and red cells were lower than normal. Zinc turnover using[66] Zinc was increased above normal, and the 24 h exchangeable pool of zinc was smaller than expected. There were no signs of liver disease or any other chronic disease that would affect zinc status except that the Egyptian subjects were infected with shistosomiasis and hookworms. Studies of populations in Egypt where these infections were absent but where the diets were similar lead to the conclusion that the growth failure and hypogonadism were indeed signs of zinc deficiency. This was proven without a doubt when zinc supplements were provided and these signs were reversed. The zinc-deficiency signs of growth failure and sexual immaturity are the result of an individual's inability to support cell division due to a lack of zinc finger proteins as well as a deficiency in the production of insulin-like growth factor and growth hormone.[77] The skin symptoms are the most obvious because skin cells turn over very rapidly (~7 days). The symptoms include a moist eczematoid dermatitis found in the nasolabial folds and around other body orifices. There is a failure in zinc-deficient individuals to replace these routinely desquamated cells. In infants and young children, inadequate zinc intake can result in abnormal CNS development[78] as well as impaired skeletal development.[79] In the latter instance, zinc deficiency results in an impaired calcium uptake probably due to a decreased synthesis of intestinal calbindin. Impaired immune response and impaired taste sensitivity also characterize the deficient state. These features again relate to the role of zinc in cell turnover. Immunity requires antibody synthesis involving zinc fingers while the taste sensation involves short-lived epithelial cells on the surface of the tongue and oral cavity. The features of zinc deficiency have been reported in infants having an autosomal-recessive mutation in one of the genes that encode the zinc-carrying metallothionine found in the enterocyte. This condition is treated with oral zinc supplements that, through mass action, provide enough zinc to the enterocyte by passive diffusion. Because only one of the metallothionine genes has mutated, this strategy overcomes the inherent zinc-deficient state. Other zinc-deficient states have been reported in severely traumatized individuals, in patients having a Roux-en-Y bypass surgery, and in patients with end-stage renal disease with or without dialysis.[80,81] In renal disease, more zinc is lost via the kidneys than normal.[80] In renal failure, excess zinc is lost through the dialysate when patients are maintained on regular dialysis treatment. Children who are anephric and on dialysis must be monitored with respect to their zinc status. Failure to do so will result in growth failure and lack of sexual maturation. Again, a zinc supplement can reverse these symptoms.

Status

Zinc status can be difficult to assess sensitively. Plasma and neutrophil zinc levels can give a static measure of status; however, these blood levels can only evaluate the amount of zinc in transport, not the functional state of the individual. Measurement of alkaline phosphatase activity is quite useful because it is a zinc-requiring enzyme and is sensitive to zinc deprivation. The level of metallothionine I in blood is also a very sensitive indicator of zinc intake adequacy.[82] Hair zinc levels have been suggested as indicators of chronic zinc status; however, hair samples are frequently contaminated by zinc-containing shampoos or zinc-containing water. Hair growth rate could also influence hair zinc content.[16] Hence, assessing zinc status using hair samples probably is not very useful. Currently, the intake recommendation is set at 2–13 mg/day depending on the life stage of the individual (see Table 14.1). Assuming that the individual consumes a wide variety of foods and that the intake recommendation for good quality protein is met, the average individual should be well nourished with respect to zinc.

COPPER

Since the bronze age, copper alloyed with tin has been used by man to fabricate a vast array of useful items. However, it has only been a few decades since it was recognized as an essential nutrient for man and other animals. In the 1920s, it was recognized that copper was needed, in addition to iron, for hemoglobin synthesis. This came about when anemic animals supplemented with iron did not improve unless copper was also provided. The pioneering work of Cartwright and his associates[83] showed the relationship between the two metals in heme biosynthesis. Other roles for copper have since been elucidated.[83–87]

Copper is a transition metal in the fourth period of the periodic table. It has a molecular weight of 63.4 and an atomic weight of 29 and two valence states, cuprous (Cu^{++}) and cupric (Cu^{+++}). There are two naturally occurring isotopes, ^{63}Cu and ^{65}Cu, and two radioisotopes, ^{64}Cu and ^{67}Cu. The former has a half-life of 12.7 h while the latter has a half-life of 62 h.

Copper is present in nearly all foods in varying amounts. Dairy products are poor sources of copper while legumes and nuts are rich in this mineral. Raisins, whole grains, beef liver, shellfish, and shrimp are excellent sources as well. Surveys of foods consumed by a variety of population groups in the United States indicate a range of intake from 0.7 to 7.5 mg/day. On low intakes, absorption is markedly more (56% of intake) than when intake is high (12% of intake). The form of copper (cuprous or cupric) is a key factor in determining the percentage of intake that is absorbed.[85,86] Zinc, tin, ascorbic acid, and iron adversely affect copper absorption.

Absorption, Metabolism, Excretion

Copper absorption takes place in the small intestine and to a limited extent in the stomach.[87–89] Copper status affects absorption; where need is great, uptake is high. The amount absorbed also depends on the food mixture consumed and on the presence of other divalent minerals, which may compete for uptake. Absorption efficiency is low with an average uptake of 12%. Copper absorption is affected (reduced) by phytate[85] and by zinc.[26,90] That which is not absorbed is excreted in the feces. Also excreted in the feces is copper transported to the intestine from the liver via the bile. About 2 mg/day is excreted via the biliary route. Copper is also excreted in the urine and lost through the skin and hair. The percent lost via the urine, biliary excretion, skin, and hair is between 12% and 43% of the intake. The daily urinary copper in the human is quite small, amounting to 10–50 μg/day. In the rat, urinary loss accounted for 2%–7% of the intake.[91]

Once copper is absorbed by the enterocyte, it passes to the blood where it is bound to either albumin or transcuprein.[92] The half-life of albumin-bound copper is on the order of 10 min. The copper is then delivered to the liver whereupon it is incorporated into an α globulin transport protein called ceruloplasmin. Ceruloplasmin can carry six atoms of copper. Blood levels of copper are about 1 mg/L while ceruloplasmin is about 150–600 mg/L. Ceruloplasmin is not only useful in transporting copper to all parts of the body, it also has enzyme activity as a ferroxidase, an amide oxidase, and as a superoxide dismutase. As a ferroxidase, it is an active participant in the release of iron from its liver storage sites to transferrin in the plasma. It is active in the conversion of iron from the ferric to ferrous state and in the linkage of the ferrous iron to apotransferrin to form transferrin, which, in turn, transports the iron to the reticulocyte for hemoglobin synthesis. Its role in iron metabolism relates to the cuprous–cupric interconversion. On average, the copper contained by the ceruloplasmin is half cuprous and half cupric.

Although ceruloplasmin may indeed be the most active of the copper transporters, other transporters also participate in the delivery of copper to the cells that use and/or store this mineral. Albumin, as mentioned, can serve in this function as can a 270 kDa protein, transcuprein and certain of the amino acids, notably histidine.[89] The liver is the major user and repositor of copper. The copper levels in the liver remain relatively constant. Biliary excretion and ceruloplasmin release are the major mechanisms used to maintain copper levels in this tissue. Ceruloplasmin has a high copper content and accounts for 70%–90% of the approximately 1 μg/mL copper in the plasma.

Transcuprein has been shown to compete with albumin at the intestine for copper yet functions in the portal circulation as a donor of copper to albumin. The existence and function of transcuprein in the maintenance of copper status have not been fully explored.

While the transport of copper in the blood has received considerable attention, its transport into the cell has not been as well studied. Copper passes through the plasma membrane via fixed membrane transporter proteins. These membrane proteins may either reversibly bind the copper or form channels through which the copper passes. The kinetics of copper transport have been studied. The K_m values are uniformly in the low micromolar range, whereas the V_{max} is highly variable depending on cell type, incubation conditions, and media used.

Function

Copper, zinc, and iron are all involved in the regulation of gene expression. Already discussed are the specific roles for zinc and iron. That of copper vis-à-vis metallothionine has been described.[12] The specific metallothionine locus (CUP1) encodes metallothionine, a 6570 molecular weight protein that binds heavy metals. The CUP1 promoter does not respond directly to copper. Rather, this is a property of an upstream activating sequence (UAS) present as a tandem sequence designated UASp and UASd located between –105 and –108 bp from the transcription start site. It would appear that transcription of the metallothionine is a function of both copper and zinc since this metal-binding protein can only be synthesized in the presence of both. This cascade-like process for the expression of the copper-responsive metallothionine is illustrated in Figure 14.7.

Using the messenger RNA differential display method, 10 other genes have been shown to have a copper response element needed for expression.[93] Seven of these had substantial homology with ferritin mRNA, fetuin mRNA, mitochondrial 12S and 16S rRNA, and with mitochondrial tRNA for phenylalanine, valine, and leucine. These homologies suggest roles for copper in mitochondrial gene expression, which in turn relate to the observation of decreased oxidative phosphorylation in copper-deficient rats.[94–96] Copper is an important component of one of the mitochondrial respiratory enzymes, cytochrome C, and serves as a cofactor for a variety of other enzymes (Table 14.6). Of the remaining RNAs identified as having a copper response element, no gene product has yet been found. It is possible that these products might be enzymes requiring copper as a cofactor or may be copper transport proteins. This would follow the paradigm of gene expression found with zinc and iron.

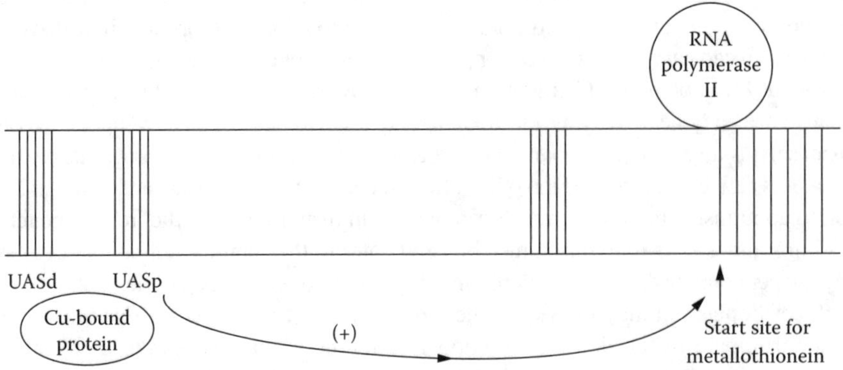

FIGURE 14.7 Copper plays a role in the expression of the gene for the cysteine-rich metallothionine by using a part of a DNA-binding protein. This protein has several zinc fingers that attach to the USSd and UASp sites. When bound it stimulates transcription.

TABLE 14.6
Enzymes Requiring Copper as a Cofactor

Cytochrome C oxidase
Lysyl oxidase
Dopamine β-hydroxylase
Tyrosine oxidase
Cytoplasmic superoxide dismutase
Amine oxidase
Monoamine oxidase
α-Amidating enzyme
Ferroxidase II
Ascorbate oxidase
Phenylalanine 4 monooxygenase
Metallothionine

Deficiency

Copper deficiency is rare in humans consuming a variety of foods. One of the major characteristics of copper deficiency is anemia and poor wound healing similar to that observed in vitamin C deficiency. The anemia is not responsive to iron supplementation. Weakness, lassitude, joint ache, osteoporosis, small petechial hemorrhaging, and arterial aneurysms can all be attributed to the vital role of copper in the synthesis of connective tissue and, in particular, collagen synthesis. Heart rupture is a frequently reported feature of copper-deficient rats.[97] Central nervous system degeneration can be related to a decline in respiratory chain activity; however, in the hierarchy of enzymes requiring copper for function, this enzyme is about the last to be affected in a copper-deficient animal. Reduced immune response has also been reported. Copper-deficient animals have been shown to have decreased T-lymphocyte and neutrophil activities.[98] Copper and chromium depletion has been shown to affect lymphocyte proliferation. Both minerals are needed simultaneously to elicit this response to a mitogen challenge.[99]

Other signs of the deficient state include elevated levels of plasma cholesterol, neutropenia, achromatism, twisted, kinky hair, and hemacytic, hypochromic anemia.[100] Copper deficiency causes elevated cholesterol levels in the blood, elevated HMG CoA reductase activity, and increased hepatic glutathione levels in rats.[101] If the rise in glutathione level is inhibited, then the hypercholesterolemia associated with copper deficiency is abolished. Heme biosynthesis is impaired in copper-deficient swine.[102] Adrenal steroidogenesis is impaired as is catecholamine synthesis in copper deficiency. The latter is due to a deficiency of the copper-containing enzyme dopamine beta-hydroxylase. Chronic diarrhea and malabsorption have been reported in infants fed copper-deficient formulas. In male rats fed purified diets, the use of pure sugars (mono and disaccharides) in a high carbohydrate diet accelerates the development of the copper-deficient state. Probably this has to do with the purity of this dietary ingredient rather than on any copper–sugar interaction at the cell or subcellular level.

Abnormal Copper Status

In normal humans, copper intake excess is rare. Although copper toxicity can develop if the exposure is high enough and long enough, the body can protect itself from occasional excess intake by lowering its absorption. The normal human should consume 0.2–1.3 mg/day of copper depending on life stage to maintain an optimal nutritional status. The estimate of an adequate dietary intake (Table 14.1) is similar to the population studies that indicate that the usual intake is between 1 and 1.5 mg/day. At intakes of 1–1.5 mg/day, no signs of deficiency have been observed. Turnlund[88] has reported that young men consuming between 0.75 and 7.53 mg/day were able to attain positive copper balance regardless of intake. Likely, the figure given for optimal intake is a little high because of the paucity of data on copper status under controlled conditions.

There are two genetic disorders that have assisted scientists in understanding the function and metabolism of copper. In one, Menkes syndrome, copper absorption is faulty. Intestinal cells absorb the copper but cannot release it into the circulation.[65,103] Parenteral copper corrects most of the condition that resembles copper deficiency, but care must be exercised in its administration. Too much can be toxic. In addition, parenterally administered copper does not reach the brain and cannot prevent the cerebral degeneration and premature death characteristic of patients with Menkes disease.

Another genetic disorder in copper status is Wilson's disease.[104–108] This condition is also associated with premature death and is due to an impaired incorporation of copper into ceruloplasmin and decreased biliary excretion of copper. This results in an accumulation of copper in the liver and brain. Early signs of Wilson's disease include liver dysfunction, neurological disease, and deposits of copper in the cornea manifested as a ring that looks like a halo around the pupil. This lesion is called the Kayser–Fleischer ring. Renal stones, renal aciduria, neurological deficits, and osteoporosis also characterize Wilson's disease. Periodic bleeding, which removes some of the excess copper, can be helpful in managing Wilson's disease as can treatment with copper chelating agents such as D-penicillamine and by increasing the intake of zinc, which interferes with copper absorption.

SELENIUM

Selenium is one of the *newer* minerals discovered during the twentieth century as being both required and toxic with a relatively narrow range of intake between the two.[2] The existence of selenium as a metal was first reported by J.J. Berzelius in 1817 and can occur in nature in a variety of forms referred to as allotropic forms. Metallic selenium is silver grey. If ground it appears black, but if ground extremely fine, it appears red. Vitreous selenium is black and shiny. Again, when powdered, it is red in color. When suspended in water, it provides a dark red liquid. In nature, selenium is frequently found in combination with lead, copper, mercury, and silver. These combinations are called selenides. Its chemistry is similar to that of sulfur. Selenium is an allotropic metal in group 6 of the fourth period of the periodic table. Its molecular weight is 78.96 and its atomic weight is 34. Although selenium has 26 isotopic forms, only five of these are naturally occurring: ^{76}Se, ^{78}Se, ^{77}Se, ^{80}Se, and ^{82}Se. Of the radioisotopes, ^{75}Se is the most useful, having a half-life of 118 days. Selenium has three valence states: Se^{++}, Se^{++++}, and Se^{++++++}. It can form selenides as described earlier, selenate, and because it will react with sulfur and oxygen will form selenomethionine, selenocystine, methylselenocysteine, and dimethyl selenide. The latter compound is quite volatile.

Although the presence of selenium in the earth's mineral matter was known, its recognition as an essential nutrient did not occur until Schwarz and Foltz[109] showed that a form of liver necrosis in rats could be cured if either vitamin E *or* selenium were administered. This report and others showed that for some purposes these two nutrients were interchangeable. It was this interchangeability that interfered with the identification of selenium as an essential nutrient. In hindsight, we now realize that selenium and vitamin E both play important roles in the detoxification of peroxides and free radicals.

Absorption, Metabolism, Excretion

Absorption is very efficient, with most of the ingested selenium absorbed readily from a variety of foodstuffs. The source of the mineral can have effects on its absorption. Figure 14.8 provides an overview of the daily selenium flux in a normal human.

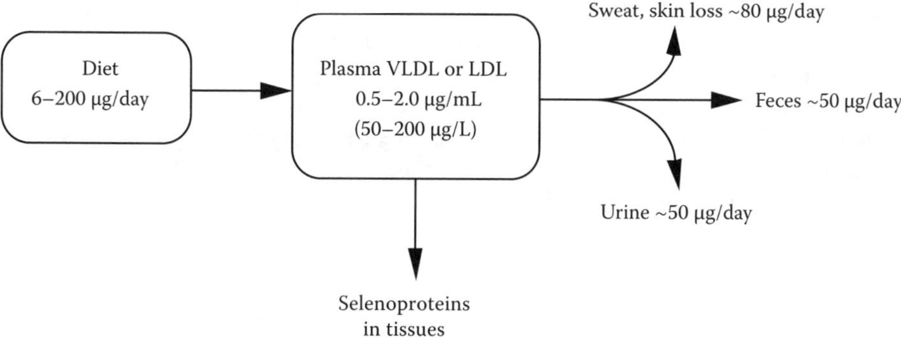

FIGURE 14.8 Daily selenium flux in a 70 kg man.

Selenium is transported from the gut on the very low and low-density lipoproteins. Red cells, liver, spleen, muscle, nails, hair, and tooth enamel all contain significant quantities of this mineral. Normal blood values for adults range from 55 to 72 μg/L. People with disorders that are characterized by increased oxidative stress to the red cell, that is, β thalassemia, diabetes, and/or smoking, tend to have slightly higher blood selenium levels, whereas pregnant and lactating women tend to have lower selenium levels. Excess (greater than 10 ppb in water or 0.05 ppm in food) intake is toxic, but unlike iron and copper that have inefficient excretory pathways, selenium is actively excreted in the urine. The urinary system functions to maintain optimal selenium status. Figure 14.9 shows how selenium is utilized. The metabolic use of selenium follows that of sulfur. It involves the formation of a selenium–sulfur bond using the SH group of either cysteine or methionine. From there it is incorporated into one of a group of proteins called selenoproteins. Under normal intake conditions (50–200 μg Se/day), about 50 μg can be found in the feces, and a similar amount is excreted in the urine. Sweat and desquamated skin cells account for another 80 μg per day. These losses can vary depending on dietary conditions. When intakes are low, losses are low, and when intakes are high there are corresponding rises in fecal and urine losses. Diets that include whole grain products, seafood, and organ meats will provide an optimal amount of selenium. In addition to these rich food sources, selenium in lesser amounts can be

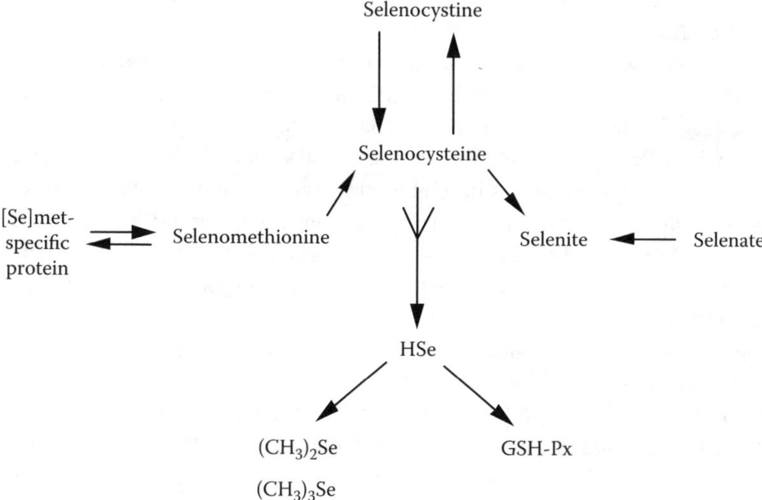

FIGURE 14.9 General scheme for selenium metabolism. Selenium is used by almost every cell type because of its vital role in glutathione peroxidase.

found in a wide variety of foods. In the United States, selenium deficiency is rare. This is not the case in China or in some parts of New Zealand and perhaps other parts of the world where the variety of foods available for consumption is severely constrained or reduced to those items produced locally. If the locality is a selenium poor area, humans as well as domestic animals may become deficient. Where there is a high selenium area, humans as well as animals may suffer from a selenium overload. Low plasma selenium concentrations have been reported to associate with poor muscle strength in older adults.[110]

Function

Selenium is an essential element in a group of proteins called the selenoproteins.[111,112] The synthesis of these proteins involves four gene products, one of which is tRNA for serine.[113,114] The synthesis of these selenoproteins involves sulfur-containing amino acids and selenium. These are joined via selenophosphate to form selenocysteine. The reaction is catalyzed by the enzyme selenophosphate synthetase. Vitamin B_6 serves as a coenzyme in this synthetic reaction. Selenocysteine in proteins is encoded by either a UGA opal codon or the TGA triplet, which is normally a stop codon. In order to read the TGA codon as selenocysteine, there must be a stem-loop structure in the 3′-untranslated region of the selenoprotein genes.[115] Although this stem-loop structure appears to be absolutely required for the incorporation of selenocysteine into a protein, documentation of this requirement is not fully complete.

Of the selenoproteins, glutathione peroxidase (GSH-PX or GPX, EC 1.11.1.9) has been the most widely studied. This enzyme catalyzes the reduction of peroxide (H_2O_2) and organic peroxides (fatty acid peroxides) in the presence of glutathione (GSH) to water and oxidized glutathione. This enzyme is an essential component of the series of reactions (shown in Figure 14.10) designed to maintain the redox state of the membrane and cell contents. Other enzymes include catalase, a peroxidase, and superoxide dismutase (SOD). Superoxide dismutase is found in both cytoplasm and mitochondria and requires different divalent ions as cofactors. Manganese, zinc, copper, and magnesium function in this respect. Glutathione peroxidase is of major importance to the red blood cell, which lacks mitochondria, the organelles that also work to maintain an optimal redox state. The red cell, because it contains the oxygen carrying hemoglobin, must regulate the redox state so that this hemoglobin can release oxygen in exchange for CO_2. In this exchange, there are opportunities for peroxide formation. These must be suppressed and glutathione peroxidase does just this.

Glutathione peroxidase is less active in deficient animals than in normally nourished animals. In fact, a decline in enzyme activity is a sensitive indicator of selenium status.[116] At least four isozymes exist, and these have been isolated and characterized. The four enzymes are numbered 1 through 4 as GPX1, GPX2, GPX3, and GPX4. Two of these, GPX1 and GPX4, are expressed in most tissues. GPX1 is found in large quantities in red blood cells, liver, and kidney, whereas GPX4 is found largely in testes. GPX2 is mainly in the gastrointestinal tract, and GPX3 is expressed mainly in kidney, lung, heart, breast, and placenta. There are species differences in the expression of these isozymes. In humans, GPX2 and 3 are expressed in the liver. In rodents, this is not the case. Rodent liver expresses only GPX1, not GPX2 or 3.

As described earlier, the active site of the selenium-dependent glutathione peroxidase contains a selenocysteine encoded by a UGA opal codon. However, not all of the isozymes are selenium dependent. There is an androgen-induced epididymal cell enzyme that shares sequence homology with GPX3 but is not selenium dependent nor does it have the UGA codon in its mRNA. The GPX2 maps to chromosome 14 while GPX3 and GPX4 map to chromosomes 5 and 19, respectively. GPX1 maps to human chromosome 3 and has sequences that are homologous to those found in chromosome 21 and the X chromosome. Glutathione peroxidase catalyzes the reduction of various organic peroxides as well as hydrogen peroxides. This reaction is shown in Figure 14.10.

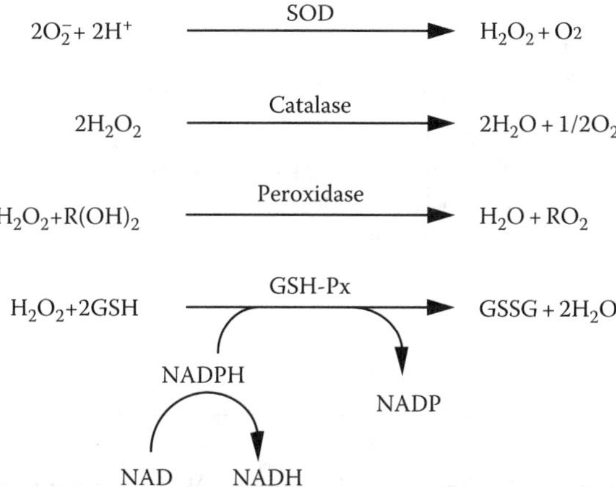

FIGURE 14.10 The reduction of oxygen radicals in the red cell. Protection from free radical attack preserves the function of the red cell membrane and hemoglobin. *Notes*: SOD, superoxide dismutase (requires Mg^{++} or Cu^{++} or Mn^{++} or Cu^{++} and zinc); GSH-Px, glutathione peroxidase (require Se); GSH, reduced glutathione; GSSG, oxidized glutathione; H_2O_2, hydrogen peroxide.

Glutathione furnishes the reducing equivalents in this reaction. Since membranes contain readily oxidizable unsaturated fatty acids, the stability of these membranes (and hence their function) is dependent on the activity of the antioxidant system of which this selenium containing enzyme is a part. If the diet is marginal in selenium but adequate in copper, iron and vitamins A, E, and C, which also serve as antioxidants, then cell damage by free radicals will be minimized. These other antioxidants can and do suppress free radical formation. While vitamin E serves an important role in suppressing free radical production, its site of action is separate from that of selenium in its role as an essential component of glutathione peroxidase. Studies of selenium deficient rats given a vitamin E supplement showed that these rats had no change in enzyme activity. Similarly, vitamin E–deficient rats show little improvement in red cell fragility with selenium supplements despite the overlap in antioxidant function of the two nutrients. The antioxidant properties of these cell components, however, are of particular interest to the pharmacologist because many drugs are, in themselves, oxidizing agents that work by disrupting the membranes of invading pathogens. The aging process as well as carcinogenesis may well be related to the adequacy of the body's antioxidant system.[117,118] Since free radicals damage cells, these cells may not be replaced at the same rate as the rate of destruction or the damage that, in turn, may make the cell vulnerable to invasion by cancer-producing viruses or agents that initiate cancer growth. Anticancer drugs, as mentioned, may be strong oxidizing agents. Normal as well as infected cells of the host will be affected by drug treatment. Should the host's antioxidant system be compromised either by nutritional deficiency or because of some genetically determined deficiency in the maintenance of intracellular redox states, cell survival and normal function will be compromised.

Several drugs have been developed that have anti-inflammatory properties and that also contain selenium. They work by catalyzing the degradation of peroxides much like glutathione peroxidase or by reducing the production of leukotriene B. Both actions serve to reduce inflammation.

Although approximately 36% of the total selenium in the body is associated with glutathione peroxidase, a number of other proteins in the body also contain this mineral. Table 14.7 provides a list of these proteins. Thirteen different selenoproteins, ranging in weight from 10 to 71 kDa, have been identified. Several of these are glutathione peroxidase isozymes and several have been isolated from a variety of cell lines. One, having thioredoxin reductase activity, has been isolated from

TABLE 14.7
Selenoproteins of Biological Importance

Cytosolic glutathione peroxidase
Phospholipid hydroperoxide glutathione peroxidase
Gastrointestinal glutathione peroxidase
Extracellular glutathione peroxidase
Selenoprotein W
Selenoprotein P
Iodothyronine deiodinase
Sperm capsule selenoprotein

human lung adenocarcinoma cells. Another, selenoprotein W, is thought to be responsible for white muscle disease when this protein is not made due to deficient selenium intake. Selenoprotein P, a protein that accumulates in plasma, may be a selenium transport protein, but its true function has yet to be elucidated. Selenium is an integral part of the enzyme, type 1 iodothyronine deiodinase, which catalyzes the deiodination of the iodothyronines notably the deiodination of thyroxine (T_4) to triiodothyronine (T_3), the most active of the thyroid hormones.[119,120] This deiodination is also catalyzed by type II and type III deiodinases, which are not selenoproteins. Whereas all the deiodinases catalyze the conversion of thyroxine to triiodothyroxine, there are differences in tissue distribution of these. While all the deiodinases catalyze the conversion of thyroxine to triiodothyronine, there are differences in the tissue distribution of these enzymes. The pituitary, brain, central nervous system, and brown adipose tissue contain types II and III, whereas type I is found in liver, kidney, and muscle. These two isozymes (II, III) contribute very little triiodothyronine to the circulation except under conditions (i.e., starvation) that enhance reverse triiodothyronine (rT_3) production. In selenium-deficient animals, type I synthesis is markedly impaired and this impairment is reversed when selenium is restored to the diet. Under these same conditions, the ratio of T_3 to T_4 is altered. There is more T_4 and less T_3 in the deficient animals, and the ratio of the two is reversed when selenium is restored. Because type II and III deiodinase also exist, these enzymes should increase in activity so as to compensate for the selenium-dependent loss of function. However, they do not do this because their activity is linked to that of the type I. When T_4 levels rise (as in selenium deficiency), this rise feeds back to the pituitary, which in turn alters (reduces) TSH release. The conversion of T_4 to T_3 in the pituitary is catalyzed by the type II deiodinase yet TSH release falls (Figure 14.11). T_4 levels are high because the type I deiodinase is less active. Whereas the deficient animal might have a T_3/T_4 ratio of 0.01, the sufficient animal would have a ratio of 0.02, a doubling of the conversion of T_4 to T_3. The effect of selenium supplementation on the synthesis and activity of the type 1 probably explains the poor growth of deficient animals.

Sunde and coworkers[121] have reported significant linear growth in deficient rats given a single selenium supplement, and this growth was directly related to the supplement-induced increase in type I deiodinase activity. In turn, the observations of changes in selenium status coincident with changes in thyroid hormone status provided the necessary background for establishing the selenium–iodine interaction that today is taken for granted. The role of selenium in the synthesis of type I deiodinase clearly explains the lack of goiter (enlarged thyroid gland) in cretins who lack both iodine and selenium in their diet. Thus, low selenium intakes impair thyroid hormone activity and there is a selenium–iodide interaction.

Selenium–Mineral Interactions

Other trace mineral interactions also exist.[12] Copper-deficient rats and mice have been shown to have reduced glutathione peroxidase activity. Copper deficiency increases oxidative stress, yet

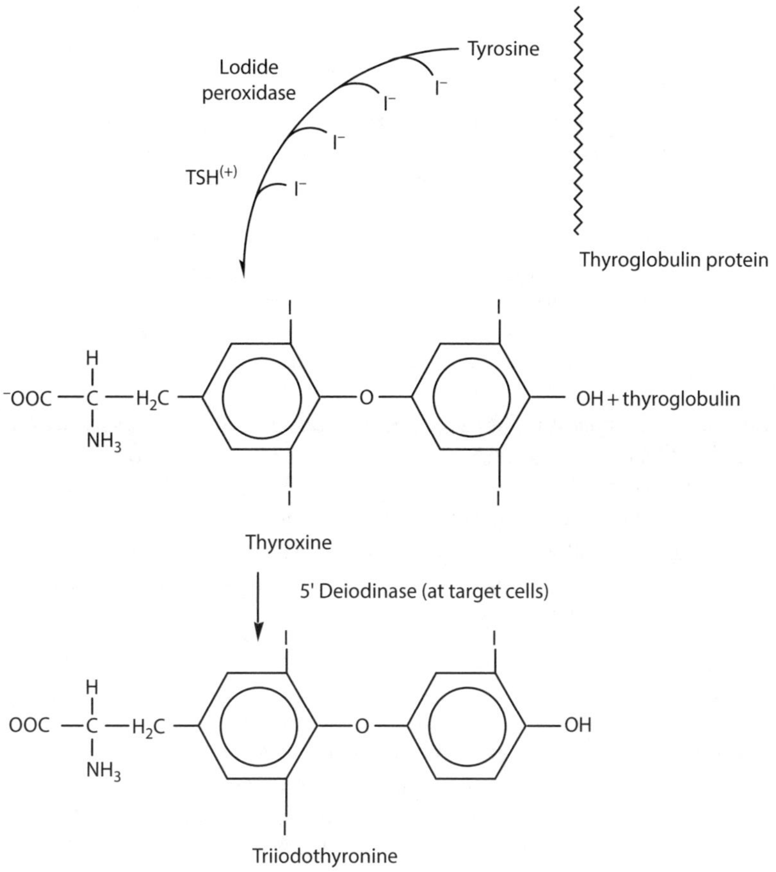

FIGURE 14.11 Feedback inhibition of TSH release.

oxidative stress affects all of the enzymes involved in free radical suppression. Even though glutathione peroxidase does not contain copper, the expression of the genes for this enzyme and for catalase is reduced in the copper-deficient animal. Note in Figure 14.10 that other trace minerals are involved as required components for SOD. Copper, zinc, magnesium, and manganese are part of the antioxidant system as is NADPH and NAD (niacin-containing coenzymes). The NAD although not usually shown as part of the system is involved because it can transfer reducing equivalents via the transhydrogenase cycle to NADP. Clearly, there are numerous nutrient interactions required for the maintenance of the optimal redox state in the cell.[122] This is important not only because it stabilizes the lipid portion of the membranes within and around the cells but also because it optimizes the functional performance of the many cellular proteins.

Deficiency

Selenium deficiency can develop in premature infants and in persons sustained for long periods of time by selenium-free enteral or parenteral solutions.[123] Symptoms characteristic of deficiency in humans include a decline in glutathione peroxidase activity in a variety of cell types,[124] fragile red blood cells, enlarged heart, cardiomyopathy, growth retardation, cataract formation, abnormal placenta retention, deficient spermatogenesis, and skeletal muscle degeneration. Some of these characteristics are shared with other species as shown in Table 14.8. In China, selenium deficiency is called Keshan disease.[14] It appears mainly in children and is marked by degenerative changes in

TABLE 14.8
Signs and Symptoms of Selenium Deficiency in Animals

Poultry: chickens, turkeys, ducks	Exudative diathesis, skeletal myopathy, encephalomalacia, pancreatic necrosis, reduced growth, reduced egg production, reduced fertility, reduced feather growth
Bovines	Reduced growth, skeletal and cardial myopathy, embryonic death, retained placenta
Equines	Skeletal myopathy, reduced performance, foals also have muscle steatitis
Ovines	Skeletal and cardial myopathy, poor growth, reduced fertility, embryonic death
Porcines	Poor growth, skeletal myopathy, *mulberry heart disease*, gastric ulcers, hepatic dysfunction
Rodents: rabbits, mice	Skeletal myopathy, erythrocyte hemolysis, testicular degeneration, fetal death, and resorption, increased hepatic malic enzyme and glutathione reductase activity

the heart muscle (cardiomyopathy). This develops in children whose intakes are less than 17 μg/day. Selenite-enriched salt has been shown to reverse this deficiency, and the time needed for this reversal in all cells depends on the half-life of the affected cells. Those cells that turn over rapidly will quickly show signs of deficiency and just as quickly show signs of reversal. Should cells that are not normally replaced quickly be affected by the deficient state, that effect will not be quickly reversed by selenium supplementation. Blood levels of selenium are not especially informative when it comes to the assessment of selenium deficiency.[125]

Toxicity

Selenium intake in excess of 400 μg/day is the upper tolerable limit for this mineral.[105,122] An intake of 750 μg/day is toxic. Toxicity does not usually occur unless the individual is exposed not only to high-diet levels but also to industrial conditions (smelters, selenium-rich smoke, etc.) that increase entry of the mineral into the body. Selenium toxicity in farm animals has been observed when the food supply for these animals consists of selenium-rich pastures and grain. Selenium toxicity in these animals is characterized by hoof loss and a neuromuscular condition known as *blind staggers*. Damage to the liver and muscle is observed as well. Excess selenium intake interferes with zinc absorption and use, reduces tissue iron stores, and increases copper level in heart, liver, and kidney. Clearly, selenium excess upsets the normal trace element balance in the body.

IODINE (IODIDE)

The essentiality of iodine has been recognized since the late 1800s. Its relationship to the production of thyroxine was not fully realized but even the ancient medical literature recommended the consumption of seaweed or burnt sponges (both of which are rich in iodine) for the treatment of goiter. Iodine deficiency used to be endemic in all but the coastal regions of the world. Presently, it is frequently observed in third world nations whose access to iodine is limited. With the advent and use of iodized salt and the development of means to process and distribute frozen seafoods, this once common nutritional disorder has all but disappeared.[126]

Iodine is a member of the halogen family that includes fluorine, chlorine, and bromine. These appear as group VII in the fifth period of the periodic table. Iodine has an atomic number of 53 and an atomic weight of 127. There are no naturally occurring isotopes, but two radioisotopes are useful in biological systems. These are ^{131}I with a half-life of 8 days and ^{125}I with a half-life of 60 days. Iodine is very labile but forms stable salts, the most common is Na I. The iodide ion has a negative one valence, I^-.

Absorption, Metabolism, Excretion

The average human in the United States consumes between 170 and 250 μg/day. The iodine is converted to the iodide ion (I^-) and is easily absorbed. Once absorbed, it circulates in the blood to all the tissues of the body. Salivary glands, the gastric mucosa, choroid plexus, and the lactating mammary gland, as well as the thyroid gland can concentrate iodine. Of the iodine consumed, 80% is trapped by the thyroid gland, which uses it for the synthesis of thyroxine.

As shown in Figure 14.12, thyroxine is synthesized through the stepwise iodination of tyrosine. The gland produces and releases thyroxine when stimulated by the pituitary thyroid-stimulating hormone (TSH). TSH acts on the tyrosine-rich thyroglobulin serving to unravel this protein to make tyrosine available for iodination via the enzyme, iodide peroxidase. First, monoiodothyronine is produced then diiodothyronine, triiodothyronine, and thyroxine are produced. TSH stimulates the thyroid to release this thyroxine, which is transported to its target tissues (all the cells of the body) by way of a transport protein called thyroid-binding protein. Upon delivery to the target cell, thyroxine is carried into the cell and deiodinated to triiodothyronine. The enzyme catalyzing this reaction is 5′ deiodinase, a selenium-containing enzyme. Triiodothyronine is the active form of the hormone having at least 10 times the activity of thyroxine. The iodine released by this deiodination is conserved and sent back into the blood stream for further use by the thyroid gland. Iodide not used or sequestered is excreted either as organic iodine in the feces or as free iodine in the urine.

The thyroid gland is stimulated to produce and release thyroxine by TSH. Thyroxine is carried to the target cells by a binding hormone. The target cells then deiodinate the thyroxine producing T_3. Figure 14.13 illustrates the endocrine pathway for thyroid hormone production, function, and excretion.

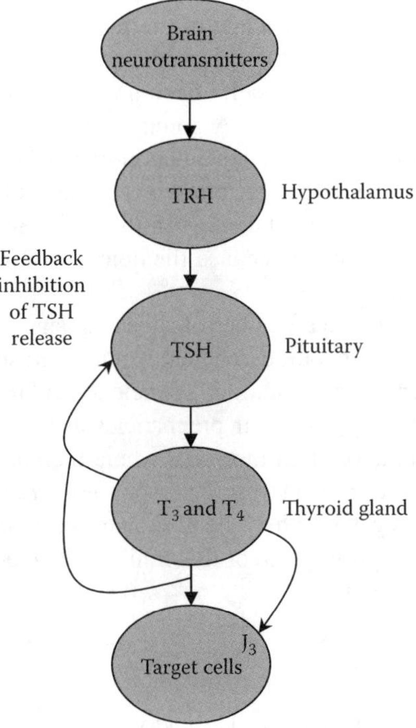

FIGURE 14.12 Schematic representation of thyroid hormone synthesis.

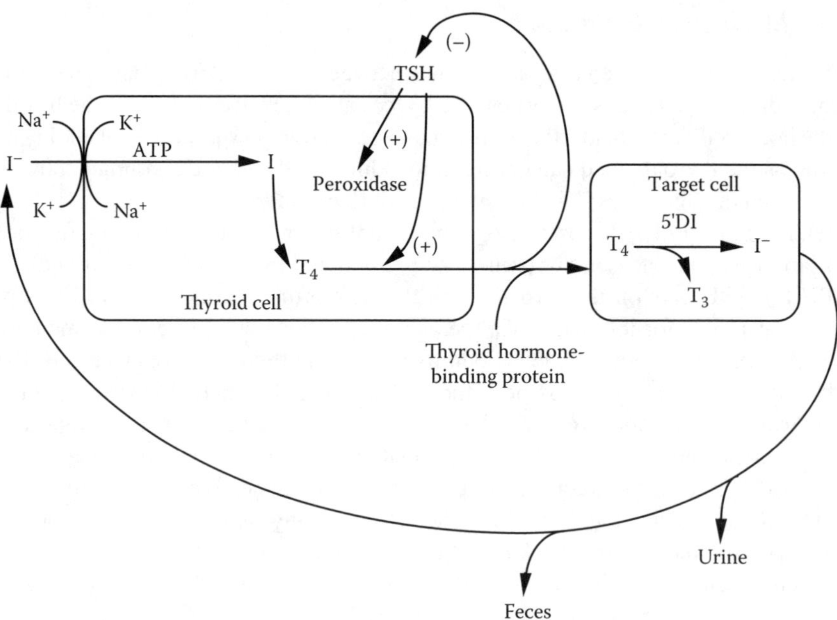

FIGURE 14.13 Overview of thyroid hormone production. TSH, thyroid-stimulating hormone from the pituitary; T_4, thyroxine; T_3, triiodothyronine; 5′DI, 5′-deiodinase.

Deficiency

The enlargement of the thyroid gland (goiter) is characteristic of iodine deficiency and is marked by a hypertrophic, hyperplasic change in the gland's follicular epithelium. These epithelial cells synthesize thyroxine, and their growth is stimulated by the pituitary hormone, thyroid-stimulating hormone (TSH). The cells become enlarged when iodine is not available to complete the thyroxine synthetic process. A goiter is not only unsightly but may also cause obstruction of the airways and damage the laryngeal nerves. The synthesis of thyroxine is the only known function of iodine. Thyroid hormone production can be influenced not only by iodine deficiency but also by selenium deficiency. In the latter instance, the active thyroid hormone, triiodothyronine, is not produced because the deiodination of thyroxine is dependent on the selenoprotein, 5′ deiodinase.

A diet deficient in iodine can cause a number of illnesses depending on the age of exposure.[127] The developing embryo or fetus of an iodine-deficient woman will suffer a neurological deficit that is quite profound. Infants and children consuming a deficient diet fail to grow normally and develop intellectually. Pregnant women may lose their pregnancies as the fetus fails to develop and dies in utero. The deficient state can develop in instances where the population subsists on a marginal iodine intake and consume a diet rich in vegetables of the *Brassica* genus (Cruciferae family). Although cabbage and related vegetables have been shown to contain goitrogens (compounds that inhibit thyroxine release by the thyroid gland or that inhibit iodine uptake by the gland), other vegetables contain these substances as well.

Need

Because iodine is conserved very efficiently and is not toxic even at 10–20 times the required intake, iodine is considered to be a benign (but essential) trace element. An intake of 1–2 μg/kg should be adequate for most adult humans. Pregnant females need slightly (10%–20%) more. Thus, the Food and Nutrition Board of the National Academy of Sciences has recommended an intake of 150 μg/day for adults, 6 μg/kg/day for infants, 5 μg/kg/day for young children, 4 μg/kg/day for older children, and 175 μg/day for pregnant and lactating females. Table 14.1 provides the details of these DRIs.

MOLYBDENUM

Molybdenum, as an essential nutrient for humans and animals, was first recognized in 1953. Its importance in relation to copper and iron was appreciated in that an excess of molybdenum interfered with copper and iron absorption. Molybdenum also interferes with the binding of copper by ceruloplasmin. In ruminants, molybdenum excess when combined with a high sulfur intake results in a copper-deficient state. The three elements (Mo, Cu, S) combine to form cupric thiomolybdate complexes. In humans, excess molybdenum intakes occur rarely. This is because most human foods that contain molybdenum also contain copper in amounts that exceed that of molybdenum.

Molybdenum is a transition metal in the fifth period of the periodic table. It has an atomic weight of 95.94 and an atomic number of 42. There are several naturally occurring isotopes ranging in weight from 92 to 100; however, Mo^{96} is the most useful in biological research. There are eight radioisotopes with weights ranging from 88 to 93. Molybdenum has four charged states: +3, +4, +5, and +6. The most common is the +6 state. Where this mineral serves as a cofactor in enzymatic reactions, it vacillates between +4 and +6.

Absorption, Excretion, Function

Molybdenum is readily absorbed from most foods. Between 40% and 100% of the ingested mineral will be absorbed by the epithelial cells of the gastrointestinal system and will be found in the blood in a protein-bound complex. A plasma concentration range of 0.5–15 μg/dL has been reported, and molybdenum may be found in very small amounts (0.1–1.0 μg/g) in most cell types. Some accumulation occurs in the liver, kidneys, bones, and skin. Molybdenum is readily excreted in the urine with small amounts excreted via the bilary route. The average intake of 300 μg/day is 1/3 to 1/5 that of copper.

Molybdenum's function is as a cofactor for the iron and flavin enzymes, xanthine oxidase, aldehyde oxidase, and sulfite oxidase. The molybdenum cofactor common to these enzymes is a pterin structure shown in Figure 14.14. This pterin is a monophosphate ester susceptible to cleavage by alkaline phosphatase.[128] One molecule of pterin phosphatase is associated with each molybdenum atom in sulfite oxidase and xanthine dehydrogenase. In situ oxidation of the pterin leads to an inactivation of sulfite oxidase. Molybdenum also serves to activate adenylate cyclase in brain, cardiac

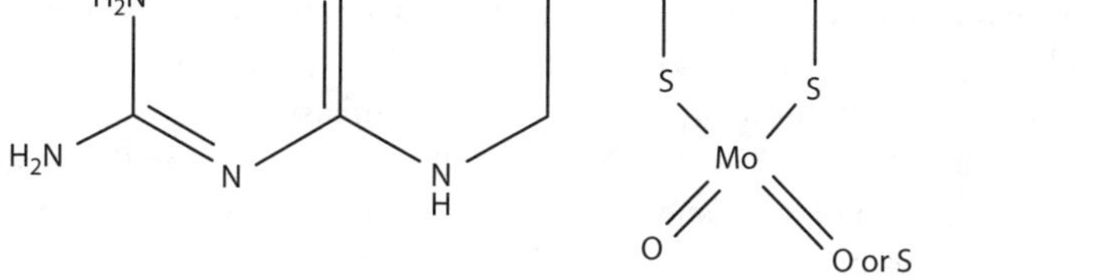

FIGURE 14.14 Pterin structure with molybdenum as part of its molecule.

and renal tissue and erythrocytes.[129] It has no effect on testicular adenylate cyclase nor does it have an effect on adenylate cyclase previously stimulated with fluoride or GTP.

Food Sources, Recommended Intake

Molybdenum is found in very small amounts in most foods. The germ of grain is a good source of this mineral; however, much of this germ is lost when the grain is milled. Table 14.1 shows the recommendations for intakes by the different age/life stage groups.

MANGANESE

Although manganese (Mn) was recognized as an essential nutrient in 1931, its ubiquitous role as a cofactor in a variety of enzymatic reactions has only recently been appreciated. Structural abnormalities in growing birds and animals are the chief symptoms of deficiency. Depression of mucopolysaccharide synthesis and decreased mitochondrial manganese superoxide dismutase activity accompany these skeletal abnormalities as does congenital ataxia due to abnormal inner ear development and abnormal brain function.[130] Biochemical abnormalities were hard to document because many of the requirements for manganese as a cofactor in a number of enzymatic reactions could be met by magnesium. Nonetheless, bone and connective tissue growth are abnormal in manganese-deficient animals. Few cases of human manganese deficiency have been reported.

Manganese, like magnesium, is a transition element. It can exist in 11 oxidation states. However, in mammalian systems, it usually exists in either the +3 or +2 state. In the +2 state, it is less easily chelated than in the +3 state. The +3 state is one that interacts with the ferric ion (Fe^{+++}); it is also the state needed for service as a cofactor in the Mn superoxide dismutase enzyme.

Absorption, Excretion, Function

Manganese is poorly absorbed through the gut. Between 2% and 15% of that ingested in the food appears in the blood. This has been traced using radioactive ^{54}Mn. As with many minerals, the route of excretion is via resecretion into the small intestine. That which is unabsorbed appears in the feces as does that which is excreted from the body via the bile. The mechanism whereby manganese is transported from the site of absorption to the site of use is not fully known. It may share transport with iron using transferrin or another protein, notably α-2-macroglobulin. Manganese circulates throughout the body at a level of 10–20 μg/L (~2 μmol/L). Widely varying blood levels of manganese have been reported. Smith et al.[114] contend that this wide variation has to do with contamination introduced by both sampling technique and analytical technique. Contamination can double the amount of manganese in the food, blood, or tissue sample. It is for this reason that balance studies to determine apparent absorption are not useful. Actually, this problem is common to many of the trace minerals. They are present in such small amounts in biological samples that extreme precautions must be taken to control contamination. Once transported from the gut to the liver, almost all of the manganese is cleared from the blood. In the liver it enters one of several pools. It can be found in the bile canaliculi from which it can be exported via the bile back into the small intestine or it can enter the hepatocytes whereupon it is used by its various organelles (lysosomes, mitochondria, nucleus), as a cofactor for several enzymes or it can remain in the cytoplasm.

Manganese is present in the bone as part of the mineral apatite, and in the lactating gland, and liver to a greater extent than in other tissues.[131] However, no tissue is free of this mineral. The turnover of manganese in the body varies depending on location. It is very short (~3 min half-life) in hepatic mitochondria and, in bone, its half-life is about an hour. The pool size likewise varies from 2 mg/kg in liver to 3.5 mg/kg in bone. As mentioned, it is an essential cofactor in a wide variety of

TABLE 14.9
Enzymes Requiring Manganese

Pyruvate carboxylase
Acetyl CoA carboxylase
Isocitrate dehydrogenase
Mitochondrial superoxide dismutase
Arginase
Glucokinase
Galactose transferase
Hydroxymethyl transferase
Superoxide dismutase

enzymatic reactions[132–134] and is essential for normal fetal and neonatal development.[135] Listed in Table 14.9 are some of the many enzymes shown to require manganese as a cofactor. Manganese and calcium share a uniport mechanism for mitochondrial transport. It can accumulate in this organelle because it is cleared very slowly. Mitochondrial manganese efflux is not sodium dependent and in fact appears to inhibit both the sodium-dependent and sodium-independent calcium efflux. This manganese effect on calcium is not reciprocal; calcium has no effect on manganese efflux.[133]

Evidence has been reported that manganese deficiency in experimental animals causes the downregulation of the mitochondrial manganese containing superoxide dismutase (SOD) at the level of the activation of transcription of the gene that encodes this protein.[132,136] Superoxide dismutases are a class of metalloproteins that catalyze the dismutation of the superoxide radical (O_2^-) to oxygen (O_2) and hydrogen peroxide (H_2O_2). These enzymes play a critical role in protecting cells against oxidative stress, particularly that produced by drugs (see Figure 14.7). Most mammalian cells contain two forms of this enzyme: one in the cytosol requiring iron or zinc and copper and the other requiring manganese. It is generally thought that the latter, present in the mitochondria, protects that organelle from potential damage by the superoxide radical that could possibly be produced through the activity of the respiratory chain. The important role of Mn SOD has been demonstrated using cell cultures. Those cultures in which the gene for this enzyme was altered or in which the enzyme was inhibited died. Apoptic cell death has been reported in cultured spinal neurons and in PC12 neuronal cells. Maintenance of mitochondrial manganese-dependent SOD is especially important if a drug is used that disrupts the control or function of the respiratory chain. Redox active drugs, for example, antibiotics, tetracycline, or pesticides, for example, paraquat, have this effect. When these compounds are given to animals or cells in culture, the activity of the manganese-superoxide dismutase increases. Interleukin-1 and tumor necrosis factor also increase the activity of this enzyme.[134] Some tumor cells respond to chemotherapeutic agents by increasing the activity of this enzyme as well. As a result, these tumors are resistant to certain cytotoxic agents. This is particularly true for melanoma cells and may explain the resistance of this cancer to many of the therapies found successful for other tumor cell types.

Food Sources, Recommended Intake

Rich food sources include nuts, whole grains, and leafy vegetables. Meats, milk, seafood, and other animal products are poor sources. The germ of grains can contain up to 14 ppm. The average diet consumed in the United States contains about 3–4 mg/day. The range of intakes suggested by the National Academy of Sciences is from 2 to 11 mg/day depending on the age and life stage of the consumers (see Table 14.1).

Toxicity

Manganese toxicity with symptoms resembling Parkinson's disease has been reported to occur in up to 25% of miners and metal mill workers in Russia, North Africa, Chile, and the former Yugoslavia. The inhalation of mineral dust in mines and mills is the main route of excess exposure.

COBALT

The discovery of cobalt as an essential nutrient for mammals was first made in Australia by animal scientists seeking to understand the pathophysiology of a wasting disease in sheep and cattle. At first, it was thought to be an iron deficiency disorder because iron supplements seemed to cure the condition. The iron supplements, however, were rather impure substances. In the mid-1930s, Underwood and associates discovered that it was not the iron per se but an impurity in the supplement that cured the condition. That impurity was cobalt.

Cobalt as an essential nutrient for humans was assumed based on the results of the aforementioned animal studies. Many human foods, especially green leafy vegetables, contain cobalt. Meats, including the organ meats, provide cobalt as a component of vitamin B_{12}. Of the free cobalt found in these foods very little is used although absorbed by the enterocyte. The results of tracer studies have shown that almost 100% of ingested cobalt appears in the urine. Very little appears in the feces and very little is retained in the tissues. As discussed in the section on vitamin B_{12} in the chapter on water-soluble vitamins, the absorption of this vitamin (and its cobalt component) is dependent on the presence of intrinsic factor in the stomach. Whereas in ruminants consumption of cobalt cures the wasting disease (pernicious anemia), it does this not because the ruminant can absorb and then use this metal but because the rumen flora can synthesize vitamin B_{12}, which in turn is absorbed. This then is the basis for understanding why vegetarians consuming large amounts of cobalt-rich green leafy vegetables are at risk for developing pernicious anemia. Vitamin B_{12} is found in foods of animal origin. Humans do not synthesize this vitamin as do the flora found in the ruminant. While vegetarians obtain sufficient cobalt, they may be vitamin B_{12} deficient. Cobalt has no other known function aside from its central action in vitamin B_{12} function.

Toxicity, Mineral Interactions

Although cobalt is readily absorbed by the enterocyte, it is just as readily excreted by the kidney. Thus, toxicity in the usual sense is not a significant problem with respect to environmental exposures. Excess cobalt (1000 times normal) can be tolerated by a variety of species with little ill effect. However, cobalt does interfere with the absorption of iron and in fact can completely block iron uptake. Symptoms of iron-deficiency anemia as well as symptoms of disturbed thyroid function (enlarged hyperplasic thyroid gland, myxedemia) and congestive heart failure have been observed when excess cobalt was consumed accidentally as a contaminant of beer. Cobalt salts were once used in the production of beer as a foaming agent. While the occasional beer would not provide toxic amounts of cobalt, regular large intakes could and have done so. Once this was recognized, this production practice was discontinued. Actually, it was not the cobalt content of the beer alone that was responsible for the toxic response. The alcohol of the beer plus the likelihood of inadequate protein, iron, and B vitamin intake were also part of the problem. Cobalt together with manganese and iodine is involved in the synthesis of thyroxine. Whether they are interacting or merely essential cofactors in thyroxine synthesis has not been satisfactorily resolved.

OTHER MINERALS

Shown in Table 14.3 are a variety of minerals that have been shown to be essential to one or more species, not necessarily man.[2] Included in this list is fluorine (fluoride), an element known to provide hardness to teeth and bones, and which also inhibits tooth decay. Arsenic, a known poison, has been shown to be essential to chickens, rats, pigs, and goats, but its biological function is not known. Animals with arsenic deficiency exhibit depressed growth, myocardial degeneration, and premature death. Boron, likewise, is an essential nutrient for rats, but its function is not known. Deficient rats have a reduced stress response that probably relates to a change in brain electrical activity. Boron–copper and boron–calcium–phosphate interactions have been reported. These interactions have to do with increased brain copper concentrations in the former and increased calcium and phosphate concentrations in the latter of boron-deprived animals.

Chromium as an essential mineral is controversial.[2,137] Early in its history it was reported to be essential for optimal peripheral insulin action with respect to glucose uptake.[138] Studies of elderly humans with noninsulin-dependent diabetes mellitus showed an improvement in glucose tolerance in about half of the subjects following a period of chromium supplementation.[139] However, chromium supplementation of subjects with established diabetes had no effect on glucose tolerance in other studies.[140–142] There is thus a question as to whether chromium has an effect on insulin-mediated glucose metabolism. In part, some of the confusion may be related to the analytical methods used for chromium analysis. These have been found inadequate.[2] Chromium has been found in bone[131] and in breast milk.[143] Whether excess chromium is toxic is also questionable because of its low availability. Chromium picolinate in a dose–response study has been shown to cause chromosome damage in vitro to hamster ovary cells.[20]

Nickel is another mineral whose function has not been defined, yet animals fed nickel-deficient diets fail to thrive. Nickel is a component of the urease enzyme family and although not found in mammalian urease has been found in ureases isolated from lower life forms. Similarly, nickel has been found associated with hydrogenases in lower life forms and in these species has a role in oxidation–reduction reactions as well as in methane formation.

Silicon has been found essential to chickens and rats and appears to be involved in bone formation.[2] Skeletal abnormalities typify silicon deficiency in these species.

Vanadium is needed by chickens for appropriate pigmentation[2]; however, whether this need is a true need or one induced by the particular diet ingredients used to compose the deficient diet is subject to discussion.

Aluminum, boron, tin, cadmium, lead, germanium, lithium, and rubidium have all been examined with respect to their essentiality. Data are lacking that document man's need for these elements. As mentioned earlier, these minerals can be toxic if exposure is great.

SUMMARY

1. The microminerals are subdivided into the trace minerals, iron, copper, and zinc and the ultratrace minerals, chromium, manganese, fluoride, iodide, cobalt, selenium, silicon, boron, vanadium, nickel, cadmium, lithium, lead, and molybdenum.
2. These nutrients are needed in very small amounts, and if intake exceeds need the excess could cause a toxic state.
3. Many of these minerals can be found in bone. Some can be found in hair.
4. Iron is an important component of hemoglobin as well as some other compounds.
5. Copper facilitates iron use and also serves as a cofactor in a number of enzyme reactions.
6. Zinc is important in gene expression as part of the zinc fingers. Zinc also is an important cofactor in a number of enzymatic reactions.
7. Fluoride serves to strengthen teeth and helps resist decay.
8. Iodide has a single purpose in serving in thyroid hormone synthesis.
9. There are interactions between the minerals. Some of these are helpful and some are not.

LEARNING OPPORTUNITIES

CASE STUDY 14.1 Cynthia Has an Automobile Accident

Cynthia is a 20-year-old college student. One night after a party at her boyfriend's fraternity, she decides to drive to her parents' home for the weekend. It is late Friday, and there was beer as well as some snack food at the party. Cynthia is not driving under the influence but being tired she was not as alert as she should have been. The driving conditions were not ideal: there had been a light misty rain and it was foggy in places. As Cynthia was traveling around a curve, an oncoming car with headlights on high suddenly appeared. Cynthia tried to escape a head-on collision but unfortunately she was unsuccessful and the two cars met head on. Fortunately, both cars were being driven cautiously and relatively slowly so neither driver was killed. Both were seriously injured. Both were transported to the local hospital by ambulance. Both suffered fractures and they both lost blood. Cynthia was worse off than the other driver. The other driver was a 35-year-old male. Analyze this situation. Why was Cynthia worse off than the male driver? What do you think contributed to her clinical condition? Playing the clinical detective what kinds of tests would you want to help you decide on the best possible course of action?

CASE STUDY 14.2 Nebraska Pioneer Women

In the late 1800s, many young couples homesteaded in the plains states of Kansas, Iowa, Nebraska, the Dakotas, and so forth. Some had migrated from the east with very few resources and very little farming experience. The land was free if you could prove it up. That is, if you lived and farmed the land you homesteaded for a set period of time. Some of these couples built dug-out homes or sod homes, cooking on an open fire, with very little cooking equipment. They ate what they grew and sometimes did not have very much to eat between harvests and the gathering of wild plants and the killing of wild animals. Those who had greater resources would have cast iron cooking pots and were able from time to time to buy needed staples.

After living out on the prairie for months at a time, the women would become unable to work and maintain their households. They became pale, listless, and weak. They would be taken into the nearby towns for rest and recuperation. After a month or two, they usually *perked up* and were able to return to their homesteads. What was going on? Describe the factors leading to the listlessness of these women? Were other members of the household similarly affected? Why or why not?

CASE STUDY 14.3 Maureen Decides to Adopt Vegetarianism

Maureen has always been a soft-hearted individual. She loves all manner of creatures and when she went away to college, she became aware of the fact that beef, lamb, chicken, and even pork chops came from living creatures and she hated the idea that these creatures were killed to provide food for her. So, she decided that she would no longer eat meat; she would only eat fruits and vegetables. She would, however, continue to enjoy small amounts of cheese, eggs, and milk.

This diet seemed to be very satisfying, but after about 6 months of vegetarianism, she began to feel less energetic than she used to feel. She decided that she should have a check-up and her doctor ordered a blood workup. He discovered that she was anemic. She had far fewer than normal red cells and many of these cells were very small or were very large immature ones. What is going on? What would you do to help Maureen recover her joy of life?

MULTIPLE-CHOICE QUESTIONS

1. Iron, copper, and zinc are
   a. Divalent ions
   b. Important to the synthesis of hemoglobin
   c. Require transporters for their absorption
   d. All of the above
2. Selenium is associated with
   a. White muscle disease
   b. Infertility
   c. Poor skin quality
   d. None of the above
3. Selenium functions in
   a. Antioxidation
   b. The enzyme, glutathione peroxidase
   c. Both a and b
   d. Neither a nor b
4. Milk and dairy products are good sources of
   a. Calcium and phosphorus
   b. Iodide and selenium
   c. Magnesium and manganese
   d. All of the above
5. Osteoporosis is
   a. Weak muscles
   b. Poor nerve conduction
   c. Thinning hair
   d. Weak, calcium-depleted bones

REFERENCES

1. Frieden, E. (1985) New perspectives on the essential trace elements. *J. Chem. Ed.* 62: 917–923.
2. Nielson, F.H. (2013) Trace mineral deficiencies. In: *Handbook of Nutrition and Food.* (C.D. Berdanier, J. Dwyer, D. Heber, eds.). Taylor & Francis, Boca Raton, FL, pp. 211–226.
3. Duncan, A., Talwar, D., McMillan, D., Stafanowicz, F., O'Reilly, D. (2012) Quantitative data on the magnitude of systemic inflammatory response and its effect on micronutrient status based on plasma measurements. *Am. J. Clin. Nutr.* 95: 64–71.
4. Fairweather-Tait, S.J. (1992) Bioavailability of trace elements. *Food Chem.* 43: 213–217.
5. Lorscheider, F.L., Vimy, M.J., Summers, A.O. (1995) Mercury exposure from silver tooth fillings: Emerging evidence questions a traditional dental paradigm. *FASEB J.* 9: 504–508.
6. Bothwell, T.H., Charlton, R.W. (1982) A general approach to the problems of iron deficiency and iron overload in the population at large. *Semin. Hematol.* 19: 54–67.
7. Herbert, V., Shaw, S., Jayatilleke, E., Stopler-Kasdan, T. (1994) Most free radical injury is iron related: It is promoted by iron, heme, holoferritin, and vitamin C and inhibited by desferoxamine and apoferritin. *Stem Cells* 12: 289–303.
8. Toyokuni, S. (1996) Iron induced carcinogenesis: The role of redox regulation. *Free Radic. Biol. Med.* 20: 553–566.
9. Conte, D., Narindrasorasak, S., Sarkar, B. (1996) In vivo and in vitro iron replaced zinc finger generates free radicals and causes DNA damage. *J. Biol. Chem.* 271: 5125–5130.
10. Kelly, E.J., Quaife, C.J., Froelick, G.J., Palmiter, R.D. (1996) Metallothionein I and II protect against zinc deficiency and zinc toxicity in mice. *J. Nutr.* 126: 1782–1790.
11. Olivares, M., Uauy, R. (1996) Limits of metabolic tolerance to copper and biological basis for present recommendations and regulations. *Am. J. Clin. Nutr.* 63: 846S–852S.
12. Chen, S.Y., Collipp, P.J., Hsu, J.M. (1985) Effect of sodium selenite toxicity on tissue distribution of zinc, iron and copper in rats. *Biol. Trace Elem. Res.* 7: 169–179.

13. Whanger, P.D. (1989) China, a country with both selenium deficiency and toxicity: Some thoughts and impressions. *J. Nutr.* 119: 1236–1239.
14. Clark, L.C. (1985) The epidemiology of selenium and cancer. *Fed. Proc.* 44: 2584–2589.
15. Mena, I., Marin, O., Fuenzalida, S., Cotzias, G.C. (1967) Chronic manganese poisoning and clinical pictures of manganese turnover. *Neurology* 17: 128–132.
16. Moser, P.B., Krebs, N.K., Blyler, E. (1991) Zinc hair concentrations and estimated zinc intakes of functionally delayed normal sized and small for age children. *Nutr. Res.* 2: 585–590.
17. Paustenbach, D.J., Finley, B.L., Kacew, S. (1996) Biological relevance and consequences of chemical or metal-induced DNA cross linking. *Proc. Soc. Exp. Biol. Med.* 211: 211–217.
18. Tsang, S.Y., Tam, S.C., Bremner, I., Burkitt, M.J. (1996) Copper-1,10-phenanthroline induces internucleosomal DNA fragmentation in HepG2 cells, resulting from direct oxidation by the hydroxyl radical. *Biochem J.* 317: 13–16.
19. Bremner, I. (1998) Manifestations of copper excess. *Am. J. Clin. Nutr.* 67: 1069S–1073S.
20. Stearns, D.M., Wise, J.P., Patierno, S.R., Wetterhahn, K.E. (1995) Chromium (III) picolinate produces chromosome damage in Chinese hamster ovary cells. *FASEB J.* 9: 1643–1648.
21. Misra, M., Athar, M., Hasan, S.K., Srivastava, R.C. (1988) Alleviation of nickel-induced biochemical alterations by chelating agents. *Fund. Appl. Toxicol.* 11: 285–292.
22. Nielsen, F.H., Zimmerman, T.J., Shuler, T.R. (1982) Interactions among nickel, copper, and iron in rats. Liver and plasma content of lipids and trace elements. *Biol. Trace Elem. Res.* 4: 125–143.
23. Spears, J.W., Hatfield, E.E., Forbes, R.M. (1977) Nickel-copper interrelationship in the rat. *Proc. Soc. Exp. Biol. Med.* 156: 140–143.
24. Fischer, P.W.F., Giroux, A., L'Abbe, M.R.L. (1984) Effect of zinc supplementation on copper status in adult man. *Am. J. Clin. Nutr.* 40: 743–746.
25. Johnson, M.A., Greger, J.L. (1985) Tin, copper, iron and calcium metabolism of rats fed various dietary levels of inorganic tin and zinc. *J. Nutr.* 115: 615–624.
26. Oestreicher, P., Cousins, R.J. (1985) Copper and zinc absorption in the rat: Mechanism of mutual antagonism. *J. Nutr.* 115: 159–166.
27. Hansen, S.L., Trakooljul, N., Liu, H.-C., Moeser, A.J., Spears, J.W. (2009) Iron transporters are differentially regulated by dietary iron, and modifications are associated with changes in manganese metabolism in young pigs. *J. Nutr.* 139: 1474–1479.
28. Christian, H.A. (1903) A sketch of the history of the treatment of chlorosis. *Med. Lab. Hist. J.* 1: 176–180.
29. Fairweather-Tait, S.J. (1987) The concept of bioavailability as it relates to iron nutrition. *Nutr. Res.* 7: 319–325.
30. Johnson, M.A. (1990) Iron: Nutrition monitoring and nutrition status assessment. *J. Nutr.* 120: 1486–1491.
31. Looker, A.C., Gunter, E.W., Johnson, C.L. (1995) Methods to assess iron status in various NHANES surveys. *Nutr. Rev.* 53: 246–254.
32. Morris, E.R. (1983) An overview of current information on bioavailability of dietary iron to humans. *Fed. Proc.* 42: 1716–1720.
33. Donovan, A., Roy, C.N., Andrews, N.C. (2006) The ins and outs of iron homeostasis. *Physiology* 21: 115–123.
34. Crichton, R.R., Charloteaux-Wauters, M. (1987) Iron transport and storage. *Eur. J. Biochem.* 164: 485–506.
35. Kuvibidila, S., Warrier, R.P., Ode, D., Yu, L. (1996) Serum transferrin receptor concentrations in women with mild malnutrition. *Am. J. Clin. Nutr.* 63: 596–601.
36. Zakim, M.M. (1992) Regulation of transferrin gene expression. *FASEB J.* 6: 3253–3258.
37. Munro, H.N., Kikinis, Z., Eisenstein, R.S. (1993) Iron dependent regulation of ferritin synthesis. In: *Nutrition and Gene Expression* (C.D. Berdanier, J.L. Hargrove, eds.). CRC Press, Boca Raton, FL, pp. 525–545.
38. Proudhon, D., Wei, J., Briat, J.F., Theil, E.C. (1996) Ferritin gene organization: Differences between plants and animals suggest possible kingdom specific selective constraints. *J. Mol. Evol.* 42: 325–336.
39. Rogers, J., Munro, H. (1987) Translation of ferritin light and heavy subunit mRNA's is regulated by intracellular chelatable iron levels in rat hepatoma cells. *Proc. Natl. Acad. Sci. USA* 84: 2277–2281.
40. Cairo, G., Castrusini, E, Minotti, G., Bernelli-Zazzara, A. (1996) Superoxidide and hydrogen peroxide-dependent inhibition of iron regulatory protein activity: A protective stratagem against oxidative injury. *FASEB J.* 10: 1326–1335.
41. Beinert, H., Kennedy, M.C. (1993) Aconitase, a two-faced protein: Enzyme and iron regulatory factor. *FASEB J.* 7: 1442–1449.

42. Price, D., Joshi, J.G. (1982) Ferritin: A zinc detoxicant and a zinc ion donor. *Proc. Natl. Acad. Sci. USA* 79: 3116–3119.
43. Sullivan, J.L. (2007) Macrophage iron, hepcidin, and atherosclerotic plaque stability. *Exp. Biol. Med.* 232: 1014–1020.
44. Nicolas, G., Chauvet, C., Viatte, L., Danan, J.L., Bigard, X., Devaux, I., Beaumont, C., Kahn, A., Vaulont, S. (2002) The gene encoding the iron regulatory peptide hepcidin is regulated by anemia, hypoxia, and inflammation. *J. Clin. Invest.* 110: 1037–1044.
45. Zimmermann, M.B., Troesch, B., Biebinger, R., Egli, I., Zeder, C., Hurrell, R.F. (2009) Plasma hepcidin is a modest predictor of dietary iron bioavailability in humans, whereas oral iron loading, measured by stable-isotope appearance curves, increases plasma hepcidin. *Am. J. Clin. Nutr.* 90: 1280–1287.
46. Roe, M.A., Collings, R., Dainty, J.R., Swinkels, D.W., Fairweather-Tait, S.J. (2009) Plasma hepcidin concentrations significantly predict interindividual variation in iron absorption in healthy men. *Am. J. Clin. Nutr.* 89: 1088–1091.
47. Mei, Z., Cogswell, M.E., Looker, A.C., Pfeiffer, C.M., Cusick, S.E., Lacher, D.A., Grummer-Strawn, L.M. (2011) Assessment of iron status in US pregnant women from the National Health and Nutrition Examination Survey (NHANES) 1999–2006. *Am. J. Clin. Nutr.* 93: 1188–1189.
48. Hunt, J.R., Zito, C.A., Johnson, L.K. (2009) Body iron excretion by healthy men and women. *Am. J. Clin. Nutr.* 89: 1792–1798.
49. Chung, B., Chaston, T., Marks, J., Srai, S.K., Sharp, P.A. (2009) Hepcidin decreases iron transporter expression in vivo in mouse duodenum and spleen and in vitro in THP-1 macrophages and intestinal caco-2 cells. *J. Nutr.* 139: 1457–1462.
50. Parke, D.V., Iannides, C., Lewis, D.F.V. (1991) The role of cytochrome P450 in the detoxification and activation of drugs and other chemicals. *Can. J. Physiol. Pharmacol.* 69: 537–549.
51. Johnson, M.A., Fischer, J.G., Bowman, B.A., Gunter, E.W. (1994) Iron nutriture in elderly individuals. *FASEB J.* 8: 609–621.
52. Hill, C.H., Ashwell, C.M., Nolin, S.J., Keeley, F., Billingham, C., Hinek, A., Starcher, B. (2007) Dietary iron deficiency compromises normal development of elastic fibers in the aorta and lungs of chicks. *J. Nutr.* 137: 1895–1900.
53. Halsted, J.A., Smith, J.C., Jr., Irwin, M.I. (1974) A conspectus of research on zinc requirements of man. *J. Nutr.* 104: 345–378.
54. Oberleas, D. (1993) Understanding zinc deficiency. *J. Texas State Nutr. Counc.* 3: 3–6.
55. Wegmuller, R., Tay, F., Zeder, C., Brnic, M., Hurrell, R.F. (2013) Zinc absorption by young adults from supplemental zinc citrate is comparable with that from zinc gluconate and higher than from zinc oxide. *J. Nutr.* 144: 132–136.
56. Failla, M., Cousins, R.J. (1978) Zinc uptake by isolated rat liver parenchymal cells. *BBA* 538: 435–444.
57. Masuoka, J., Saltman, P. (1994) Zinc (II) and copper (II) binding to serum albumin. *J. Biol. Chem.* 269: 25557–25561.
58. Lupo, A., Cesaro, E., Montano, G., Zulo, D., Izzo, P., Costanzo, P. (2013) KRAB-zinc finger proteins: A repressor family displaying multiple biological functions. *Curr. Genomic.* 14: 268–278.
59. Wei, S., Zhang, L., Zhou, X., Du, M., Hausman, G.J., Bergen, W.G., Zan, L., Dodson, M.V. (2013) Emerging roles of zinc finger proteins in regulating adipogenesis. *Cell Mol. Life. Sci.* 70: 4569–4584.
60. Billings, T., Parvanov, E.D., Baker, C.L., Walker, M., Paigen, K., Petkov, P.M. (2013) DNA binding specificities of the long zinc-finger recombination protein PRDMS. *Genome Biol.* 24: 14–35.
61. Wu, H., Yang, W-P., Barbas, C.F. (1995) Building zinc fingers by selection: Toward a therapeutic application. *Proc. Natl. Acad. Sci. USA* 92: 344–348.
62. Cousins, R.J., Leinart, A.S. (1988) Tissue specific regulation of zinc metabolism and metallothionein genes by interleukin 1. *FASEB J.* 2: 2884–2890.
63. Dalton, T., Fu, K., Palmiter, R.D., Andrews, G.K. (1996) Transgenic mice that overexpress metallothionine-I resist zinc deficiency. *J. Nutr.* 126: 825–833.
64. Durnam, D.M., Palmiter, R. (1981) Transcriptional regulation of the mouse metallothionine-I gene by heavy metals. *J. Biol. Chem.* 256: 6712–6716.
65. Kelly, E.J., Palmiter, E.D. (1996) A murine model of Menkes disease reveals a physiological function of metallothionein. *Nat. Genet.* 13: 219–222.
66. Palmiter, R.D. (1994) Regulation of metallothionein genes by heavy metals appears to be mediated by a zinc sensitive inhibitor that interacts with a constitutively active transcription factor MTF-1. *Proc. Natl. Acad. Sci. USA* 91: 1219–1223.
67. Reyes, J.G. (1996) Zinc transport in mammalian cells. *Am. J. Physiol.* 270: C401–C410.

68. Shay, N.F., Cousins, R.J. (1993) Dietary regulation of metallothionein expression. In: *Nutrition and Gene Expression* (C.D. Berdanier, J.L. Hargrove, eds.). CRC Press, Boca Raton, FL, pp. 507–523.
69. Kanoni, S. et al. (2011) Total zinc intake may modify the glucose-raising effect of a zinc transporter (SLC30A8) variant: A 14-cohort meta analysis. *Diabetes* 60: 2407–2416.
70. Castro, C.E., Kaspin, L.C., Chen, S-S., Nolker, S.G. (1992) Zinc deficiency increases the frequency of single strand DNA breaks in rat liver. *Nutr. Res.* 12: 721–736.
71. Fung, E.B., Kwiatkowski, J.L., Huang, J.N., Gildengorin, G., King, J.C., Vichinsky, E.P. (2013) Zinc supplementation improves bone density in patients with thalassemia: A double-blind, randomized, placebo-controlled trial. *Am. J. Clin. Nutr.* 98: 960–971.
72. Bao, B., Prasad, A.S., Beck, F.W.J., Fitzgerald, J.T., Snell, D., Singh, T., Cardozo, L.J. (2010) Zinc decreases C-reactive protein, lipid peroxidation, and inflammatory cytokines in elderly subjects: A potential implication of zinc as an atheroprotective agent. *Am. J. Clin. Nutr.* 91: 1634–1641.
73. Song, Y., Leonard, S.W., Traber, M.G., Ho, E. (2009) Zinc deficiency affects DNA damage, oxidative stress, antioxidant defenses and DNA repair in rats. *J. Nutr.* 139: 1626–1631.
74. Song, Y., Chung, C.S., Bruno, R.S., Traber, M.G., Brown, K.H., King, J.C., Ho, E. (2009) Dietary zinc restriction and repletion affects DNA integrity in healthy men. *Am. J. Clin. Nutr.* 90: 321–328.
75. Sheline, C.T., Shi, C., Takata, T., Zhu, J., Zhang, W., Sheline, J., Cai, A.-L., Li, L. (2012) Dietary zinc reduction, pyruvate supplementation or zinc transporter-5 knockout attenuates β-cell death in nonobese diabetic mice, islets and insulinoma cells. *J. Nutr.* 142: 2119–2127.
76. Prasad, A.S. (1984) Discovery and importance of zinc in human nutrition. *Fed. Proc.* 43: 2829–2834.
77. McNall, A.D., Etherton, T.D., Fosmire, G.J. (1995) The impaired growth induced by zinc deficiency in rats is associated with decreased expression of the hepatic insulin-like growth factor I and growth hormone receptor genes. *J. Nutr.* 125: 874–879.
78. Keen, C.L., Taubeneck, M.W., Daston, G.P., Rogers, J.M., Gershwin, M.E. (1993) Primary and secondary zinc deficiency as factors underlying abnormal CNS development. *Ann. N.Y. Acad. Sci.* 678: 37–47.
79. Emery, M.P., O'Dell, B.L. (1993) Low zinc status in rats impairs calcium uptake and aggregation of platelets stimulated by fluoride. *Proc. Soc. Exp. Biol. Med.* 203: 480–484.
80. Mahajan, S.K., Prasad, A.S., Rabbani, P., Briggs, W.A., McDonald, F.D. (1982) Zinc deficiency: A reversible complication of uremia. *Am. J. Clin. Nutr.* 36: 1177–1183.
81. Ruz, M., Carrasco, F., Ropjas, P., Codoceo, J., Inostroza, J., Basfi-fer, K., Csendes, A. et al. (2011) Zinc absorption and zinc status are reduced after Roux-en-Y gastric bypass: a randomized study using supplements. *Am. J. Clin. Nutr.* 94: 1004–1011.
82. Reeves, P.G. (1995) Adaptation responses in rats to long term feeding of high zinc diets: Emphasis on intestinal metallothionein. *J. Nutr. Biochem.* 6: 48–54.
83. Hart, E.B., Steenbock, H., Wasddell, J., Cartwright, G. (1928) Iron in nutrition. VII. Copper as a supplement to iron for hemoglobin building in the rat. *J. Biol. Chem.* 77: 797–812.
84. Frieden, E. (1983) The copper connection. *Semin. Hematol.* 20: 114–117.
85. Sandstead, H.H. (1982) Copper bioavailability and requirements. *Am. J. Clin. Nutr.* 35: 809–814.
86. Johnson, M.A., Kays, S.E. (1990) Copper: Its role in human nutrition. *Nutr. Today* January/February: 6–14.
87. Fields, M., Craft, N., Lewis, C., Holbrook, J., Rose, A., Reiser, S., Smith, J.C. (1986) Contrasting effects of the stomach and small intestine of rats on copper absorption. *J. Nutr.* 116: 219–2228.
88. Turnlund, J.R., Keyes, W.R., Anderson, H.L., Acord, L.L. (1989) Copper absorption and retention in young men at three levels of dietary copper by use of the stable isotope ^{65}Cu. *Am. J. Clin. Nutr.* 49: 870–878.
89. Weiss, K.C., Linder, M.C. (1985) Copper transport in rats involving a new plasma protein. *Am. J. Physiol.* 249: E77–E88.
90. Fischer, P.W.F., Giroux, A., L'Abbe, M.R. (1981) Effect of dietary zinc on intestinal copper absorption. *Am. J. Clin. Nutr.* 34: 1670–1675.
91. Linder, M., Roboz, M. (1986) Turnover and excretion of copper in rats as measured with ^{67}Cu. *Am. J. Physiol.* 251: E551–E555.
92. Harris, E.D. (1991) Copper transport: An overview. *Proc. Soc. Exp. Biol. Med.* 196: 130–146.
93. Wang, Y.R., Wu, J.Y.J., Reaves, S.K., Lei, K.Y. (1996) Enhanced expression of hepatic genes in copper deficient rats detected by the messenger RNA differential display method. *J. Nutr.* 126: 1772–1781.
94. Hoshi, Y., Hazeki, O., Tamura, M. (1993) Oxygen dependence of redox state of copper in cytochrome oxidase in vitro. *J. Appl. Physiol.* 74: 1622–1627.
95. Johnson, W.T., Dufault, S.N., Newman, S.M. (1995) Altered nucleotide content and changes in mitochondrial energy states associated with copper deficiency in rat platelets. *J. Nutr. Biochem.* 6: 551–556.

96. Matz, J.M., Saari, J.T., Bode, A.M. (1995) Functional aspects of oxidative phosphorylation and electron transport in cardiac mitochondria of copper deficient rats. *J. Nutr. Biochem.* 6: 644–652.
97. Wildman, R.E.C., Hopkins, R., Failla, M.L., Medeiros, D.M. (1995) Marginal copper restricted diets produce altered cardiac ultrastructure in the rat. *Proc. Soc. Exp. Biol. Med.* 210: 43–49.
98. Hopkins, R.G., Failla, M. (1995) Chronic intake of a marginally low copper diet impairs in vitro activities of lymphocytes and neutrophils from male rats despite minimal impact on conventional indicators of copper status. *J. Nutr.* 125: 2658–2668.
99. Rhee, Y.S., Burnham, B.K., Stoecker, B.J., Lucas, E. (2004) Effects of chromium and copper depletion on lymphocyte reactivity to mitogens in diabetes prone BHE/Cdb rats. *Nutrition* 20: 274–279.
100. Klevay, L.M., Inman, L., Johnson, L.K., Lawler, M., Mahalko, J.R., Milne, D.B., Lukaski, H.C., Bolonchuk, W., Sandstead, H.H. (1984) Increased cholesterol in plasma in a young man during experimental copper deficiency. *Metabolism* 33: 1112–1118.
101 Kim, S., Chao, P.Y., Allen, K.G.D. (1992) Inhibition of elevated glutathione abolishes copper deficiency cholesterolemia. *FASEB J.* 6: 2467–2471.
102. Lee, G.R., Cartwright, G.E., Wintrobe, M.M. (1968) Heme biosynthesis in copper deficient swine. *Proc. Soc. Exp. Biol. Med.* 127: 977–981.
103. Prohaska, J.R. (1986) Genetic diseases of copper metabolism. *Clin. Physiol. Biochem.* 4: 87–93.
104. Reed, V., Williamson, P., Bull, P.C., Cox, D.W., Boyd, Y. (1995) Mapping the mouse homologue of the Wilson disease gene to mouse chromosome 8. *Genomics* 28: 573–575.
105. Yang, G.Q., Wang, S., Zhou, R., Sun, S. (1983) Endemic selenium intoxication of humans in China. *Am. J. Clin. Nutr.* 37: 872–881.
106. DiDonato, M., Narindrasorasak, S., Forbes, J.R., Cox, D.W., Sarkar, B. (1997) Expression, purification and metal binding properties of the N-terminal domain from the Wilson disease putative copper-transporting ATPase (ATP7B). *J. Biol. Chem.* 272: 33279–33282.
107. Yang, X.L., Miura, N., Kawarada, Y., Petrukhin, K., Gilliam, T.C., Sugiyama, T. (1997) Two forms of Wilson disease protein produced by alternative splicing are localized in distinct cellular compartments. *Biochem. J.* 326: 897–902.
108. Ke, B.-X., Llanos, R.M., Mercer, J.F.B. (2008) ATP7A transgenic and nontransgenic mice are resistant to high copper exposure. *J. Nutr.* 138: 693–697.
109. Schwartz, K., Foltz, C.M. (1957) Selenium as an integral part of factor 3 against dietary necrotic degeneration. *J. Am. Chem. Soc.* 79: 3292–3293.
110. Lauretani, F., Semba, R., Bandinelli, S., Ray, A.L., Guralnik, J.M., Ferrucci, L. (2007) Association of low plasma selenium concentrations with poor muscle strength in older community-dwelling adults: The InCHIANTI study. *Am. J. Clin. Nutr.* 86: 347–352.
111. Yeh, J.-Y., Beilstein, M.A., Andrews, J.S., Whanger, P.D. (1995) Tissue distribution and influence of selenium status on levels of selenoprotein W. *FASEB J.* 9: 392–396.
112. Burk, R.F. (1989) Recent developments in trace element metabolism and function: Newer roles of selenium in nutrition. *J. Nutr.* 119: 1051–1054.
113. Burk, R.F. (1991) Molecular biology of selenium with implications for its metabolism. *FASEB J.* 5: 2274–2279.
114. Stadtman, T.C. (1987) Specific occurrence of selenium in enzymes and amino acid tRNAs. *FASEB J.* 1: 375–379.
115. Bermano, G., Nicol, F., Dyer, J.A., Sunde, R.A., Beckett, G.J., Arthur, J.R., Hesketh, J.E. (1996) Selenoprotein gene expression during selenium-repletion of selenium deficient rats. *Biol. Trace Elem. Res.* 51: 211–223.
116. Levander, O.A., DeLoach, D.P., Moris, V.C., Moser, P.B. (1983) Platelet glutathione peroxidase activity as an index of selenium status in rats. *J. Nutr.* 113: 55–63.
117. Floyd, R.A. (1990) Role of oxygen free radicals in carcinogens and brain ischemia. *FASEB J.* 4: 2587–2597.
118. Tamura, T., Stadtman, T.C. (1996) A new selenoprotein from human lung adenocarcinoma cells: Purification, properties and thioredoxin reductase activity. *Proc. Natl. Acad. Sci. USA* 93: 1006–1011.
119. Arthur, J.R., Nicol, F., Beckett, G.J. (1993) Selenium deficiency, thyroid hormone metabolism and thyroid hormone deiodinases. *Am. J. Clin. Nutr.* 57: 236S–239S.
120. Beckett, G.J., Nicol, F., Rae, P.W.H., Beech, S., Guo, Y., Arthur, J.R. (1993) Effects of combined iodine and selenium deficiency on thyroid hormone metabolism in rats. *Am. J. Clin. Nutr.* 57: 240S–243S.
121. Thompson, K.M., Haibach, H., Sunde, R.A. (1995) Growth and plasma triiodothyronine concentrations are modified by selenium deficiency and repletion in second generation selenium deficient rats. *J. Nutr.* 125: 864–873.

122. Cheng, W.H., Fu, Y.X., Porres, J.M., Ross, D.A., Lei, X.G. (1999) Selenium-dependent cellular glutathione peroxidase protects mice against a pro-oxidant-induced oxidation of NADPH, NADH, lipids and protein. *FASEB J.* 13: 1467–1475.
123. Cohen, H.J., Brown, M.R., Hamilton, D., Lyons-Patterson, J., Avessar, N., Liegey, P. (1989) Glutathione peroxidase and selenium deficiency in patients receiving home parenteral nutrition: Time course for development of deficiency and repletion of enzyme activity in plasma and blood cells. *Am. J. Clin. Nutr.* 49: 132–139.
124. Lai, C.C., Huang, W-H., Askari, A., Klevay, L.M., Chiu, T.H. (1995) Expression of glutathione peroxidase and catalase in copper-deficient rat liver and heart. *J. Nutr. Biochem.* 6: 256–262.
125. Robberecht, H., Deelstra, H. (1994) Factors influencing blood selenium concentration values. *J. Trace Elem. Electrolytes Health Dis.* 8: 129–143.
126. Wilber, C.G. (1980) Toxicology of selenium: A review. *Clin. Toxicol.* 17: 171–230.
127. Boyages, S. (1993) Iodine deficiency disorders. *J. Clin. Endo. Metab.* 77: 587–591.
128. Maberly, G.F. (1994) Iodine deficiency disorders: Contemporary scientific issues. *J. Nutr.* 124: 1473S–1478S.
129. Rajagopalan, K.V., Johnson, J.L., Hainline, B.E. (1982) The pterin of the molybdenum factor. *Fed. Proc.* 41: 2608–2612.
130. Richard, J.M., Swislocki, N.I. (1979) Activation of adenylate cyclase by molybdate. *J. Biol. Chem.* 254: 6857–6860.
131. Wolinsky, I., Klimis-Tavantzis, D.J., Richards, L.J. (1994) Manganese and bone metabolism. In: *Manganese in Health and Disease* (D.J. Klimis-Tavantzis, ed.). CRC Press, Inc., Boca Raton, FL, pp. 115–120.
132. Smith, J.C., Anderson, R.A., Ferretti, R., Levander, O.A., Morris, E.R., Roginski, E.E., Veillon, C., Wolf, W.R., Anderson, J.B., Mertz, W. (1981) Evaluation of published data pertaining to mineral composition of human tissue. *Fed. Proc.* 40: 2120–2125.
133. Borrello, S., DeLeo, M.E., Galeotti, T. (1992) Transcriptional regulation of MnSOD by manganese in the liver of manganese deficient mice and during rat development. *Biochem. Int.* 28: 595–561.
134. Gavin, C.E., Gunter, K.K., Gunter, T.E. (1990) Manganese and calcium efflux kinetics in brain mitochondria. *Biochem. J.* 266: 329–334.
135. Hirose, K., Longo, D.L., Oppenheim, J., Matsushima, K. (1993) Overexpression of mitochondrial manganese superoxide dismutase promotes the survival of tumor cells exposed to interleukin 1, tumor necrosis factor, selected anticancer drugs and ionizing radiation. *FASEB J.* 7: 361–368.
136. Hurley, L.S. (1981) Roles of trace elements in fetal and neonatal development. *Phil. Trans. R. Soc. Lond.* 294: 145–152.
137. Santiard-Baron, D., Aral, B., Ribiere, C., Nordmann, R., Sinet, P.-M., Caballos-Picot, I. (1995) Quantitation of Mn-SOD mRNA's by using a competitive reverse-transcription polymerase chain reaction. *Redox Rep.* 1: 185–189.
138. Stoecker, B.J. (1996) Chromium. In: *Present Knowledge in Nutrition* (E.E. Eckhard, L.J. Filer, eds.). ILSI Press, Washington, DC, pp. 344–352.
139. Mertz, W. (1993) Chromium in human nutrition: A review. *J. Nutr.* 123: 626–633.
140. Potter, J.F., Levin, P., Anderson, R.A., Freiberg, J.M., Andres, R., Elahi, D. (1985) Glucose metabolism in glucose-intolerant older people during chromium supplementation. *Metabolism* 34: 199–204.
141. Offenbacher, E.G., Rinko, C.J., Pi-Sunyer, X. (1985) The effects of inorganic chromium and brewer's yeast on glucose tolerance, plasma lipids, and plasma chromium in elderly subjects. *Am. J. Clin. Nutr.* 42: 454–461.
142. Rabinowitz, M.B., Gonick, H.C., Levin, S.R., Davidson, M.B. (1983) Clinical trial of chromium and yeast supplements on carbohydrate and lipid metabolism in diabetic men. *Biol. Trace Min. Res.* 5: 449–466.
143. Engelhardt, S., Moser-Veillon, P.B., Mangels, A.R., Patterson, K.Y., Veillon, C. (1990) Appearance of an oral dose of chromium (^{53}Cr) in breast milk. In: *Breast Feeding, Nutrition, Infection and Infant Growth in Developed and Emerging Countries* (S.A. Atkinson, L.A. Hanson, R.K. Chandra, eds.). ARTS Biomedical Publishing, St. John's Newfoundland, Canada, pp. 484–487.

Appendix

TABLE A.1
Websites for Information from Health-Oriented Organizations

Organization	Web Address
Nutrition	www.ASN.org
Physiology	www.aps.org
Heart disease	www.americanheart.org/presenter.jhtml?identifier=1477
	www.pediheart.org
Diabetes mellitus	www.diabetes.org
	www.jdfr.org
Genetic diseases	www.mansfieldct.org/schools/mms/staff/hand/Gendisease.htm
	www.cdh.org/healthinformation.aspx?pageld=P02505
	www.genetics.org.uk
	www.nlm.nih.gov/medlineplus/rarediseases.html
	www.research.jax.org/index.html
Crohn's disease	www.ccfa.org/reuters/geneticlink
Kidney disease	www.kidneyhealth.org/genetic.html
Pompe's disease	www.agsdus.org/html/typeiipompe.html
Tay Sach's disease	www.kumac.edu/gec/support/tay-sach.html
Celiac disease	www.celiaccenter.org/faq.asp
Huntington's disease	www.hdny.org/genetic.html
Parkinson's disease	www.parkinson's.org
Cystic fibrosis	www.cff.org
	www.nim.nih.gov/medlineplus/cysticfibrosis.html

TABLE A.2
Nutrition-Related Web Resources

Nutritional effects on chronic alcoholism	
http://www.britannica.com/EBchecked/topic/422916/nutritional-disease/247876/Alcohol	Single article with links to related topics such as fetal alcohol syndrome, pancreatitis, and thiamine deficiency.
http://www.niaaa.nih.gov/	Links to research and informational papers on many aspects of diet and alcohol consumption.
Food allergies and food intolerance	
http://www.fda.gov/Food/	Links to papers on allergies and intolerances.
https://www.facebook.com/AmericanAcademyofAllergyAsthmaandImmunology?sk=wall	Good site for pubic/professional interaction. Must be on Facebook and "like" AAAAI.
http://www.aaaai.org/conditions-and-treatments/allergies/food-allergies.aspx	Good overview of food allergies in general with links to specific topics related to food allergies and intolerance.
http://www.nhs.uk/Conditions/food-allergy/	Good overview of food allergies and intolerances. UK based.
http://www.niaid.nih.gov/pages/default.aspx?wt.ac=tnHome	Links to Bioinformatics, Translational research tools, Biological materials.
http://www.nutrition.gov/nutrition-and-health-issues/food-allergies-and-intolerances	Clearing house site with links to FDA, NIH, and FDA many connection to specific topics.
http://www.foodallergy.org/	Slanted toward nonprofessionals.
Nutrition and immune function	
http://www.ajcn.org/	This site is for researchers. Use the search button to look for immune function.
Making a nutritional assessment (clinical)	
http://fnic.nal.usda.gov/dietary-guidance/dietary-assessment	Links to Super tracker, Nutrition analysis tool, Several calorie trackers, Fat screener.
http://apps.medsch.ucla.edu/nutrition/dietassess.htm	Includes several assessment checklists.
Metabolic syndrome (overweight and fatty liver)	
http://www.heart.org/HEARTORG/Conditions/More/MetabolicSyndrome/Metabolic-Syndrome_UCM_002080_SubHomePage.jsp	Includes a risk assessment checker, good explanations associated with treatment and symptoms.
http://www.nhlbi.nih.gov/health/health-topics/topics/ms/	National heart lung and blood institute site with links to many areas associated with metabolic syndrome.
http://www.nlm.nih.gov/medlineplus/metabolicsyndrome.html	Lots of links to associated topics and diseases. Very complete site.
Malnourished child	
http://kidshealth.org/parent/growth/feeding/hunger.html	
http://www.bapen.org.uk/	Definitions of malnutrition with a malnutrition *calculator* and tracking malnutrition. Although based in the United Kingdom, may be of interest to dietetic professionals.
Failure to thrive	
http://kidshealth.org/parent/growth/growth/failure_thrive.html#cat162	
http://www.ncbi.nlm.nih.gov/pubmedhealth/PMH0001986/	Definition of failure to thrive and possible causes along with links to assessment and treatment options.
Pediatric nutrition	
http://www.eatright.org/	Information about supporting normal growth and development.
http://www.bcm.edu/cnrc/	
http://www.familyfoodzone.com/	

(*Continued*)

TABLE A.2 (*CONTINUED*)
Nutrition-Related Web Resources

Childhood obesity	
http://www.cdc.gov/nccdphp/dnpao/index.html http://win.niddk.nih.gov/index.htm http://www2.aap.org/obesity/ http://www.med.umich.edu/1libr/yourchild/obesity.htm http://www.aafp.org/afp/990215ap/861.html	These sites provide information on childhood obesity, consequences, and treatment options.
Eating disorders	
http://www.nationaleatingdisorders.org/ http://www.helpguide.org/mental/anorexia_signs_symptoms_causes_treatment.htm http://kidshealth.org/teen/your_mind/mental_health/eat_disorder.html http://my.clevelandclinic.org/healthy_living/weight_control/hic_the_psychology_ofeating.aspx http://www.recoveryconnection.org/eating-disorders/	All of these sites list and describe various eating disorders from too little food to ingestion of too much food. There are assessments for evaluating diet distortions.
Nutrition and oral health	
http://www.mouthhealthy.org/Home/az-topics/d/diet-and-dental-health	American Dental Association site. Good review of topic, site deals with nutrition at all lifestages.
Protein nutrition and muscle mass (appetite)	
http://www.eatright.org/	Various topics including suggested means of providing nutrients for building muscles under "nutrition for men" tab.
Macro and micronutrient supplementation	
http://familydoctor.org/familydoctor/en/prevention-wellness/food-nutrition/nutrients/dietary-supplements-what-you-need-to-know.html	Subtopics include calcium supplementation and antioxidant needs.
http://fnic.nal.usda.gov/food-composition/individual-macronutrients-phytonutrients-vitamins-min	Links for many common vitamins and minerals as well as other related topics in nutrition (see Chapter 1).
Bioactive food components	
http://www.eufic.org/article/en/artid/Nutrient-bioavailability-food/	
http://ec.europa.eu/research/biosociety/food_quality/projects_en.html	Contains an A–Z list of project relative to obtain maximum nutrient value from foods.
Herbal supplements	
http://nccam.nih.gov/health/supplements/wiseuse.htm	Site discusses safety and efficacy factors related to mass produced herbal supplements.
http://fnic.nal.usda.gov/dietary-supplements/herbal-information	Clearing house with links to the American Academy of Physicians and various university research sites.
http://fnic.nal.usda.gov/food-composition/individual-macronutrients-phytonutrients-vitamins-minerals/phytonutrients	Clearing house with links to several search engines with information about nutrient supplementation.
Nutrition and disease	
http://www.nestlehealthscience.com.au/	Multiple topics including nutrition and cancer, Crohn's disease, dysphagia, malnutrition, pediatrics, weight management and wound care.
http://fnic.nal.usda.gov/diet-and-disease	

(*Continued*)

TABLE A.2 (*CONTINUED*) Nutrition-Related Web Resources

Nutrition and renal disease	
http://kidney.niddk.nih.gov/index.aspx	Multiple links related to kidney and urologic diseases. In addition, links to chronic kidney disease nutrition management learning modules.
Nutrition and cardiovascular disease	
http://fnic.nal.usda.gov/diet-and-disease/heart-health	Links to dietary guidelines, children's education, cholesterol education program.
Nutritional disorders of the GI tract	
http://diabetes.niddk.nih.gov/	
http://digestive.niddk.nih.gov/	
http://fnic.nal.usda.gov/diet-and-disease/digestive-diseases-and-disorders	This is a clearing house site with links to other clearing house pages as well links for specific section of the GI tract and diseases or structural problems that affect those areas.
Nutrition and diabetes	
http://fnic.nal.usda.gov/consumers/eating-health/diabetes-and-prediabetes	Clearing house site with links to the American Diabetes Association, NIH, and various university research topics.
Nutritional management of the bariatric surgery patient	
http://www.nlm.nih.gov/medlineplus/weightlosssurgery.html	Many articles and videos associated with weight loss surgery.
Nutritional management of the frail elderly	
http://www.howtocare.com/diet.htm	Links to subjects that most of us do not think about!
Enteral and parenteral nutrition support (hospitalized patient)	
http://guideline.gov/browse/by-organization.aspx?orgid=100	Links to subtopic papers. This site is recommended for health professionals.
http://www.fda.gov/Food/GuidanceComplianceRegulatoryInformation/GuidanceDocuments/MedicalFoods/ucm054048.htm	Defining and discussion of *medical foods* FDA guidance document.
Nutrition and cancer (prevention and treatment)	
http://www.carolinawell.org/healthyliving	Use the link for healthy living/healthy behaviors.
http://www.cancer.org/Treatment/SurvivorshipDuringandAfterTreatment/NutritionforPeoplewithCancer/index	There are multiple inter-related topics related to food choices and exercise for during and after cancer treatment.
http://fnic.nal.usda.gov/diet-and-disease/cancer	This is a clearing house site with multiple links to the National Cancer Institute, the American Cancer Society and the Centers for Disease Control. These sites have specific information about nutrition and physical exercise as a means of preventing cancer and suggested guidelines for nourishing the cancer patient.
http://www.cancer.gov/cancertopics/pdq/supportivecare/nutrition/HealthProfessional/page3	
Nutrition and age-related eye disease	
http://www.lighthouse.org/eye-health/	This site covers everything from eye structure to common problems of the eye to diseases affecting the eye to nutrition as a preventative for eye problems. Click on the prevention tab then nutrition and eye health.

(*Continued*)

TABLE A.2 (*CONTINUED*)
Nutrition-Related Web Resources

Macular degeneration	
http://www.macular.org/nutrition/index.html	This is a *single-article* site but has some good overall information concerning this topic.
http://www.umm.edu/altmed/articles/macular-degeneration-000104.htm	This is a *single-article* site but with good information and references for further reading.
Glaucoma	
http://www.glaucoma.org/treatment/nutrition-and-glaucoma.php	General information focusing on diet as a preventative measure to eye disease.
http://www.umm.edu/altmed/articles/glaucoma-000069.htm	Information on complementary medicine associated with glaucoma.
Cataracts	
http://www.ars.usda.gov/research/publications/publications.htm?seq_no_115=207417	This is one of a cluster of sites associated with the USDA. It specifically links research publications and may not be appropriate for a nonscience reader.
Nutrition and CNS health	
http://www.ars.usda.gov/is/ar/archive/aug07/aging0807.htm	Single-article site on "Food for the Aging Mind".
Nutrition and skin Nothing but commercial sites found	
Nutrition and skeletal health	
http://fnic.nal.usda.gov/consumers/eating-health/osteoporosis-and-bone-health	This is a clearing house site with links to the National Osteoporosis Foundation, clinical treatment groups, and various university research groups.
Drug/nutrient interactions	
http://edis.ifas.ufl.edu/he776	Single-article site but has the chart of common nutrient drug interactions. Good definitions and guidelines.

TABLE A.3
Prefixes and Suffixes Used in Medical Terms

Prefix	Example	Meaning
Pre—before	Prenatal	Period before birth
Peri—around	Perinatal	Period around birth
Epi—above, upon	Epidermis	Outermost layer of skin
Hypo—under, below	Hypodermic	Under the skin
Hyper—above	Hyperglycemic	Above normal blood sugar
Infra—under, below	Infracostal	Below the ribs
Sub—under, below	Subdural	Below the dura mater
Inter—between	Intercostals	Between the ribs
Post—behind	Posterior	Back part of anatomical point
Retro—backward, behind	Retroversion	Tipping backward
Bi—two	Bilateral	Two sides
Diplo—two	Diplococcus	Two attached bacterial cells
Hemi—one half	Hemiplegia	Paralysis of one body side
Macro—large	Macrophage	Large cell
Micro—small	Microscope	Instrument for magnification
Ab—from, away from	Abduction	Movement away from center line of body
Ad—toward	Adduction	Movement toward the center line of the body
Circum—around	Circumduction	Movement in a circular direction
a—without, not	Aphagic	Not eating
Anti—against	Antibacterial	Against bacteria
Contra—not	Contraindicated	Not recommended
Brady—slow	Bradycardia	Slow heart rate
Tachy—rapid	Tachycardia	Rapid heart rate
Dys—bad, painful	Dystocia	Difficult childbirth
Homeo—same	Homeostasis	Maintenance of sameness
Eu—good, normal	Eupnea	Normal breathing
Mal—bad	Malnutrition	Any disturbance in adequate intakes of nutrients
Pseudo—false	Pseudostratified	False appearance of cell layers

TABLE A.4
Types of Immune Diseases

Type	Problem	Example
I	Excess IgE production	Food allergies, environmental allergies
II	Loss of antigen recognition specificity; inadequate suppressor T cells	Autoimmune diabetes, psoriasis, rheumatoid arthritis
III	Leaky cell membranes allowing soluble cell components to act as antigens	Lupus, adverse response to some drugs, glomerulonephritis, arthritis, rash, pleurisy
IV	Loss of helper cells	Tuberculosis; AIDS

TABLE A.5
Websites for Information on Food Intake

Use	Web Address
Food composition	http://www.nal.usda.gov/fnic/foodcomp/data/foods,82nutrients
Foods from India	http://www.unu.edu/unupress/unupbooks/80633Eoi.htm
Foods from Europe	Cost99/EUROFOODS:Inventory of European Food Composition food.ethz.ch/cost99db-inventory.htm
Foods, developing nations	www.fao.org/DOCREP/WOO73e/woo73eO6htm
Other food data	www.arborcom.com/frame/foodc.htm
Foods from McDonald's restaurants	www.mcdonalds.com
Food intake recommendations: DRI	www.nap.edu and www.nal.usda.gov/fnic/etext/000105.html
Dietary guidelines	www.health.gov/dietary guidelines
Food pyramid	www.mypyramid.gov/tips resources/menus.html

TABLE A.6
Pathogens That Can Cause Food-Borne Illness

Pathogen	Symptoms or Disease
Bacteria	
Enterohemorrhagic *Escherichia coli*	Hemorrhagic colitis, hemolytic uremic syndrome, and thrombocytopenic purpura
Salmonella (several species)	Prolonged and spiking fever, abdominal pain, diarrhea, and headache
Campylobacter species (*C. jejuni* and *C. coli*)	Enteritis: abdominal cramps, diarrhea headache, and fever lasting up to 4 days
Shigella (several species)	Diarrhea containing bloody mucus, lasts 1–2 weeks
Yersinia enterocolitica	Acute enteritis, enterocolitis, mesenteric lymphadenitis, terminal ileitis
Vibrio (three species) (*V. parahaemolyticus*, *V. vulnificus*, and *V. cholera*)	Gastroenteritis. When *V. cholera* is the agent, severe diarrhea, fever, dehydration, potentially fatal if fluids and electrolytes are not replaced
Aeromonas hydrophila	Watery diarrhea, mild fever
Listeria monocytogenes	Listerosis; potentially fatal to the elderly, pregnant women, and fetuses
Staphylococcus aureus	Nausea, vomiting, diarrhea, and abdominal pain
Clostridium botulinum	Paralysis due to a neurotoxin
Clostridium perfringens (five types)	Produces an enterotoxin that causes diarrhea
Bacillus cereus	Induces vomiting, nausea, and watery stools
Brucella (six species)	Causes brucellosis
Helicobacter pylori	Causes stomach ulcers that are responsive to antibiotics
Viruses	
Hepatitis A virus	Nausea, abdominal pain, jaundice, fever
Norwalk-like viruses	Nausea, vomiting, diarrhea
Rotavirus	Fever, vomiting, diarrhea
Avian influenza virus	Systemic infections, fever
Molds	
Aspergillus species	Can produce aflatoxins that may cause cancer
Penicillium species	Can produce a toxin that causes disease
Fusarium graminearum	Produces a toxin that causes anorexia, nausea, vomiting, diarrhea, dizziness, convulsions
Parasites	
Giardia lamblia (*G. intestinalis*)	Cramps, nausea, diarrhea, weight loss, anorexia
Entamoeba histolytica	Abdominal pain, fever, vomiting, diarrhea, bloody stool
Trichinella spiralis	Two phases: First—abdominal pain, fever, vomiting, diarrhea; Second—edema, myalgia, difficulty in breathing, thirst, profuse sweating, chills, weakness, prostration
Cryptosporidium parvum	Profuse watery diarrhea, abdominal pain, nausea, vomiting
Cyclospora cayetanesis	Watery diarrhea, nausea, vomiting, myalgia, weight loss
Toxoplasma gondii	Fever, headache, muscle pain, lymph node swelling, abortion in pregnant women
Anisakis species (threadworms)	Epigastric pain, nausea, vomiting
Taenia species (tape worms)	Nausea, epigastric pain, nervousness, insomnia, anorexia, weight loss, digestive disturbances, weakness, dizziness
Diphyllobothrium latum (large tape worm)	Nausea, epigastric pain, diarrhea, pernicious anemia

Glossary

Throughout this text, the reader may find terms or expressions that are unfamiliar. Scientists in this hybrid field of nutrition–biochemistry–genetics–physiology sometimes *speak in code*. They adopt a text-shorthand that is known to them but seldom explained to the uninitiated. It is for this reason that a list of definitions for these abbreviations and terms is provided. This glossary can also serve as a review for the reader whose background preparation for a course in advanced nutrition may be a bit *rusty*. Some of the terms are medical ones, some are abbreviations common to biochemistry and/or biotechnology, and still others are relevant to the epidemiology of nutrition-related diseases.

Abscess: A circumscribed collection of pus.

Acarbose: A drug that inhibits α-glucosidase, an enzyme important to the digestion of starch.

Acetaldehyde: An aldehyde formed from the oxidation of ethanol; can be converted to acetate and then to acetyl CoA.

Acetaldehyde dehydrogenase: An enzyme that catalyzes the conversion of acetaldehyde to acetate.

Acetaminophen: An over-the-counter (OTC) drug that reduces headache, fever, and/or inflammation. Trade names include aspirin-free Anacin, Tylenol, Apacet, and others.

Acetoacetate: A four-carbon compound found in large amounts in the uncontrolled insulin-dependent diabetic. It is a normal end product of fatty acid oxidation and can be further metabolized and used as fuel by normal tissues. Its further metabolism yields carbon dioxide and water.

Acetone: A three-carbon ketone found in normal tissues and blood. It can accumulate if the citric acid cycle is not working properly. Levels of acetone are high in the uncontrolled insulin-dependent diabetic and can be toxic.

Acetonemia: Higher than normal levels of acetone in the blood. Normal levels can be between 3 and 20 mg/mL. In the uncontrolled insulin-dependent diabetic individual, acetone levels can significantly exceed 20 mg/mL.

Acetonuria: Higher than normal (1 mg/L/24 h) levels of acetone in the urine.

Acetyl CoA: A two-carbon metabolic intermediate that is the starting substrate for fatty acid synthesis. It is also the end product of fatty acid degradation (fatty acid oxidation). When joined to oxaloacetate, it enters the citric acid cycle as citrate and the CoA portion of the molecule is removed for use in other reactions.

Acetylcholine: A neurotransmitter released by a calcium-dependent process in response to the arrival of an action potential. Acetylcholine initiates changes in ion permeability that occur at the neuromuscular junction. Acetylcholine is hydrolyzed by acetylcholine esterase. The choline is then reused.

Achlorhydria: Absence of hydrochloric acid in the stomach.

Acid–base balance: Minute-to-minute regulation of the hydrogen ion concentration (pH) in the body; accomplished through the action of the bicarbonate buffering system, the phosphate buffering system, and the action of body proteins as buffers.

Acidic amino acids: Amino acids having two carboxyl groups in their structures. These amino acids are aspartic and glutamic acids.

Acidosis: When the blood pH falls below 7.4 acidosis develops.

Acroderma enteropatica: A rare genetic disease characterized by an inability to absorb zinc.

Acrolein: An oxidation product of excessively heated fats.

Acromegaly: Disease that results from excess growth hormone production and release from the anterior pituitary.

ACTH: Adrenocorticotropin hormone. Hormone released by the anterior pituitary that stimulates the release of the adrenal cortical steroid hormones (cortisol, corticosteroid, hydrocortisone, dehydroepiandrosterone, aldosterone).

Active site: That part of an enzyme or hormone or carrier or other substance to which a substrate binds.

Activity increment: The energy needed to sustain body activities.

Actuarial data: Information used to create mortality tables and life expectancy tables.

Acylation: The addition of an acyl group (carbon chain) to a substrate.

Adenine: A purine base that is an essential component of the genetic material, DNA.

Adenyl cyclase: The enzyme responsible for the conversion of ATP to cyclic AMP, an important second messenger for hormones that stimulate catabolic processes.

ADH: Antidiuretic hormone, also called vasopressin, produced by the posterior pituitary plays a role in water conservation by the body. It stimulates water reabsorption by the renal tubules.

Adhesions: Fibrous bands of material that connect two surfaces that are normally separate.

Adipocytes: Cells that store fat.

Adiponectin: Hormone secreted by adipocytes and acting as an insulin-sensitizing hormone.

Adipsia: Lack of thirst sensation.

ADP: Adenosine diphosphate. A metabolite of ATP. Energy is released when ATP releases a phosphate group (Pi) and becomes ADP.

Aerobic metabolism: Metabolic reactions that require oxygen.

Aflatoxins: Contaminants of food produced by molds.

Age-adjusted death rate: The number of deaths in a specific age group for a given calendar year divided by the population of that same age group and multiplied by 1000.

AIDS: Acquired Immune Deficiency Syndrome. A disease that results when a specific virus (HIV) attacks elements of the immune system rendering it unable to respond to incoming antigens or infective agents.

Albumin: A small molecular weight protein found in blood and sometimes in urine.

Alcohol: A hydrocarbon containing a hydroxyl group (–OH) attached to one of the carbons in the carbon chain.

Aldehyde: A carbon compound containing a –C=O group.

Aldosterone: A steroid hormone produced by the adrenal cortex that acts on the cells bordering the distal tubules of the kidney stimulating them to reabsorb sodium.

Aliphatic: A chain of carbon atoms with associated hydrogen and/or hydroxyl groups.

Aliphatic amino acids: Amino acids that consist of a chain of carbon atoms. These include alanine, cysteine, glycine, isoleucine, leucine, methionine, serine, threonine, and valine.

Alkalosis: A condition where the blood pH rises above 7.4.

Allele: Any one of a series of different genes that may occupy the same location (locus) on a specific chromosome in the nuclear DNA.

Allergens: Substances capable of eliciting an immunological response.

Allosterism: The binding of an inhibitor or activator to an enzyme at a site removed from the active site of that enzyme.

Alopecia: Loss of hair.

Alveoli: Cells in the lungs responsible for O_2/CO_2 exchange.

Amide bond (peptide bond): A bond involving an amino ($-NH_3$) group.

Amino acids: Simple organic nitrogenous compounds that are the building blocks of proteins.

Aminoacidopathy: Inborn errors (mutations in specific base sequences for specific gene products) resulting in inadequate utilization of one or more amino acids.

Aminotransferases (transaminases): Enzymes that catalyze the transfer of an amino group ($-NH_2-$ or $-NH_3$) from one carbon chain to another.

AMP: Adenosine monophosphate. Metabolite of ADP. Energy is released when ADP releases a phosphate group (Pi) to become AMP.
Amphipathic: The characteristic of a compound containing both polar and nonpolar groups. This allows the compound to be soluble in both polar and nonpolar solvents. Water is a polar solvent; chloroform is a nonpolar solvent.
Amphoteric: The characteristic of a compound that allows it to have either an acidic or a basic function depending on the pH of the solution.
Amylase: An enzyme that catalyzes the cleavage of glucose molecules from amylose (starch).
Amylin: A 37-amino acid peptide co-secreted with insulin; it serves as a satiety signal.
Amylopectin: A branched chain polymer of glucose found in plants.
Amylose: A straight chain polymer of glucose also found in plants.
Anabolism: The totality of reactions that account for the synthesis of the body's macromolecules.
Androgens: Male sex hormones.
Android obesity: A form of obesity where fat stores accumulate over the shoulders and abdominal area. Sometimes referred to as the *apple* shape.
Anemia: Below normal amounts of hemoglobin and/or red blood cells.
Aneurism: A bulge in the vascular tree (usually arterial).
Angina pectoris: Chest pain due to lack of oxygen supplied to the heart muscle.
Angiotensin: The natural substrate for renin.
Angiotensin converting enzyme (ACE): The enzyme responsible for converting angiotensin I to angiotensin II in the kidney.
ANH: Atrial natriuretic hormone. The hormone that counteracts ADH.
Anosmia: Loss of the sense of smell.
Anoxia: Lack of oxygen in blood or tissues.
Antecedents: Events that precede or causally linked to an event.
Anthropometry: Measurement of body features, that is, weight, height, etc.
Antibiotics: Drugs that inhibit growth of (or kill) pathogens.
Antibody: Proteins produced by the B cells and T cells (parts of the body's immune system) that in turn react with antigens. Each antigen has a specific antibody that senses and reacts to it. In autoimmune disease, there is a loss in antigen specificity and antibodies react to groups of similar proteins some of which may be the body's own protein.
Anticoagulants: Compounds that interfere with blood clotting.
Anticodon: A sequence of three bases in the transfer RNA, which is complimentary to that in the messenger RNA.
Anticoding strand: A strand of DNA that is used as a template to direct the synthesis of RNA that is complementary to it.
Antigen: A compound external (usually) to the body that elicits the synthesis of antibodies specific to its structure.
Antioxidants: Agents that prevent or inhibit oxidation reactions.
Anus: Opening at the posterior end of the digestive tract.
Apoenzyme: The inactive part or *backbone* of an enzyme protein.
Apoprotein: Carrier proteins that carry specific compounds such as lipid or vitamins or some other material requiring a carrier.
Apoptosis: Programmed cell death.
Apparent digestibility: Nutrients may not be completely available from foods that are consumed. To determine availability, the amount of the nutrient in the feces is subtracted from the amount of the nutrient in the ingested food.
Apparent digested energy (DE): Energy in the food consumed less the energy in the feces: DE=IE–FE.
Arachidonic acid: Long-chain fatty acid having 4 double bonds and 20 carbons.

Archimedes principle: An object's volume when submerged in water equals the volume of the water it displaces. If the mass and volume are known, the density can be calculated.

Aromatic amino acids: Amino acids that have a ring structure. Included are phenylalanine, tyrosine, and tryptophan.

ARS: Autonomously replicating sequence; the origin of replication in yeast.

Arteriography: A method of examining the major arteries using x-rays and an infusion of a radiopaque dye solution.

Aseptic: Sterile; absence of pathogens.

Atherogenic: Producing or inducing atherosclerosis.

Atherosclerosis, Arteriosclerosis: A progressive degenerative condition occurring within the vascular tree and resulting in occlusions and loss of elasticity of the vessel.

ATP: Adenosine triphosphate. The energy-rich compound that is produced by oxidative phosphorylation in the mitochondria. ATP can also be produced by substrate phosphorylation.

ATPase: A group of enzymes that catalyze the removal or addition of a single phosphate group to the high-energy compound containing adenine.

Atrophy: Reduced size of an organ, tissue, or cell.

Attenuated: Weakened or lessened activity of a given biologically active compound.

Autocrine system: A variation of the paracrine system where the hormone secreting cell and the target of the hormone are located in the same cell.

Autoimmunity: The destruction of self through the development of antibodies to the body's own proteins.

Autonomic nervous system: The system that includes portions of the brain, spinal cord, and adrenals and that serve to regulate the synthesis and release of epinephrine enkephalins, and norepinephrine.

Autosomal recessive trait: A genetic trait that will express itself only if the individual inherits two identical copies of the same gene (one from each parent).

Autoxidation: Reaction of an organic compound with elemental oxygen under mild conditions.

B cells: Lymphocytic cells produced in the bone marrow that are not processed further by the thymus gland.

ß Alanine: A naturally occurring form of alanine, which is not incorporated into protein but which is an essential component of coenzyme A, pantothenic acid, and carnosine.

ß-Carotene: Precursor of active vitamin A.

ß Cells: Cells in the islets of Langerhans in the endocrine pancreas that release insulin upon a glucose signal.

ß Hydroxybutyrate, ß hydroxybutyric acid: Included in the group of compounds called ketone bodies.

ß Oxidation: Process in the mitochondria for the oxidation of fatty acids.

Bacteriophage: Bacteria eater.

Bariatrics: A medical term referring to the management of people who are overfat or obese.

Baroreceptors: Sensory nerve endings in the walls of the auricles of the heart, carotid artery sinus, vena cava, and aortic arch that respond to changes in pressure.

Basal energy expenditure (BEE): Estimated energy used by the body at rest in a fasting state to maintain essential body functions. The BEE is then adjusted for activity, injury or disease, and thermic effect of food to predict the total daily energy expenditure. This is then used to estimate the energy intake requirement.

Basal metabolism (basal metabolic rate, BMR): The minimum amount of energy needed to maintain the activity of metabolic processes occurring in the body. When rate is used, an element of time is added.

Basic amino acids: Amino acids whose side chains have positively charged amino groups. These are histidine, lysine, and arginine.

BCAA: Branched chain amino acids. These are valine, leucine, and isoleucine.

Betaine: Precursor of choline.

Bicarbonate: Any salt containing HCO_3; bicarbonate in the blood is indicative of the alkali reserve.

Bile acids: Cholic and chenodeoxycholic acid synthesized by the liver from cholesterol.

Bile pigments: Breakdown products of the heme portion of hemoglobin, myoglobin, and the cytochromes (bilirubin, biliverdin, and heme) excreted by way of bile.

Bile salts: Anionic forms of bile acids.

Bioavailability: Quantity of nutrient available to the body after absorption.

Biopsy: The removal of a tiny tissue sample.

Biogenic amines: Compounds formed when amino acids are decarboxylated.

BMI: Body mass index = body weight (kg)/height $(cm)^2$.

Bombesin: A 14-amino acid peptide hormone found in the central nervous system, the thyroid gland, lung, adrenal, and skin and which has a broad spectrum of action.

Brown adipose tissue (BAT): Highly vascularized adipose tissue with mitochondria-rich adipocytes.

BTU: British thermal unit. Amount of energy needed to raise the temperature of one pound of water one degree Fahrenheit.

Buffer: A compound that resists a change in hydrogen ion concentration in solution.

Bulimia: Habitual self-induced vomiting. Frequently accompanies anorexia nervosa.

Cachexia: Tissue wasting as in disease or overwhelming trauma or starvation.

Calculus: Synonym for gallstones or kidney stones; complex mineral precipitants.

cAMP: Cyclic AMP. Cyclic 3′5′ adenosine monophosphate—a second messenger for catabolic hormone effects. Produced when adenyl cyclase acts on ATP.

Cancer: A group of diseases characterized by abnormal growth of cells which, because it is uncontrolled, subsume the normal functions of vital organs and tissues.

Candidate gene: A gene, if mutated, that is suspected to play a causal role in a clinical syndrome.

Cap: The structure at the 5′ end of eukaryotic mRNA, introduced after transcription by linking the terminal phosphate of the 5′ GTP to the terminal base of the mRNA. The added G and sometimes other bases are methylated.

Carbohydrate: Polyhydroxy aldehydes or ketones and their derivatives.

Carbonyl group: An aldehyde (–CH=O) group or ketone (–C=O) group; a group that characterizes aldehydes and ketones.

Carboxylase: An enzyme that catalyzes the addition of a carboxyl group to a carbon chain. This enzyme class usually requires thiamin as thiamin pyrophosphate (TPP) as a coenzyme.

Carboxylation: The addition of a carboxyl (–COOH) group to a carbon chain.

Carcinogenesis: The process of developing cancer.

Cardiomyopathy: Structural or functional disease of the heart muscle (the myocardium).

Cardiovascular disease: A group of diseases characterized by a diminution of heart action.

Cariogenesis: The process of tooth decay.

Carnosine: A dipeptide synthesized from ß alanine and histidine. Found in muscle where it activates myosin ATPase. Carnosine also serves to buffer the acidic state that develops in working muscle.

Carotenes, Carotinoids: A group of yellow-orange pigments some of which can be hydrolyzed to active vitamin A. α, β, and γ carotene are considered provitamins because they can be converted to active vitamin A. The carotenes also have an antioxidant function.

Carrier: A substance, usually a protein, which binds to a substrate and transports it from its point of origin to its point of use.

Catabolism: The totality of those reactions that reduce macromolecules to usable metabolites, carbon dioxide, and water.

Catalase: An enzyme that catalyzes the conversion of peroxide to water and oxygen; this is a key enzyme in the cytoplasmic-free radical suppression system.

Catalyst: A substance, usually a protein, in living (or nonliving) systems that enhances or promotes a chemical reaction without being a reactant. Enzymes are catalysts.

Catecholamines: Neurotransmitters (epinephrine, dopamine, and norepinephrine) that are produced in the adrenal medulla from tyrosine. These hormones are instrumental in orchestrating the *fight or flight* response to stress conditions.

Cation: A positively charged ion.

CDC: Centers for Disease Control; an agency of the Department of Health and Human Services.

cDNA: A single-stranded DNA molecule that is complementary to an mRNA and is synthesized from it by the action of reverse transcription.

CDP: Cytidine diphosphate. A nucleotide consisting of cytosine (a pyrimidine), ribose, and two high-energy phosphate groups.

Cecum: A blind appendage of the intestinal tract located at the juncture of the small and large intestine. Also called the appendix.

Cellulose: A structural polysaccharide found primarily in plants and composed of glucose units linked together with ß 1,4 bonds.

Cephalin: A phospholipid, similar to lecithin, present in the brain.

Cerebroside: A complex lipid in nerve and other tissues. A cerebroside is a sphingolipid.

Cerebrovascular accident: Also referred to as a stroke; sudden circulatory impairment in one or more blood vessels that supply the brain.

Cerebrovascular disease: Similar to cardiovascular disease in that the vascular tree of the brain has developed atherosclerotic lesions that restrict or occlude the blood supply to this organ.

Ceruloplasmin: A copper-containing globulin in blood plasma with a molecular weight of 150,000 and 8 copper atoms. It catalyzes the oxidation of amines, phenols, and ascorbic acid.

Chelate, chelation: A combination of metal ions chemically held within a ring of heterocyclic structures by bonds from each of these structures to the metal. Iron is held by heme in this fashion as part of the hemoglobin structure.

Chimeric molecule: A molecule of DNA or RNA or protein containing sequences from two different species.

Chloride shift: Part of the system that maintains the blood acid–base balance. Chloride and bicarbonate ions exchange across the erythrocyte plasma membrane and is called the shift.

Cholecholithiasis: Obstruction of the common bile duct; presence of a stone in the duct.

Cholecystitis: Inflammation of the gallbladder.

Cholecystokinin (CCK): A hormone released from duodenal cells and that stimulates the gall bladder to contract and release bile into the duodenum.

Cholelithiasis: Presence or formation of gallstones.

Cholestasis: Arrest of bile excretion.

Cholesterol: A four-ringed structure in the nonsaponifiable lipid class that is an important substrate for steroid hormone synthesis.

Chondrocytes: Cartilage precursor cells or cartilage cells.

Chorionic gonadotropin: A heterodimeric glycoprotein hormone of 57 kDa consisting of a noncovalent bound α (92-amino acid residues) and a distinctive ß (134-amino acid residues) subunit found in the blood of pregnant females. The major function of this hormone is to stimulate the production of progesterone by the corpus luteum.

Chromaffin cells: Cells in the adrenal medulla and also the kidney, ovary, testis, heart, and gastrointestinal tract. Similar cell types are found in the carotid and aortic bodies. In the adrenal medulla, these cells produce epinephrine.

Chromosomes: When DNA is extracted from the cell nucleus, it is not one continuous strand. Rather, it breaks up into fairly predictable arrangements called chromosomes.

Chromosome walking: The sequential isolation of clones carrying overlapping sequences of DNA, allowing large regions of the chromosomes to be spanned. Walking is often performed in order to reach a locus of interest.

Chyle: A turbid white or yellow fluid, taken up by the lacteals in the process of lipid digestion and absorption.

Chylomicron: Fat-protein complex formed to carry absorbed dietary fats from the intestine to other tissues. Not normally found in the blood of a fasting individual.

Chyme: The semifluid mass of partly digested food extruded from the stomach into the duodenum of the small intestine.

Cilia, Cilium: Hair-like processes extending out from the surface of epithelial cells.

Citrate: An intermediate in the citric acid cycle; the essential starting metabolite for fatty acid synthesis in the cytosol.

Citric acid cycle (Kreb's Cycle): A cycle found in mitochondria that produces reducing equivalents for use by the respiratory chain and that also produces carbon dioxide.

Clone: A large number of cells or molecules that are identical to a single parental cell or molecule.

CMP: Cytidine monophosphate. A nucleotide consisting of cytosine (a pyrimidine), ribose, and one high-energy phosphate group.

CoA, Coenzyme A: A coenzyme containing the vitamin, pantothenic acid. CoA forms a thio ester bond with acetyl and acyl groups and with amino acids and facilitates their metabolism.

CoQ, Coenzyme Q: A coenzyme also called ubiquinone. It serves as an essential component of the respiratory chain and transfers electrons between the flavoproteins and the cytochromes.

Coding strand: A strand of DNA with the same sequences as mRNA.

Codon: A sequence of three bases (triplet) that specifies a particular amino acid in the sequence of reactions that comprise protein synthesis. Amino acids can have more than one codon.

Cofactor: An essential ingredient for an enzyme catalyzed reaction. Cofactors are usually minerals.

Competitive inhibition: Inhibition of an enzymatic reaction that occurs when a substance, closely related to the substrate, binds to the active site of the enzyme yet is not catalyzed by it.

Complementary base pairs: The pairing of purine and pyrimidine bases of the DNA. Adenine is paired with thymine and cytosine with guanine. These pairs are linked together via hydrogen bonds that form the cross-links between the two strands of DNA for the double helix typical of the nuclear genetic material. In RNA, adenine pairs with uracil.

Concordance: The chance that an identical disease will occur in related family members.

Consensus sequence: An idealized sequence in which each position represents the base most often found when many actual sequences are compared.

Constitutive genes: Genes that are expressed as a function of the interaction of RNA polymerase with the promoter, without additional regulation; sometimes called housekeeping genes in the context of describing functions expressed in all cells at a low level.

Corepressor: A small molecule that triggers repression of transcription by binding to a regulator protein.

Cori cycle: A cycle that occurs between the red blood cell, kidneys, muscle, platelets, and the liver and that helps maintain a normal blood glucose level in the face of changes in lactate production.

Cosmid: A plasmid into which the DNA sequences from bacteriophage lambda that are necessary for the packaging of DNA (cos sites) have been inserted; this permits the plasmid DNA to be packaged in vitro.

Coupled reaction: Two reactions that have a common intermediate that transfers electrons or reducing equivalents or some other element from one set of reactants to another.

C-peptide: When proinsulin is cleaved to form active insulin, the fragment removed is the c-peptide.

Creatine: A metabolite in muscle that is synthesized from glycine and arginine and that can be phosphorylated to form creatine phosphate.

Creatine phosphate: A high-energy compound in muscle that has a higher phosphate group transfer potential than ATP. It acts as a reservoir for phosphate so that the muscle can maintain a steady level of ATP to support muscle contraction. It also serves this function in nerve so that a steady supply of ATP for nerve conduction is provided.

Creatine phosphokinase (creatine kinase): Enzyme in skeletal muscle, cardiac muscle, and in brain tissue that catalyzes the transfer of high-energy phosphate from phosphocreatine to ADP to make ATP.

Creatinine: The urinary excretion product of creatine breakdown.

Crenation: Shriveling of the cell.

Crude fiber: The residue of plant food left after extraction by dilute acid and alkali.

CTP: Cytidine triphosphate. A nucleotide consisting of cytosine (a pyrimidine), ribose, and three high-energy phosphate groups.

Cyclooxygenase: Two forms exist, COX I and COX II. Enzyme responsible for the formation of eicosanoids particularly those that act as inflammatories. COX I is a constitutive enzyme present in most cell types and works under noninflammatory conditions. COX II is inducible in cells as part of an inflammatory response to injury or irritation. COX II is the target of several prescription anti-inflammatory drugs useful in the treatment of arthritis.

Cytidine: A nucleotide consisting of cytosine (a pyrimidine) and ribose.

Cytochromes: Electron carriers in the respiratory chain and elsewhere. All cytochromes have a heme prosthetic group that contains iron. The iron fluctuates between the +2 and +3 states. The cytochrome P-450 enzymes are important to the detoxification processes in the body.

Cytokines: A family of peptide hormones produced mainly by macrophages and lymphocytes. Some cytokines are produced by the brain, adipose tissue, and other cell types.

Cytoplasm: Cell sap; the medium in which the organelles of the cell are suspended.

Cytosine: A pyrimidine base found in the genetic material, DNA and RNA.

Cytotoxic agents: Chemicals that destroy specific cells; streptozotocin is an example. This agent destroys the insulin-producing ß cells of the pancreas.

Daily reference intake (DRI): Revised guidelines for the intakes of nutrients including fats, carbohydrates, proteins, energy, and micronutrients. These guidelines are designed to prevent chronic disease and encompass several types of recommendations including the Recommended Dietary Allowance (RDA) by the Food and Nutrition Board (National Academy of Sciences) that provide guidance for the prevention of deficiency diseases.

DE: Digestive energy. The energy of food after the costs (and losses) of digestion are subtracted.

Deaminase: An enzyme that catalyzes the removal of an amino group from a carbon chain.

Deamination: The process of amino group removal.

Decarboxylase: An enzyme that catalyzes the removal of a carboxy group from a carbon chain.

Decarboxylation: The reaction in which a carboxyl group is removed.

Degrade: To reduce large molecules to smaller ones.

Dehydratases: Enzymes that catalyze the removal of a molecule of water from a carbon chain. These enzymes frequently require pyridoxine as a coenzyme.

Dehydration: The process of water removal.

Dehydrogenases: Enzymes that catalyze the removal of reducing equivalents (hydrogen ions) from carbon chains.

Dehydrogenation: Removal of hydrogen ions; catalyzed by a group of enzymes called dehydrogenases.

Delta (Δ): Change. The Greek symbol is Δ.

ΔG°: Free energy that is available to do work.

$\Delta G^{\circ\prime}$: Standard free energy of biochemical reactions.

Densitometry: Measurement of body density.

Deoxyadenosine: A nucleoside containing adenine (a purine) and deoxyribose.

Deoxycytidine: A nucleoside containing cytosine (a pyrimidine) and deoxyribose.

Deoxyguanine: A nucleoside containing guanine (a purine) and deoxyribose.

Deoxyribonucleic acid (DNA): The genetic material in the nucleus and mitochondria.

Dermatitis: Inflammation of the skin.

Detoxification: Removal of toxic properties of a substance; metabolic conversion of pharmacologically active compounds to nonactive compounds.
Deuterium: A hydrogen isotope having twice the mass of the common hydrogen atom.
Deuterium oxide: Heavy water that contains two molecules of deuterium and one of oxygen.
DEXA: Dual-energy x-ray absorptiometry. It is a method used to estimate bone density and soft tissue composition.
Dextran: A glucose polymer.
Dextrose: Synonym of glucose.
Diacylglycerol (diglyceride): A lipid having two fatty acids esterified to glycerol; also called diglyceride.
Diet-induced thermogenesis (DIT): A rise in heat production associated with the consumption of food. This energy loss represents the energy cost of the processing of food for metabolic use.
Diffusion: A uniform distribution of solutes on both sides of a permeable membrane.
Dipeptide: Two amino acids linked together by a peptide bond.
Direct calorimetry: The measurement of heat produced by a body through the use of a calorimeter.
Disaccharide: A carbohydrate containing two sugar (saccharide) units. Sucrose, mannose, and lactose are common disaccharides in the human diet.
Distal: Away from the center of the body.
Distention: The condition of being expanded or extended beyond normal.
Disulfide bridge: A bond containing two sulfur molecules.
Diuresis: Urine excretion in excess of normal.
Diuretics: Pharmaceutical agents that increase urinary water loss.
Diurnal variation: Cyclical changes in one or more features of the body over a 24 h period.
Duodenum: The first 12 in. of the small intestine of the human.
Edema: Excess accumulation of water in the body, particularly in the periphery.
Eicosanoids: A group of hormone-like compounds synthesized from arachidonic acid.
Electrolyte: An electrically charged particle.
Electron donor: In an electron acceptor/donor pair, the electron donor gives or donates electrons to the acceptor. An electron donor is a reducing agent.
Elongation factors: Proteins that associate with ribosomes cyclically during the addition of each amino acid to the amino acid chain.
Embolism: Obstruction of a blood vessel by blood clot or foreign body.
Embryo: The initial stage of development of the fertilized egg; usually the first 12 weeks in human pregnancy.
Emulsion: A mixture of fat and water held together by an agent that has a lipophilic and a hydrophilic portion of its structure. Bile salts serve as emulsifying agents facilitating lipid digestion and absorption.
Endocytosis: The process of forming a vesicle within the secreting cell of material the cell will release upon appropriate signaling.
Endonuclease: An enzyme that cleaves internal bonds in DNA or RNA.
Endorphin: A peptide produced in the brain that has sedative properties. ß endorphin stimulates prolactin release.
Endothelin: A 21-amino acid peptide that is a potent vasoconstrictor.
Energetic efficiency: The percentage of the intake energy that the body traps energy in the high-energy bond and subsequently stores that energy or uses it to synthesize body components.
Enhancer element: A cis-acting base sequence that binds one or more promoters. It can function in either orientation and in any location (upstream or downstream) relative to the promoter region.
Enteral nutrition: The provision of nutrients in a solution infused via a nasogastric tube.
Enterocyte: Absorptive cells lining the gastrointestinal tract.

Epithelium: The layer of cells that provide the surface covering of the body; the nonvascular cell layer of skin, gastrointestinal tract, and respiratory tract.

ER: Endoplasmic reticulum.

ESADDI: Estimated safe and adequate daily dietary intakes. Refers to those nutrients for which there are indications of essentiality but for which the database is insufficient to make valid recommendations for intakes.

Ester: A compound containing an oxygen linkage (–O–); the product of the condensation of an acid and alcohol with the loss of a molecule of water.

Etiology: The study of the causes of disease.

Excinuclease: An enzyme that is involved in nucleotide exchange/repair of DNA.

Exocrine cells: Cells that produce secretions into the surrounding environment.

Exon: The sequence of bases used to transcribe mRNA.

Exonuclease: An enzyme that cleaves nucleotides from either the 3′ or 5′ ends of DNA or RNA.

Extracellular: Outside of the cell, as in serum that surrounds the blood cells.

Extravascular: Outside the vascular system as the fluids that are between the cells in the tissues or between the capillaries and the cells they supply.

Facilitated transport: Transport against a concentration gradient using a carrier but that is not energy or sodium dependent.

FAD, FMN: Flavin adenine dinucleotide, flavin mononucleotide. Coenzymes that carry reducing equivalents (H^+) in reactions of intermediary metabolism. Riboflavin is an essential component of these nucleotides.

Fatty acids: Carbon chains having a carboxyl group at one end and a methyl group at the other end.

Fecal energy (FE): The gross energy of the feces.

Feces: Excrement discharged from the bowel via the anus; contains undigested food, intestinal secretions, intestinal flora, and desquamated intestinal cells.

Fetus: An unborn child; stage of development of a human from embryo to birth or from about 12 weeks postfertilization to full gestational age (approximately 40 weeks).

Fibroblasts: Progenitor cells that can differentiate into other more specific cells.

Fibrous plaque: Lipids that collect on a fibrous network within or on the arterial walls during the atherogenic process creating a projection into the lumen of the vessel and impeding flow.

Fingerprinting: The use of restriction fragment LPs or repeat sequences of DNA to establish a unique pattern of DNA fragments for an individual.

Flatulence: Release from the anus of gases (methane, sulfur dioxide, etc.) produced in the large intestine through the action of intestinal flora on food residue. If the gas is not released, intestinal distention and discomfort result.

FMN: Flavin mononucleotide. A nucleotide coenzyme containing riboflavin.

Footprinting: A technique for identifying the site on DNA bound by proteins that protect certain bonds from attack by nucleases.

Free energy: Energy not trapped or used further; usually dissipated as heat.

Free radicals: Very reactive products of the autooxidation of unsaturated fatty acids. Some amino acids also may be radicalized.

FSH: Follicle stimulating hormone.

GABA: Gamma amino butyric acid. A neurotransmitter formed through the decarboxylation of glutamic acid. It is an inhibitory neurotransmitter that quiets excited neurons.

Galanin: A 30-amino acid peptide found in the neurons of the gastrointestinal submucosa. It can inhibit the release of somatostatin, insulin, pancreatic polypeptide, and neurotensin.

Gaseous products of digestion (GPE): Combustible gases that are products of digestion/fermentation in the gastrointestinal tract. Especially important in the calculation of energy balance of ruminant animals.

Gastrin: A small peptide hormone produced by gastric cells. Gastrin stimulates the parietal cells to release hydrochloric acid.

GDP: Guanosine diphosphate. A dephosphorylated form of GTP important in the activation of substances participating in the biosynthesis of proteins.
Gene: Carrier of the genetic codes for specific protein components of an organism.
Genotype: The inherited characteristic of an organism.
Geophagia: The eating of dirt; an abnormal appetite.
Ghrelin: Hormone secreted by the stomach that stimulates food intake.
GIP: Gastric inhibitory peptide. A peptide hormone inhibiting gastric motility and acid secretion.
Gynoid obesity: Excess body fat deposited mainly on the hips and thighs; sometimes referred to as the *pear* form of obesity.
Hairpin: A double helical stretch formed by base pairing between neighboring complementary strands of a single strand of DNA or RNA.
Half-life: The time required for half of the amount of a given substance to disappear or be degraded.
HANES (NHANES I, II, III, OR HHANES): Health and Nutrition Examination Survey sponsored by the U.S. Centers for Disease Control, a unit of the U.S. Public Health Service.
HcE: Heat of thermal regulation; additional heat due to the body's need to maintain body temperature below or above their zone of thermic neutrality.
HdE: Heat of activity; the additional heat, above that of maintenance, produced by physical activity.
HfE: Heat of fermentation; same as GdE; energy lost due to the production of gases by the ruminal bacteria.
HiE: Heat increment also abbreviated **HI**; the increase in heat produced as a result of activities.
HrE: Heat of product formation; heat associated with the biosynthesis of metabolic products.
HwE: Heat produced in association with the production of waste products.
Heat shock protein: A 90 kDa protein involved in gene transcription.
Hematocrit: Volume of erythrocytes packed by centrifugation in a given volume of blood.
Hematopoiesis: The production of blood cells.
Heme: The protein portion of hemoglobin that holds iron and is responsible for the carriage and release of oxygen by red blood cells.
Heme iron: Iron held by heme.
Hemoglobin (Hb): The iron containing protein in red blood cells that carries oxygen to the periphery and carbon dioxide back to the lungs for excretion.
Heterozygote: An individual carrying two different copies of a gene for a given characteristic.
Heterodimerization: The polymerization of two unlike compounds to DNA.
Histones: Conserved DNA binding proteins that protect the DNA from damage.
HLA genes: Genes that encode elements of the immune system.
HMG CoA: 3-Hydroxy-3-methylglutaryl coenzyme A. A metabolic intermediate in cholesterol synthesis.
Homodimerization: The binding of two identical compounds to DNA.
Homozygote: An individual carrying two identical copies of a gene for a particular gene product.
Hybridization: The specific reassociation of complementary strands of nucleic acids.
Hydroxylation: The addition of a hydroxyl (–OH) group to a compound.
Hyperlipidemia: Abnormally high levels of lipids in the blood.
Hypermetabolism: Higher than normal rates of metabolism.
Hypertension: High blood pressure; systolic/diastolic reading higher by 20% of normal (120/80).
Hypertrophy: Increased cell size.
Ileum: The last third of the small intestine
Incidence: The number of new events or cases of a disease in a population within a specified time period.
Indirect calorimetry: Estimation of energy need based on oxygen consumption.
Infarct: Death of local tissue fed by obstructed vein or artery.
Initiation factors: Proteins that associate with the small subunit of ribosomal RNA that play a role in the initiation of the assemblage of amino acids into an amino acid chain.

Insert: An additional length of base pairs introduced artificially.

Insulitis: Inflammation of the pancreatic islets.

Intron: The sequence of bases in a gene that are transcribed but removed by mRNA editing before the mRNA leaves the nucleus.

Inverted repeats: Two copies of the same sequence of DNA repeated in opposite orientation on the same molecule; adjacent inverted repeats constitute a palindrome.

Intercellular compartment: The water that surrounds cells and is contained in the intracellular space. Plasma is part of this compartment and surrounds the red blood cells in the blood.

Interstitial fluid: Fluid located between cells and in some body cavities such as joints, pleura, and the gastrointestinal tract.

Interstitial spaces: Space between tissues.

Intracellular compartment: Body water compartment consisting of fluids within the cells.

Intravascular: Within the vascular tree. An intravascular (i.v.) injection is one where the substance is injected into a vein.

Ion: An element with either a positive or negative charge.

IRS-1: A 131 kDa intracellular protein essential for most of insulin's intracellular actions.

Ischemia: Impaired blood flow causing oxygen and nutrient deprivation resulting in pain and, if severe, death of some or all parts of the tissue.

Islets of Langerhans: Endocrine clusters of cells embedded in the exocrine pancreas; responsible for the secretion of glucagon, somatostatin, amylin, insulin, and probably some other small hormones.

ISF (interstitial fluid): Fluid surrounding the extravascular cells providing a medium for passage of nutrients to and from cells.

Isoprenoids: Members of the steroid class of compounds. Isoprenoids include the carotenes and ubiquinone.:

IU (international unit): An amount defined by the International Conference for Unification of Formulae.

Jejunum: The middle third of the small intestine.

Joule: A unit of energy in the metric system.

Kinetic energy: Mechanical energy.

Km: Michaelis constant. The substrate concentration that produces half maximal velocity of the reaction. The affinity of the enzyme for its substrate determines Km. If the affinity is high, the reaction will proceed very quickly. If two enzymes work on the same substrate, the one with the greater affinity will be more active and have a higher Km.

Labile: Easily degraded; unstable.

Lean body mass: LBM; that fraction of the body exclusive of stored fat. This fraction is considered to be the active metabolic fraction.

Leptin: A cytokine produced by the adipocyte that signals satiety.

LH: Leutinizing hormone—released by the pituitary and serves to stimulate estrogen and progesterone production in females and testosterone in males.

Lumen: Interior aspect of a vessel.

M (μ): Greek letter prefix that indicates 10^{-6} fraction of a liter or gram.

Macrophages: Large mononuclear cells that phagocytosize foreign compounds and neutralize them.

Magnetic resonance imaging (MRI): A technology allowing the imaging of a body without radiation hazard.

MAO: Monoamine oxidase. A copper-containing enzyme that catalyzes the removal of oxygen from epinephrine, tyramine, and serotonin, inactivating them and reducing neuronal activity. Inhibitors of MAO are valuable drugs for treating depression.

MCV: Mean corpuscular volume. The ratio of the volume of packed cells to the volume of the blood sample; an indirect measure of the number of red blood cells in the blood sample.

Mean: Average value for a group of values.
Median: Value where half the values fall below and half fall above this value.
Menopause: Cessation of estrus cycles.
Messenger RNA (mRNA): A single strand of purine and pyrimidine bases synthesized in the nucleus so that its base sequence complements DNA.
Metabolic water: Water formed as a result of metabolic reactions.
Metabolizable energy (ME): The energy in the food less that lost in feces, urine, and combustible gases.
Microsatellite marker: A dispersed group of 2–5 base sequences that are repeated up to 50 times. May occur at 50–100000 locations in the genome. Used in linkage analysis.
Microsatellite polymorphism: Heterozygosity of a certain microsatellite marker in an individual.
Milliequivalent: A measurement of the concentration of electrolytes in solution. It is determined by multiplying the milligrams per liter by the valence of the chemical and dividing by the molecular weight of the substance: mEq/L = (mg/L). Valence⁄molecular weight. A measurement of the osmotic activity of a solution that is determined by dividing the milliequivalent value by its valence.
mRNA: Messenger RNA; short-lived species of RNA that carries the code for the synthesis of specific gene products to the ribosomes.
Morbidity: Illness leading to death.
Mortality: Cause of death.
MOTILIN: A gastrointestinal hormone that plays a role in controlling the motility of the small intestine during periods without food.
Na^+K^+ PUMP: An energy-dependent pump that operates to keep Na^+ on the outside of cells and K^+ on the inside of cells.
NAD, NADH, NADP, NADPH: Niacin-containing coenzymes that function as carriers for hydrogen ions in dehydrogenase catalyzed reactions.
National Center for Health Statistics (NCHS) (U.S.): An agency that collects data on the causes of death and disease in the United States as well as in other nations.
National Research Council (NRC): A division of the U.S. National Academy of Sciences established in 1916 to promote the effective utilization of scientific and technical resources.
National Science Foundation (NSF) (U.S.): A U.S. government funding organization for the basic sciences.
Nationwide Food Consumption Survey (NFCS) (U.S.): Data collected by scientists in the US Department of Agriculture to document the kinds and amounts of food consumed in the United States.
Neuropeptide Y: A small peptide hormone released by the GI tract and by the central nervous system having a possible role in food intake regulation.
Nucleosome: The basic structural subunit of chromatin, consisting of ~200 bp of DNA and an octomer of histones.
Null mutation: A mutation that completely eliminates the function of the gene usually because it has been eliminated.
Nutrient density: The nutrient composition of food expressed in terms of nutrient quantity per 100 kcal.
Obesity: Excess accumulation of body fat (more than 20% of the body as fat).
Odds ratio (OR): A good approximation of the relative risk.
Olfaction: The sense of smell.
Oligonucleotide: A short, defined sequence of nucleotides joined together in the typical phosphodiester linkage.
Oliguria: Decreased urine production.
Oncogene: A gene related to cancer.
Oncotic pressure: The pressure exerted by the plasma proteins on the walls of the vascular system.

Oocyte: An egg produced by the ovary.
Oogenesis: The production of oocytes (eggs) by the ovary of the female.
Open reading frame: A series of triplets coding for amino acids without any termination codons.
Ophthalmia: Inflammation of the conjunctiva (membrane that lines the eyelid) of the eye.
Opioid receptors: Structures on the surface of neuronal cells that mediate the function of opiates.
ORI: The origin of replication in prokaryotes.
Orthostatic hypotension: Hypotension that results from standing and often associated with dehydration.
Osmolality: Quantity of solutes per liter of solution that contributes to the pressure of that solution on a membrane.
Osmoreceptors: Structures in the hypothalamus that detect changes (elevations) in blood tonicity. When tonicity is increased, a signal is generated that inhibits water loss and water uptake into the blood.
Osmosis: The passage of solvents across a membrane so as to equalize the concentrations of solutes on each side of the membrane.
Osmotic effect: The effects of solutes on water passage.
Osmotic pressure: The pressure that must be applied to prevent the passage of a solvent.
Ossification: The process of bone formation.
Osteoarthritis: Degenerative bone and joint disease due to wear and tear; age-associated.
Osteoblasts: Bone-forming cells.
Osteocalcin: A protein whose synthesis is dependent on vitamin K and that acts to promote mineral deposition in bone.
Osteoclasts: Cells responsible for bone remodeling. These cells mobilize bone mineral.
Osteomalacia: A condition characterized by a weakening and softening of the bone and in which the bending of long bones can develop. Associated with vitamin D deficiency.
Osteopenia: Decreased bone mass.
Osteoporosis: Disease in which the bone loses its mineral content and becomes porous; associated with aging, particularly in females lacking estrogen.
Oxidase: An enzyme group responsible for oxygen removal; catalyzes oxidation/reduction reactions using oxygen as the electron acceptor.
Oxidation: The removal of electrons using oxygen as the electron acceptor.
Oxidation/reduction: Reactions in which electrons are lost by one reactant and gained by another.
Oxidative deamination: The removal of an amino group together with the loss of electrons that are accepted by oxygen.
Oxidative decarboxylation: The removal of a carboxyl group together with the loss of electrons accepted by oxygen.
Oxidative phosphorylation (OXPHOS): Two processes whereby water and ATP are synthesized simultaneously. One, respiration, joins hydrogen and oxygen ions to make water, and the other, ATP synthesis, uses some of the energy so released to synthesize ATP. These coupled processes occur in the mitochondria of the cell.
Parenteral nutrition: Nutritional support furnished through the vascular system.
Passive diffusion: A process for the passage of solutes across a membrane that does not involve a carrier or energy.
PEP: Phosphoenopyruvic acid, a key metabolite in gluconeogenesis.
PEPCK: Phosphoenolpyruvate carboxykinase; the rate-limiting enzyme in gluconeogenesis.
PGI, PGE: Prostaglandins in the I or E series.
pH: The numerical representation of the hydrogen ion concentration in a solution. A low pH represents an acid solution while a high pH represents a basic or alkaline solution. Physiological pH is 7.4.
Phenotype: A category or group to which an individual is assigned based on one or more inherited characteristics; the overt expression of the genotype.

Phosphatase: An enzyme that catalyzes the removal of a phosphoryl group from a substrate.

Physiological fuel value: The energy provided by food with a correction for the energy lost through digestion and absorption.

PLP: Pyridoxal phosphate.

Polyunsaturated fatty acid (PUFA): A fatty acid having more than one double bond.

PP-Fold: Polypeptide fold hormones: polypeptide Y (PYY), pancreatic polypeptide (PP) and neuropeptide Y (NPY). NPY serves as a neurotransmitter. All three have a role (inhibitory) in food intake as well as other functions.

Polyadenylation: The addition of a sequence of polyadenylate to the 5′ end of a eukaryotic RNA after its transcription.

Polymerase chain reaction (PCR): An enzymatic method for repeated copying of DNA.

Postprandial: After a meal.

Precision: No random errors in the measurements. Also referred to as reproducibility.

Prevalence: The number of existing cases of X in a given population at a given time.

Primosome: The mobile complex of helicase and primase that is involved in DNA replication.

Probe: A molecule used to detect the presence of a specific fragment of DNA or RNA.

Prokaryotes: Single-cell organisms.

Promoter: A region of DNA involved in binding RNA polymerase and various regulatory factors to initiate the transcription of RNA.

Prosthetic group: A nonprotein component of an enzyme (or other body protein) that is necessary to the activity of that enzyme or protein.

Proton: A particle in the nucleus of an atom that has a positive charge.

Proximal: Toward the center of the body.

P/S ratio: The ratio of polyunsaturated fatty acids to saturated fatty acids.

Pseudogene: An inactive segment of DNA arising from the mutation of parental genes; an artifact of gene isolation.

PTH: Parathyroid hormone.

Purine: A nitrogenous base that is an essential structural unit of DNA and RNA. Includes adenine and guanine.

PVN: Paraventricular nucleus in the hypothalamus.

Pyrimidines: A group of nitrogenous bases needed for DNA and RNA structures. Includes cytosine, thymine, and uracil.

RBC: Red blood cell. Erythrocyte.

RBP: Retinol binding protein.

Reading frame: One of the three possible ways of reading a nucleotide sequence as a series of triplets.

Receptor: A general term applied to any protein in any part of the body that binds to a specific compound and allows that compound to do its job.

Recombinant DNA: DNA isolated and/or synthesized in the laboratory.

Recovered energy (RE): RE; commonly called energy balance; that portion of the feed energy retained as part of the body or voided as a useful product.

Regression equation: A statistical method for calculating the causal relationship of an independent variable to a dependent variable.

Replication: Duplication of the genetic code.

Reporter gene: A coding unit whose product is easily detected; may be connected to any promoter of interest so that the expression of that gene can be monitored.

RER: Rough endoplasmic reticulum.

Respiratory quotient (RQ): The ratio of carbon dioxide exhaled to oxygen consumed.

Restriction enzyme: An endonuclease enzyme that causes cleavage of both strands of DNA at highly specific sites dictated by base sequence.

Restriction fragment length polymorphism (RFLP): Inherited differences in sites for binding restriction enzymes.

Reverse transcription: RNA-directed synthesis of DNA catalyzed by reverse transcriptase.

RIA: Radioimmunoassay.

Ribonuclease: An enzyme that catalyzes the destruction of RNA.

Ribonucleic acid (RNA): A single strand of nucleosides having ribose instead of deoxyribose and uracil in place of thymine. There are three types of RNA—messenger RNA, transfer RNA, and ribosomal RNA. Messenger RNA serves as the template for the order of amino acids of the particular protein being synthesized. Transfer RNA carries these amino acids, and ribosomal RNA serves as the docking place on the ribosome for the messenger RNA.

Ribosome: The organelle of the cell where protein synthesis occurs.

RBP: Retinol binding protein.

RDA: Recommended daily dietary allowance; a term that has been replaced by DRI.

SAM: S-adenosylmethionine. A principal methyl donor.

SER: Smooth endoplasmic reticulum

Sex-linked trait: A genetic characteristic carried on either the X or the Y chromosome.

SGOT: Serum glutamate-oxaloacetate transaminase. A vitamin B6–dependent enzyme whose level in the serum rises after muscle damage, particularly after a heart attack.

SGPT: Serum glutamate-pyruvate transaminase. Another vitamin B6–dependent enzyme.

SI units: Standard units for expressing biological values.

Signal: The end product observed when a specific sequence of DNA or RNA is detected by autoradiography. This term is also applied to the transmission or intercellular and intracellular reactions that occur once a hormone binds to its cognate receptor on the surface of the cell.

Signal transduction: The process by which a receptor interacts with a ligand at the surface of the cell and then transmits a signal to trigger a series of reactions within that cell.

Sines: Short interspersed sequences.

Skinfold thickness: A double fold of skin and underlying tissue that can be used to estimate body fat stores.

SnRNA: A small nuclear RNA. This family of RNAs is best known for its role in splicing and other RNA-processing reactions.

SOD: Superoxide dismutase.

Southern blotting: A method for transferring DNA from an agarose gel to a nitrocellulose filter on which DNA can be detected by a suitable probe.

Specific dynamic action (SDA): Heat production resulting from the metabolism of food.

Splicing: The removal of introns from RNA accompanied by the joining of the exons.

Splicisome: The macromolecule complex responsible for precursor mRNA slicing. The splicisome consists of at least five small nuclear RNAs and many proteins.

Stable isotope: An isotope that is nonradioactive. K^{40} is a stable isotope.

Sticky ended DNA: Complementary single strands of DNA that protrude from opposite ends of a DNA duplex or from the ends of different duplex molecules.

Stool: Feces.

Stroke: Blockage or rupture of blood vessel(s) supplying the brain with resulting loss of consciousness, paralysis, and other symptoms. Apoplexy is a common term for stroke.

Supine: Lying on one's back.

Symptoms: Signs or indications of disease.

T_3: Triiodothyronine. The most active of the thyroid hormones.

T_4: Thyroxine. The form of thyroid hormone released by the thyroid gland to the blood.

T-Cells: Cells of the immune system that originated from the thymus gland.

Tandem: Describes multiple copies of the same sequence that lie adjacent to each other in gene.

Targeted mutation: (knockout): An animal that has a specific gene altered or deleted at a specific location.

TBF: Total body fat.

TBG: Thyroid hormone binding globulin; protein that carries the thyroxine from the thyroid gland to its target tissue.

TBW: Total body water.

TDP, TPP: Thiamin-containing coenzyme required for decarboxylation reactions.

Thymidine phosphate (TMP, TDP, TTP): A nucleotide consisting of thymine (a pyrimidine base) deoxyribose and 1, 2, or 3 phosphate groups.

Thymine: A pyrimidine base in DNA.

TPN: Total parenteral nutrition. A method of providing all nutrient needs through a solution infused into a large blood vessel.

TSH: Thyroid-stimulating hormone. A hormone released by the pituitary that stimulates the thyroid gland to make and release thyroxine.:

Translation: The synthesis of protein using the message for amino acid sequence carried by messenger RNA. Occurs on the ribosomes.

Translocases: Proteins that move smaller molecules through a membrane.

tRNA: Transfer ribonucleic acid. Form of nucleic acid responsible for transferring specific amino acids to specific sites on the mRNA in the process of protein synthesis.

Tritium ($^3H^+$): Radioactive hydrogen.

TXA_2: Thromboxane A2. An eicosanoid involved in stimulating platelet aggregation.

Ubiquinone: Coenzyme Q, an electron carrier that is part of the respiratory chain in the mitochondria.

UMP, UDP, UTP: Uridine mono-, di-, or triphosphate. A high-energy compound essential to glycogen synthesis.

Uracil: Pyrimidine base used in DNA.

Uridine: Uracil with a ribose group attached.

VIP: Vasoactive peptide. A neuropeptide originating in the neurons of the gastrointestinal system.

VLDL: Very low-density lipoprotein. A lipid–protein complex involved in the transport of lipids from the liver and gut to storage sites.

Western blot: A method for transferring protein to a nitrocellulose filter on which the protein can be detected by an antibody.

Xeropthalmia: Vitamin A deficiency.

Index

A

B

C

D

E

N

O

P

T